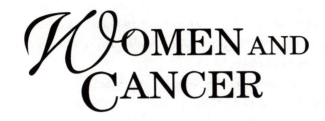

WOMEN AND CANCER

JONES AND BARTLETT SERIES IN ONCOLOGY

American Cancer Society's Consumers Guide to Cancer Drugs, Wilkes/Ades/Krakoff

American Cancer Society's Patient Education Guide to Oncology Drugs, Wilkes/Ades/Krakoff

Biotherapy: A Comprehensive Overview, Rieger

Blood and Marrow Stem Cell Transplantation, Second Edition, Whedon

Cancer and HIV Clinical Nutrition Pocket Guide, Second Edition, Wilkes

Cancer Chemotherapy: A Nursing Process Approach, Second Edition, Barton-Burke/Wilkes/Ingwersen

Cancer Nursing: Principles and Practice, Fifth Edition, Yarbro et al.

Cancer Symptom Management, Second Edition, Yarbro et al.

Cancer Symptom Management, Patient Self-Care Guides, Second Edition, Yarbro et al.

Chemotherapy Care Plans Handbook, Second Edition, Barton-Burke/Wilkes/Ingwersen

A Clinical Guide to Cancer Nursing, Fourth Edition, Groenwald et al.

A Clinical Guide to Stem Cell and Bone Marrow Transplantation, Shapiro et al.

Clinical Handbook for Biotherapy, Rieger

Comprehensive Cancer Nursing Review, Fourth Edition, Groenwald et al.

Contemporary Issues in Breast Cancer, Hassey Dow

Contemporary Issues in Prostate Cancer: A Nursing Perspective, Held-Warmkessel

Fatigue in Cancer: A Multidimensional Approach, Winningham/Barton-Burke

Handbook of Oncology Nursing, Third Edition, Johnson/Gross

HIV Homecare Handbook, Daigle

HIV Nursing and Symptom Management, Ropka/Williams

Homecare Management of the Bone Marrow Transplant Patient, Third Edition, Kelley et al.

Medication Errors: Causes, Prevention and Risk Management, Cohen

Memory Bank for Chemotherapy, Third Edition, Preston/Wilfinger

Oncology Nursing Review, Yarbro et al.

Oncology Nursing Society's Instruments for Clinical Nursing Research, Second Edition, Frank-Stromborg

Pocket Guide to Breast Cancer, Hassey Dow

Pocket Guide for Women and Cancer, Moore et al.

Quality of Life: From Nursing and Patient Perspectives, King/Hinds

2000 Oncology Nursing Drug Handbook, Wilkes/Ingwersen/Barton-Burke

Women and Cancer: A Gynecologic Oncology Nursing Perspective, Second Edition, Moore-Higgs et al.

SOCIETY OF GYNECOLOGIC NURSE ONCOLOGISTS

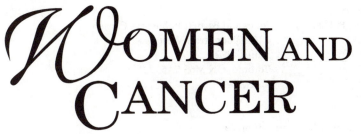

WOMEN AND CANCER

A Gynecologic Oncology Nursing Perspective

SECOND EDITION

Giselle J. Moore-Higgs, ARNP, MSN, AOCN
Editor in Chief

Lois A. Almadrones, RN, MS, FNP, MPA

Lynn M. Gossfeld, RN, MSN

JoAnn Huang Eriksson, RN, MS, AOCN

Beth Colvin Huff, MSN, RN

JONES AND BARTLETT PUBLISHERS

Sudbury, Massachusetts

BOSTON   LONDON   TORONTO   SINGAPORE

World Headquarters
Jones and Bartlett Publishers
40 Tall Pine Drive
Sudbury, MA 01776
978-443-5000
info@jbpub.com
www.jbpub.com

Jones and Bartlett Publishers Canada
2100 Bloor Street West
Suite 6-272
Toronto, ON M6S 5A5
CANADA

Jones and Bartlett Publishers International
Barb House, Barb Mews
London W6 7PA
UK

Senior Acquisitions Editor: Greg Vis
Production Editor: Linda S. DeBruyn
Director of Manufacturing: Therese Bräuer
Editorial, Design, and Production Service: Nesbitt Graphics, Inc.
Cover Design: Judy Arisman, Arisman Design
Typesetting: Nesbitt Graphics, Inc.
Printing and Binding: Malloy Lithography
Cover photo credit: © Tomonori Taniguchi/Photonica

Library of Congress Cataloging-in-Publication Data
Society of Gynecologic Nurse Oncologists' women and cancer : a gynecologic oncology nursing perspective / edited by Giselle J. Moore-Higgs et al.—2nd ed.
    p. cm. — (Jones and Bartlett series in oncology)
    Includes bibliographical references and index.
    ISBN 0-7637-1166-7
    1. Generative organs, Female—Cancer—Nursing. 2. Cancer in women—Nursing. I. Title: Women and cancer. II. Series. III. Moore-Higgs, Giselle J. IV. Society of Gynecologic Nurse Oncologists.
    [DNLM: 1. Genital Neoplasms, Female—Nurses' Instruction. WP 145 S678 2000]
RC280.G5 S65 2000
    616.99'465 21—dc21   99-040657

Printed in the United States of America
03 02 01 00   10 9 8 7 6 5 4 3 2

The selection and dosage of drugs presented in this book are in accord with standards accepted at the time of publication. The authors, editor, and publisher have made every effort to provide accurate information. However, research, clinical practice, and government regulations often change the accepted standard in this field. Before administering any drug, the reader is advised to check the manufacturer's product information sheet for the most up-to-date recommendations on dosage, precautions, and contraindications. This is especially important in the case of drugs that are new or seldom used.

CONTENTS

PREFACE

In 1979, Richard Boronow, MD, suggested establishing a nursing organization to foster education and communication among nurses interested in gynecologic oncology. With the commitment of ten dedicated nurses, the Society of Gynecologic Nurse Oncologists was established the same year. The first symposium was held in Colorado in 1982. From these small beginnings, the SGNO has grown to become an international organization. The Society is a nonprofit organization of registered nurses dedicated to the advancement of patient care, education, and research in the field of gynecologic oncology.

Continuing advances in our profession make heavy demands on us to increase knowledge and skills in clinical situations, develop new insights and techniques in psychosocial intervention, and achieve up-to-date understanding of professional issues. The Society of Gynecologic Nurse Oncologists responds to these needs by disseminating the most current information at our annual symposium and through our quarterly journal.

It was during a planning session for the symposium in 1990 that a new idea evolved: a presymposium workshop dedicated to the needs of nurses new to the field of gynecologic oncology. Today the workshop provides the opportunity for experienced nurses to share knowledge and skills, as well as expound on some of the special needs of women with cancer, such as sexuality and infertility. After conducting several workshops, the Society had developed a substantial syllabus, and requests for copies were received from all over the country. Thus the idea for this book was born, proposed, and accepted by the Society. The purpose of *Women and Cancer* is to provide a textbook for nurses who specialize or have an interest in gynecologic oncology. Each chapter was developed in such a manner that nurses in the outpatient clinic or office, at the bedside, and in an advanced practice role have a reference that addresses the specific needs of this patient population.

The SGNO is very proud to present the second edition of this book. Several chapters have been extensively revised to narrow their focus or to explore the treatments available for women with a gynecologic malignancy. In addition, we have added three new chapters to enhance the book.

Chapters 1 and 2 provide extensive examination of the issues of screening, detection, and management of preinvasive disease. This material provides a foundation for

Chapters 3 through 10, which are devoted to specific gynecologic and breast malignancies. The format of the chapters consists of a review of the anatomy and physiology of the organ involved, the natural history of the disease, diagnostic procedures, and treatment considerations. In addition, each chapter has a comprehensive section highlighting the nursing care issues identified with the disease, including a cluster of nursing diagnoses.

The treatment modalities of chemotherapy, biotherapy, and radiation therapy are addressed in Chapters 11 through 13 using a similar format.

Chapters 14 and 15 address the psychosocial issues of sexuality/infertility in women with cancer and the spirituality issues that become salient to patients following diagnosis.

Chapter 16 examines controversial issues in breast cancer care. Chapter 17 provides an overview of HIV disease in women and its impact on gynecologic malignancies. Chapter 18 explores the issues surrounding complementary and alternative medicine and the role of nursing in guiding patients to select appropriate therapies.

CONTRIBUTING AUTHORS

Lois A. Almadrones, RN, MS, FNP, MPA
Clinical Nurse Specialist
Memorial Sloan-Kettering Cancer Center
New York, New York

Anita Axiak, RN, BSN, OCN
Brachytherapy Nurse Clinician
William Beaumont Hospital
Royal Oak, Michigan

Jacqueline Balon, RN, MSN, OCN
Nurse Practitioner
Karmanos Cancer Institute
Detroit, Michigan

Connie L. Birk, RN, BSN, OCN
Gynecologic Nurse Oncologist
Gynecologic Oncology Associates
Newport Beach, California

Debra M. Brown, RN, BSN, OCN
Radiation Oncology
William Beaumont Hospital
Royal Oak, Michigan

Linda W. Carter, MSN, RN, AOCN
Home Care Nurse
University of Pittsburgh Shadyside
    Home Care
Pittsburgh, Pennsylvania

Mary Lou Cullen, RNP, MS
Pittsford, New York

JoAnn Huang Eriksson, RN, MS, AOCN
Oncology/Medicine Clinical Nurse Specialist
Evanston Northwestern Healthcare
Evanston Hospital
Evanston, Illinois

Sheryl Redlin Frazier, RN
Gynecologic Oncology Nurse
Vanderbilt University Medical Center
Nashville, Tennessee

Mitzi Fudge, RN, ADN, MSN
Vanderbilt University Medical Center
Nashville, Tennessee

Lynn M. Gossfeld, RN, MSN
West Dundee, Illinois

Randolph E. Gross, MS, RN, CS, AOCN
Nurse Clinician
Memorial Sloan-Kettering Cancer Center
New York, New York

Beth Colvin Huff, MSN, RN
Nurse Practitioner
Department of Obstetrics and Gynecology
Vanderbilt University Medical Center
Nashville, Tennessee

Margaret Anne Lamb, PHD, RN
Associate Professor
School of Health and Human Services,
    Department of Nursing
University of New Hampshire
Durham, New Hampshire

Linda C. Lewis, RN, BSN
Radiation Oncology Case Manager
William Beaumont Hospital
Royal Oak, Michigan

Suzy Lockwood-Rayermann, RN, MSN
Instructor
Texas Christian University–Harris College of
    Nursing
Ft. Worth, Texas

Giselle J. Moore-Higgs, ARNP, MSN, AOCN
Nurse Practitioner and Clinic Coordinator
Department of Radiation Oncology
University of Florida College of Medicine
Gainesville, Florida

Susan Nolte, RN, MSN, CRNP
Clinical Nurse Specialist/Nurse Practitioner
Gynecologic Oncology
Abington Memorial Hospital
Abington, Pennsylvania

James C. Pace, RN, DSN, MDIV, ANP-CS
Associate Professor of Adult Health Nursing;
    Adult Nurse Practitioner
Nell Hodgson Woodruff School of Nursing
Emory University
Atlanta, Georgia

Bridget M. Paniscotti, RN, BSN
Case Manager
Monmouth Medical Center, An Affiliate of
    Saint Barnabas Health Care System
Long Branch, New Jersey

Kimberly A. Schmit-Pokorny, RN, MSN, OCN
Manager/Case Manager
University of Nebraska Medical Center
Omaha, Nebraska

Alice Spinelli, RN, ANP, OCN
Nurse Practitioner
Gynecologic Oncology Associates, PA
Miami, Florida

Susan Vogt Temple, RN, MSN, ETN
Program Administrator–Developmental
    Therapeutics
Washington University School of Medicine
Washington University in St. Louis
St. Louis, Missouri

Janet Ruth Walczak, MSN, RN, CRNP
Nurse Practitioner
Johns Hopkins Oncology Center
Baltimore, Maryland

Teresa C. Wehrwein, PHD, RN, CNAA
Director, Education and Practice
Henry Ford Health System
Detroit, Michigan

Jane Duffy-Weisser, RN, ANP, CS
Nurse Practitioner, Gynecologic Oncology
Memorial Sloan-Kettering Cancer Center
New York, New York

Lois A. Winkelman, RN, MS
Clinical Nurse Specialist
Rush Medical Center Department of
    Gynecologic Oncology
Chicago, Illinois

To our gynecologic oncology nurse colleagues
AND
*To the women who, through their experience with a
gynecologic malignancy, continue to teach us how to care*

CHAPTER 1

Screening and Prevention of Gynecologic Malignancies

Susan A. Nolte, RN, MSN, CRNP

Janet R. Walczak, RN, MSN, CRNP

✳ INTRODUCTION

In 1999, an estimated 256,000 women in the United States will be diagnosed with breast/gynecologic malignancies and 70,500 will die of these diseases.[1] How many of these deaths could be avoided through early detection? Estimates indicate that early detection via screening for breast and cervical cancer alone could result in a 3% reduction in cancer deaths.[2] To promote early cancer detection, the National Cancer Institute (NCI), Division of Cancer Prevention and Control, has directed in its Cancer Control Objectives for the Nation: 1985–2000, that health care providers educate patients on the value of cancer screening and recommend the use of established screening procedures. Nurses are in a key position to carry out this directive, thus promoting the NCI's ultimate goal of a 50% reduction in cancer mortality by the year 2000.[3]

This chapter focuses on the screening and early detection of breast and gynecologic malignancies. Its aim is to provide a foundation for understanding the high-risk factors related to the development of breast and gynecologic cancers as well as strategies directed toward the screening and prevention of these malignancies.

✳ PRINCIPLES OF SCREENING

Screening, as defined by the United States Commission on Chronic Illness, is the identification of unrecognized disease by the easy application of tests, examinations, or other procedures. Screening tests separate out apparently healthy persons who probably have a disease from those who probably do not.[4] The American Cancer Society (ACS) has adopted the definition of screening as the search for disease in asymptomatic people. An asymptomatic person does not have symptoms or does not recognize the symptoms as being related to the disease.[5] In terms of outcomes, the objective of screening for a particular cancer is to reduce the complications and mortality rate for that cancer among the persons screened.[6]

It is important to emphasize that a positive screening test does not establish a definitive diagnosis, but rather indicates the need for further diagnostic tests. Early detection refers to efforts directed at the diagnosis of cancer in an early stage and should not be confused with cancer screening, which is one of the strategies used to achieve this goal.[7]

Relative Risk

A frequent measure of association of risk status is determined by relative risk. Relative risk (RR) is defined as the disease rate in the exposed population divided by the disease rate in the unexposed population.[8] This measure gives the relative disease risk between two populations (e.g., those with a positive family history versus no family history of disease) and is helpful in comparing risk groups.

Diseases Suitable for Screening

Effective cancer screening should be directed toward diseases that meet criteria appropriate for screening and early detection. Several characteristics of diseases suitable for screening have been identified.[6,9,10] First, the disease should have serious consequences and be an important cause of morbidity, disability, or mortality. In addition, the disease must have treatments that are both sufficiently effective and more effective when applied to disease early rather than after symptoms have appeared. Furthermore, the natural history of the disease should be known and must include a detectable preclinical phase that has a high prevalence among the persons screened. In some diseases, such as cancer of the cervix, a detectable precancerous phase also exists, affording an opportunity for primary as well as secondary prevention. The natural history of disease and the duration of the preinvasive and preclinical phases with respect to the reliability of screening are illustrated in Figure 1.1.[9] The small vertical arrows represent implied time frames during which screening is advantageous. Clearly, the presence of a preinvasive phase and/or a long preclinical phase provides a greater opportunity for screening.

Screening Tests

The essential features of screening tests have been discussed by many authors.[5,9,11] The ACS[12] stresses four essential aspects of screening tests: effectiveness, benefit/risk ratio, cost-effectiveness, and feasibility.

To be effective, a screening test should have both high sensitivity and specificity. Test sensitivity is the likelihood that a test will be positive among people who truly have a disease. Specificity represents the likelihood that a test will be negative among people who do not have a disease. Sensitivity and specificity for Papanicolaou (Pap) smears, for example, have been estimated at 67% and 60%, respectively, whereas for mammography they are 85% and 80%, respectively.[9] Sensitivity and specificity can vary from setting to setting owing to improper technique and test application, subop-

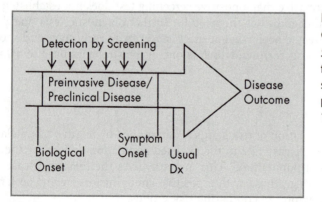

FIGURE 1.1. Natural history of disease in relation to screening. *Source:* Modified with permission from Hulka, B. (1988). Cancer screening: Degrees of proof and practical application. *Cancer, 62,* 1777.

timal laboratory practice, and degree of clinical expertise. Nurses and nurse practitioners can play a major role in the accuracy of screening techniques such as Pap smear and pelvic and breast examinations.[13]

Screening tests should be safe, relatively painless, and beneficial. The benefits of cancer screening, such as improved prognosis, less radical treatment, lower costs, and the psychological benefit of negative test results, must be weighed against the potential risk. For example, the benefit of screening mammography clearly outweighs the risk from the minimal amount of radiation exposure, estimated to be less than 0.5 rad to each breast per screening examination.[9] In fact, the risks of radiation-induced cancer with modern mammographic techniques are considered to be extremely low, if any.[5] However, the positive and negative effects of screening on quality of life are being questioned. False-positive results may lead to unnecessary diagnostic procedures as well as increased cost, discomfort, and anxiety.[11]

The cost of screening tests must be reasonable in terms of expected outcomes. Cancer detection tests are not analyzed for their cost-effectiveness in the sense that a dollar value is placed on human life. Rather, cost-effectiveness is analyzed in such a way that the maximum benefit of early detection with available resources is achieved while costs, risks, and inconvenience are reduced.[5]

Finally, recommended screening tests must meet feasibility criteria, such as ease of administration and acceptability to patients as well as to those performing the tests.

Guidelines for Screening

Guidelines for screening have been established by several organizations, including the ACS, Canadian Task Force, American College of Obstetricians & Gynecologists (ACOG), and the National Cancer Institute (NCI). But an important issue is the degree of cancer detection guidance these organizations provide. Consequently, screening practices may vary, and the need for uniform guidelines from all major health professional organizations is apparent.

American Cancer Society

The ACS first published cancer screening guidelines for asymptomatic persons in 1980.[12] The original guidelines later incorporated changes related to the detection of cervical, endometrial, and breast cancers. These guidelines have served as the "gold standard" for cancer detection. However, the ACS cautions that their guidelines are intended to detect early cancer in asymptomatic persons on an individual basis.[12] Current recommendations for screening for breast and gynecologic malignancies in asymptomatic women are presented in Table 1.1.

Canadian Task Force

The Canadian Task Force on the Periodic Health Examination was established in 1976 to determine how periodic health examinations might enhance or protect the health of the Canadian population. The goal of the task force, which consisted of clinicians and scientists, was to develop guidelines for standard recommendations that

TABLE 1.1

American Cancer Society Guidelines for Early Detection of Breast and Gynecologic Cancer in Asymptomatic Women

Test or procedure	Age	Frequency
Breast Self-Exam	20 & over	Every month
Breast Clinical Exam	20–39 >40	Every 3 years Every year
Mammography*	40 & over	Every year
Pap Test	Sexually active (or age 18)	Annual Pap test. After >3 consecutive satisfactory normal exams, may be performed at physician discretion.
Pelvic Exam	18 & over	Every year
Endometrial Tissue Sample	At menopause if at high risk**	At menopause

*Screening mammography should begin by age 40.
**History of infertility, obesity, failure to ovulate, abnormal uterine bleeding, or unopposed estrogen or Tamoxifen therapy.
Source: Adapted with permission from American Cancer Society (1999). *Cancer facts and figures—1999* (ACS Publication 5008.99), pp. 7–31. Atlanta: American Cancer Society.

would prevent specific diseases and promote health. The task force had six major objectives: to identify significant disabling conditions or behaviors that could be prevented; to consider evidence for the benefit of early detection or prevention of these conditions; to define high-risk groups; to design health protection "packages"; to make recommendations on procedure frequency and the appropriate provider of this "package"; and to develop evaluation measures that would permit recurring assessment and improvement of the recommended health plan.[14] The recommendations of the task force, which are considered minimal standards, included interventions for aspects of general health as well as for cancer. Current recommendations of the Canadian Task Force specific to breast and gynecologic cancers are presented in Table 1.2.[14–17]

American College of Obstetricians & Gynecologists

In 1985, ACOG developed a task force to review methods of screening for cancer in women and to provide guidelines for screening for gynecologic malignancies as well as other malignancies for which women are at high risk. At that time, ACOG guidelines were at variance with the guidelines of other organizations, specifically the

TABLE 1.2

Canadian National Task Force Guidelines for Screening for Breast and Gynecologic Cancer

Screening for Breast Cancer

Maneuver	Effectiveness	Recommendation
Clinical examination and mammography, women aged 50–69 years	Routine clinical examination and mammography reduces mortality from breast cancer. Optimum frequency of screening has not been determined.	Good evidence for screening aged 50–69 years annually by clinical examination and mammography (A)
Clinical examination and mammography, women aged 40–49 years	Routine clinical examination and mammography has not consistently been shown to reduce mortality from breast cancer.	Contradictory evidence regarding benefits and risks of clinical examination and mammography but fair evidence to exclude from periodic health examination of asymptomatic women aged 40–49 years (D)
Teaching breast self-examination (BSE)	Increased survival and other indicators of early detection demonstrated but studies subject to bias.	Inadequate evidence that the practice of BSE improves survival; insufficient evidence to include or exclude from the periodic health examination (C)

Screening for Cervical Cancer

Maneuver	Effectiveness	Recommendation
Papanicolaou smear* *Annual screening is recommended following initiation of sexual activity or age 18. After 2 normal smears screen every 3 years until age 69. Consider increasing frequency for women with risk factors; age of first sexual intercourse < age 18, many sexual partners or consort with many partners, smoking, low socioeconomic status.	Cervical smears reduce the risk of developing invasive carcinoma of the cervix in women who have been sexually active.	Fair evidence to include in PHE of sexually active women (B)

A. There is good evidence to support the recommendation that the condition be specifically considered in a periodic health examination.

B. There is fair evidence to support the recommendation that the condition be specifically considered in a periodic health examination.

C. There is insufficient evidence to include or exclude from the periodic health examination.

D. There is fair evidence to exclude from the periodic health examination.

Source: Adapted with permission from Canadian Task Force on the Periodic Health Examination (1994) Canadian guide to clinical preventive health care. Ottawa: Canadian Communications Group, 620-31.

recommendations for Pap smear screening. Experts from the ACS and NCI were invited to address the ACOG task force, which ultimately led to a unified recommendation for the frequency of cervical cytology screening among these organizations. ACOG guidelines were revised in 1993, and again in 1997 to include annual general health counseling and check-ups as well as guidelines for suggested cancer screening.[18] ACOG cancer screening guidelines for cervical, breast, endometrial, and ovarian cancer are set forth in Table 1.3.

TABLE 1.3

American College of Obstetricians & Gynecologists Suggested Cancer Screening Guidelines

General Health Counseling and Cancer Check-up	All women should have a general health evaluation annually or as appropriate, to include evaluation of risk for cancer* and evaluation to detect signs of premalignant or malignant conditions.[†]
Cervical Cancer	All women who are or who have been sexually active or who have reached age 18 should undergo an annual Pap test and pelvic examination. After a woman has had three or more consecutive satisfactory annual examinations with normal findings, the Pap test may be performed less frequently on low-risk women at the discretion of her physician.
Breast Cancer	It is suggested that mammography be performed every 1–2 years for women aged 40–50 years and annually for women over 50 years.
Endometrial Cancer	Screening all women for endometrial cancer and its precursors is neither cost-effective nor warranted.
Ovarian Cancer	No techniques that have proved effective in reducing the disease-specific mortality of ovarian cancer are currently available.
Colorectal Cancer	After age 50, a digital rectal examination should accompany the pelvic examination; annual fecal occult blood tests should be performed, and sigmoidoscopy should be performed every 3–5 years.
Lung Cancer	No available techniques are currently suitable for routine screening.

*Evaluation of risk for cancer includes questions about high-risk habits (smoking, excessive sunlight exposure, drug use, sexual practices, etc.), evaluation of family history of cancer, and review of symptoms pertinent to each organ system (e.g., abnormal vaginal bleeding, rectal bleeding, change in moles).

[†]The examination should include skin, lymph nodes, thyroid gland, oral cavity, breasts, external and internal genitalia, anus, and rectum.

Source: Reprinted with permission from American College of Obstetricians and Gynecologists. Routine cancer screening (Technical Bulletin No. 185). Washington, DC: ACOG © 1997.

TABLE 1.4

National Cancer Institute Working Guidelines for
Early Cancer Detection

Condition	Guidelines
Breast Cancer	Encourage monthly breast self-exam Clinical breast exam at time of periodic examination >40, mammogram every 1–2 years
Cervical Cancer	All women who are or have been sexually active, or who have reached age 18, should have an annual Pap test and pelvic exam. After a woman has had three or more consecutive normal annual examinations, the Pap test may be performed less frequently at the discretion of her physician.

Source: National Cancer Institute (1998). *Cancer Facts: Screening Mammograms.* NCI NIH 5.28 (9/15/98): 1–6.

National Cancer Institute

In 1987, NCI, in consultation with many professional medical organizations including the ACS, developed early cancer detection guidelines for several cancers. NCI emphasized that their recommendations would be considered "working guidelines" based on a particular patient's background, medical history, and circumstances. These guidelines are subject to modification as new evidence becomes available.[19,20] For example, in 1993 the NCI released a statement regarding breast cancer screening that altered their 1987 working guidelines.[21] Current NCI working guidelines for screening women for breast and cervical malignancies are presented in Table 1.4.

✳ BREAST CANCER

The breast is a leading site of cancer among women in the United States regardless of race and ethnicity. White, Hawaiian, and African American women have the highest incidence rates per 100,000 population (111.8, 105.6, and 95.4, respectively) and Korean, American Indian, and Vietnamese have the lowest (28.5, 31.6, and 37.5, respectively).[23] It was estimated that 175,000 new cases would be diagnosed in the United States in 1999.[1] Overall incidence increased about 2% a year since the beginning of the 1970s but plateaued since 1987 at approximately 107 per 100,000 women. Some of the recent increase can be attributed to greater utilization of mammography, which can diagnose cancers before they become clinically apparent; however, reasons for long-term increases, particularly in postmenopausal woman, are not known and need to be investigated.[22]

Breast cancer is second only to lung cancer as the leading cause of cancer deaths among women in most racial and ethnic groups in the United States. African American women have the highest mortality rate (31.4 per 100,000) followed by white (27.0) and Hawaiian (25.0) women.[23] It is anticipated that 43,300 women will die in 1999 from breast cancer.[1] Mortality has remained stable over the past fifty years until recently when data show a decline that is most apparent in younger women, white women, and African American women.[24] This can be partially explained by increases in screening and detection and improved treatment modalities.[24]

Population at Risk

Multiple risk factors have been defined for breast cancer, which include age, family history of breast cancer, genetic predisposition, endocrine factors, exogenous hormones, diet, weight, benign breast conditions, and history of breast cancer (Table 1.5).[22, 25] Age may be the single most important risk factor; a woman's risk of developing breast cancer increases over her lifetime. Although young women in their 20s and 30s may have breast cancer, it is more common after menopause. While only one in 227 women from birth to 39 years will develop breast cancer, one in 25 women 40 to 59 years and 1 in 15 women 60 to 79 years will develop the cancer. Overall lifetime percentage of population to develop breast cancer is 12.52%, or one in eight women.[1] Age-specific incidence rates show a slight plateau around age 50, then a sharper increase. Contrary to these data is the fact that Asian women do not have this increase in incidence in the postmenopausal years; the incidence for them peaks in the fourth decade of life, and at a level below that of their Western counterparts.[22]

Height, weight, and body mass have all been described as being related to breast cancer. In a prospective study of Norwegian women, after adjusting for other risk factors, there was a gradual increase in risk associated with increasing height, and an inverse relationship between body mass index and breast cancer risk in the premenopausal years. In postmenopausal women, there appeared to be an increase in risk associated with obesity.[26] The associations of decreased risk in obese premenopausal women and a modest increased risk in obese postmenopausal women have also been previously described by others.[27,28,29] In addition, obesity was associated not only with increased risk in another large study of Norwegian women, but also with increased mortality. That is, a 20% increase in mortality was observed if the woman was

TABLE 1.5
Risk Factors for Breast Cancer

Age	Diet
Family history	Weight
Genetic predisposition	Benign breast disease
Endocrine factors	History of breast cancer
Exogenous hormones	

obese before diagnosis.[30] In a Dutch study, the increased risk from obesity in post-menopausal women was related to waist-to-hip ratio rather than body mass index. Women whose weight was concentrated in the abdomen rather than hips were at increased risk.[31]

A family history of breast cancer in a first-degree relative (mother, sister, or daughter) increases risk by up to 80% over the woman who has no first-degree relatives with breast cancer. The risk is even greater if any of the first-degree relatives has had bilateral disease.[22] The relative risk of breast cancer in a woman whose mother has had breast cancer is 1.8, and 2.5 if a sister has had breast cancer. The relative risk is magnified to 5.6 if both have had breast cancer.[32] However, there are more recent data that demonstrate improved survival in premenopausal women with a family history of breast cancer.[33]

Mutations in the BRCA1 and BRCA2 genes account for 5–10% of all breast cancer cases. Women with this mutation have an approximate lifetime risk of 85% of developing breast cancer. About 1 in 200 to 400 women have the BRCA1 mutation. Women with the mutation are usually from families in which there are multiple cases of breast cancer, primarily in younger women. Cumulative risk from BRCA1 mutations increases from 3.2% at age 30 to 85% at age 70 which represents a 20-fold greater risk over women of average risk. In addition, if a woman who is positive for the BRCA1 mutation has breast cancer, she has a 64% risk of developing cancer in the other breast by age 70 and a cumulative risk for ovarian cancer of 44% by the same age. Women with BRCA2 mutations have a similar risk profile.[34] Testing for this mutation is currently limited to high-risk families.[35,36]

Many endocrine factors are known to be associated with increased risk for breast cancer. These factors include age at menarche, age at menopause, parity, and age at first full-term pregnancy.[25,37,38] One issue related to age at menarche and age at menopause is the number of years that a woman menstruates. Women who menstruate for more than thirty years are at higher risk than those who menstruate for fewer than thirty years. For women who experience a natural menopause, risk is two times greater for women who are over 55 years than for women who are under 44 years of age at menopause. Women who have an induced menopause at ages 50–55 have a relative risk of 1.34, compared with a relative risk of 0.77 in women with menopause induced before age 45. Although it appears that an early induced menopause may significantly reduce risk, there are no data from a prospective randomized trial to substantiate this. And the subsequent increased risk for other health conditions related to an early menopause may negate any positive benefit for breast cancer risk.[37,38]

Age at menarche and, more important, time that normal menstrual cycles are established relate to risk for breast cancer. If menarche occurs before age 13, the risk is about two times that if menarche is after age 13. To compound this finding, if normal menstrual cycles are established before age 13, the relative risk is 3.7, while the relative risk is 1.0 if menarche is after age 13 and regular cycles are established after five years.[25,39]

Risk is directly related to increased age at first full-term pregnancy. That is, it is hypothesized that the number of ovulatory cycles before the first pregnancy is important in determining the woman's total lifetime risk of developing breast cancer.[39] The older a woman is when she has her first full-term pregnancy, the greater the number of ovulatory cycles before pregnancy, and possibly the greater the risk of developing breast cancer. And if a woman's first pregnancy is before the age of 19 or between the ages of 30 and 34, her risk is about half that of the woman who is nulliparous. Risk is highest when the first full-term pregnancy is after age 35.

Exogenous hormone use has also been associated with breast cancer risk. There have been numerous studies evaluating the relationship between oral contraceptive use and breast cancer, and postmenopausal estrogen use and breast cancer. In a meta-analysis,[36] there was no statistically significant association of oral contraceptive use and breast cancer. The length of oral contraceptive use did not seem to be associated with increased risk. However, a slightly increased risk seemed to be associated with women diagnosed with breast cancer before the age of 45 who used oral contraceptives for more than ten years. This risk may be greatest if the period of use is for more than four years before the first pregnancy.[22,25,40,41]

Use of estrogens after menopause has also been the subject of many studies, with often contradictory results. One meta-analysis[42] indicated an increased risk of less than 10% from use of postmenopausal estrogen therapy, and this risk had questionable statistical significance. In another meta-analysis,[43] there was no increase in risk when all women from all studies were included. However, when the analysis controlled for duration of use, the relative risk was 1.3 for use longer than 15 years. Increasing risk with increasing length of hormone replacement therapy in addition to level of endogenous estrogen has also been demonstrated.[38,44] In addition, risk was greatest for those women who had a family history of breast cancer with a relative risk of 3.4. There was no risk association identified for sequencing postmenopausal estrogen replacement therapy with progestins. In the Nurses' Health Study, there was no increase in risk observed in twelve years of follow-up of current users, and no decrease in risk for women who took estrogen and progestins sequentially.[45]

Multiple dietary factors have been implicated as risk factors for breast cancer. These include fat, alcohol, and vitamins. It has long been conjectured that geographic differences in breast cancer incidence may be related to dietary influences, particularly fat intake. However, data on the relationship between fat and breast cancer risk have been conflicting.[46–49] One reanalysis of twelve case-control studies[50] and a recent study in Italy[51] concluded that dietary fat is related to increased risk of breast cancer. Conversely, there have been reported decreases in risk in southern European countries where the diet is high in olive oil. It has been proposed that the protective effect may be from a component of the olive oil and not from uptake of oleic acid in body tissues.[52]

Alcohol intake has also been demonstrated to increase risk of developing breast cancer.[53] In the Nurses' Health Study, Willett et al.[54] attempted to quantify this risk. They found that risk increased with increasing number of drinks per day. Relative risk for an average of less than 25% of a drink per day was 1.0, and 1.5 for an average of more than one drink per day. A meta-analysis of studies relating alcohol intake to risk also showed that relative risk increases with increasing alcohol intake.[55]

Other dietary components that have been evaluated are vitamins. Vitamin A, including dietary supplements of the vitamin, has been associated with a decrease in risk,[56] but no association has been seen with vitamin C or beta carotene.

A history of biopsies showing benign breast disease has been associated with breast cancer risk. Proliferative disease has been reported to increase risk of developing breast cancer, with highest risk seen in women who had atypical hyperplasia on previous biopsies.[57] The Nurses' Health Study replicated this research and found a relative risk of 3.7 for women with atypical hyperplasia and a relative risk of 1.6 for women with proliferative changes without atypia. The risk was even greater for premenopausal women and women with a family history of breast cancer.[58] These data are further supported by recent data from the case-controlled study of the Breast Cancer Detection Demonstration Project, which concluded that women with atypical hyperplasia had 4.3 times the breast cancer risk of women without proliferative disease. They further concluded that atypical hyperplasia is a reliable indicator of breast cancer risk.[59]

Finally, history of a previous breast cancer increases the woman's risk for developing a second cancer in the same or contralateral breast. There is a 0.5 to 1% risk during each year of follow-up for developing a cancer in the contralateral breast, and the probability of developing a breast cancer in the ipsilateral breast is approximately the same. The risk is similar if the woman has a history of carcinoma in situ of the breast.[25]

Screening Methods

Breast cancer meets the criteria of a disease appropriate for screening and early detection discussed earlier in this chapter. No one would argue that breast cancer has serious consequences and can cause significant morbidity and mortality. Certainly, the ability to diagnose breast cancer in its earliest stages, when the disease may not be clinically evident, is an important factor in survival. There are three modalities involved in screening for breast cancer: breast self-examination (BSE), clinical breast examination, and mammography. Regular monthly breast self-examination has been associated with early detection of small tumors, when survival benefit is greatest.[60,61] Up to 90% of all breast cancers are first discovered by women themselves, and about a fourth are found in the interval between annual mammograms or clinical breast examinations.[62,63]

In a large controlled clinical trial by the Health Insurance Plan of Greater New York (HIP) completed in the 1960s, mortality from breast cancer significantly decreased with annual mammography in patients over 50 years.[64] Later studies have confirmed this benefit.[65,66,67] Lesions of less than 1 cm can be detected with mammography, thus chance of survival is enhanced. There is less documented benefit of mammography for women between 40 and 49 years, but there is increasing evidence to support annual mammographic screening for women over 40 particularly if the test is performed in the first two weeks of the menstrual cycle when breast tissue is less dense.[68,69]

Annual physical examination of the breasts by a health professional is an important component of early detection. However, it should be done in combination with mammography, since mammography has an overall accuracy rate of 85% for detecting abnormalities. The two examinations are complementary—both are needed to adequately assess and screen asymptomatic women.[19,70]

Compliance with the three methods of breast cancer screening has also been investigated. While breast self-examination is easily accomplished by the woman without any equipment, compliance rates for monthly BSE have been reported to be only 15 to 40%.[71] Possible causes for low compliance have been reported to be forgetfulness, lack of competence in performing the examination, the complexity of the procedure, embarrassment, and lack of awareness of the effects of breast surgery on femininity and options of breast reconstruction.[72,73,74] Perceived risks that have been identified with breast self-examination that may affect compliance include anxiety experienced when some women examine their own bodies; potential risk of false-negative results, giving women at risk false reassurance; and false-positive results that incur expensive, time-consuming, and unnecessary diagnostic tests.[13,71,75]

In one study, Kurtz et al. found compliance with the American Cancer Society guidelines was 59% for breast self-examination, 71% for mammography, and 92% for clinical breast examination.[72] These rates are higher than others have reported,[76,77,78] but still demonstrate compliance problems with breast self-examination and mammography. While 98% of the sample had been taught breast self-examination, only 65% reported performing it according to a specific procedure, and only about half actually performed it monthly.

Barriers to and facilitators for compliance have also been defined. Perceived barriers included discomfort from the three types of examination, difficulty scheduling the mammogram at convenient times, and lack of knowledge of breast self-examination. Facilitators included desire for control over health and perceived efficacy of all three, perceived importance for mammography and clinical breast examination, and flexible scheduling of appointments. It is of note that cost was not perceived as a barrier to screening.[72,79]

Nurses need to incorporate these findings into comprehensive gynecologic educational programs for screening and detection (Table 1.6). Specific information about the importance of and need for breast self-examination and mammography must be stressed. A detailed procedure for performing breast self-examination (Figure 1.2), as well as supervised opportunities to practice, need to be provided. The benefits and efficacy of the screening tests also need to be discussed and reinforced. Finally, women need to be informed that timing of the tests during the menstrual cycle and reduction in caffeine intake have been correlated with decreased pain during mammography and clinical examination.[70]

The American Cancer Society recommends that women 40 and older have an annual mammogram and clinical breast exam performed by a health care professional at about the same time. A clinical physical examination of the breast is recommended every 3 years for women 20 to 39 years of age and annually for women over age 40. Breast self-examination should be performed monthly from age 20 onward.[24]

The NCI recommends regular mammograms (every 1 to 2 years) for women 40 years and older. Women who are at increased risk should discuss the initiation and frequency of mammograms with their health care provider.[80] The NCI also recommends monthly breast self-examination and consultation with a health professional on BSE technique.[81]

TABLE 1.6	
Client Information Needs: Screening Modalities	
Mammography	Avoid use of powder, deodorant, or perfume prior to test Schedule test after menses Advise that some discomfort may occur during test Advise to reduce caffeine intake prior to test
Breast Self–Exam	Perform exam at same time every month, preferably after menses in premenopausal women Instruct client regarding proper technique per NCI guidelines (Fig. 1.2)
Pap Smear	Proper timing of test prior to or after menses Refrain from intercourse for 48–72 hours prior to test Adequate preparation—no intravaginal medication, douching, or tampon use for 48–72 hours prior to test Advise that a small amount of vaginal spotting may occur
CA-125	Have blood test done at nonovulatory time Emphasize that false-positive test may occur
Ultrasound	Schedule test following menses Explain difference between vaginal probe and abdominal ultrasound
Endometrial Biopsy	Advise that minor discomfort and cramping may occur Consult with health care provider regarding premedication with nonsteroidal anti-inflammatory agents

Vulvar Exam	Instruct monthly self vulvar exam according to Sandella guidelines:[255]
	  Use mirror
	  Choose comfortable position such as sitting on bed with knees bent; standing beside toilet with one foot resting on the lid; sitting in bathtub or on edge of toilet seat
	  Observe entire vulva and examine for symmetry
	  Gently push back hood of clitoris, separate lips, and examine inner parts (urinary opening, vagina, skin between vagina and anus)
	  Feel for lumps or thickening

Controversial Issues

While there are still discussions about issues related to screening mammography (e.g. at what age to begin, what age to stop, and frequency), most groups are now recommending regular screening for women over 40 years. The controversy now seems to be related to issues of genetic testing: when to test women for BRCA1 and BRCA2 gene

BREAST SELF-EXAMINATION

Breast self-examination should be done once a month so you become familiar with the usual appearance and feel of your breasts. Familiarity makes it easier to notice any changes in the breast from one month to another. Early discovery of a change from what is "normal" is the main idea behind BSE. The outlook is much better if you detect cancer in an early stage.

If you menstruate, the best time to do BSE is 2 or 3 days after your period ends, when your breasts are least likely to be tender or swollen. If you no longer menstruate, pick a day such as the first day of the month, to remind yourself it is time to do BSE.

Here is one way to do BSE:

1. Stand before a mirror. Inspect both breasts for anything unusual such as any discharge from the nipples or puckering, dimpling, or scaling of the skin.

The next two steps are designed to emphasize any change in the shape or contour of your breasts. As you do them, you should be able to feel your chest muscles tighten.

2. Watching closely in the mirror, clasp your hands behind your head and press your hands forward.

3. Next, press your hands firmly on your hips and bow slightly toward your mirror as you pull your shoulders and elbows forward.

Some women do the next part of the exam in the shower because fingers glide over soapy skin, making it easy to concentrate on the texture underneath.

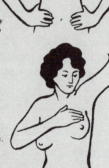

4. Raise your left arm. Use three or four fingers of your right hand to explore your left breast firmly, carefully, and thoroughly. Beginning at the outer edge, press the flat part of your fingers in small circles, moving the circles slowly around the breast. Gradually work toward the nipple. Be sure to cover the entire breast. Pay special attention to the area between the breast and the underarm, including the underarm itself. Feel for any unusual lump or mass under the skin.

5. Gently squeeze the nipple and look for a discharge. (If you have any discharge during the month— whether or not it is during BSE—see your doctor.) Repeat steps 4 and 5 on your right breast.

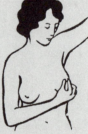

6. Steps 4 and 5 should be repeated lying down. Lie flat on your back with your left arm over your head and a pillow or folded towel under your left shoulder. This position flattens the breast and makes it easier to examine. Use the same circular motion described earlier. Repeat the exam on your right breast.

FIGURE 1.2. Breast self-examination.

Source: Reproduced with permission from National Cancer Institute (1992a). Breast exams: What you should know (NCI Publication No. 93–2000). Bethesda, MD: National Cancer Institute.

mutations and when to start screening women who have the BRCA1 or BRCA2 mutation. Genetic testing is not for everyone. While it is focused on women who have a strong family history of breast cancer, particularly those diagnosed at early ages, not all of these women take advantage of the testing. Some women may find that knowing that they have the mutation is helpful in future planning, while others may be overwhelmed by the knowledge. Additionally, maintaining or ensuring confidentiality of the results is an important issue since it is unknown how this information may be used for negative purposes for the woman and her offspring (i.e., by insurers or employers). Because there are no absolute prevention strategies to offer these women with the genetic mutation, the knowledge may be more academic than useful. While some recommend early screening for women with the mutation beginning at age 25 to 35, there is controversy as to the sensitivity and specificity of the mammogram in this younger population.[82] (See Table 1.7 on screening recommendations for women with the BRCA1 and BRCA2 mutations).

Prevention

Methods for preventing breast cancer focus on reducing risk by intervening in those factors that can be changed. Information on risk-reducing behaviors is an important aspect of the health education for any woman and is particularly important for the high-risk woman (Table 1.8). Diet alterations to prevent obesity, to reduce fat and alcohol intake, and to increase ingestion of raw vegetables, especially carrots, and vitamin A intake, may reduce the risk and thus prevent the development of breast cancer.[83] Prophylactic mastectomies are an option advocated for women at high risk, that is, those with a strong family history of breast cancer. This approach is associated with

TABLE 1.7	
Guidelines for Early Detection for BRCA1 and BRCA2 Mutation Carriers (CGSC)	
Condition	*Guidelines*
Breast Cancer	Monthly breast self-exam beginning at age 18–21 Clinical breast exam: annual or semiannual beginning at age 25–35 Annual mammography beginning at age 25–35
Ovarian Cancer	Annual or semiannual TVS ideally with addition of color flow Doppler beginning at age 25–35 Annual or semiannual CA-125

Source: Burke et al, Recommendations for follow-up care of individuals with an inherited predisposition to cancer II. BRCA1 and BRCA2. *JAMA,* 277(12), 997–1003.

TABLE 1.8

Client Information Needs: Risk-Reducing Behaviors

Primary cancer	Risk-reducing behaviors

Breast Cancer	Maintain normal body weight
	Reduce dietary fat and alcohol intake
	Increase dietary intake of vitamin A
	Practice monthly breast self-examination
	Have annual breast examination by health care professional
	Have mammogram as appropriate for age and risk
	High risk:
	    Chemoprevention with tamoxifen
	    Prophylactic mastectomies
	    Genetic screening as available

Cervical Cancer	Have annual Pap smear Limit sexual activity in the teen years Limit number of sexual partners Develop safe sexual practices by using barrier contraception: diaphragm and condom Health education before girls become sexually active regarding risks of sexual contact; safe sexual practices and disease prevention methods; and purpose, need, and frequency of Pap testing and pelvic examinations Stop smoking: referral to smoking cessation program, prescription for medical treatment Increase dietary intake of vitamin A Seek prompt treatment of cervical intraepithelial neoplasia

Ovarian Cancer	Have annual pelvic examination
	Reduce dietary fat intake
	Increase dietary intake of vitamin A
	Use oral contraceptives for birth control
	Eliminate use of talc-containing products for genital hygiene
	High risk:
	    Screening with transvaginal ultrasound and CA-125
	    Prophylactic oophorectomies if childbearing completed

Endometrial Cancer	Have annual pelvic examination Sequence progesterone with estrogen replacement therapy Use oral contraceptives for birth control Modify diet for weight control; reduce total weight if overweight If diabetic, have regular medical check-ups for control of diabetes Seek timely medical evaluation for abnormal uterine bleeding Consider treatment of endometrial hyperplasia with progestins, or hysterectomy if childbearing completed

TABLE 1.8 *(continued)*

Client Information Needs: Risk-Reducing Behaviors

Primary cancer	Risk-reducing behaviors
Vulvar Cancer	Have annual vulvar and pelvic examination Perform monthly self-examinations of vulva Modify diet for weight control; reduce total weight Stop smoking: referral to smoking cessation program, prescription for medical treatment If diabetic, have regular medical check-ups for control of diabetes Seek prompt medical attention for vulvar irritation or genital warts Have prompt treatment of intraepithelial neoplasia of the vulva Develop safe sexual practices by using barrier contraception (condom, diaphragm), limit number of sexual partners
Vaginal Cancer	Have annual pelvic examination Seek prompt treatment of cervicovaginal intraepithelial neoplasia Use of water or vinegar for douching if necessary Seek prompt medical attention for HPV infection or genital warts Develop safe sexual practices by using barrier contraception (condom, diaphragm), limit number of sexual partners

personal and ethical concerns as well as medical concerns and is obviously not the ideal method of prevention for the general population.

Another focus in prevention is that of chemoprevention. Because of evidence that estrogen stimulation is related to the development of breast cancer, it is hypothesized that methods to interrupt that stimulation may prevent breast cancer. Tamoxifen has been identified as a potential chemopreventive agent because of data from clinical trials demonstrating increased survival and decreased incidence of a second breast cancer with its use. Reduction of cell proliferation in breast tissue is the goal of chemoprevention, and tamoxifen, as an anti-estrogen, can potentially achieve this in normal breast tissue.[25]

To determine if tamoxifen can reduce the risk or prevent breast cancer in high-risk women over 35, the National Surgical Adjuvant Breast and Bowel Project initiated the Breast Cancer Prevention Trial in May 1992. The aim of this trial was to randomize 16,000 women to receive either tamoxifen 20 mg daily or a placebo. In September 1997, 13,388 women were randomly assigned in the trial. Because of the strength of the risk reduction demonstrated in the accrued sample, the trial was closed early to patient entry. The data showed that invasive breast cancer risk was reduced by 49% overall with the greatest reduction in women 60 years and older. Noninvasive breast cancer risk was decreased by 50%. Despite adverse effects seen such as increased endometrial cancer, stroke, pulmonary embolism, and deep venous thrombosis in the tamoxifen-treated group, it was concluded that the benefit outweighed the risks. Tamoxifen is an appropriate agent for prevention of breast cancer in many women at high risk for the disease. A new trial will compare tamoxifen with raloxifene, a new selective estrogen-receptor modulator, to determine if raloxifene can prevent breast cancer without some of the side effects of tamoxifen such as increasing the risk of endometrial cancer.[84]

The association of dietary intake of phytoestrogens derived from plants, such as soy, and reduction of breast cancer, and the use of suppressor genes BRCA1 and BRCA2, or the development of similar agents to prevent or treat breast cancer are also being investigated. Further research is needed to understand if there is a role for these modalities in prevention.[85]

✖ CERVICAL CANCER

The ACS estimated that in 1999, approximately 12,800 women would be diagnosed with cervical cancer and that 4,800 women would die from this disease.[1] The incidence of cervical cancer has decreased worldwide, largely due to use of the Pap test. However, it is still a major cause of cancer mortality in developing countries. Conversely, the incidence of precancerous lesions, cervical intraepithelial neoplasia (CIN), has risen dramatically owing to increased screening as well as a true increase in incidence. The median age for the occurrence of cervical cancer is 45 to 50 years, while the median age for CIN is in the third decade.

Population at Risk

Numerous epidemiologic studies have identified a positive association between squamous cervical cancer and multiple social and physical characteristics (Table 1.9). The frequency and length of exposure to these risk factors increases the risk of developing cervical cancer. High-risk factors include sexual habits (early coitus, multiple partners), male sexual partners (multiple partners, penile cancer, venereal disease), genital infection (human papilloma virus), chemical carcinogens (cigarette smoking, oral contraceptives), immunosuppression (in organ transplant recipients), and social status (low socioeconomic class).

TABLE 1.9	
Risk Factors for Cervical Cancer	
Intercourse at an early age	Cigarette smoking
Multiple sexual partners	Oral contraceptive use
Male partner risk factors	Immunosuppression
Human papilloma virus infection	Low socioeconomic status

Squamous cancer of the cervix appears to be a "venereal" disease, since the association of this cancer risk with sexual behavior has been the most consistent epidemiological finding. The two critical sexual determinants of risk include early age at first intercourse and lifetime number of sexual partners.[86] The sexual behavior of the male partner has also been found to affect the risk of cervical cancer. In a study by Zunzunegui et al.,[87] the husbands of women with cervical cancer had more sexual partners, had intercourse at an earlier age, and had a greater history of venereal disease than husbands of women without cervical cancer. Women married to men who previously had wives with cervical cancer are also at a greater risk for the development of cervical cancer.[88] Studies have demonstrated that wives of men with penile cancer are also at increased risk.[89,90]

The strong association between cervical cancer and sexual activity suggests that a sexually transmitted infectious organism may be an etiologic agent. In recent years the role of viruses as etiologic agents has been suggested. Initially, herpes simplex virus type II (HSV-2) received the emphasis, but currently human papilloma virus (HPV) is suggested as exerting an etiologic role in the genesis of cervical cancer.[91,92,93] Clearly HPV is an insufficient cause of cervical cancer, since HPV infection is also found in a substantial proportion of disease-free women. Therefore, other risk factors may be responsible for the progression of HPV to invasive cancer.

Cigarette smoking has been implicated as a risk factor for cervical cancer, especially squamous cell carcinoma. Cotinine and nicotine have been shown to exert mutagenic activity in the cervical mucus of smokers.[94] Cigarette smoking produces a local immunosuppression in cervical epithelium, which may increase the likelihood of the development of HPV-induced neoplastic transformation.[95] In a case control study, women who reported ever having regularly smoked cigarettes had a 50% elevated risk compared with nonsmokers. Women who smoked 40 or more cigarettes per day, as well as those who smoked for 40 or more years, had significant twofold excess risks.[96]

The relationship between oral contraceptive use and cervical neoplasia has been studied extensively. Early studies failed to demonstrate an association between pill use and cervical abnormalities,[97,98] but recent studies have found positive relationships. In a case control study of invasive cervical cancer in five geographic areas of the United States, pill users were found to have a 50% excess risk. Risks were highest among users of high-estrogen pills, and associations were observed for both adenocarcinomas and squamous cell carcinomas.[99] Further evidence that the pill is related to invasive cervical cancer was reported by the World Health Organization (WHO) Collaborative Study of Neoplasia and Steroid Contraceptives. In this study, after extensive control of confounding variables such as sexual activity and cancer history, an increased risk was noted with any use of the pill, with the greatest increase in users for 5 or more years.[100] The mechanism of action of oral contraceptives on the cervical epithelium is unclear. There is evidence that cervical tissue is subject to a variety of proliferative changes resulting from oral contraceptive use; however, further studies are needed to address this question. In contrast to hormonal contraceptives, several studies have demonstrated that users of barrier methods, such as diaphragm and condom, are at a lower cervical cancer risk.[101,102]

Immunosuppression has been identified as a risk factor for cervical neoplasia. Women who are iatrogenically immunosuppressed due to medical conditions or organ transplant have a greater incidence of cervical as well as other anogenital malignancies. In a study, women who had undergone renal transplants were shown to have an incidence of cervical cancer five times higher than that of age-matched controls.[103] The progressive immunosuppression associated with HIV infection has prompted concern regarding its impact on the potential for cervical neoplasia in HIV-positive women. Feingold et al.[104] reported a 49% incidence of HPV infection in HIV-infected women, compared to 25% in HIV-negative women. The progression of HPV infection to the development of cervical neoplasia in HIV-positive women has been shown to be related to the degree of immunosuppression.[105] More rapid progression of cervical intraepithelial neoplasia to cervical cancer and a poorer response to therapy has been noted in HIV-positive women.[106]

It has been demonstrated that cervical cancer predominantly affects women in lower socioeconomic classes. The risk among women in the lowest social classes is approximately five times that among those in the highest classes.[107] The role that social class exerts is unclear but may be related to poor diet or inadequate health care.

Screening Methods

Pelvic examination and the Papanicolaou (Pap) smear are the primary screening tools for cervical cancer. The success of the Pap test is so well established that there is no doubt about its clinical usefulness. However, issues related to frequency and what errors impede its sensitivity require clarification.

Recommended guidelines for Pap smear screening are listed in Tables 1.1 to 1.4. ACS, ACOG, and NCI recommend initial Pap smear screening in women who have been sexually active or who have reached 18. After a woman has had three or more consecutive satisfactory annual exams, the Pap test may be performed less frequently at the discretion of the physician. The Canadian Task Force recommends Pap smear screening frequency based on age and risk factors (Table 1.2). Objection to the guidelines for Pap testing center on insistence that it be performed annually. In a 1989 survey of physicians' attitudes and practices in early cancer detection, 82% of 1,629 physicians surveyed indicated that Pap test screening should be done annually, regardless of risk factors.[108] There are some very practical problems in advising women to have less frequent Pap smear screening. That is, an assessment of a woman's screening history should be based on verification of past Pap smear reports and frequency. Several studies have demonstrated that self-reported information on Pap smears is often inaccurate.[109,110,111] Women were likely to report more frequent and more recent smears than could be documented and inconsistent or incorrect Pap smear results as well. Thus, it is crucial that before less frequent screening is recommended, evidence for these negative consecutive annual tests be firmly documented.[112] Nurses should encourage women to learn the results of their tests in order to assume responsibility for their own health.[113]

There is general agreement that annual or more frequent screening be carried out in high-risk women. This group includes women who begin sexual activity prior to age 20, who have had multiple sexual partners or who have had a partner who has had multiple sexual partners, those with sexually transmitted diseases (particularly HPV or HSV), those who have CIN, and those who smoke.[114] It is estimated that a substantial proportion of women fall into these high-risk categories. Thus it is essential for nurses to obtain a thorough sexual, social, and physical history at each visit to determine risk category changes and appropriate screening intervals. Elements of the history should include questions specific to high-risk factors for cervical cancer, such as age at first intercourse, number of sexual partners, history of HPV infection, male partners' sexual history, birth control methods, and smoking history.

The growing number of women with HIV infection are potentially at risk for cervical cancer. Careful and frequent Pap smear screening to ensure prompt follow-up for those HIV-positive women in whom abnormalities are detected have been advocated.[115,116] Vermund et al.[117] recommended yearly Pap smear and gynecologic examinations for women at high risk for HIV and screening every six months for women with symptomatic HIV infection or CD4 cell counts <200/mm^3. The CDC recommends that HIV-positive women should have a Pap smear as part of their initial evaluation. A Pap smear should then be obtained twice in the first year after diagnosis of HIV infection and, if the results are normal, annually thereafter.[118]

Pap Smear Technique and Interpretation

An optimal Pap smear requires sampling of the entire transformation zone of the cervix, including epithelium from the endocervical canal as well as epithelium from the ectocervix. Sampling of the endocervical canal requires the use of a small, narrow brush or a saline-moistened, cotton-tipped applicator. Advantages of the brush include its ability to trap fewer cells in its network than the cotton applicator, and its smaller size, enabling sampling in women who have a narrow or stenotic cervical os. The use of a small, narrow brush has consistently demonstrated superiority over the cotton swab in obtaining endocervical cells.[119,120] Use of the brush in pregnancy is not recommended at this time, although no adverse effects on pregnancy outcome were noted in a recent study.[121] Sampling of the ectocervix requires use of a spatula that is placed in the cervical os and rotated 360 degrees. Samples should be spread out uniformly over the slide and should be fixed immediately with an aerosol fixative or similar product.

For many years, cervical cytologic smears were reported according to the original Papanicolaou classification. This system utilized numerical classes from I (normal) to V (invasive cancer). This classification was later revised to the CIN system in an attempt to better distinguish precancer phases from cancer. The most recent attempt to standardize Pap smear technology involves the Bethesda System,[122,123] which was introduced to replace both the numerical Papanicolaou and CIN class designations and promote precise communication regarding cytologic results. This system includes three main categories: (1) a statement of specimen adequacy, (2) a general categorization of normal or abnormal, and (3) descriptive diagnoses. Epithelial cell abnormalities are divided into low- and high-grade groups. Low-grade squamous intraepithelial lesion (SIL) includes mild dysplasia/CIN I and human papilloma virus lesions, and high-grade SIL includes moderate dysplasia/CIN II and severe dysplasia or carcinoma in situ/CIN III. The Bethesda System also includes an evaluation of hormonal state, infection, reactive and reparative changes, and glandular cell components.

It is a common assumption that the Pap test is a precise tool of cancer detection and that no errors in its interpretation can be tolerated. This is not the case. The rate of smear failure for invasive cancer has been shown to be 24 to 50%.[124,125] Numerous demonstrations of cervical smear failure in the presence of precancerous lesions have also been reported.[124,126,127] The false-negative rate for the Pap smear may be attributed to sampling technique, interpretation error, and patient factors.

Meticulous technique in obtaining a Pap smear is essential in reducing false-negative results. To avoid contamination of the cell sample with foreign material, excess cervical mucus should be gently removed with a dry, cotton-tipped applicator, and use of lubricants must be avoided. To prevent air-drying artifact, the smear must be fixed rapidly. (Refer to Chapter 2 for more information on Pap smear technique.)

To minimize interpretation errors, Koss recommends several procedures to improve quality control.[128] The Centers for Disease Control recommends rescreening 10% of all negative smears to issue a license for interstate commerce. Other possible methods of quality control include a reasonable, regulated workload for cytotechnologists to prevent "fatigue" error (mandatory in California only), competency examination (mandatory in New York State only), and continuing education through seminars and postgraduate workshops. It is evident that there is room for improvement in the area of quality control.

Patient preparation is an important variable in improving the reliability of Pap smear screening (Table 1.6). Women should be instructed to refrain from coitus, tampon use, douching, or intravaginal medication use for forty-eight to seventy-two hours before the Pap appointment. The appointment should be scheduled at an appropriate time, preferably in the first half of the menstrual cycle before ovulation but after completion of menses. The Pap smear ideally should not be taken at menses or if the woman is experiencing any bleeding, since the presence of blood interferes with accurate interpretation.

Nursing has a critical role in the promotion and adequacy of Pap smear screening. This role, discussed by Ginsburg,[129] is twofold and includes consumer advocacy for wellness and education of other health care professionals. Consumer advocacy includes counseling regarding the Pap smear procedure, timing of test, high-risk behaviors, test results, and screening intervals. The acute need for education regarding Pap smear screening was demonstrated in a study of women attending an inner-city sexually transmitted disease (STD) clinic. Thirty-three percent of these women did not know the purpose of a Pap smear. Of the 67% who stated that they did know, only 30% accurately stated that a Pap smear is used to detect cancer.[130] Ginsburg also suggested that education of other health professionals include an in-service program for office staff on screening techniques, quality control issues, and timing of appointments.[129] The nurse should also request information from the laboratory concerning protocols for maintaining quality control and assurance.

Nurse practitioners (NPs) can have a substantial impact on the accuracy of Pap smear screening. In a recent Australian study comparing Pap smears collected by NPs versus medical practitioners, women screened by NPs were more likely to be older, of non–English-speaking background, and to have had fewer smears collected previously.[131] The quality of the smears collected by the NPs did not differ from the smears obtained by medical practitioners.[131] In a two-year study examining the relationship between various levels of experience and the ability to obtain adequate Pap smears, nurse practitioners had the second highest rating in the first year and the highest percentage of successful smears in the second year when compared with first- to fourth-year residents and attending staff.[132] In a study of 149 rural black women, those seeing a nurse practitioner were more likely to accurately report frequency of past Pap smears compared to those seeing gynecologists and family practitioners.[110] Koss states that well-trained paramedical staff may perform better Pap smears than most untrained physicians.[128] Clearly, nurse practitioners are in an ideal position to promote Pap smear screening, to provide accurate sampling of all populations, and to provide counseling and education to women and other health professionals regarding all aspects of prevention and screening for cervical cancer.

Controversial Issues

Controversy exists regarding the need for Pap smear screening in elderly women. However, cervical cancer remains an important health problem into old age. The Canadian Task Force recommends no further screening in women over age 60 who have had repeated satisfactory smears without significant atypia (Table 1.2). Earlier ACS guidelines recommended screening up to age 65, but based on recent evidence that the Pap test may be useful for women over that age, revised guidelines now have no upper age limit.[5] To promote decreased morbidity and mortality for cervical cancer, Medicare coverage was extended in 1990 to include triennial Pap smear screening in this population. And Mandelblatt et al. caution that recommended screening intervals may need to be adjusted as data regarding the transit time of CIN to invasive cancer in elderly women become available.[133]

Other screening tools, aside from the conventional Pap test, may detect cervical neoplasia, although their role in routine screening is controversial. These tools include colposcopy, cervicography, self-administered cervical cancer screening, automated cytology, and ThinPrep.

The combined use of the Pap smear and colposcopy has been shown to improve the accuracy of cervical cancer detection. Colposcopy requires the application of acetic acid to the cervix, followed by careful microscopic evaluation of the entire transformation zone. Colposcopic screening requires considerable expertise, time, and expense; thus it is not practical as a routine screening test. At present, the primary role of colposcopy is in evaluating women with abnormal Pap smears. Efforts directed at improving screening with acetic acid visualization of the cervix without colposcopy are not helpful in detecting cervical abnormalities.[134]

Cervicography, a newer diagnostic method, provides permanent documentation of cervical patterns. After the application of acetic acid, a cervicograph camera is used to take photographs of the cervix. The cervicogram can be taken by a nurse or physician and sent to an expert for evaluation. Cervicography offers the diagnostic accuracy of combined colposcopy and cytology with minimal added expense.[135] A comparison of the Pap smear versus the cervicogram demonstrated higher sensitivity but lower specificity with the cervicogram in detecting cervical neoplasia.[136] Cervicography is not recommended at this time as a routine screening tool.

Self-administered cervical cancer screening offers the possibility of reaching women in areas that lack access to health care, as well as those who object to Pap smear screening for various reasons. An evaluation of the self-administered device, MY-PAP, in 1,151 women identified 78% of high-grade lesions, 97% of invasive cancers, but only 53% of low-grade lesions.[137] However, comparable results between the standard Pap smear and the vaginal cytopipette were noted in 107 Danish women.[138] No one could argue against the traditional administration of a conventional Pap smear, which provides consultation with a health care provider in addition to visual and manual examinations. Thus self-administered techniques, rather than replace the Pap smear and pelvic examination, provide options to those women not reached though standard screening methods. However, at this time, MY-PAP is not FDA approved or commercially available.

A solution to the Pap smear false-negative rate, the tedious nature of slide analysis, and the decreasing number of cytotechnology graduates lies in the potential of automated examination of the Pap smear. The NCI states that a satisfactory automated instrument must have a false-negative rate of 5% or less.[139] Recent studies have demonstrated the efficacy of automated devices for cervical cytology that meet NCI criteria.[140,141] But clinical trials are needed to examine the role, advantages, disadvantages, and medical-legal issues of automated cytology.

A new method of cytology preparation, the ThinPrep process, has been developed. This method requires direct transfer of cells into a preservative solution, gentle dispersion, homogenization of the cell population, collection on a polycarbonate filter, followed by transfer to a glass slide. Clinical trials have demonstrated that this method is more sensitive for the detection of cervical abnormalities than the conventional Pap smear method.[142] Increased diagnostic accuracy, with the potential to reduce false-negative cervical cytology, is an important advantage of the ThinPrep method.[142]

Prevention

Squamous cervical cancer is a potentially preventable disease due to the long preinvasive stage and the availability of effective screening techniques. The fact that cervical cancer still accounts for over 4,900 deaths per year in the United States emphasizes the need for nursing strategies directed at primary and secondary prevention. Nurses are in a key position to promote routine Pap smear screening to all women.

Primary prevention strategies (Table 1.7) could include education of women, especially adolescents, regarding the risk of early sexual activity, number of sexual partners, and HPV infection. The integration of cervical cancer information in health classes for adolescents by school nurses may be helpful.[143] Sexual abstinence would be ideal but difficult to achieve. The use of barrier/condom contraception should be promoted. Safe sex guidelines and HIV preventive strategies have been compiled and may also be appropriate in the prevention of cervical neoplasia.[144] Information regarding the purpose, need, and frequency of Pap smear screening may promote better compliance with screening efforts.

Women should be advised of the health risks of cigarette smoking, including the increased risk of cervical cancer. Nursing strategies directed toward smoking cessation could include the use of educational materials, counseling smokers to help them quit, referral to smoking cessation programs, and medical treatment such as nicotine gum or the patch.

Vitamin A (transretinoic acid) has been shown to be capable of preventing epithelial cell changes. That retinoids have the capability of preventing the progression of precancerous lesions to malignant disease supports the concept that they may play a role in the prevention of cervical neoplasia.[145,146] Based on limited data, it is reasonable, from a prevention standpoint, to encourage women to include adequate amounts of vitamin A in their diets.

OVARIAN CANCER

Carcinoma of the ovary is responsible for 46% of all gynecologic cancers and is the most common fatal gynecologic malignancy.[1] In the United States, the overall probability of a woman developing ovarian cancer is estimated to be 1 in 70, and it is estimated that 1 of every 100 women will die of the disease.[147] Ovarian cancer has its major impact on postmenopausal women, with the greatest incidence in women 55 to 59 years of age. There has been little appreciable reduction in the mortality from ovarian cancer in the last twenty years, probably related to the advanced stage at the time of diagnosis and the lack of effective screening modalities.

Population at Risk

The exact etiology of ovarian cancer is not known. However, age, environmental, dietary, reproductive, endocrine, hereditary, chemical, and viral risk factors have been identified as potentially causative (Table 1.10).[148] Ovarian cancer risk increases with age and the incidence peaks in the eighth decade.

TABLE 1.10

Risk Factors for Ovarian Cancer

Age	Endocrine factors
Environment	Family history
Diet	Chemical exposure
Reproductive factors	Viral exposure

That an environmental factor or factors may be implicated in increasing risk is suggested by the fact that the highest incidence of ovarian cancer occurs in industrialized countries, particularly in northern and western Europe and North America. Japan, with its low incidence of ovarian cancer, is the one exception.[149] Further, indication of a possible environmental link is supported by the fact that first- and second-generation Japanese women in the United States have incidence rates of ovarian cancer approximating those of white women born in the United States.[148]

The major dietary difference among people in industrialized nations is in their intake of meat and animal fat. In a study by Cramer et al.,[150] women above the highest quartile of animal fat consumption had a twofold increase in ovarian cancer compared with those below the lowest quartile. Milk, when it is a vehicle for animal fat consumption, has been shown to increase ovarian cancer risk. Daily consumption of multiple glasses of whole milk has resulted in a threefold increase in ovarian cancer risk, whereas reported intake of 2% milk has been associated with reduced risk.[151] No association between ovarian cancer and the consumption of coffee, alcohol, or tobacco has been found. A diet rich in vitamin A has been suggested to reduce the risk of ovarian cancer.[152]

Reproductive factors have been suggested as playing a role in either the causation or prevention of ovarian cancer. Several studies have indicated that pregnancy and use of oral contraceptives are protective against its development. Early age at first pregnancy,[153] number of pregnancies,[154] and number of incomplete pregnancies[155] have also been demonstrated to reduce risk. The protection afforded by oral contraceptives against ovarian cancer risk is well established. The most impressive study reported by the Cancer and Steroid Hormone Study[156] demonstrated that the decrease in risk was directly related to the duration of oral contraceptive use and that this lower risk proved to be a long-term effect. A quantitative assessment of oral contraceptive use and risk of ovarian cancer revealed a 36% risk reduction from ever use, and a 50% decrease in risk after five years of use.[157]

Whittemore et al.[158] reported that inability to conceive, possibly due to some form of hormonal or endocrine abnormality, was an underlying high-risk factor. In this study, nulliparous women who had ovulatory cycles and unprotected sexual relations for ten or more years had a twofold risk of developing ovarian cancer compared with women who did not have two or more years of unprotected sexual intercourse without pregnancy.

Two theories have been offered to explain the decreased incidence of ovarian cancer associated with oral contraceptive use and pregnancy, and the increased incidence in women who are unable to conceive. Gardner proposed that repetitive high levels of gonadotropin acting on the ovary due to the inability of the ovarian/pituitary feedback mechanism to inhibit excretion of high levels of it results in ovarian cancer.[159] This theory may explain why infertile women are at increased risk for ovarian cancer. If true, then perhaps hyperstimulation of the ovary by fertility drugs may also increase risk. The association between ovulation-inducing agents and ovarian cancer in infertile women was first suggested in two case reports.[160,161] And Whittemore et al.[162] reported that women who had used fertility drugs had almost three times the risk of developing ovarian cancer over women with no history of infertility. Further research is warranted to explore the possible role of fertility drugs in the etiology of ovarian cancer. The second theory, the "incessant ovulation theory" proposed by Fathalla,[163] suggests that continuous ovulation causes repeated trauma to the ovary and may lead to the development of ovarian cancer. Thus a decrease in ovulation resulting from pregnancy or oral contraceptive use can exert a protective effect.

Despite increased attention to the genetic predisposition to ovarian cancer, it is important to note that genetic factors account for only 5 to 10% of all ovarian cancer cases.[164] Familial ovarian cancer is transmitted as an autosomal dominant trait with variable penetration through maternal or paternal lineage. Three types of families that have demonstrated this mode of genetic transmission include: site-specific ovarian cancer families,[165] breast-ovarian cancer families,[166] and hereditary nonpolyposis colorectal cancer (Lynch syndrome II) families.[167] Ovarian cancer in each of these syndromes is characterized by early age of onset;[168] predominance of the serous type of tumor, with a trend toward more poorly differentiated adenocarcinomas; and a high percentage of bilateral ovarian involvement.[169,170] It is estimated that the risk of female offspring developing ovarian cancer in these autosomal-dominant familial syndromes may be as high as 50% in first-degree female relatives.[171]

The recent identification of BRCA1 and BRCA2 mutations has confirmed the existence of hereditary ovarian cancer patterns. Mutations of the BRCA1 gene are responsible for the majority of cases of familial breast-ovarian cancer syndrome. It is estimated that a female BRCA1 mutation carrier has 40–60% lifetime risk of developing ovarian cancer in contrast to the 1–3% incidence of ovarian cancer in the general population.[172] It is estimated that a female BRCA2 mutation carrier has an estimated 10–20% lifetime risk of developing ovarian cancer.[172]

The Familial Ovarian Cancer Registry was established in 1981 at the Roswell Park Cancer Center to collect reports of familial ovarian cancer and to evaluate epidemiologic characteristics, chromosomal analysis, and biochemical markers in women with these syndromes.[170] After the 1989 death of well-known comedienne Gilda Radner to familial ovarian cancer, the registry was renamed the Gilda Radner Familial Ovarian Cancer Registry.

Chemicals, including talc and asbestos, have been implicated in the causation of ovarian cancer. Until 1977, most talc powders contained asbestos, and there is sufficient evidence to support the translocation of particulate matter from the vagina to the ovaries.[173,174] However, there are conflicting reports on the role of talc in causing ovarian cancer. Several epidemiologic studies have demonstrated a genital talc–ovarian cancer association,[175,176,177] whereas Whittemore et al.[158] failed to demonstrate any such link.

There are conflicting and speculative reports on the association between viral infection and increased risk of ovarian cancer. Mumps virus is known to have an affinity for the gonads as well as the parotid gland, and ovarian cancer patients have been shown to have a decreased incidence of clinical mumps.[178] However, Menczer et al.[179] reported a higher incidence of subclinical mumps, demonstrated by the presence of positive serologic evidence, in women with ovarian cancer. Rubella infection between the ages of 12 and 18 has also been suggested as a risk factor, but confirmatory studies are lacking.[180]

Screening Methods

There is little doubt concerning the need for screening and early detection of ovarian cancer.(See Table 1.7.) It fulfills some of the disease criteria appropriate for screening: it is a major cause of mortality, and survival rates of early stage disease are significantly higher than those of advanced stage disease. However, the low incidence of ovarian cancer when compared to other cancers, the lack of a preinvasive phase, and the relatively short preclinical phase pose problems for effective screening.

Periodic pelvic examination is currently the only standard method of surveillance for ovarian cancer. (ACS guidelines regarding frequency of pelvic examination are outlined in Table 1.1.) Most would agree that a bimanual rectovaginal examination should be part of the annual physical, even though it is not very effective in early detection of ovarian cancer. For example, in a study of 23,635 women in Australia, pelvic examination resulted in detection of only six primary ovarian cancers.[181] It has also been estimated that in 10,000 routine examinations, only one case of ovarian cancer would be identified.[182] The Pap smear is not a useful tool for screening and early detection and, in one study, was positive in only 26% of women with ovarian cancer, primarily those with ascites and advanced disease.[183] Thus the 1994 NCI Consensus Development Conference on Ovarian Cancer concluded that all women should have a comprehensive family history taken by a health care professional knowledgeable in the risks associated with ovarian cancer and should continue to undergo annual rectovaginal pelvic examination as part of routine medical care.[184]

Controversial Issues

Much controversy exists regarding the use of current screening modalities, the appropriateness of mass screening, as well as the screening of high-risk populations. But at this time there are no available techniques, other than pelvic examination, suitable for routine screening.[18,182]

Presently, serum tumor markers and ultrasonography in conjunction with pelvic examination are being investigated as possible ovarian cancer screening tests. The screening test most widely discussed in the literature is the serum tumor marker CA-125. CA-125 is an antigenic determinant defined by monoclonal immunoglobulin antibody (OC125). This antigenic determinant is associated with a high molecular weight glycoprotein that is expressed in coelomic epithelium during embryonic development.[185]

Serum levels of CA-125 have been reported to be elevated in >80% of patients with epithelial ovarian cancer and to reflect the clinical course of the disease.[186,187] High CA-125 levels have also been associated with poor prognosis.[188] Furthermore, the frequency of elevated serum CA-125 is directly related to extent of disease and histologic type of tumor: CA-125 is elevated in only 50% of early Stage I disease and is

TABLE 1.11	
Disorders Associated with	
Elevation of Serum CA–125	
Malignancies	*Other disorders*
Ovary	Benign ovarian tumors
Pancreas	Salpingitis
Liver	Pregnancy
Lung	Endometriosis
Gastrointestinal	Menstruation
Colorectal	Cirrhosis
Breast	Renal failure
Esophagus	Hepatitis
	Pancreatitis

expressed less often in mucinous type tumors.[189] But CA-125 levels may be elevated in other malignancies and other benign pathological and physiological states (Table 1.11).[190–196] Thus the use of CA-125 as a sensitive primary screening test for ovarian cancer is limited.

The specificity of CA-125 as a screening method for ovarian cancer has also been investigated. In a study of 5,500 healthy women, elevated CA-125 levels were detected in 175 (3.1%). On the basis of clinical examination and ultrasound, twelve women underwent exploratory laparotomy, and six ovarian cancers were detected.[197] A study of 4,000 postmenopausal volunteers in England detected only one case of ovarian cancer out of 70 women with elevated CA-125 levels.[198] In both of these studies, the specificity of CA-125 was 97% with an extremely low yield. Extremely high specificity is an essential requirement for any screening test for ovarian cancer. It has been estimated that a screening test with a 99.6 specificity would still result in nine false-positive tests for each case of ovarian cancer.[199] Therefore, the current 97% specificity of CA-125 used alone precludes its use as a primary screening modality.

The use of other tumor markers in conjunction with CA-125 has been suggested in an attempt to improve screening techniques.[199,200] A combination of other tumor-associated antigens and CA-125 achieved higher sensitivity and specificity for the detection of advanced ovarian cancer, but still missed a significant number of early cases.[201,202] Thus use of multiple tumor marker assays in combination still poses serious limitations. Clearly other approaches are needed.

The use of abdominal sonography as a screening method for ovarian cancer has been suggested by Campbell et al.[203] These investigators screened 5,500 asymptomatic pre- and postmenopausal women for ovarian cancer with abdominal ultrasound. A total of 326 women (from 338 abnormal scans) underwent laparotomy, resulting in a diagnosis of early stage ovarian cancer in five women. But since abdominal sonography requires a full bladder for accurate identification of pelvic structures, the exam is uncomfortable and not time-efficient. Furthermore, the ovaries are difficult to visualize in obese women due to increased body fat.

The use of transvaginal sonography (TVS) for ovarian cancer screening is more comfortable, time-efficient since it does not require a full bladder, and more accurate due to the shorter distance between the vaginal transducer and the ovaries. In a study of 1,000 women 40 years or older, TVS was carried out to investigate the efficacy of this technique as a screening method. Thirty-one women had abnormal sonograms. Of the twenty-four women who underwent exploratory laparotomy, one woman was diagnosed with metastatic ovarian carcinoma from a primary colon cancer that had been in remission for two years.[204] It has been suggested that TVS is more effective in postmenopausal women, in whom variation in ovarian size during different phases of the menstrual cycle is avoided. But in a study of 1,300 asymptomatic, postmenopausal women, ovarian cancer was detected in only two women.[205]

Adjunctive methods to increase the specificity of TVS are being evaluated. These include Doppler flow sonography and the morphology index. Doppler flow sonography is a noninvasive technique for evaluating the blood flow and vasculature of ovarian tumors. (It is known that malignant ovarian tumors have increased vascularity and altered blood flow.) Preliminary studies have suggested the ability of Doppler flow studies to differentiate benign from malignant ovarian tumors, thus possibly enhancing the value of sonography in screening for ovarian cancer.[206,207] However, in one study, transvaginal Doppler sonography was not shown to be superior to TVS, magnetic resonance imaging (MRI), or CA-125 in the differentiation of malignant from benign ovarian tumors.[208] A morphology index, based on specific sonographic characteristics of benign versus malignant ovarian tumors, has been developed and may help predict the risk of malignancy in a woman with a tumor identified by TVS.[209]

To recommend the use of CA-125 and ultrasound as mass screening tests for ovarian cancer is premature at this time. Creasman and DiSaia point out the exorbitant expense and consequences of such testing.[182] To screen the 43,000,000 women in the United States aged 45 years or older with pelvic ultrasound and CA-125 would increase health care costs by more than $13 billion per year without any guarantee of lowering the death rate from ovarian cancer. Furthermore, this total cost does not include the morbidity and possible mortality resulting from unnecessary surgical evaluations for false-positive diagnostic findings.

However, clinical trials are needed to establish the effectiveness and utility of ovarian cancer screening techniques in high-risk groups such as women with a documented pelvic mass, postmenopausal women, and women with a genetic risk for ovarian cancer. It has been suggested that CA-125 or ultrasound may be helpful screening tools in predicting benign versus malignant pathology in women with a documented pelvic mass. An elevated CA-125 level, by itself, was not shown to sufficiently distinguish benign from malignant masses, although CA-125 level was more predictive in women over age 50.[194] Abdominal sonography has been shown to be a sensitive, but not specific, method for evaluating adnexal masses in postmenopausal women, but missed 6% of malignant ovarian tumors in one series.[210] Sensitivity for CA-125 in combination with ultrasound in women with ovarian masses was increased, with the greatest sensitivity noted in postmenopausal women.[211] Thus the use of screening techniques may have an important role in the preoperative evaluation of women, especially postmenopausal women, with ovarian masses. The use of ultrasound has also been suggested for the woman whose pelvic examination is suboptimal, such as obese women and others with problems that preclude an adequate examination.[212]

The screening of women at high genetic risk for ovarian cancer remains controversial but may best involve extensive surveillance. A detailed maternal/paternal family history, of at least three generations and detailing the pedigree occurrence of ovarian cancer and other integral syndrome tumors, is required to identify high-risk women. The challenge to nursing to identify women with a positive family history and to provide effective education to these women is essential. Fitzsimmons et al.[213] suggest that each oncology patient is a potential member of a hereditary cancer family and should be assessed for family cancer history. Due to the early onset of hereditary forms of ovarian cancer, screening, if done, should be initiated by age 30.[214] Furthermore, for women with a documented family history, Piver et al. suggest the use of pelvic ultrasound with CA-125 levels in combination with frequent pelvic examination.[215] However, until prospective studies have established the effectiveness of screening in this population, guidelines cannot be absolute.[216] Nursing strategies directed at high-risk women who request screening should include education regarding timing and the implications of CA-125 and ultrasound (Table 1.6).

Several conclusions regarding screening of high-risk women were made at the 1994 NCI Consensus Development Conference on Ovarian Cancer. There is currently no evidence to support routine screening in women with one first-degree relative with ovarian cancer; however, participation in clinical trials is an appropriate option. Women with two or more first-degree relatives should be counseled by a specialist regarding their individual risks despite no conclusive data that screening benefits these women. However, women with a hereditary ovarian cancer syndrome should undergo at least annual rectovaginal pelvic examination, CA-125 determinations, and transvaginal ultrasound until childbearing is completed or until age 35, at which time prophylactic bilateral oophorectomy is recommended.[184]

A task force organized by the Cancer Genetics Studies Consortium (CGSC) convened to provide recommendations for cancer surveillance and risk reduction for individual carrier mutations of BRCA1 and BRCA2 genes. Recommendations for ovarian cancer surveillance include annual or semiannual screening with TVS with color flow Doppler and serum CA-125 levels, beginning at age 25–35 years for BRCA1 mutation carriers. Screening is also an option for BRCA2 mutation carriers, but their lower risk reduces the likelihood of benefit in this group.[217]

Prevention

Despite the fact that the exact etiology of ovarian cancer is unknown, several potential prevention strategies are possible, based on current epidemiological and genetic data (Table 1.8). These strategies include prophylactic oophorectomy, oral contraceptive use, diet modifications, and elimination of genital chemical (talc, asbestos) exposure.

Attention has been drawn to the prevention of ovarian cancer by prophylactic oophorectomy. Some authorities advocate routine prophylactic oophorectomy in all women undergoing hysterectomy or other abdominal surgery after a certain age.[218] This recommendation is based on reports of ovarian cancer in women who have undergone prior hysterectomy with ovarian conservation ranging from 1 to 14%.[219] ACOG cautions that elective oophorectomy at the time of hysterectomy for benign disease is a complex decision and should take into account the woman's age, parity, risk factors, menstrual status, family and personal history, likelihood of postoperative follow-up and cultural factors; thus the decision should be highly individual and dogmatic recommendations are not appropriate.[220] Nurses are in a key position to assist women in this decision-making process by providing information and counseling regarding the potential benefits and consequences of oophorectomy.

The role of prophylactic oophorectomy in women with family risk factors is controversial as it may not offer total protection from ovarian cancer. In one study, three women from ovarian cancer–prone families who had previously undergone prophylactic oophorectomy developed intra-abdominal carcinomatosis that was indistinguishable from ovarian cancer.[221] Numerous case reports have provided further evidence of this occurrence, suggesting that epithelial ovarian cancer may arise from any tissue originally derived from coelomic epithelium.[222,223,224] Currently there are no standard recommendations regarding prophylactic oophorectomy in the prevention of ovarian cancer in familial-high-risk women. Physicians at the Gilda Radner Familial Ovarian Cancer Registry recommend prophylactic oophorectomy by age 35 for women who have two or more first-degree relatives with ovarian cancer.[225] Lynch et al.[214] suggest that prophylactic oophorectomy is a viable option in carefully selected women with unequivocally high genetic risk for ovarian cancer, if they have completed childbearing, although the long-term physiologic and psychological effects must also be considered. The conclusions of the NIH Consensus Development Conference on Ovarian Cancer are that women with hereditary ovarian cancer syndrome should undergo prophylactic bilateral oophorectomy when childbearing is complete, or by age 35.[184] The CGSC concluded that there is insufficient evidence at this time to recommend for or against prophylactic oophorectomy for women with a known genetic mutation.[217]

The protective effect of oral contraceptives on the development of ovarian cancer is well established. In fact, it has been suggested that such prevention appears to be more effective in lowering the incidence and death rates of ovarian cancer than are currently available screening tests and therapies.[182] Nurses should include this benefit of oral contraceptives when providing birth control counseling to women, regardless of ovarian cancer risk factors. At this time, it may be prudent to encourage women with high-risk factors to take oral contraceptives after a careful analysis of potential risks and benefits.

All women should be counseled regarding the beneficial effects of a low-fat, high–vitamin A diet on ovarian cancer prevention, especially since the benefits of such a diet on the prevention of other cancers is also well established. Nurses should provide education to women regarding genital hygiene, with emphasis on the avoidance of perineal exposure to talc. For women with a BRCA1 or BRCA2 mutation, the CGSF endorses lifestyle modifications that have a broad range of health benefits, without the risk of pharmacological or procedural intervention, even though the benefit in ovarian cancer reduction is not established.[217] These lifestyle modifications include adoption of low-fat, high-fiber diets, adequate vegetable and fruit intake, regular exercise, and avoidance of carcinogenic agents such as cigarettes.[217]

ENDOMETRIAL CANCER

Endometrial cancer is the predominant gynecologic cancer and the fourth most common cancer in women. It was estimated that 36,100 new cases of endometrial cancer would be diagnosed in 1999 and that approximately 6,300 women would die of this disease. Incidence rates have been stable for ten to fifteen years at 21 per 100,000. The overall five-year survival rate for all stages of endometrial cancer is 83%, with survival for localized disease about 94%, regional disease 68%, and distant disease at time of diagnosis 26%.[24] Although the majority of patients are diagnosed in early stages, when cure is possible, there remains the need for better screening and detection for the population of women at risk for this disease.

Population at Risk

Risk factors for endometrial cancer have been well defined and include age, obesity, polycystic ovarian syndrome, parity, diabetes, hypertension, use of unopposed estrogen therapy or tamoxifen, adenomatous hyperplasia, and history of breast cancer (Table 1.12).[24,114,226,227]

Postmenopausal women are at the greatest risk for endometrial cancer; the average age at diagnosis is 61 years. However, about a fourth of the cases occur in premenopausal women, and 5% are diagnosed before the age of 40.[114,228]

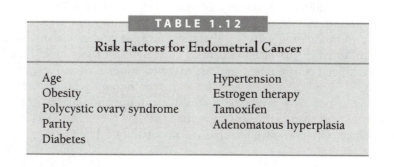

TABLE 1.12

Risk Factors for Endometrial Cancer

Age	Hypertension
Obesity	Estrogen therapy
Polycystic ovary syndrome	Tamoxifen
Parity	Adenomatous hyperplasia
Diabetes	

Obesity has long been associated with the development of endometrial cancer. Risk in women who are greater than twenty pounds overweight increases three- to tenfold.[227,229] Distribution of body fat also seems to be a factor. There has been a 5.8-fold increase in risk reported if the pattern of distribution is concentrated in the upper body and abdomen.[230] Abnormalities in endogenous estrogen production or metabolism that are associated with obesity may account for this increased risk. More specifically, androgens are converted to estrogen in fat tissue where it is then stored and slowly released. Since sex hormone–binding globulin is diminished in obese postmenopausal women, there are increased circulating levels of the active form of free estrogen, estradiol. Thus the elevated risk for obese postmenopausal women may be explained by the increased endogenous estrogens and lack of progesterone that can result in endometrial proliferation.[231] In addition, it is not uncommon for obese woman to have anovulatory menstrual cycles and irregular bleeding as a result of the lack of progesterone, which then permits unopposed estrogen proliferation of the endometrium.[228,232,233] Contrary to these data, however, Abeler and Korstad reported that obesity could not be substantiated as a significant risk factor.[234]

Other hormonal and reproductive factors play an important role in the development of endometrial cancer. Endogenous estrogen production associated with polycystic ovary syndrome has been identified as one such factor. Endometrial proliferation associated with this syndrome can be reversed with clomiphene citrate, progesterone, or with wedge resection of the ovary.[228,235] Late menopause (after age 52) and nulliparity have also been associated with endometrial cancer, and the association of parity and risk has recently been further defined by Parazzini et al.[231] In a case-control study of nearly 2,500 women, parous women had a 30% lower risk than did nulliparous women. While there was no evidence to show that risk decreased with increasing number of births, risk did significantly diminish with the number of spontaneous and induced abortions. There was no association of age at first birth with endometrial cancer, but there was a decrease in risk with increasing age at last birth. The effects of these factors seemed to be greater in the premenopausal years and tended to flatten out in later years. These data suggest a limited protective effect of pregnancy and a carcinogenetic role of the reproductive factors of late menopause, nulliparity, and polycystic ovary syndrome.

Diabetes, or at least an abnormal glucose tolerance, has been associated with risk for endometrial cancer,[114] but the exact nature of the relationship is unclear. The overall endocrine imbalance that is related to obesity, diabetes, hypertension, and reproductive factors may play the operative role in risk elevation.

Use of unopposed estrogen therapy, that is, estrogen without progesterone, was first implicated in the development of endometrial cancer in 1975, and the relative risk has since been reported as four to seven times greater for women on estrogen therapy.[236,237,238] Women who take estrogen therapy without progestins for more than three years have a relative risk of developing endometrial cancer of 5.7, while women who take progestins for more than ten days per month have a relative risk similar to those who take no hormones (relative risk of 1.1).[239]

Tamoxifen use has recently been identified with endometrial cancer. While it acts as an antiestrogen on breast tissue, tamoxifen has been shown to act as a weak estrogen on endometrial tissue, inducing endometrial proliferation. Thus in women using tamoxifen long term for breast cancer, cases of endometrial cancer have been identified.[240] The potential relationship is such that the risk of endometrial cancer is discussed in detail with each participant in tamoxifen trials, and pelvic examinations are included in the surveillance tests.

Endometrial hyperplasia is another hormone-related risk factor. Increased estrogens, whether endogenous or exogenous, are associated with the development of endometrial hyperplasia; however, it is not known whether the hyperplasia is a precursor for endometrial cancer if there is no atypia present.[228]

Screening Methods

There remains no good screening test for endometrial cancer. The pelvic exam enables the clinician to detect only an abnormally sized uterus. Even though the Pap smear is an effective screen for cervical cancer, it detects only an occasional endometrial cancer if the vaginal pool is sampled. Cytologic evaluation is neither a sensitive nor a specific test for endometrial cancer because of the difficulty of analyzing aspirate containing bloody and, often, endocervical material. In order to adequately screen for endometrial cancer, tissue needs to be sampled, and so an endometrial biopsy needs to be performed.[114,229] While this is a sensitive and specific test, having a 90% accuracy rate, it is not without morbidity and should be reserved for high-risk women. But the advantage of endometrial biopsy over the traditional dilatation and curettage is that it can be performed safely in the office setting without anesthesia.[228]

The current recommendation for screening for endometrial cancer from the American Cancer Society and the American College of Obstetricians and Gynecologists is an annual pelvic exam and Pap smear (Tables 1.1 and 1.3). However, sampling of the endometrium is neither cost effective nor indicated in the general population and is not required before or during hormone replacement therapy in the asymptomatic woman.[241]

Controversial Issues

The frequency and method of screening a woman with endometrial hyperplasia and the frequency of performing endometrial biopsy in a high-risk woman have not been well defined. Gronroos et al.[242] reported data to support regular screening of asymptomatic diabetic women over 45 years of age by aspiration sampling of the endometrium. They did not support mass screening because of the low yield of endometrial pathology in the population at large. Some clinicians question the value of endometrial biopsy prior to the initiation of estrogen replacement therapy unless the patient is symptomatic.[228,243] Additional data are needed to determine the optimal interval and frequency for endometrial biopsy.

Prevention

While hysterectomy provides the most reliable method of preventing endometrial cancer, it is an excessive approach that would gain little support due to the potential morbidity and mortality associated with any surgery and general anesthesia. Thus the major focus of prevention is on reduction of risk, which is facilitated through intensive health education on risk-reducing behaviors (Table 1.8).

Certainly the addition of progestins to the estrogen replacement regimen reduces endometrial proliferation and reduces the risk of endometrial cancer to that of the woman taking no estrogen therapy.[244,245] Similarly, oral contraceptives have a protective effect on the endometrial surface by reducing the amount of monthly proliferation and sloughing.[246] The timely assessment and treatment of abnormal uterine bleeding can also prevent the development of endometrial cancer. Anovulatory cycles causing abnormal bleeding can be treated with progestins. Endometrial hyperplasia also can be treated with progestins or with hysterectomy. Diet modification to reduce total body weight may reduce the risk of developing endometrial cancer.[228] Finally, while no one would promote smoking as a means of preventing endometrial cancer, it has been reported to be associated with a reduction in risk.[247]

✖ VULVAR CANCER

Carcinoma of the vulva accounts for only 5% of all gynecologic cancers and is the fourth most common cancer of the female genital tract.[1] Invasive vulvar cancer is predominantly a disease of elderly women; the incidence is highest in the seventh decade. In its preinvasive stage, vulvar intraepithelial neoplasia (VIN) appears to be on the rise, with the majority of these lesions occurring in younger, premenopausal women.

Population at Risk

The etiology of vulvar malignancy is not clear. Several risk factors for vulvar cancer have been suggested, including advanced age, chronic vulvar inflammatory disorders, vulvar intraepithelial neoplasia, history of vulvar HPV infection, history of other neoplasia of the lower genital tract, cigarette smoking, obesity, diabetes, and environmental factors (Table 1.13).

Carcinoma of the vulva is most frequently associated with intraepithelial abnormalities such as lichen sclerosis, severe atypia as seen in VIN, and vulvar HPV infection. Lichen sclerosis is a benign inflammatory disease of unknown etiology resulting in patchy white changes on the vulva with associated pruritus. It is most common in postmenopausal women and is responsive to topical testosterone cream. Controversy exists over the malignant potential of lichen sclerosis with research results demonstrating the coexistence of lichen sclerosis with carcinoma ranging from little or no association to 60%.[248,249,250] Lessana-Leibowitz et al.[249] suggest that this discrepancy

TABLE 1.13
Risk Factors for Vulvar Cancer

Age	Cigarette smoking
Chronic vulvar inflammatory disorders	Obesity
Lower genital tract neoplasia	Diabetes
HPV Infection	Environmental Factors

may reflect the beneficial effects of treatment of lichen sclerosis, as the majority of cases in their study with coexistent lichen sclerosis and carcinoma of the vulva had not been diagnosed or treated previously.

Vulvar intraepithelial neoplasia has been associated with vulvar cancer, although the actual percentage of VIN that evolves into invasive cancer is not known. Cancers associated with VIN lesions are more likely to occur in younger women and are frequently associated as well with other factors, such as HPV infection and immunosuppression.[251,252]

The relationship of HPV in association with vulvar cancer has produced a disparity of results, specifically related to the age of the population under study. In one study, genital warts were associated with a fifteenfold excess risk of vulvar cancer, thus emphasizing the link between vulvar cancer and a sexually transmitted disease.[253] Other studies, though, have demonstrated a relatively low incidence (23% and 28%) of HPV in association with vulvar cancer, especially in older women.[254,255] These conflicting results suggest that, from an epidemiologic perspective, vulvar cancer may encompass more than one distinct risk group. Vulvar carcinoma may have diverse pathogenesis resulting in different subsets of cancers, such as that seen in the older woman with chronic inflammation versus the younger woman with preexisting VIN or HPV.

The occurrence of multiple primary cancers in the female lower genital tract is widely recognized. From 2 to 38% of women with vulvar cancer are reported to develop another primary lower genital tract malignancy, most commonly involving the cervix.[256] Approximately 20% of women with vulvar cancer had an in situ or invasive squamous cancer of the cervix at least five years earlier.[257] This apparently high risk of multiple primaries supports the suggestion of a common carcinogenic stimulus affecting multiple sites in the squamous epithelium of the lower genital tract.[258]

Personal characteristics such as smoking, obesity, and diabetes have been inconsistently recognized as risk factors. The association of vulvar cancer with cigarette smoking has been established.[250,259] But particularly noteworthy in a study by Brinton et al.[253] was the further elevation of risk with both long-term and high-intensity smoking, and the significant interaction between smoking and a history of genital warts. In a survey of forty-five women with vulvar cancer, cigarette smoking was found in over half (57.8%) of the sample.[260] However, no association was found between cigarette smoking and vulvar cancer in an Italian case-control study.[261] Cigarette smoking has been shown to be a carcinogen, cancer promoter, and immunosuppressant that may have a synergistic effect with HPV. Thus the role of cigarette smoking in vulvar cancer requires further study.

A relationship between diabetes and obesity and vulvar cancer has been reported by some[262,263] but refuted by others.[250,253,261] Nevertheless, the often chronic vulvar dermatitis and pruritus associated with diabetes and obesity may present a fertile field for the development of cellular disturbances that may lead to neoplasia.

Finally, occupation as a maid or in the laundry, cleaning, or garment services or on tobacco farms has been shown to increase risk, suggesting that the vulva may be more sensitive to exposure to environmental carcinogens than other cutaneous sites.[250,264,265]

Screening Methods

There are no specific guidelines for the routine screening for vulvar cancer. Screening may be accomplished by visual inspection of the entire perineum for symmetry, color changes, inflammation, and lesions; and palpation of the Bartholin's and Skene's glands. ACS guidelines regarding frequency of pelvic examination, although not specific for screening for vulvar cancer, are outlined in Table 1.1. More frequent screening may be warranted in young women with a history of lower genital intraepithelial neoplasia, HPV infection, and in older women with lichen sclerosis. Colposcopy, using the application of 1% toluidine solution to the vulva with resultant uptake by abnormal areas, and vulvar biopsy are not screening techniques but may be employed in women with vulvar symptoms.

Prevention

Nursing intervention directed at smoking cessation, preventing exposure to HPV infection, weight reduction in obese women, good glucose control in diabetic women, prompt evaluation and treatment of any vulvar irritation or genital warts, and protection from potential occupational hazards may be beneficial risk reduction strategies (Table 1.8).

Nurses should encourage all women, and especially those with vulvar cancer risk factors, to have annual gynecological examinations and provide instruction for the performance of monthly self-examination of the vulva (Table 1.6) and good hygienic practices. A brochure such as "Vulvar Self-Examination," by Sandella,[266] may be helpful.

✳ VAGINAL CANCER

Primary carcinoma of the vagina is a rare neoplasm, accounting for only 1 to 2% of all gynecologic malignancies. Most vaginal neoplasms are metastatic from adjacent organs such as the cervix, vulva, or endometrium.

TABLE 1.14	
Risk Factors for Vaginal Cancer	
DES exposure	History of abnormal Pap smear
Low socioeconomic level	Previous hysterectomy
HPV infection	Vaginal trauma
Vaginal discharge/irritation	

Population at Risk

Potential risk factors for primary and metastatic vaginal cancer include low socio-economic level, history of genital HPV infection, vaginal discharge or irritation, history of abnormal Pap smear, previous hysterectomy for malignant or premalignant disease, and vaginal trauma (Table 1.14).[253] Another risk factor, the association between the incidence of clear cell adenocarcinoma of the vagina and prenatal diethylstilbestrol (DES) exposure, is discussed in Chapter 2.

Screening Methods

Pap smear and pelvic examination, although specific for cervical cancer screening, can be used for screening for vaginal cancer as well. (Recommended guidelines for Pap screening are listed in Tables 1.1 to 1.4.) Women who have had hysterectomies should not automatically be excluded from screening programs. First, prior to the 1960s, many women had partial hysterectomies that left the cervix intact, indicating the need for continued Pap smear screening in these women. Also, since women who have had a hysterectomy for malignant or premalignant disease are at increased risk for vaginal cancer, vaginal cytologic screening is necessary in these women. Even though the cost-effectiveness of vaginal cytologic screening after removal of the cervix for benign disease has not been demonstrated, ACOG recommends periodic cytologic evaluation of the vagina at minimum intervals of three to five years in these women.[267] The reason for the prior surgery and the presence or lack of an intact cervix is the best guide to the need for Pap surveillance.[133] Specific screening guidelines for DES-exposed women are detailed in Chapter 2.

✳ NURSING IMPLICATIONS

Nurses are in a key position to promote screening and prevention of breast and gynecologic malignancies. The encouragement of risk-reducing behaviors is crucial to the prevention of cancer in women. Risk reduction strategies for breast and gynecologic malignancies are detailed in Table 1.7. Screening modalities should be carried out

---

TABLE 1.15

Diagnostic Cluster

NURSING DIAGNOSIS
1. Potential altered health maintenance related to insufficient knowledge of basic reproductive female anatomy, cancer prevention, and screening recommendations
2. Anxiety related to insufficient knowledge about screening techniques, uncertainty about outcomes, and possible cancer diagnosis

---

after relevant client education to optimize their efficacy and promote understanding of each technique. (See Table 1.15.)

✺ REFERENCES

1. Landis, S.H., Murray, T., Bolden, S., Wingo, P.A. (1998). Cancer statistics, 1998. *CA Cancer J Clin, 48*(1), 6–29.
2. National Cancer Institute (1990). Cancer Statistics Review 1973–1987 (NCI Publication No. 90–2789). Bethesda, MD: National Cancer Institute.
3. National Cancer Institute (1980). Cancer control objectives for the nation: 1985–2000 (NCI Monograph, NIH Publication 86–2880). Bethesda, MD: National Cancer Institute.
4. United States Commission on Chronic Illness (1957). *Chronic Illness in the United States,* vol. 1 (p. 267). Cambridge, MA: Harvard University Press.
5. Fink, D. (1991). *Guidelines for Cancer-related Checkup* (ACS 91–50M, No. 3347-PE). Atlanta: American Cancer Society.
6. Cole, P., & Morrison, A.S. (1980). Basic issues in population screening for cancer. *J Natl Cancer Inst, 64,* 1263–1272.
7. Miller, D.G. (1986). Cancer prevention? Steps you can take. In A.I. Holleb, ed., *The American Cancer Society Cancer Book* (pp. 15–40). Garden City, NY: Doubleday.
8. Fraumeni, J.F., Hoova, R.N., Devesa, S.S., & Kinler, L.J. (1993). Epidemiology of cancer. In V.T. Devita, S. Hellman, & S.A. Rosenberg, eds., *Cancer: Principles & Practice* (pp. 166–167). Philadelphia: Lippincott.
9. Hulka, B. (1988). Cancer screening: Degrees of proof and practical application. *Cancer, 62,* 1776–1780.
10. Wilson, J., & Jungner, G. (1968). Principles and practices of screening for disease (Public Health Paper 34 (pp. 26–39). Geneva: World Health Organization.
11. Shapiro, S. (1992). Goals of screening. *Cancer, 70*(5), 1252–1258.
12. American Cancer Society (1980). Guidelines for the cancer-related checkup: Recommendations and rationale. *CA Cancer J Clin, 30,* 4–50.
13. Olson, S.J., & Frank-Stromborg, M. (1991). Cancer screening and early detection. In S.B. Baird, R. McCorkle & M. Grant, eds., *Cancer Nursing: A Comprehensive Textbook* (pp. 190–218). Philadelphia: Saunders.
14. Canadian Task Force (1979). The periodic health examination. *Can Med Assoc J, 121,* 1193–1254.
15. Canadian Task Force (1982). Cervical cancer screening programs: Summary of the 1982 Canadian Task Force report. *Can Med Assoc J, 127,* 581–589.
16. Canadian Task Force (1986). The periodic health examination II: 1985 update. *Can Med Assoc J, 134,* 724–729.
17. Canadian Task Force on the Periodic Health Examination (1994). Canadian guide to clinical preventive health care. Ottawa: Canadian Communications Group, 620–631.
18. American College of Obstetricians and Gynecologists Committe on Gynecologic Practice (1997, September). Routine cancer screening ACOG Committee (Opinion No. 185). Washington, DC.).
19. Smart, C.R., Chu, K.C., Conley, V.L., et al. (1993). Cancer screening and early detection. In J.F. Hol-

land, E. Frei III, R.C. Bast, et al., eds., *Cancer Medicine*, 3rd ed. (pp. 408–431). Philadelphia: Lea & Febiger.

20. National Cancer Institute. (1987). Working guidelines for early cancer detection: Rationale and supporting evidence to decrease mortality (NCI Sec. 27). Bethesda, MD: Early Detection Branch Division of Cancer Prevention and Control.

21. National Cancer Institute (1993, December). Breast cancer screening (Memo, NCI Press Office). Bethesda, MD: National Cancer Institute.

22. Colditz, G.A. (1993). Epidemiology of breast cancer: Findings for the Nurses' Health Study. *Cancer, 71*(4), 1480–1489.

23. Parker, S.L., Davis, J.K., Wingo, P.A., et al. (1998). Cancer statistics by race and ethnicity. *CA, 48*(1), 31–48.

24. American Cancer Society (1998). *Cancer Facts and Figures–1998* (ACS Publication 5008.98), pp. 7–31. Atlanta: American Cancer Society.

25. Henderson, I.C. (1993). Risk factors for breast cancer development. *Cancer, 71* (suppl. 6), 2127–2140.

26. Vatten, L.J., & Kvinnsland, S. (1992). Prospective study of height, body mass index, and risk of breast cancer. *Acta Oncol, 31*(2), 195–200.

27. London, S.J., Colditz, G.A., Stampfer, M.J., et al. (1989). A prospective study of relative weight, height, and the risk of breast cancer. *JAMA, 262*(20), 2853–2858.

28. Tretli, S. (1989). Height and weight in relation to breast cancer morbidity and mortality: A prospective study of 570,000 women in Norway. *Int J Cancer, 44*(1), 23–30.

29. Willett, W.C., Browne, M.L., Baine, C., et al. (1985). Relative weight and risk of breast cancer among premenopausal women. *Am J Epidemiol, 122*(5), 731–740.

30. Tretli, S., Haldorsen, T., & Ottestad, L. (1990). The effect of premorbid height and weight on the survival of breast cancer patients. *Br J Cancer, 62*(2), 299–303.

31. Kaaks, R., VanNoord, P.A., DenTonkelaar, I., et al. (1998). Breast cancer incidence in relation to height, weight, and body fat distribution in the Dutch "DOM" cohort. *Int J Cancer, 76*(5): 647–651.

32. Bain, C., Speizer, F.E., Rosner, B., Belanger, C., & Hennekens, C.H. (1980). Family history of breast cancer as a risk indicator for the disease. *Am J Epidemiol, 111*(3), 301–308.

33. Mohammed, S.N., Smith, P., Hodgson, S.V., et al. (1998). Family history and survival in premenopausal breast cancer. *Br J Cancer, 77*(12), 2252–2256.

34. Nasser, B.A., Ludman, M.D., Costa, M.T., et al.

(1998). More on breast cancer guidelines. *CMAJ, 158*(11): 1429–1430.

35. Biesecker, B.B., Boehnke, M., Calzone, K., et al. (1993). Genetic counseling for families with inherited susceptibility to breast and ovarian cancer. *JAMA, 269*(15), 1970–1974.

36. King, M.C., Rowell, S., & Love, S.M. (1993). Inherited breast and ovarian cancer: What are the risks? What are the choices? *JAMA, 269*(15), 1975–1980.

37. Henderson, B.E. (1989). Endogenous and exogenous endocrine factors. *Hematol Oncol Clin North Am, 3*(4), 577–598.

38. Colditz, G.A. (1997). Hormone replacement therapy increases risk of breast cancer. *Ann NY Acad Sci, 833*: 129–136.

39. Henderson, B.E., Pike, M.C., & Casagrande, J.T. (1981). Breast cancer and oestrogen window hypothesis. *Lancet, 2,* 363–364.

40. Romieu, I., Berlin, J.A., & Colditz, G. (1990). Oral contraceptives and breast cancer: Review and meta-analysis. *Cancer, 66*(11), 2254–2263.

41. Romieu, I., Willett, W.C., Colditz, G.A., Stampfer, M.J., Rosner, B., Hennekens, C.H., & Speizer, F.E. (1989). A prospective study of oral contraceptive use and the risk of breast cancer in women. *J Natl Cancer Inst, 81*(17), 1313–1321.

42. Dupont, W.D., & Page, D.L. (1991). Menopausal estrogen replacement therapy and breast cancer. *Arch Intern Med, 151*(1), 67–72.

43. Steinberg, K.K., Thacker, S.B., Smith, J., et al. (1991). A meta-analysis of the effect of estrogen replacement therapy on the risk of breast cancer. *JAMA, 265*(15), 1985–1990.

44. Colditz, G.A. (1998). Relationship between estrogen levels, use of hormone replacement therapy, and breast cancer. *J Natl Cancer Inst, 90*(11): 814–823.

45. Colditz, G.A., Stampfer, M.J., Willett, W.C., et al. (1992). Type of postmenopausal hormone use and risk of breast cancer: Twelve year follow-up of the Nurses' Health Study. *Cancer Causes Control, 3*(5), 433–439.

46. Albanes, D. (1987). Total calories, body weight, and tumor incidence in mice. *Cancer Res, 47*(8), 1987–1992.

47. Mettlin, C. (1984). Diet and the epidemiology of human breast cancer. *Cancer, 53*(3), 605–611.

48. Prentice, R.L., Kakar, R., Hursting, S., et al. (1988). Aspects of the rationale for the Women's Health Trial. *J Natl Cancer Inst, 80*(11), 802.

49. Willett, W. (1989). The search for the causes of breast and colon cancer. *Nature, 338*(6214), 389–394.

50. Howe, G.R., Hirohata, T., Hislop, T.G., et al. (1987). Dietary factors and risk of breast cancer:

Combined analysis of twelve case-control studies. *J Natl Cancer Inst, 82*(4), 561–569.

51. D'Avanzo, B., Negri, E., Gramenzi, A., et al. (1993). Fats in seasoning and breast cancer risk: An Italian case-control study. *Eur J Cancer, 27*(4), 420–423.

52. Simonsen, N.R., Fernandez-Crehut, N.J., Martin-Moreno, J.M., et al. (1998). Tissue stores of individual monosaturated fatty acids and breast cancer: The EURAMIC study. European Community Multicenter Study on antioxidants, myocardia infarction, and breast cancer. *Am J Clin Nutr, 68*(1): 134–141.

53. Howe, G.R., Rohan, T., Decarli, A., et al. (1991). The association between alcohol and breast cancer risk: Evidence from the combined analysis six dietary case-control studies. *Int J Cancer, 47*(5), 707–710.

54. Willett, W., Stampfer, M.J., Colditz, G.A., et al. (1987). Moderate alcohol consumption and risk of breast cancer. *N Engl J Med, 316*(19), 1174–1180.

55. Longnecker, M.P., Berlin, J.A., Orza, M.J., & Chalmers, T.C. (1988). A meta-analysis of alcohol consumption in relation to risk of breast cancer. *JAMA, 260*(5), 652–656.

56. Hunter, D.J., Stampfer, M.J., Colditz, G.A., et al. (1991). A prospective study of consumption of vitamins A, C, and E and breast cancer risk (abstract). *Am J Epidemiol, 134*(7), 715.

57. Dupont, W.D., & Page, D.L. (1985). Risk factors for breast cancer in women with proliferative breast disease. *N Engl J Med, 312*(3), 146–151.

58. London, S.J., Connolly, J.L., Schnitt, S.J., & Colditz, G.A. (1992). A prospective study of benign breast disease and risk of breast cancer. *JAMA, 267*(7), 941–944.

59. Dupont, W.D., Parl, F.F., Hartman, W.H., et al. (1993). Breast cancer risk associated with proliferative breast disease and atypical hyperplasia. *Cancer, 71*(4), 1258–1265.

60. Greenwald, P., Nasca, P.C., Lawrence, C.E., et al. (1978). Estimated effect of breast self-examination and routine physician examinations on breast cancer mortality. *N Engl J Med, 299*(6), 271–273.

61. Huguley, C.N., & Brown, R.L. (1981). The value of breast self-examination. *Cancer, 47*(5), 989–995.

62. Carlile, T., & Hadaway, E. (1985). Screening for breast cancer. In B.A. Stoll, ed., *Screening and Monitoring of Cancer* (pp. 135–152). New York: Wiley.

63. Taber, L., Fagerberg, C.J.G., Gad, A., et al. (1985). Reduction in mortality from breast cancer after mass screening with mammography. *Lancet, 1,* 829–832.

64. Thier, S.O. (1977). Breast cancer screening: A view from outside the controversy. *N Engl J Med, 297*(19), 1063–1065.

65. Collette, H.J.A., Day, N.E., Rombach, J.J., & De-Waard, F. (1984). Evaluation of screening for breast cancer in a nonrandomized study (the Dom project) by means of a case-control study. *Lancet, 1*(8388), 1224–1226.

66. Palli, D., Del Turco, M.R., Buiatti, E., et al. (1986). A case-control study of the efficacy of a nonrandomized breast cancer screening program in Florence (Italy). *Int J Cancer, 38*(4), 501–504.

67. Verbeek, A.L.M., Hendriks, J.H.C.L., Holland, R., et al. (1985). Mammographic screening and breast cancer mortality: Age specific effects in Nijmegen Project, 1975–82. *Lancet, 1,* 865–886.

68. Reichle, J.L. (1998). Benefits of screening mammography: A review for the primary care physician. *South Med J, 91*(6): 510–7.

69. White, E., Velentgas, P., Madelson, M.T., et al. (1998). Variation in mammographic breast density by time in menstrual cycle among women aged 40 to 49 years. *J Natl Cancer Inst 90* (12): 906–910.

70. Nielsen, B.B. (1991). Breast cancer screening. *Semin Oncol Nurs, 7*(3), 161–165.

71. O'Malley, M., & Fletcher, S. (1987). Screening for breast cancer with breast self-examination: A critical review. *JAMA, 257*(16), 2196–2203.

72. Kurtz, M.E., Given, B., Given, C.W., & Kurtz, J.C. (1993). Relationships of barriers and facilitators to breast self-examination, mammography, and clinical breast examination in a worksite population. *Cancer Nurs, 16*(4), 251–259.

73. Morra, M.E., & Blumberg, B.D. (1991). Women's perceptions of early detection in breast cancer: How are we doing? *Semin Oncol Nurs, 7*(3), 151–160.

74. Rutledge, D.N., & Davis, G.T. (1988). Breast self-examination compliance and the health belief model. *Oncol Nurs Forum, 15*(2), 175–179.

75. Holliday, H., Roebuck, E.J., & Doyle, P.J. (1983). Initial results from a program of BSE. *Clin Oncol, 9*(1), 11–16.

76. Billings, K. (1986). Status of mammography in breast cancer screening. *Postgrad Med, 79*(6), 89–95.

77. Champion, V. (1991). The relationship of selected variables to breast cancer detection behaviors in women 35 and older. *Oncol Nurs Forum, 18*(4), 733–739.

78. Taylor, S., Lichtman, R., Wood, J., et al. (1984). Breast self-examination among diagnosed breast cancer patients. *Cancer, 54*(11), 2528–2532.

79. Elwood, M., McNoe, B., Smith, T., et al. (1998). Once is enough . . . why some women do not continue to participate in a breast cancer screening programme. *NZ Med J, 111*(1066): 180–183.

80. NCI (1998). *Cancer Facts: Screening Mammograms.* NCI NIH 5.28, (9/15/98): 1–6.

81. National Cancer Institute (1992a). Breast exams: What you should know (NCI Publication No. 93–2000). Bethesda, MD: National Cancer Institute.

82. Burke, W., Daly, M., Garber, J., et al. (1997). Recommendations for follow-up care of individuals with an inherited predisposition to cancer. II BRCA1 and BRCA2. *JAMA, 277*(12), 997–1003.

83. Franceschi, S., Parpinel, M., LaVecchia, C., et al. (1998). Role of different types of vegetables and fruit in the prevention of cancer of the colon, rectum, and breast. *Epidemiology, 9*(3), 338–341.

84. Fisher, B., Costantino, J.P., Wickerman, D.L., et al. (1998). Tamoxifen for prevention of breast cancer: Report of the National Surgical Adjuvant Breast & Bowel Project P-1 Study. *J Natl Cancer Inst, 90*(18), 1371–1388.

85. Ingram, D., Sanders, K., Kolybaba, M., & Lopez, D. (1997). Case control study of phyto-oestrogens and breast cancer. *Lancet, 30*(9083), 990–994.

86. Franco, E.L. (1991). Viral etiology of cervical cancer: A critique of the evidence. *Review of Infectious Disease, 13,* 1195–1206.

87. Zunzunegui, M.V., King, M.C., Coria, C.F., & Charlet, J. (1986). Male influence on cervical cancer risks. *Am J Epidemiol, 123,* 302–307.

88. Kessler, I.I. (1974). Cervical cancer epidemiology in historical perspective. *J Reprod Med, 12,* 173–185.

89. Graham, S., Priore, R., Graham, M., et al. (1979). Genital cancer in wives of penile cancer patients. *Cancer, 44,* 1870–1874.

90. Smith, P.G., Kinlen, L.J., White, G.C., Adelstein, A.M., & Fox, A.J. (1980). Mortality of wives of men dying with cancer of the penis. *Br J Cancer, 41,* 422–428.

91. Koss, L.G. (1987). Cytologic and histologic manifestations of human papillomavirus infection of the female genital tract and their clinical significance. *Cancer, 60,* 1942–1950.

92. Syrjanen, K.J., & Syrjanen, S.M. (1985). Human papilloma virus (HPV) infections related to cervical intraepithelial neoplasia (CIN) and squamous cell carcinoma of the uterine cervix. *Ann Clin Res, 17,* 45–56.

93. Walker, J., Bloss, J.D., Shu-yuan, L., et al. (1989). Human papillomavirus genotype as a prognostic indicator in carcinoma of the uterine cervix. *Obstet Gynecol, 74*(5), 781,785.

94. Sasson, I.M., Haley, N.J., Hoffman, D., et al. (1985). Cigarette smoking and neoplasia of the uterine cervix: Smoke constituents in cervical mucus (letter). *N Engl J Med, 312,* 315–316.

95. Barton, S.E., Jenkins, D., Cuzick, J., et al. (1988). Effect of cigarette smoking on cervical epithelial immunity: A mechanism for neoplastic change (letter). *Lancet,* 652–654.

96. Brinton, L.A., Schairer, C., Haenszel, W., et al. (1986). Cigarette smoking and invasive cervical cancer. *JAMA, 255*(23), 3265–3269.

97. Boyce, J.G., Lu, T., Nelson, J.H., & Fruchter, R.G. (1977). Oral contraceptives and cervical carcinoma. *Am J Obstet Gynecol, 128,* 761–766.

98. Fuertes-de la Haba, A., Pelegrinam, I., Bangdiwalam, I.S., & Hernandez-Cibes, J.J. (1973). Changing patterns in cervical cytology among oral and non–oral contraceptive users. *J Reprod Med, 10,* 3–10.

99. Brinton, L.A., Huggins, G.R., Lehman, E.F., et al. (1986). Long term use of oral contraceptives and risk of cervical cancer. *Int J Cancer, 38,* 339–344.

100. WHO Collaborative Study of Neoplasia and Steroid Contraceptives (1985). Invasive cervical cancer and combined oral contraceptives. *Br Med J, 290,* 961–965.

101. Melamed, M.R., Koss, L.G., Flehinger, B.J., Kelisky, R.P., & Dubrow, H. (1969). Prevalence rates of uterine cervical carcinoma in situ for women using the diaphragm or contraceptive oral steroids. *Br Med J, 3,* 195–200.

102. Wright, N.H., Vessey, M.P., Kenward, B., McPherson, K., & Doll, R. (1978). Neoplasia and dysplasia of the cervix uteri and contraception: A possible protective effect of the diaphragm. *Br J Cancer, 38*(2), 273–279.

103. Penn, I. (1986). Cancers of the anogenital region in renal transplant recipients: Analysis of sixty-five cases. *Cancer, 58*(3), 611–616.

104. Feingold, A.R., Vermund, S.H., Burk, R.D., et al. (1990). Cervical cytologic abnormalities and papillomavirus in women infected with human immunodeficiency virus. *J Acquire Immune Defic Syn, 3*(9), 896–903.

105. Schafer, A., Friedman, W., Mielke, M., et al. (1991). The increased frequency of cervical dysplasia–neoplasia in women infected with the human immunodeficiency virus as related to the degree of immunosuppression. *Am J Obstet Gynecol, 164*(2), 593–599.

106. Maiman, M., Fruchter, R.G., Serur, R., et al. (1990). Human immunodeficiency virus and cervical neoplasia. *Gynecol Oncol, 38,* 377–382.

107. Brinton, L.A., & Fraumeni, J.F. (1986). Epidemiology of uterine cervical cancer. *J Chronic Dis, 39*(12), 1051–1065.

108. American Cancer Society (1990). 1989 survey of physicians' attitudes and practices in early cancer detection. *Cancer, 40,* 77–101.

109. Bowman, J.A., Redman, S., Dickinson, J.A., et al.

(1991). The accuracy of Pap smear utilization self-report: A methodological consideration in cervical screening research. *Health Ser Res, 26*(1), 97–107.

110. Sawyer, J.A., Earl, J.A., Fletcher, R.H., Daye, F.F., & Wynn, J.M. (1989). Accuracy of women's self-report of their last Pap smear. *Am J Public Health, 79*(8), 1036–1037.

111. Walter, S.D., Clarke, E.A., Hatcher, J., & Stitt, L.W. (1988). A comparison of physician and patient reports of Pap smear histories. *J Clin Epidemiol, 41,* 401–410.

112. Boyce, J.G., & Fruchter, R.G. (1993). Deciding on the interval between Pap smears. *Contemp OB/GYN-NP, 4,* 13–21.

113. White, L.N. (1986). Cancer prevention and detection: From 20 to 65 years of age. *Oncol Nurs Forum, 13*(2), 59–64.

114. White, L.N. (1993). An overview of screening and early detection of gynecologic malignancies. *Cancer, 71*(4), 1400–1405.

115. Schrager, L.K., Friedland, G.H., Maude, D., et al. (1989). Cervical and vaginal squamous cell abnormalities in women infected with human immunodeficiency virus. *J Acquire Immune Defic Syn, 2,* 570–575.

116. Provencher, D., Valme, B., Averette, H.E., et al. (1988). HIV status and positive Papanicolaou screening: Identification of a high risk population. *Gynecol Oncol, 31,* 184–188.

117. Vermund, S., Keley, K.F., Klein, R.S., et al. (1991). High risk of human papillomavirus infection and cervical squamous intraepithelial lesions among women with symptomatic human immunodeficiency virus infection. *Am J Obstet Gynecol, 165*(2), 392–400.

118. Center for Disease Control (1998). *MMWR,* January 23.

119. Koonings, P.P., Dickinson, K., d'Ablaing, G., & Schlaerth, J.B. (1992). A randomized clinical trial comparing the cytobrush and cotton swab for Papanicolaou smears. *Obstet Gynecol, 80,* 241–245.

120. Murata, P.J., Johnson, R.A., & McNicoll, K.E. (1990). Controlled evaluation of implementing the cytobrush technique to improve Papanicolaou smear quality. *Obstet Gynecol, 75,* 690–695.

121. Orr, J.W., Barrett, J.M., Orr, P.F., Holloway, R.W., & Holimon, J.L. (1992). The efficacy and safety of the cytobrush during pregnancy. *Gynecol Oncol, 44,* 260–262.

122. Broder, S. (1992). Rapid communication: The Bethesda System for reporting cervical/vaginal cytologic diagnoses—Report of the 1991 Bethesda workshop. *JAMA, 267*(14), 1892.

123. National Cancer Institute (1989). The 1988 Bethesda System for reporting cervical/vaginal cytologic diagnoses developed and approved at a National Cancer Institute workshop, Bethesda, Maryland, USA, December 12–13, 1988. *J Reprod Med, 34*(10), 779–785.

124. Coppleson, L.W., & Brown, B. (1974). Estimation of the screening error rate from the observed detection rates in repeated cervical cytology. *Am J Obstet Gynecol, 119*(7), 953–958.

125. van der Graaf, Y., Vooijs, G.P., Gaillard, H.L., & Go, D.M. (1987). Screening errors in cervical cytology screening. *Acta Cytology, 31,* 434–438.

126. Ferenczy, A. (1986). Screening for cervical cancer: A renewed plea for annual smears. *Contemp Obstet Gynecol, 28,* 93–108.

127. Richart, R.M., & Vaillant, H.W. (1965). Influence of cell collection techniques upon cytologic diagnoses. *Cancer, 18,* 1474–1478.

128. Koss, L.G. (1989). The Papanicolaou test for cervical cancer detection: A triumph and a tragedy. *JAMA, 26*(5), 737–743.

129. Ginsberg, C.K. (1990). Exfoliative cytologic screening: The Papanicolaou test. *J Obstet Gynecol Nurs, 20*(1), 40–46.

130. Horn, J.E., McQuillan, G.M., Ray, P.A., & Hook, E.W. (1990). Reproductive health practices in women attending an inner-city STD clinic. *Sex Transm Dis, 17*(3), 133–137.

131. Mitchell, H. (1993). Pap smears collected by nurse practitioners: A comparison with smears collected by medical practitioners. *Oncol Nurs Forum, 20*(5), 807–810.

132. Lee, D., Patrissi, G.A., & Kaminski, P.F. (1988). Accuracy of Papanicolaou smears: Art or science? *J Reprod Med, 33*(10), 795–798.

133. Mandelblatt, J., Schechter, C., Fahs, M., & Muller, C. (1991). Clinical implications of screening for cervical cancer under Medicare. *Am J Obstet Gynecol, 164*(2), 644–651.

134. VanLe, L., Broekhuizen, F.F., Janzer-Steele, R., et al. (1993). Acetic acid visualization of the cervix to detect cervical dysplasia. *Obstet Gynecol, 81*(2), 293–295.

135. Stafl, A. (1981). Cervicography: A new method for cervical cancer detection. *Am J Obstet Gynecol, 139*(7), 815–821.

136. Tawa, K., Forsythe, A., Cove, K., et al. (1988). A comparison of the Papanicolaou smear and the cervigram: Sensitivity, specificity, and cost analysis. *Obstet Gynecol, 71*(2), 229–235.

137. Geven, F.T., & Jones, H.W. (1992). Self-administered cervical cancer screening. *Clin Obstet Gynecol, 35*(1), 3–12.

138. Fischer, S. (1992). Inexpensive population screening for abnormal cells from the uterine cervix and valid results using the vaginal cytopipette. *Gynecol Oncol, 46,* 62–64.

139. Herman, C.J., & Bunnag, B. (1976). Goals of the

cytology automation program of the National Cancer Institute. *J Histochem Cytochem, 24,* 2–5.

140. Hutchinson, M.L., Cassin, C.M., & Ball, H.G. (1991). The efficacy of an automated preparation device for cervical cytology. *Am J Clin Pathol, 96,* 300–305.

141. van Driel-Kulker, A.M.J., & Ploem-Zaaijer, J.J. (1989). Image cytometry in automated cervical screening. *Anal Cell Pathol, 1,* 63–77.

142. Sheets, E.E., Constantine, N.M., Dinisco, S., et al. (1995). Colposcopically directed biopsies provide a basis for comparing the accuracy of thin prep and Papanicolaou smears. *J Gynecol Tehcniques, 1*(1), 27–33.

143. Yoder, L., & Rubin, M. (1992). The epidemiology of cervical cancer and its precursors. *Oncol Nurs Forum, 19*(3), 485–493.

144. Nolte, S., Sohn, M.A., & Koons, B. (1993). Prevention of HIV infection in women. *J Obstet Gynecol Nurs, 22*(2), 128–134.

145. Chu, E.W., & Malmgren, R.A. (1965). An inhibitory effect of vitamin A on the induction of tumors of the forestomach and cervix in the Syrian hamster by carcinogenic polycylic hydrocarbons. *Cancer Res, 25,* 884–885.

146. Weiner, S.A., Surwit, E.A., Graham, U.E., & Meystens, F.L. (1986). A phase I trial of topically applied transretinoic acid in cervical dysplasia: Clinical efficacy. *Invest New Drugs, 4,* 241–244.

147. Barber, H.R.K. (1986). Ovarian cancer. *Cancer, 36*(3), 149–184.

148. Piver, M.S., Baker, T.R., Piedmonte, M., & Sandecki, A.M. (1991). Epidemiology and etiology of ovarian cancer. *Semin Oncol, 18*(3), 177–185.

149. Kolstad, P., & Beechman, J.C. (1974). Epidemiology of ovarian neoplasia. *Proceedings of the American-European Conference on the Ovary* (pp. 364–366). Mortreaux, Switzerland: Exerpta Medica Int. Congress Series.

150. Cramer, D.W., Welch, W.R., Hutchinson, G.B., Willett, W., & Scully, R. (1984). Dietary animal fat in relation to ovarian cancer risk. *Obstet Gynecol, 63*(6), 833–838.

151. Mettlin, C.J., & Piver, S.M. (1990). A case-control study of milk drinking and ovarian cancer risk. *Am J Epidemiol, 132*(5), 871–876.

152. Byers, T., Marshall, J., Graham, S., et al. (1983). A case control study of dietary and nondietary factors in ovarian cancer. *J Natl Cancer Inst, 71* (4), 681–686.

153. Joly, D.J., Lilienfeld, A.M., Diamond, E.I., & Bross, I.D.J. (1974). An epidemiologic study of the relationship of reproductive experience to cancer of the ovary. *Am J Epidemiol, 99,* 190–209.

154. Kvale, G., Heuch, I., Nilssen, S., & Beral, V. (1988). Reproductive factors and risk of ovarian cancer: A prospective study. *Int J Cancer, 42,* 246–251.

155. Negri, E., Francheschi, S., LaVecchia, C., & Parazzini, F. (1992). Incomplete pregnancies and ovarian cancer risk. *Gynecol Oncol, 47,* 234–238.

156. The Cancer and Steroid Hormone Study of the Centers for Disease Control and the National Institute of Child Health and Human Development (1987). Combination oral contraceptive use and the risk of endometrial cancer. *JAMA, 257*(6), 796–800.

157. Hankinson, S.E., Colditz, G.A., Hunter, D.J., et al. (1992). A quantitative assessment of oral contraceptive use and risk of ovarian cancer. *Obstet Gynecol, 80*(4), 708–714.

158. Whittemore, A.S., Wu, M.L., Paffenbarger, R.S., et al. (1988). Personal and environmental characteristics related to epithelial ovarian cancer II. Exposures to talcum powder, tobacco, alcohol, and coffee. *Am J Epidemiol, 128,* 1228–1240.

159. Gardner, W.U. (1948). Hormonal imbalances in tumorigenesis. *Cancer Res, 8,* 397–411.

160. Atlas, M., & Menczer, J. (1982). Massive hyperstimulation and borderline carcinoma of the ovary. *Acta Obstet Gynecol Scand, 61,* 261–263.

161. Bamford, P.N., & Steele, S.J. (1982). Uterine and ovarian carcinoma in a patient receiving gonadotrophin therapy (Case report). *Br J Obstet Gynecol, 89,* 962–964.

162. Whittemore, A.S., Harris, R., Itnyre, J., & Collaborative Ovarian Cancer Group (1992). Characteristics relating to ovarian cancer risk: Collaborative analysis of twelve United States case-control studies. *Am J Epidemiol, 136*(10), 1184–1203.

163. Fathalla, M.F. (1971). Incessant ovulation: A factor in ovarian neoplasia. *Lancet, 2,* 163.

164. Schildkraut, J.M., & Thompson, W.D. (1988). Familial ovarian cancer: A population-based case-control study. *Am J Epidemiol, 128,* 456–466.

165. Lynch, H.T., Albano, W.A., Black, L., et al. (1981). Familial excess of cancer of the ovary and other anatomic sites. *JAMA, 245,* 261–264.

166. Lynch, H.T., Harris, R.E., Guirgis, H.A., et al. (1978). Familial association of breast/ovarian carcinoma. *Cancer, 41,* 1543–1548.

167. Lynch, H.T., Kimberling, W.J., & Albano, W.A. (1985). Hereditary nonpolyposis colorectal cancer parts I & II. *Cancer, 56,* 939–951.

168. Lynch, H.T., Bewtra, C., & Lynch, J.F. (1986). Familial ovarian cancer. *Am J Med, 81,* 1073–1076.

169. Fraumeni, J.F., Grunday, G.W., & Creagan, E.T. (1975). Six families prone to ovarian cancer. *Cancer, 36,* 364–369.

170. Piver, M.S., Mettlin, C.J., Tsukada, Y., et al. (1984). Familial ovarian cancer registry. *Obstet Gynecol, 64*(2), 195–199.

171. Heintz, A.P.M., Hacker, N., & Lagasse, L.D. (1985). Epidemiology and etiology of ovarian cancer: A review. *Obstet Gynecol, 66*(1), 127–135.

172. Weber, B.L. (1996) Genetic testing for breast cancer. *Sci Am Sce Med, 3*(1), 12–21.

173. Egli, G.E., & Newton, M.D. (1961). The transport of carbon particles in the female reproductive tract. *Fertil Steril, 12,* 151–155.

174. Venter, P.F., & Iturralde, M. (1979). Migration of particulate radioactive tracer from the vagina to the peritoneal cavity and ovaries. *S Afr Med J, 55,* 917–919.

175. Booth, M., Becal, V., & Smith, P. (1989). Risk factors for ovarian cancer. A case-control study. *Br J Cancer, 60,* 592–598.

176. Harlow, B.L., Cramer, D.W., Bell, D.A., & Welch, W.R. (1992). Perineal exposure to talc and ovarian cancer. *Obstet Gynecol, 80*(1), 19–26.

177. Rosenblatt, K.A., Szklo, M., & Rosenshein, N.B. (1992). Mineral fiber exposure and the development of ovarian cancer. *Gynecol Oncol, 45,* 20–25.

178. West, R.O. (1966). Epidemiologic study of malignancies of the ovary. *Cancer, 19,* 1001–1007.

179. Menczer, J., Modan, M., & Ranon, L. (1979). Possible role of mumps virus in the etiology of ovarian cancer. *Cancer, 43,* 1375–1379.

180. McGowan, L., Parent, L., Lednar, W., & Norris, H.J. (1979). The woman at risk for developing ovarian cancer. *Gynecol Oncol, 7*(3), 325–344.

181. Garrett, W.J. (1970). On the reduction of cancer mortality: Graham Crawford's experiment, 1949–1969. *Med J Aust, 1*(25), 1239–1243.

182. Creasman, W.T., & DiSaia, P.J. (1991). Screening in ovarian cancer. *Am J Obstet Gynecol, 165*(1), 7–10.

183. Takashina, T., Ono, M., Kanda, Y., et al. (1988). Cervicovaginal and endometrial cytology in ovarian cancer. *Acta Cytol, 32*(2), 159–162.

184. National Institutes of Health. (1994). Ovarian cancer: Screening, treatment, and follow-up. *NIH Consensus Statement 12*(3), 1–30.

185. Kabawat, S.E., Bast, R.C., Bhan, A.K., et al. (1983). Tissue distribution of a coelomic epithelium–related antigen recognized by the monoclonal antibody OC125. *Lab Invest, H8,* 42A.

186. Bast, R.C., Klug, T.L., St. John, E., et al. (1983). A radioimmunoassay using a monoclonal antibody to monitor the course of epithelial ovarian cancer. *N Engl J Med, 309*(15), 883–887.

187. Makar, A.P.H., Kristensen, G.B., Kearn, J., et al. (1992). Prognostic value of pre- and postoperative serum CA–125 levels in ovarian cancer: New aspects and multivariate analysis. *Obstet Gynecol, 79*(6), 1002–1010.

188. Rustin, G.J.S., Gennings, J.N., Nelstrop, A.E., et al. (1989). Use of CA-125 to predict survival of patients with ovarian cancer. *J Clin Oncol, 7*(11), 1667–1671.

189. Zurawski, V.R., Knapp, R.C., Einhorn, N., et al. (1988). An initial analysis of preoperative serum CA-125 levels in patients with early stage ovarian cancer. *Gynecol Oncol, 30,* 7–14.

190. Haga, Y., Sakamoto, K., Egami, H., et al. (1986a). Clinical significance of serum CA-125 values in patients with cancers of the digestive system. *Am J Med Sci, 292*(1), 30–34.

191. Haga, Y., Sakamoto, K., Egami, H., et al. (1986b). Evaluation of serum CA-125 values in healthy individuals and pregnant women. *Am J Med Sci, 292*(1), 25–29.

192. Jacobs, I., & Bast, R.C. (1989). The CA-125 tumor-associated antigen: A review of the literature. *Hum Reprod, 4*(1), 1–12.

193. Ruibal, A., Encabo, G., Martinez-Miralles, E., et al. (1984). CA-125 seric levels in nonmalignant pathologies. *Bulletin Cancer, 71*(2), 145–148.

194. Vasileu, S.A., Schlaerth, J.B., Campeau, J., & Morrow, P.C. (1988). Serum CA-125 levels in preoperative evaluation of pelvic masses. *Obstet Gynecol, 71*(5), 751–756.

195. Bergman, J.F., Beaugrand, M., Labadie, H., Bidart, J.M., & Bohoun, C. (1986). CA-125 (ovarian tumor-associated antigen) in ascitic liver diseases. *Clin Chim Acta, 155,* 163–166.

196. Kuzuya, K., Nozaki, M., & Chihara, T. (1986). Evaluation of CA-125 as a circulating tumor marker for ovarian cancer. *Acta Obstet Gynecol Japan, 38,* 949–957.

197. Einhorn, N., Sjovall, K., Knapp, R., et al. (1992). Prospective evaluation of the specificity of serum CA-125 levels for detection of ovarian cancer in a normal population. *Obstet Gynecol, 80*(1), 14–18.

198. Jacobs, I.J., & Oram, D.A. (1989). Potential screening tests for ovarian cancer. In F. Sharp, W.P. Mason & R.E. Leake, eds., *Ovarian Cancer* (pp. 197–205). London: Chapman & Hall Medical.

199. Jacobs, I.J., Oram, D.H., & Bast, R.C. (1992). Strategies for improving the specificity of screening for ovarian cancer with tumor-associated antigens CA-125, CA 15-3, and TAG 72. 3. *Obstet Gynecol, 80*(3), 396–399.

200. Einhorn, N., Knapp, R.C., Bast, R.C., & Zurawski, V.R. (1989). CA-125 assay used in conjunction with CA-15-3 and TAG-72 assays for discrimination between malignant and nonmalignant diseases of the ovary. *Acta Oncol, 28,* 655–657.

201. Cole, L.A., Nam, J.H., Chambers, J.T., & Schwartz, P.E. (1990). Urinary gonadotropin fragment: A new tumor marker. *Gynecol Oncol, 36,* 391–394.

202. Inoue, M., Fujita, M., Nakazawa, A., et al. (1992).

Sialyl-Tn, Sialyl Lewis Xi, CA-19-9, CA-125, carcinoembryonic antigen, and tissue polypeptide antigen, in differentiating ovarian cancer from benign tumors. *Obstet Gynecol, 79*(3), 434–439.

203. Campbell, S., Bhan, V., Roysten, P., et al. (1989). Transabdominal ultrasound screening for early ovarian cancer. *Br Med J, 299,* 1365–1366.

204. van Nagell, J.R., Higgins, R., Donaldson, E.S., et al. (1990). Transvaginal sonography as a screening method for ovarian cancer. *Cancer, 65,* 573–577.

205. van Nagell, J.R., DePriest, P.D., Puls, L.E., et al. (1991). Ovarian cancer screening in asymptomatic postmenopausal women by transvaginal sonography. *Cancer, 68,* 458–462.

206. Bourne, T., Campbell, S., Steer, C., et al. (1989). Transvaginal colour flow imaging: A possible new screening technique for ovarian cancer. *Br Med J, 299,* 1367–1370.

207. Weiner, Z., Thaler, I., Beck, D., et al. (1992). Differentiating malignant from benign ovarian tumors with transvaginal color flow imaging. *Obstet Gynecol, 79*(2), 159–162.

208. Hata, K., Hata, T., Manabe, A., et al. (1992). A critical evaluation of transvaginal Doppler studies, transvaginal sonography, magnetic resonance imaging, and CA-125 in detecting ovarian cancer. *Obstet Gynecol, 80*(6), 922–926.

209. Sassone, A.M., Timor-Tritsch, I.E., Artner, A., et al. (1991). Transvaginal sonographic characterization of ovarian disease: Evaluation of a new screening system to predict ovarian malignancy. *Obstet Gynecol, 78*(1), 70–76.

210. Luxman, D., Bergman, A., Sagi, J., & David, M.P. (1991). The postmenopausal adnexal mass: Correlation between ultrasonic and pathologic findings. *Obstet Gynecol, 77*(5), 726–728.

211. Finkler, N.J., Benacerraf, B., Lavin, P.T., et al. (1988). Comparison of serum CA-125, clinical impression, and ultrasound in the preoperative evaluation of ovarian masses. *Obstet Gynecol, 72*(4), 659–664.

212. Sparks, J.M., & Vasna, R.E. (1991). Ovarian cancer screening. *Obstet Gynecol, 77*(5), 787–792.

213. Fitzsimmons, M.L., Conway, T.A., Madsen, N., et al. (1989). Hereditary cancer syndrome: Nursing's role in identification and education. *Oncol Nurs Forum, 16*(1), 87–94.

214. Lynch, H.T., Albano, W.A., Lynch, J.F., et al. (1982). Surveillance and management of patients at high genetic risk for ovarian cancer. *Obstet Gynecol, 59*(5), 589–596.

215. Piver, M.S., Baker, T.R., Jishi, M.F., et al. (1993). Familial ovarian cancer. *Cancer, 71* (suppl. 2), 582–588.

216. American College of Obstetricians and Gynecologists. (1992). Genetic risk and screening techniques for epithelial ovarian cancer. *ACOG Committee Opinion 117,* 1–3.

217. Burke, W., Daly, M., Garber, J., et al. (1997). Recommendations for follow-up care of individuals with an inherited predisposition to cancer II. BRCA1 and BRCA2. *JAMA, 227*(12), 997–1003.

218. Sightler, S.E., Boike, A.M., Estape, R.E., & Averette, H.E. (1991). Ovarian cancer in women with prior hysterectomy: A fourteen-year experience at the University of Miami. *Obstet Gynecol, 78,* 681–684.

219. McGowan, L. (1987). Ovarian cancer after hysterectomy. *Obstet Gynecol, 69*(3), 386–389.

220. American College of Obstetricians and Gynecologists (1987). Prophylactic oophorectomy. *ACOG Technical Bulletin, 111,* 1–4.

221. Tobacman, J.K., Tucker, M.A., Kase, R., et al. (1982). Intra-abdominal carcinomatosis after prophylactic oophorectomy in ovarian cancer–prone families. *Lancet, 2,* 795–797.

222. Chen, K.T.K., Schooley, J.L., & Flam, M.S. (1985). Peritoneal carcinomatosis after prophylactic oophorectomy in familial ovarian cancer syndrome. *Obstet Gynecol, 66*(suppl. 3), 938–994.

223. Kemp, G.M., Gwang-Jeng, H., & Andrews, M.C. (1992). Papillary peritoneal carcinomatosis after prophylactic oophorectomy. *Gynecol Oncol, 47,* 395–397.

224. Weber, A.M., Hewett, W.J., Gajewski, W.H., & Curry, S.L. (1992). Serous carcinoma of the peritoneum after oophorectomy. *Obstet Gynecol, 80*(3), 558–560.

225. Kerlikowske, K., Brown, J.S., & Grady, D.G. (1992). Should women with familial ovarian cancer undergo prophylactic oophorectomy? *Obstet Gynecol, 80*(40), 700–707.

226. Friedlander, M., & Segekov, E. (1992). Risk factors, epidemiology, screening, and prognostic factors in female genital cancer. *Curr Opin Oncol, 4*(5), 913–922.

227. Parazzini, F., La Vecchia, C., Bocciolone, L., & Franceschi, S. (1991a). The epidemiology of endometrial cancer. *Gynecol Oncol, 41*(1), 1–16.

228. DiSaia, P.J., & Creasman, W.T. (1993). *Clinical Gynecologic Oncology* 4th ed. (pp. 156–193). St. Louis, MO: Mosby.

229. Ferency, A. (1987). Methods for detecting endometrial carcinoma and its precursors. In H.J. Buchsbaum & J.J. Sciarra, eds., *Gynecology and Obstetrics* 4th ed. Philadelphia: Harper & Row.

230. Elliott, E.A., Matnoski, G.M., Rosenshein, N.B., Grumbine, F.C., & Diamond, E.L. (1990). Body fat patterning in women with endometrial cancer. *Gynecol Oncol, 39*(3), 253–258.

231. Parazzini, F., La Vecchia, C., Negri, E., et al. (1991b). Reproductive factors and risk of endometrial cancer. *Am J Obstet Gynecol, 164*(2), 522–527.

232. Ewertz, M., Shou, G., & Boice, J.D., Jr. (1988). The joint effect of risk factors on endometrial cancer. *Eur J Cancer Clin Oncol, 24*(2), 189–194.

233. MacMahan, B. (1974). Risk factors for endometrial cancer. *Gynecol Oncol, 2*(2–3), 122–129.

234. Abeler, V.M., & Korstad, K.E. (1991). Endometrial adenocarcinoma in Norway: A study of a total population. *Cancer, 67*(12), 3093–3103.

235. Fu, Y.S., Gambone, J.C., & Berek, J.S. (1990). Pathophysiology and management of endometrial hyperplasia and carcinoma. *West J Med, 153*(1), 50–61.

236. Harlap, S. (1992). The benefits and risks of hormone replacement therapy: An epidemiologic overview. *Am J Obstet Gynecol, 166*(6), 1986–1992.

237. Smith, D.C., Prentice, R., & Thompson, D.J. (1975). Association of exogenous estrogen and endometrial carcinoma. *N Engl J Med, 293*(23), 1164–1167.

238. Ziel, H.K., & Finkle, W.D. (1975). Increased risk of endometrial carcinoma among users of conjugated estrogens. *N Engl J Med, 293,* 1167–1170.

239. Voigt, L.F., Weiss, N.S., Chu, J., et al. (1991). Progestogen supplementation of oestrogens and risk of endometrial cancer. *Lancet, 338,* 274–277.

240. Fornander, T., Rutqvist, L.E., Cedermark, B., et al. (1989). Adjuvant tamoxifen in early breast cancer: Occurrence of new primary cancers. *Lancet, 1,* 117–120.

241. American College of Obstetricians and Gynecologists, Committee on Gynecologic Practice (1997), September). *Routine Cancer Screening.* ACOG Committee Opinion #185, Washington, D.C.

242. Gronroos, M., Salmi, T.A., Vuento, M.H., et al. (1993). Mass screening for endometrial cancer directed in risk groups of patients with diabetes and patients with hypertension. *Cancer, 71*(4), 1279–1282.

243. Averette, H.E., Steren, A., & Nguyen, H.N. (1993). Screening in gynecologic cancers. *Cancer, 72*(suppl.3), 1043–1049.

244. Hulka, B.S. (1987). Replacement estrogens and risk of gynecologic cancers and breast cancer. *Cancer, 60*(8), 1960–1964.

245. Persson, I., Adami, H.O., Bergkvist, L., et al. (1989). Risk of endometrial cancer after treatment with oestrogens alone or in conjunction with progestogens: Results of a prospective study. *Br J Med, 298*(6667), 147–151.

246. The Cancer & Steroid Hormone Study of the Centers for Disease Control and the National Institute of Child Health and Human Development (1987). The reduction in risk of ovarian cancer associated with oral contraceptive use. *N Engl J Med, 316*(11), 650–655.

247. Franks, A.L., Kendrick, J.S., Tyler, C.W., Jr. (1987). The cancer and steroid hormone study group: Postmenopausal smoking, estrogen, and the risk of endometrial cancer. *Am J Obstet Gynecol, 156*(1), 20–23.

248. Hart, W.R., Norris, H.J., & Helwig, E.B. (1975). Relation of lichen sclerosis et atrophicus of the vulva to development of carcinoma. *Obstet Gynecol, 45* (4), 369–377.

249. Lessana-Leibowitz, M., Pelisse, M., & Moyal-Barracco, M. (1990). Lichen sclerosis, invasive squamous cell carcinoma, and human papillomavirus. *Am J Obstet Gynecol 162*(6), 1633–1644.

250. Mabuchi, K., Bross, D.S., & Kessler, I.I. (1985). Epidemiology of cancer of the vulva. *Cancer, 55,* 1843–1848.

251. Bloss, J.D., Liao, S.Y., Wilczynski, S.P., et al. (1991). Clinical and histologic features of vulvar carcinomas analyzed for human papillomavirus status: Evidence that squamous cell carcinoma of the vulva has more than one etiology. *Hum Pathol, 22,* 711–718.

252. Zaino, R.J., Husseinzadeh, N., Nahhas, W., & Mortel, R. (1982). Epithelial alterations in proximity to invasive squamous carcinoma of the vulva. *Int J Gynecol Pathol, 1,* 173–184.

253. Brinton, L.A., Nasca, P.C., Mallin, K., et al. (1990). Case-control study of cancer of the vulva. *Obstet Gynecol, 75*(5), 859–866.

254. Anderson, W.A., Franquemont, D.W., Williams, J., Taylor, P.T., & Crum, C.P. (1991). Vulvar squamous cell carcinoma and papilloma viruses: Two separate entities. *Am J Obstet Gynecol, 165*(2), 329–336.

255. Rusk, D., Sutton, G.P., Look, K.Y., & Roman, A. (1991). Analysis of invasive squamous cell carcinoma of the vulva and vulvar intraepithelial neoplasia for the presence of human papillomavirus DNA. *Obstet Gynecol, 77*(6), 918–922.

256. Choo, Y.C., & Morley, G.W. (1980). Double primary epidermoid carcinoma of the vulva and cervix. *Gynecol Oncol, 9,* 325–333.

257. Hacker, N.F. (1989). Vulvar cancer. In N.F. Hacker & J.S. Berek, eds., *Practical Gynecologic Oncology* (pp. 391–424). Baltimore: Williams & Wilkins.

258. Marcus, S.L. (1960). Multiple squamous cell carcinomas involving the cervix, vagina, and vulva: The theory of multicentric origin. *Am J Obstet Gynecol, 80,* 802–812.

259. Newcomb, P.A., Weiss, N.S., & Daling, J.R. (1984). Incidence of vulvar carcinoma in relation to menstrual, reproductive, and medical factors. *J Natl Cancer Inst, 73,* 391–396.

260. Moore, G. (1990). Risk factors in vulvar carcinoma (unpublished Master's thesis). Gainesville: University of Florida.

261. Parazzini, F., La Vecchia, C., Garsia, S., et al. (1993). Determinants of invasive vulvar cancer risk: An Italian case-control study. *Gynecol Oncol, 48*, 50–55.

262. Japaze, H., Garcia-Buneul, R., & Woodruff, J.D. (1977). Primary vulvar neoplasia: A review of in situ and invasive carcinoma 1935–1972. *Obstet Gynecol, 49*(4), 404–411.

263. O'Mara, B.A., Byers, T., & Schoenfeld, E. (1985). Diabetes mellitus and cancer risk: A multisite case-control study. *J Chronic Disease, 38*(5), 435–441.

264. Gerrard, E.A. (1932). Epithelioma vulvae as an occupational disease among cotton operatives. *Trans North Engl Obstet Gynaecol, 65*.

265. Way, S. (1960). Carcinoma of the vulva. *Am J Obstet Gynecol, 79*, 692–697.

266. Sandella, J. (1987). Vulvar self-examination. *Oncol Nurs Forum, 14*(6), 71–73.

267. American College of Obstetricians and Gynecologists. (1984). Cervical cytology evaluation and management of abnormalities. *ACOG Technical Bulletin, 81*, 1–5.

Preinvasive Diseases of the Cervix, Vulva, and Vagina

Alice Spinelli, RN, ANP, OCN

✖ INTRODUCTION

Intraepithelial neoplasia of the lower genital tract encompasses a wide spectrum of premalignant lesions of the cervix, vulva, and vagina. Preinvasive disease and other related conditions are seen with increasing frequency, perhaps because of increased screening as well as a true increase in incidence. Precancerous lesions are becoming a disease of young, sexually active women in the reproductive age group.[1] The average age of a patient with carcinoma in situ is ten to fifteen years younger than the average age of patients with invasive cancer of the cervix.[2] Considering such a natural history, screening can be an effective tool in controlling the incidence of invasive cancer of the uterine cervix. In fact, it has been estimated that annual Pap smear testing reduces a woman's chance of dying of cervical cancer from 4/1000 to about 5/10,000—a difference of almost 90%.[2]

Pathology

Intraepithelial neoplasia, also referred to as *dysplasia,* is a term used to describe premalignant changes of epithelial tissue. The term cervical intraepithelial neoplasia (CIN), was proposed by Richart in 1973,[3] to define the spectrum of intraepithelial changes that precede invasive cervical cancer. These changes were classified into three grades: CIN I (mild dysplasia) represents involvement of less than one-third of the thickness of the epithelium; CIN II (moderate dysplasia) represents one-third to two-thirds involvement; and CIN III (severe dysplasia and carcinoma in situ) represents two-thirds to full-thickness involvement but with no involvement of the underlying stroma (Figures 2.1 and 2.2).[1] The difference between preinvasive disease (intraepithelial neoplasia) and invasive disease is that preinvasive disease does not penetrate the basement membrane so there is no stromal invasion. Intraepithelial neoplasia of the vulva and vagina is categorized and graded in a similar fashion.

✖ CERVICAL INTRAEPITHELIAL NEOPLASIA

Intraepithelial neoplasia of the cervix occurs predominantly in young women, with the peak age of incidence in the early 30s (Table 2.1),[4] in contrast with the average age of 50 years for women with invasive cervical cancer.[1] It is not unusual to discover CIN in women in their late teens and early 20s. In an analysis of approximately 800 women with the diagnosis of CIN at the Duke University Medical Center, it was noted that 30% were 20 years of age or younger at the time of diagnosis. More than 95% of the patients had intercourse by the age of 20, and one-half had been sexually active by 16 years of age. More than one-half of these patients had the diagnosis of CIN established within five years of the beginning of their sexual activity.[2] Thus screening young women early, when they seek contraception or other medical attention, is extremely important and should be done on a routine basis.

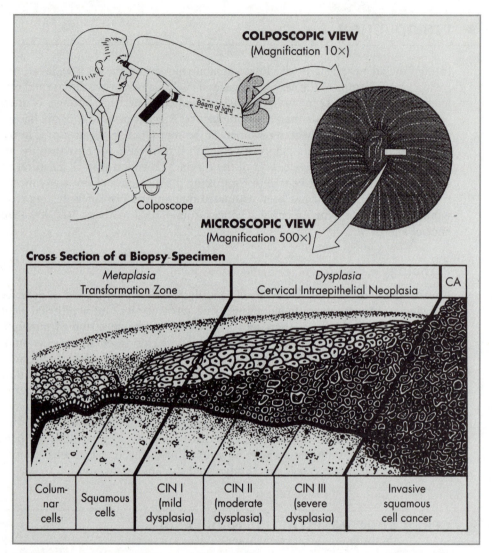

COLPOSCOPIC VIEW
(Magnification 10×)

Beam of light

Colposcope

MICROSCOPIC VIEW
(Magnification 500×)

Cross Section of a Biopsy Specimen

Metaplasia Transformation Zone		Dysplasia Cervical Intraepithelial Neoplasia			CA
Colum-nar cells	Squamous cells	CIN I (mild dysplasia)	CIN II (moderate dysplasia)	CIN III (severe dysplasia)	Invasive squamous cell cancer

FIGURE 2.1. Colposcopist's view of the cervix.

Source: Reproduced with permission from Waye, R.D. (1990). *The Pap Smear and Your Cervix.* Chicago: Medfax-Sentinel.

Diethylstilbestrol (DES) Exposure

In the late 1940s, diethylstilbestrol (DES) was used during pregnancy to prevent complications such as threatened abortion or prematurity. Though many studies disputed the efficacy of DES in these situations, it continued to be prescribed through the 1960s. It was first noted in 1971 that young women whose mothers took DES during pregnancy were at increased risk of developing clear cell adenocarcinoma of the

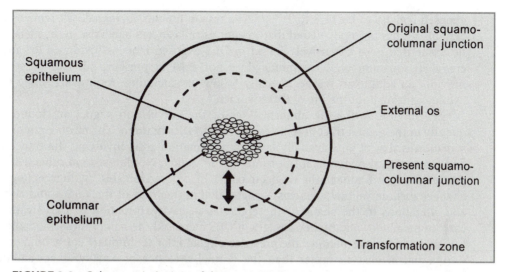

FIGURE 2.2. Colposcopist's view of the cervix undergoing metaplasia.

Source: Reprinted with permission from Barter, J. (1984). *Gynecologic Oncology Review Notes.* Washington DC: Division of Gynecologic Oncology, Georgetown University.

vagina.[4] Fortunately, however, the feared epidemic never materialized. Of approximately 3 million females with in utero DES exposure, as few as 1.4 per 10,000 cases of clear-cell adenocarcinoma have been reported.[11] Although it is anticipated that the vast majority of DES-exposed associated adenocarcinomas have been identified, history of DES exposure is important in the follow-up of these patients as adenocarcinoma could still appear in the future.[2]

In addition, research has clearly demonstrated that DES-exposed females are at an increased risk of developing CIN (relative risk 2).[12] Prevalence rates of squamous cell neoplasia in the general female population between adolescence and 30 years of age range between 4 and 7%, while various studies indicate the prevalence rate in DES-

TABLE 2.1	
Transition Time of CIN	
Stages	*Mean Years*
Normal to mild-moderate dysplasia	1.62
Normal to moderate-severe dysplasia	2.20
Normal to carcinoma in situ	4.51

Source: Reprinted with permission from DiSaia, P.J., & Creasman, W.T. (1997). *Clinical Gynecologic Oncology* 4th ed. St. Louis, MO: Mosby Year Book, Inc.

exposed females to be 11.3 to 18%.[13] The reason for this increased risk remains uncertain.[12] It has been postulated that squamous cell cancers may arise in the metaplastic tissue that is so extensively found in DES-exposed females. Evidence for an increase in squamous cell carcinoma does not exist at present, but this possibility provides an additional reason for close follow-up, including routine screening with cytology, throughout the life of these women.[2]

Several non-neoplastic abnormalities of the cervix and vagina are found frequently in the genital tract of females exposed to DES in utero. The most common observation is that of an unusually large transformation zone involving the ectocervix and frequently also significant portions of the vagina. Nordquist (and others) noted extension of the T-zone to the vagina in 63.8% of exposed females.[13] Other teratogenic changes include vaginal adenosis, structural abnormalities of the vagina and cervix, and alterations in the shape of the endometrial cavity. Initiation of DES treatment early in pregnancy and higher dosages of DES increased the risk of these anomalies.[4]

Vaginal adenosis denotes the presence of glandular (columnar) epithelium in the vagina and ectocervix rather than the normal presence of squamous epithelium.[4] It occurs in approximately 35 to 40% of women exposed.[13]

Structural abnormalities of the vagina and cervix include transverse ridges, cervical collars, cervical hood, cockscomb cervix, and pseudopolyp. Malformation of the endometrial cavity (T-shaped uterus) can be identified on hysterosalpingogram and has implications for infertility. These structural abnormalities are seen in approximately 25% of women exposed.[4]

Papanicolaou Screening

Cytologic screening for intraepithelial neoplasia was first demonstrated by Papanicolaou in 1943, and its subsequent application in routine screening has resulted in a significant decrease in the incidence of invasive cervical cancer. The Pap smear involves obtaining a sampling of cells from the cervix and vagina for cytologic review. While it is an effective screening tool, the diagnosis of neoplasia requires tissue for histologic study, obtained by biopsy. When screening patients, it is prudent to recognize that false-negative results do not occur infrequently and any inconsistencies or abnormal findings should be pursued despite a negative Pap smear.

Cervical neoplasia usually is discovered at the transformation zone (T-zone), and the presence of endocervical cells ensures that the T-zone has been sampled (Table 2.2). The transformation zone is the area of the cervix that was originally covered with columnar epithelium, and, through metaplasia, has undergone replacement by squamous epithelium. The outer border of the T-zone is the original squamocolumnar junction and the inner border the existing squamocolumnar junction. The transformation process (Figure 2.2) begins during puberty, when hormonal influence causes a significant decrease in the vaginal pH. The exposed columnar cells undergo metaplasia, and this dynamic area is the transformation zone. The subsequent squamocolumnar junction moves proximally toward the endocervix. The precise location of the T-zone may be influenced by puberty, DES exposure in utero, pregnancy, parity,

TABLE 2.2		
Factors Contributing to Optimal Cytology Sampling		
Examination Techniques	*Office Process*	*Quality Control*
1. Prelabel slide. 2. Insert speculum of appropriate temperature without lubricant 3. Carefully remove excess. mucous or blood from cervix. 4. Retrieve cells from squamous epithelium, transformation zone (squamo-columnar junction), and endo cervical epithelium.- 5. Obtain sample with endocervical brush, and Ayre spatula. 6. Place sample on clean strokes. 7. Rapidly fix specimen with laboratory choice of cytology fixative.	1. Protect slide in a cytology collection kit. 2. Document patient clinical information on cytology form. 3. Log specimens in a recording system. 4. Arrange laboratory transport.	1. Verify evaluations by trained cytotechnologists. 2. Verify that abnormal smears are reviewed by a pathologist. 3. Assess laboratory quality control measures. 4. Request clarification for any unclear reports. 5. Interpret screening results. 6. Implement appropriate follow-up.

Source: Adapted with permission from Woodward, J. (1990). The triple C approach to the detection of cervical cancer. *Nurse Practitioner Forum,* 1(1), 32.

menopause and other factors and is therefore individualized. The T-zone is best visualized with colposcopy. Proper technique in obtaining the Pap smear usually results in a satisfactory sampling of the T-zone.

The procedure for obtaining an adequate Pap smear begins with patient education, which includes: no samples taken while menstruating, no intercourse for forty-eight hours beforehand, and no douching or use of intravaginal creams for forty-eight hours beforehand.

Technique

1. With the patient in the lithotomy position, place the speculum into the vagina and position properly so that the cervix is completely visible.

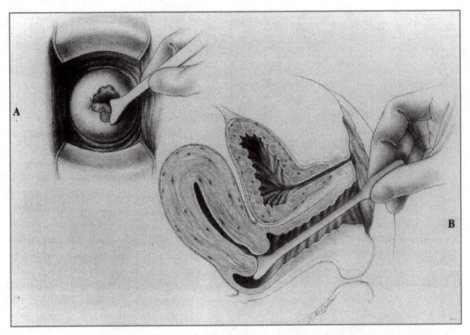

FIGURE 2.3. A. Scrape of endocervix with spatula. **B.** Scrape of exocervix with spatula.
Source: Reproduced with permission from Herbst, A.L. (1992). Intraepithelial neoplasia of the cervix. In A.L. Herbst, D.R. Mishell, Jr., M.A. Stenchever, & W. Droefemueller, eds., *Comprehensive Gynecology* 2nd ed. (p. 837). St. Louis, MO: Mosby Year Book, Inc.

2. Use a wooden or plastic spatula to scrape the ectocervical and endocervical exfoliated cells (Figure 2.3). An endocervical brush should then be inserted and a sampling obtained by rotating the brush 1/4–1/2 turn in the same direction (Figure 2.4). The absence of endocervical cells results in an inadequate or unsatisfactory Pap smear, as endocervical brushes have yielded better results than the spatula alone in obtaining endocervical cells.[4] Many commercial brushes are available and provide superior results to the cotton swab (Figure 2.5). If a cotton swab is used instead, it must first be moistened to prevent absorption of the cells into the cotton. Separate smears from the vagina may also be obtained.
3. Place the specimen(s) on a glass slide and fix immediately, either in 90% alcohol or sprayed with fixative. It is important to hold the fixative more than 12 inches from the smear and not to permit the specimen to air-dry before fixing. If using the ThinPrep® Pap test, the spatula and brush must be vigorously swirled into the PreservCyt® Solution vial ten times to release the material.[5]
4. In completing the cytology form to be submitted with the specimen, relevant information regarding the patient's history must be noted, such as last menstrual period (LMP), pregnancy, history of hysterectomy, CIN, condyloma, or radiation therapy.

FIGURE 2.4. Obtaining cells from the endocervix using a cytobrush.

Source: Reprinted with permission from Stenchever, M.A. (1992). History and examination of the patient. In A.L. Herbst, D.R. Mishell, Jr., M.A. Stenchever, & W. Droefemueller, eds., *Comprehensive Gynecology* 2nd ed. (p. 155). St. Louis, MO: Mosby Year Book, Inc.

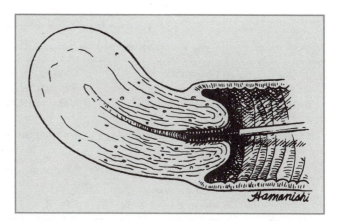

5. Make the patient aware that light spotting and/or mild cramping may occur as a result of the examination.

Bethesda System

The Bethesda System for reporting cervical/vaginal cytologic diagnosis was developed as evolving cytopathologic advances rendered the Papanicolaou System less useful in guiding treatment (Table 2.3).

In 1988, the Division of Cancer Prevention and Control at the National Cancer Institute convened a workshop of distinguished expert consultants "to review existing terminology and to recommend effective methods of reporting."[6] The Bethesda System was revised at a second NCI-sponsored workshop in 1991, when the following recommendations were unanimously approved:

1. The cytopathology report is a medical consultation.
2. The Papanicolaou classification for reporting consultations is not acceptable in the modern practice of diagnostic cytopathology.
3. The Bethesda System should serve as a guideline for cytopathology reports of cervical/vaginal specimens.[7]

FIGURE 2.5. Commercial brushes for endocervical sampling.

Source: Reproduced with permission from Herbst, A.L. (1992). Intraepithelial neoplasia of the cervix. In A.L. Herbst, D.R. Mishell, Jr., M.A. Stenchever, & W. Droefemueller, eds., *Comprehensive Gynecology* 2nd ed. (p. 837). St. Louis, MO: Mosby Year Book, Inc.

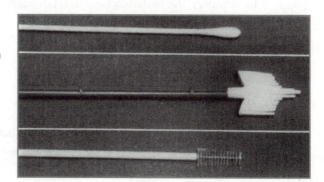

	TABLE 2.3		
	Comparison of Pap Smear Classifications		
Numerical System	Dysplasia Cytologic Classification	Cervical Intraepithelial Neoplasia (CIN)	Bethesda System
Class I	Negative; squamous metaplasia	No designation	Negative
Class II	Atypical squamous cells	No designation	Atypical squamous cells
Class III	Mild dysplasia	CIN I	Low-grade SIL
	Moderate dysplasia	CIN II	High-grade SIL
Class IV	Severe dysplasia	CIN III	High-grade SIL
	Carcinoma in situ		
Class V	Invasive cancer	Invasive cancer	Invasive cancer

Source: Adapted with permission from Yoder, L., & Rubin, M. (1992). The epidemiology of cervical cancer and its precursors. *Oncology Nursing Forum, 19*(3), 485–493.

Under the Bethesda System a new diagnostic term was added. It is squamous intraepithelial lesion (SIL), which may be either a low- or a high-grade neoplastic lesion. The phrase "cellular changes associated with HPV" (i.e., koilocytosis) is added to the report of either low-grade SIL (LGSIL) or high-grade SIL (HGSIL) when appropriate.[8] The category of low-grade SIL includes condyloma in addition to CIN I. The classification "atypical cells of undetermined significance" (ASCUS), was also introduced to categorize lesions with cells presenting abnormal nuclear characteristics but without changes suggestive of koilocytotic atypia or CIN[8] (Table 2.3). In addition to these diagnostic changes, a report should include a written statement of the adequacy of the diagnostic specimen as well as a general categorization of the diagnosis, such as "normal" or "further action required."[8]

In summary, the Bethesda System report contains three main categories:

1. A statement of adequacy of the specimen
2. A general categorization of the diagnosis
3. A descriptive diagnosis

The goal of Pap screening and subsequent patient management is to reduce the morbidity and mortality associated with cervical neoplasia. It is hoped that this goal can be realized through use of the Bethesda System, which was developed to facilitate communication between the cytopathologist and the clinician and thereby permit better correlation of cytologic, colposcopic, and histologic findings.[8]

✳ VULVAR INTRAEPITHELIAL NEOPLASIA

Although vulvar cancer is an uncommon tumor, the incidence of vulvar intraepithelial neoplasia (VIN) has increased recently. The incidence of VIN in the United States has increased from 1.2 to 2.1 per 100,000 women in the last 20 years. The trend is most significant in white women under 35 years of age, in whom the incidence has nearly tripled. This increase may be due to changes in sexual behavior that have put women at higher risk of HPV (human papilloma virus) infection and other sexually transmitted diseases and to increased smoking among younger women.[9] The risk of VIN transformation to malignancy is 5%.[10]

Despite the increase in the incidence of VIN, the rate of invasive vulvar cancer remains stable. This may be due to the liberal use of vulvar biopsy and subsequent early diagnosis, the possibility that VIN does not develop into cancer or that many of the squamous cell carcinomas of the vulva, especially those found in older women, are not HPV related and therefore are not preceded by VIN.[10]

✳ VAGINAL INTRAEPITHELIAL NEOPLASIA

Vaginal intraepithelial neoplasia (VAIN) is much less common than intraepithelial neoplasia of the cervix and vulva. The increased risk of VAIN after treatment for CIN or squamous cell neoplasia of the vulva illustrates the increased risk of squamous cell neoplasia arising anywhere in the lower genital tract in at-risk women. Additional risk factors include prior radiation therapy of the genital tract, immunosuppressive therapy in transplant patients, and chemotherapy in patients undergoing treatment for malignant disease.[4] The predisposing factors in the development of VAIN are probably the same as for CIN.[1]

✳ HUMAN PAPILLOMA VIRUS

In the 1970s ZurHausen first postulated the etiologic potential of HPV in CIN and cervical cancer.[14] In the late 1970s Meiser described a new virus-induced condylomatous lesion of the cervix, and the presence of intranuclear HPV in koilocytotic cells associated with CIN was noted.[4] (Koilocytosis is the histologic appearance of cells with perinuclear halos consistent with HPV infection.)

Human papillomavirus (HPV) is a tumor-producing virus with more than 70 identified strains, many of which produce the common epidermal warts on hands, feet, and knees. More than 20 of these strains are anogenital and sexually transmitted. The most common form of HPV infection is genital warts or condyloma.[15] HPV is thought to be transmitted sexually by skin-to-skin contact, facilitating integration of the virus at sites of microtrauma.[12] The identification of the more than 20 genital strains, along with their characteristics and potential oncogenicity, is the most recent advancement in the research connecting HPV and cervical cancer.[15] Particularly over recent years, a steady accumulation of diverse molecular and epidemiologic evidence has firmly implicated HPV infection in the etiology of anogenital intraepithelial neoplasia. Oncogenic HPV infection is now accepted as the major initiating factor for premalignant epithelial proliferations on the cervix, vulva, vagina, penis, and anus.[16] HPV infection was recognized as the major cause of cervical cancer by the World Health Organization (WHO) in 1992.[17]

Due to the multiple site or multicentric nature of HPV infections, women with visible external lesions or vulvar warts often have vaginal and cervical HPV infections as well. Greenberg et al. found that 68% of women with vulvar condyloma also had cervical and vaginal lesions. Kulski et al. studied the presence of HPV in cell scrapings of the cervix and vulva of 128 women with CIN and/or HPV infection of the cervix and found that subclinical papillomavirus infections of the vulva frequently coexist with CIN and HPV infections of the cervix.[18]

HPV is the most prevalent sexually transmitted disease. It is estimated that approximately 28% of sexually active women (or approximately 30 million) have been infected with the virus. There are 1 to 3 million new cases of genital HPV per year.[15] Data from the International Biological Study on Cervical Study Group found HPV DNA detected in 93% of cancer specimens from women in 22 countries and analyzed by the PCR technique.[19] (PCR, polymerase chain reaction, is a virological test allowing for identification of the presence of HPV DNA and specific DNA strains or types.) Similarly, HPV DNA has been detected by PCR in up to 94% of women with preinvasive disease (CIN) and in up to 46% of women with cytologically normal tissue.[20]

Despite the prevalence of HPV, screening of healthy populations suggests most HPV exposure results only in latent infection.[16] By definition, latent HPV infection implies the presence of HPV DNA as determined by molecular investigative techniques (e.g., PCR) and by the absence of epithelial cell abnormalities by cytology, histology, or colposcopy.[21] In other words, the presence of HPV DNA often occurs without evidence of disease and may never result in neoplasia. Some low-grade lesions (LGSIL) may spontaneously regress. The difference between the high prevalence of HPV infection (11–80%) in young healthy women and the low incidence of cervical neoplasia, as well as the low rate of progression of untreated CIN lesions, supports the hypothesis that HPV may be a necessary but insufficient factor for cervical neoplasia. While HPV is the most important risk factor for cervical neoplasia, the presence of other cofactors seems to be necessary for the development of disease.[20] Cofactors that may be important for the development of disease include: immunosuppression, early age at first coitus, multiple sex partners, cigarette smoking, vitamin deficiencies, hormonal status, and presence of other sexually transmitted diseases.[15,20]

HPV DNA Typing

Triaging treatment of abnormal Papanicolaou (Pap) smears involves differentiating low-grade squamous intraepithelial lesions (LGSIL), high-grade squamous intraep-

TABLE 2.4	
High and low risk types of HPV[20]	
High Risk	16, 18, 31, 45, and 56
Intermediate Risk	31, 33, 35
Low Risk	6, 11

ithelial lesions (HGSIL), and invasive cancer. The potential of LGSIL to persist or to progress to a higher-grade lesion appears to depend largely on its association with specific types of HPV.[21] The most common HPV types detected in cervical lesions are those classified as high-risk HPV types (including 16, 18, 31, 45, and 56), intermediate-risk types (including types 33, 35, 39, 51, and 52), and low-risk types (including types 6, 11, 42, 43, and 44).[20] LGSILs associated with HPV types such as 6 and 11 are at no or low risk for developing into invasive cancer; HPV types such as 31, 33, and 35 are at intermediate risk for developing into a higher-grade lesion. (Table 2.4). HPV 16 and HPV 18 put the patient at a high level of risk for developing invasive cancer. Typically, HGSIL contains high and intermediate oncogenic risk HPV's such as 16 and 18 (52%) and 31, 33, 35, 39, 51, and 52 (23%), respectively. Over 95% of invasive squamous cell carcinomas contain HPV DNA, mainly types 16 and 18.[21]

HPV 16 is the most common genital HPV type associated with cervical carcinoma and has been studied most extensively.[17] HPV 18 appears to be associated with rapidly progressive lesions in young women. Kurman, Schiffman, and Lancaster noted a deficit of HPV 18 in CIN compared to cancer, but no significant difference in the distribution of HPV 16 in CIN compared to cancer. These authors postulated that the deficit of HPV 18 in CIN could represent a rapid transit time through the preinvasive phase.[22] A study by Lorincz, Reid, Jenson, et al. found HPV 18 to be detected 2.6 times more frequently in women with invasive cancer that occurred within one year of a negative Pap smear and concluded that the presence of HPV 18 was a poor prognostic factor.[23, 24]

Clinical Application of Routine HPV DNA Typing

The role of HPV DNA testing in screening or diagnosis remains unclear. Whereas Kurman in 1991 stated ". . . HPV typing should not currently play a role in the screening or management of a patient with an abnormal cytology smear,"[8] evolving technologic advances in HPV DNA testing may soon challenge this opinion.

The current, acceptable triage approach to management of a minor-grade, abnormal Pap smear (ASCUS or LGSIL) is to repeat the Pap smear in 3-6 months. If ASCUS or LGSIL persists, and the patient falls into a low-risk category (reliable for follow-up, no past history of SIL, no history of HIV or immunosuppression), she may continue to be followed with Pap tests at 6-month intervals for up to 2 years to determine whether her lesion will remain persistent or regress. High-risk patients should be colposcoped at once and, if appropriate, treated to prevent the development of invasive disease.[21] The possible use of modern HPV DNA testing into triage schemes of women with minor-grade cytologic atypia recently has been suggested as one of the options for managing women with ASCUS and LGSIL smears. According to this HPV-based triage approach, only women with minor-grade smears who test positive for high-oncogenic-risk HPV DNA would be referred for colposcopy. HPV-negative women and those with a clinically normal cervix would have colposcopy deferred. This would theoretically reduce the number of women referred for colposcopy and may eliminate overtreatment and associated costs. Further cost reduction may be achieved if HPV DNA testing is performed without a repeat smear. In this triage protocol, HPV DNA is assayed using ThinPrep smears.[21] Cox, Lorincz, and Schiffman (1995) showed that colposcopic referrals could have been safely reduced by 58% by referring only those women with ASCUS cytology who were also positive for HPV DNA.[25]

Although the benefits of incorporating HPV DNA testing with current screening practice is apparent, prudent clinical management should continue to pursue the most reliable, cost-effective means of caring for women with HPV.

HPV Infections and Abnormal Pap Smears During Pregnancy

The high incidence of HPV in pregnancy may be due to temporary immunosuppression and increased levels of sex steroid hormones. That is, existing lesions may enlarge and proliferate during pregnancy. Previously subclinical disease may become visible during pregnancy because of alterations in the immune system and a marked increase in general vascularity throughout the body. Pregnancy is known to be associated with depression of selective aspects of cell-mediated immunity that permit fetal retention but may also interfere with resistance to infections, including HPV-induced infections. A significant proportion of HPV-associated lesions enlarge during pregnancy but spontaneously regress after delivery.[26]

Kiguchi et al. suggest higher regression rates following detection in pregnant women than in nonpregnant women.[27] The precise reason is not known, but two explanations are offered:

1. The low-grade intraepithelial changes, particularly those with mild dysplasia recorded during pregnancy, may represent cytologic changes that occur as a consequence of pregnancy itself.
2. Intraepithelial lesions may be removed during the trauma of vaginal delivery.[3]

As a rule, CIN is not treated during pregnancy unless a cone biopsy is indicated to rule out invasive disease. In patients with CIN, an initial cytologic and colposcopic exam, which may be followed by interval exams throughout pregnancy, is recommended. The goal of colposcopic evaluation during pregnancy is to rule out invasive cancer. Cervical biopsy is performed with discretion to minimize the risk of interrupting the pregnancy. Endocervical curettage (ECC) is rare unless invasive cancer involving the cervical canal is suspected.

HPV Infections Among HIV-Infected Women

Cervical neoplasms are more frequently found among immunosuppressed and HIV-infected women than in the general population.[28] Initially it was unclear whether the frequent detection of coincident HPV and HIV infections was simply the result of shared risk factors and exposures, or whether the two viruses interact in as yet unexplained ways either to facilitate their mutual transmission or to alter the natural history of anogenital HPV infections. The New York Cervical Disease Study (NYCDS) is a prospective study of the gynecologic manifestations of HIV infection. In this study, both low-grade CIN and high-grade CIN were detected at higher rates among HIV-seropositive women than among HIV-seronegative controls.[29]

With results of recent studies, it is now clear HIV infection and HIV-induced immunosuppression alter the natural history of anogenital HPV infections and are specific risk factors for the development of CIN, as well as other anogenital neoplasias. The Centers for Disease Control and Prevention has included high-grade squamous intraepithelial neoplasia (HGSIL), including cervical carcinoma in situ, as part of the classification of HIV and designated invasive cervical cancer as an AIDS case-defining illness in the 1993 Expanded Surveillance Cancer Definition of AIDS.[30]

Several studies have found that the prevalence of HPV infection increases with increasing levels of immunosuppression. Wright and Sun, using NYCDS data, found latent HPV infections and clinically expressed HPV infections (e.g., CIN), increase as the CD4+ T-lymphocyte count decreases. While the ratio of latent HPV infections to clinically expressed HPV infection is approximately 8:1 in the anogenital tract of women in the general population, this ratio was reduced to 3:1 in HIV-seropositive women with CD4+ T-lymphocyte counts < 500 cells/μl. It was further reduced to 1:1 in women with CD4+ T-lymphocyte counts < 200 cells/μl. [29]

Although an "epidemic of invasive cervical cancer" has not yet developed in this population, the high prevalence of cervical cancer precursors in HIV-infected women may result in the development of more cases of invasive cancer as these women live longer with profound immunosuppression.[29] Authorities agree HIV-positive women should receive close monitoring for anogenital neoplasia, yet there is no consensus on the frequency and type of monitoring. While initial studies raised concerns of a higher false-negative Pap smear result rate in this population, additional studies suggest Pap smears perform similarly in HIV-infected and HIV-uninfected women.[29] Based on the findings of these more recent studies, the Centers for Disease Control and Prevention has recommended that HIV-infected women be monitored closely for cervical disease as described in Table 2.5.[31]

In addition to cervical disease, HIV-infected women have an increased incidence of other anogenital neoplasias, including vulvar intraepithelial neoplasia (VIN). Abercrombie and Korn found women infected with HIV were 29 times more likely to have VIN than a comparison group of self-identified HIV-negative women. HIV-infected women also have a higher recurrence rate of (anogenital) dysplasias compared with women without HIV, yet the most effective mode of treatment for these women has not yet been determined.[32] Clinical trials are ongoing to compare the effectiveness of the various stan-

TABLE 2.5
CDC Guidelines for HIV-Infected Women[31]
After obtaining a complete history of previous cervical disease, HIV-infected women should have a comprehensive gynecologic examination, including a pelvic examination and Pap smear as part of their initial evaluation. A Pap smear should be obtained twice in the first year after diagnosis of HIV infection and, if the results are normal, annually thereafter. If the results of the Pap smear are abnormal, care should be provided accordingly. Women who have a cytological diagnosis of HGSIL or squamous cell carcinoma should undergo colposcopy and directed biopsy. HIV infection is not an indication for colposcopy in women who have normal Pap smears.

dard modes of treatment for cervical dysplasia (observation, cryotherapy, loop excision, and cold knife cone).[32]

The need for close monitoring of HIV-infected women for HPV-associated neoplasias poses a challenge to clinicians caring for these women. Life circumstances including homelessness, poverty, lack of health insurance, lack of social support systems, childcare issues, substance abuse, and concomitant illnesses may compromise their compliance with recommended treatment and follow-up care. Providing adequate patient education about HPV infection, dysplasia, procedures that may be performed, treatment options, as well as involving the patient in treatment decisions is key to a successful therapeutic experience.[10]

✖ ASSESSMENT

Detailed History

A thorough patient history should be the basis of any clinical evaluation. Components of a history obtained in screening for intraepithelial neoplasia of the lower genital tract should reflect the following known risk factors:

- Age at first intercourse
- Number of past and present sexual partners
- Contraceptive history
- History of sexually transmitted diseases
- History of immunosuppression, including HIV-induced
- In utero DES exposure
- History of cigarette smoking
- Prior Pap smear history and treatment for any vulvar, vaginal, or cervical lesions such as condyloma
- Prior history of cancer or cancer therapy (radiation, chemotherapy, surgery)

Items to include in the history of a patient with condyloma should include:

- Onset of lesion
- Course of infection
- Associated symptoms: vaginal discharge, pruritus, postcoital or other irregular vaginal bleeding
- Lesions in sexual partners (Studies have shown that approximately two-thirds of male consorts of women with condylomas are infected, yet the majority have subclinical disease.)[33]

Physical Assessment

Pelvic Examination

Vulva.   Careful inspection and palpation of the vulva, including the groin nodes, mons, and perianal area is the most productive screening technique for VIN. A magnifying glass may be helpful. Condyloma usually appears as soft, pink to white, raised lesions with multiple fingerlike projections resembling cauliflower (Figure 2.6).. The most common symptoms of VIN are vulvar pruritis, burning, or dyspareunia. A previous history of vulvar condyloma, VIN, CIN, VAIN (vaginal intraepithelial neoplasia), anal intraepithelial neoplasia, or cancers of the lower genital tract should raise suspicion and lead to a thorough examination of the vulva.[10]

The most common sites of development are those that are abraded during intercourse, such as the posterior introitus and labia minora. Warts may remain small and

FIGURE 2.6. The appearance of condyloma acuminatum.

Source: Reproduced with permission from Friedrich, E.G. (1983). *Vulva Disease* 2nd ed. (p. 195). Philadelphia: W.B. Saunders.

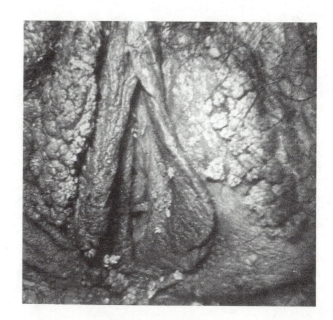

localized, or spread and coalesce. As the lesions extend on to nonmucosal areas, they tend to become more keratotic.[33]

When lichen sclerosis is present, there is usually a diffuse whitish change to the vulvar skin. The skin often appears thin, and there may be scarring and contracture. In addition, fissuring of the skin is often present, accompanied by excoriation secondary to itching. Areas of squamous hyperplasia also appear as whitish lesions in general, but the tissues of the vulva appear thickened and the process tends to be more focal or multifocal than diffuse. A biopsy is necessary to establish the diagnosis.[4]

The appearance of VIN is variable and may include white, red, blue, or brown pigmented lesions. Atypical or therapy-resistant vulvar condyloma and hyperpigmented lesions must be viewed with a high degree of suspicion and a biopsy specimen taken. To diagnose VIN and rule out invasive cancer, an adequate biopsy procedure, often utilizing a dermal punch biopsy, must be carried out with local anesthesia (Figure 2.7). Evaluation of the cervix and vagina with Pap smear and colposcopy is also important because of the high incidence of concomitant cervical and vaginal neoplasia.[1]

Non-Neoplastic Epithelial Disorders of the Vulva

Non-neoplastic epithelial disorders of the vulva now have newer terminology that replaces the old dystrophy designation as discussed below. Mixed disorders can occur, and both conditions should be reported.[2] Lichen sclerosis is typical in clinical presentation, with pale, thin, and sometimes shiny and wrinkled appearance. Itching is a common symptom. Biopsy confirms the diagnosis. The usual treatment of topical testosterone has been very successful.[2]

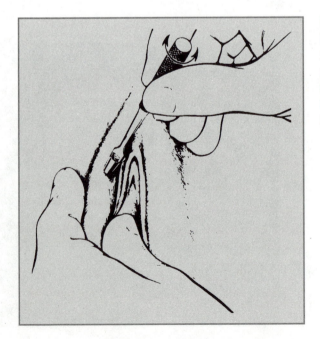

FIGURE 2.7. Diagnostic punch biopsy.

Source: Reproduced with permission from Friedrich, E.G. (1983). *Vulva Disease* 2nd ed. (p. 64). Philadelphia: W.B. Saunders.

Squamous cell hyperplasia typically presents with a thickened, hyperplastic, elevated, white keratinized surface that is very difficult to distinguish clinically from VIN. Biopsy should be done before treatment is initiated.[2]

Vagina.   Approximately one-third of women with vulvar condyloma also have vaginal lesions. The lesions vary in size and often are undetectable without colposcopy. Vaginal condylomas are more commonly distributed on the upper and lower thirds of the vaginal walls. Most are asymptomatic, although discharge, pruritus, and postcoital bleeding may be present with extensive infection. Spontaneous regression of vaginal condylomas is not uncommon.[33] With the increasing incidence of VAIN, obtaining vaginal smears with routine Pap smear screening is essential. This need becomes even more crucial in women who have undergone hysterectomy or radiation therapy for cervical neoplasia. Many women require education regarding the need for vaginal Pap smears following hysterectomy.

Cervix.   Gross inspection of the cervix on speculum examination may reveal obvious tumors, suspicious lesions, bleeding or a friable cervix, abnormal discharge, or other cervical abnormalities. Obtain a Pap smear. Further intervention is dependent on physical findings and cytologic reports. Generally, it is recommended that all women with high-grade SIL (HGSIL) be referred for colposcopic evaluation. Women with abnormal Pap smear results demonstrating ASCUS or LGSIL should be referred as indicated earlier in this chapter.

Colposcopic Examination

The colposcope is a magnifying instrument used to identify those abnormal cervical areas that require further evaluation (see Figure 2.1). Developed in the 1920s, colposcopy preceded the Pap smear as an initial screening tool, but it has been replaced by the Pap smear so it is no longer indicated for routine screening. The high-risk site requiring evaluation by colposcopy is the T-zone.

To evaluate the T-zone, the cervix is cleaned with 2 to 5% acetic acid solution to remove cervical mucus and accentuate abnormal patterns. Colposcopy facilitates the identification of abnormal areas and the delineation of the squamocolumnar junction. The colposcopic examination is categorized as satisfactory if the entire squamocolumnar junction is visualized and inconclusive if not.[1] In about 10 to 15% of patients, the T-zone is located inside the endocervical canal and cannot be visualized. This is often true in postmenopausal women.[34] The presence of white epithelium with or without atypical vessel pattern suggests CIN and is graded based on degree of abnormality. The recognition of abnormal colposcopic findings is not specific enough for a final diagnosis, and biopsy for histologic confirmation is necessary.[1]

An endocervical curettage (ECC) is usually performed to evaluate the endocervical canal when colposcopy is unsatisfactory. Patients may experience mild pelvic cramping for a few minutes as a result of the biopsy. They may also experience light spotting up to 24 to 48 hours following the biopsy. The patient should be taught to anticipate these possibilities to prevent confusion or anxiety. Most patients referred for colposcopy are not familiar with the procedure and they often experience considerable fear awaiting the appointment. Taking a few minutes to explain the significance of an abnormal Pap smear and what to expect from the colposcopy and biopsy procedure may allay anticipatory anxiety.

✖ TREATMENT

Selecting the most appropriate treatment option for the patient with intraepithelial neoplasia of the lower genital tract depends on several factors, including

- Anatomic site
- Grade and extent/severity of lesion(s)
- Primary treatment versus recurrence
- Pregnancy
- Adequacy of colposcopic evaluation
- Age
- Desire for fertility
- Cost

Treating intraepithelial neoplasia produces a stable remission in about 85% of patients even though such lesions are usually surrounded by subclinical disease.[33] Successful treatment of condyloma remains elusive. Resolution rates are approximately 70% overall, and recurrence rates in the general population may be as high as 25-50%.[35] No therapy is 100% effective and the benefit–risk ratio should be explained to the patient so that she is fully informed and can make a reasonable decision concerning her therapy and well-being.[2]

Condyloma Acuminata

Podophyllin Resin

Podophyllin has been the mainstay of external wart management since 1942.[33] The Centers for Disease Control recommends that application to external lesions not exceed 0.5 ml and be limited to 10 cm or less per session.[36] After the initial application, the patient is reexamined and retreated at weekly intervals if necessary. The patient should be instructed to wash the treated area in 2–4 hours following each application. If no significant improvement is noted after one month, alternative treatments should be considered. However, most successfully treated lesions respond in two to four days. Cure rates vary from 22 to 98%.[33]

Podophyllotoxin Topical 0.5% Solution or Gel (Podofilox)

One of the most common and established forms of ablative therapy for genital warts is the use of podophyllin resin. But because of the potential toxicities of this medication when given in high concentrations, and the variability in concentration of the active ingredient, podophyllin resin has been reserved for physician-administered therapy. Podophyllotoxin is one of the active lignans present in crude podophyllin resin and has shown activity in concentrations of 0.5 to 10.0% in treatment of genital HPV infection. The ability to administer a defined, consistent concentration of a chemical ingredient has allowed patient-administered therapy as a means of treating genital warts. Kirby et al. reported podophyllotoxin 0.5% solution to be effective in treating penile warts and well tolerated in a self-administered regimen. It also offers potential advantages in safety and cost over podophyllin resin therapy of genital warts.[37]

Podophyllotoxin is applied to external condyloma twice daily for three consecutive days. Treatment is then held for four days, and the cycle is repeated for up to four consecutive weeks. Patient instructions should include the following:

- Burning on application should be anticipated, but excessive burning, pain, or swelling should be reported.
- Wash hands after every use.
- Avoid sexual intercourse on treatment days.

Topical 5% Imiquimod Cream

Imiquimod's mechanism of action is unknown. It is a potent inducer of interferon alpha and other cytokines, including tumor necrosis factor alpha and interleukin-6, and is believed to act as an immune response enhancer. As with Podofilox, it has the advantage of patient administration. Recommended application is at bedtime on three alternating days per week until clear or 16 weeks.[38] The patient should be instructed to wash off the treated area the following morning, minimizing the risk of an inflammatory reaction with mild–moderate pain. Edwards, Ferenczy, and Eron (1998) found a complete wart clearance rate in women of 72% compared with 33% in men, with an overall rate of 50%. During a 12-week follow-up period, 13% whose lesions had completely cleared had a recurrence of at least one lesion in the treated area.[39]

Trichloroacetic Acid (TCA)

Trichloroacetic acid is applied much like podophyllin, usually in an 80 to 90% solution in water, but is not washed off. It can be used on vulvar, vaginal, perineal, and perianal lesions. Trichloroacetic acid is also safe to use during pregnancy, and no systemic effects are known. Because TCA is less toxic than podophyllin, it can be applied up to three times per week, although intervals for treatment are usually weekly.[33]

Unlike podophyllin, which tends to cause burning or irritation several hours after treatment, TCA usually produces marked burning on application to external lesions. Because TCA is strongly acidic, a solution of sodium bicarbonate should be on hand to neutralize accidental spills on normal skin. Dusting the area with talc or baking soda following treatment may be practiced to remove unreacted acid.[33] Because of the usual need for frequent applications and discomfort associated with treatment, counseling and education efforts are essential to maximize compliance in these patients, who are often quite young.

5-Fluorouracil

5-Fluorouracil (5FU) is an antimetabolite that prevents nucleic acid synthesis. It is used as a 5% cream to treat extensive intravaginal HPV infections, VAIN, and urethral condyloma in men. The cure rate may be over 80%.[33]

Treatment regimens vary from 1 to 2.5 grams at bedtime for five consecutive nights, to applications twice weekly for four to six weeks. A vaginal tampon should be introduced after application or on arising, as the cream can cause vulvitis and urethritis. These side effects can be prevented by coating the vulva with petrolatum or zinc oxide.[33]

DiSaia and Creasman recommend the following technique. One-quarter applicator of 5% 5FU cream is inserted high in the vagina after the patient is in bed. Tampons are not used. This is done every night for seven to ten days, followed by a ten- to fourteen-day rest period, and then the application cycle is repeated. This regimen usually allows an adequate treatment time without causing the patient to experience the extreme local reaction that can occur with prolonged use. Weekly insertion of one-third of an applicator (1.5 gm) deep in the vagina at bedtime for ten consecutive weeks has also been shown to be efficacious. Compliance appears to be fairly high.[33]

Dimethylether Cryosurgery

Dimethylether is a new cryosurgical treatment for external genital condyloma. It has been used in Europe to treat many types of warts. The clinician applies dimethylether from a small hand-held canister. The epidermis is frozen and separates from the basement membrane, with subsequent growth of healthy skin in approximately two weeks. Gaydos, Lambe, Schwartz, and Krall, in a small prospective pilot study, demonstrated the dimethylether method of treatment to appear to be comparable to the published response rates of three standard methods: TCA, podophyllin, and standard cryotherapy. No complications such as depigmentation, blistering, or scarring were seen.[40] Advantages of this method include patient tolerance and cost-effectiveness.

Interferon

Interferon has antiviral properties and can now be produced by recombinant DNA techniques. It has been used in the treatment of extensive or recalcitrant anogenital warts. Results have been promising in some clinical trials, with lesions either reducing in size or completely resolving after a series of intramuscular or intralesional injections. Side effects can include fever, chills, headache, myalgia, fatigue, nausea, and vomiting. But these problems often recede as treatment continues.[33]

Reid however, criticizes intralesional use of interferon, stating, "The practicality of this regimen is doubtful for several reasons: only a few papillomas can be injected during one course of treatment; there is no effect on either uninjected lesions or the subclinical reservoir; and at least a third of initial successes will develop new warts in adjacent areas."[41] Interferon is not routinely recommended because of its cost and the high frequency of systemic adverse side effects.[38]

Laser Therapy

Laser therapy is reserved for extensive, resistant condyloma. See "Laser Vaporization" later in this chapter.

Intraepithelial Neoplasia

Treatment of intraepithelial neoplasia can be either ablative or excisional (Table 2.6). Excision preserves tissue for histologic examination and is indicated when further diagnostic information is required.

Observation

Observation is appropriate in a highly select patient population. If the lesion is small and of low histologic grade (i.e., CIN I), spontaneous regression may occur. Syrjanen and Syrjanen cite spontaneous regression rates of CIN I-II in from 23 to 54% of women with HPV-6 and -11.[42] None of the HPV-16 or -18 lesions regressed. The patient should be followed with repeat examination, including Pap smear, for CIN lesions and colposcopy at three- to six-month intervals.[1] Patient compliance to follow-up is an important consideration in selecting this method of management.

Ablative Therapies

Electrocautery. Electrocautery has been used for many years in the treatment of CIN. Success rates of 100% for CIN I and II, and 87% for CIN III have been reported. Despite these successes, there are several disadvantages: discomfort, potential for significant scarring (which has fertility implications), and possible need for anesthesia

TABLE 2.6	
Conservative Treatment for CIN	
Method (Based on Single Treatment)	*Failures*
Electrocoagulation	47/1734 (2.7%)
Cryosurgery	540/6143 (8.7%)
Laser	119/2130 (5.6%)
Cold Coagulators (CIN III)	110/1628 (6.8%)
LEEP	95/2185 (4.3%)

Source: Reprinted with permission from DiSaia, P.J., & Creasman, W.T. (1997). *Clinical Gynecologic Oncology* 4th ed. St. Louis, MO: Mosby Year Book, Inc.

and outpatient surgery.[1] These disadvantages make electrocautery almost obsolete in light of other effective treatment options.

Cryotherapy. Cryotherapy is often used to treat CIN. The freezing process results from rapid expansion of fluid, usually CO_2 or nitrous oxide, into a probe, which is placed against the cervix. Contact is enhanced by placing water-soluble lubricating jelly on the tip of the probe. Once the gas is released from the probe, an ice ball begins to form and is usually complete in three to five minutes. Either a single- or double-freezing technique may be used.[4] Use of a *freeze-thaw-refreeze cycle* will increase the reliability of cell death, particularly when machines that produce suboptimal rates of cooling are used.[43]

The process is well tolerated in the outpatient setting, and no anesthesia is required. Cramping during the procedure is the most commonly reported discomfort.[1] Patients should be advised of a profuse watery vaginal discharge after cryotherapy, usually persisting for about two weeks. Patients should also be given the following postoperative instructions:

1. Nothing per vagina for two to three weeks (no vaginal intercourse, tampons, swimming, douching, or baths)
2. Initial follow-up appointment in three months for repeat colposcopy and Pap smear. The importance of complying with follow-up must be stressed to the patient. There should be documentation that such instructions were given. Initial treatment cure rates are approximately 90%.[4]

The advantages of cryotherapy are a high success rate with a low incidence of cervical stenosis and subsequent impairment of fertility. In addition, treatment is performed on an outpatient basis and is therefore economical.

A potential disadvantage to cryosurgery is that the squamocolumnar junction (SCJ) may move to the endocervix after treatment and not be completely visible on colposcopy.[1] An additional disadvantage is increased risk of false-negative Pap smears following cryosurgery in cases of high-grade lesions, possibly because the squamocolumnar junction moves toward the endocervix after cyrotherapy. As cryosurgery treats to a depth of approximately 2 mm, CIN that may exist deep in the epithelial crypts can escape treatment and thus go undetected following regrowth of the epithelium.[43]

Laser Vaporization. The term *laser* is an acronym for "light amplification by stimulated emission of radiation." The carbon dioxide laser beam is invisible but usually guided by a second laser that emits visible light.[2] Laser therapy is used as treatment for intraepithelial neoplasia of the vulva, vagina, and cervix, including extensive or resistant condyloma. The laser is used with the colposcope, providing the added advantage of visualizing the transformation zone during treatment of the cervix and therefore minimizing trauma to normal tissue. The objective is to lase the entire

T-zone. The energy from the laser beam is absorbed by water, with resultant vaporization of the target tissue. Patient instructions are similar to those for cryosurgery.

Different degrees of power density are available, and recommendations vary depending on tissue site and depth. Most reports express the treatment mode as a power density, that is, watts per square centimeter. Current practice is to carry therapy to a depth of 5–7 mm and to use a power density of 600 w/cm^2. Treatment is more effective at higher densities; however, the complications of bleeding and cramping are also related to power density and depth of treatment.[4] General anesthesia, paracervical block, and/or oral antiprostaglandins are used at the discretion of the clinician.

Healing in the laser crater is usually complete in four to six weeks, and the site is covered with metaplastic squamous tissue within two months. A particular advantage of the laser is that the T-zone is more likely to remain visible colposcopically after treatment than is true with cryosurgery.[4] Baggish et al., summarizing the results from 3,070 women treated by laser vaporization over ten years, reported that 94% were free of disease at one year.[44]

Postoperative bleeding can occur up to two weeks following laser conization of the cervix. It is usually light, but occasionally heavy bleeding can occur. Light bleeding can usually be controlled with rest or chemical cauterization (Monsel's solution). Heavy bleeding may require electrocautery, suturing, or vaginal packing, but such measures are rarely necessary.

Follow-up teaching postconization should include advising the patient to:

- Expect brownish discharge or light bleeding for one to several days post-treatment. A watery discharge may persist for two to three weeks.
- Report heavy bleeding or fever.
- Take nothing per vagina for two weeks.
- Minimize activity (including not returning to work) for 48 hours. No strenuous activity for one week.
- Make a follow-up appointment in two weeks to assess healing, and three months for repeat colposcopy and Pap smear. The patient must be advised of the importance of keeping this appointment so that treatment response can be evaluated.
- Use mild analgesics as needed. Mild pelvic cramping may occur during the first twenty-four hours. Narcotic analgesics are usually not required.[44]

The vaginal discharge associated with laser therapy is less likely to be malodorous and generally persists only half as long as the discharge associated with cryotherapy. The excessive discharge following cryotherapy results from sloughing of necrotic tissue, which does not occur with the vaporization of tissue in laser therapy.[45]

Laser treatment of VAIN can result in single-treatment cure rates ranging from 73 to 90%. Disease-free status has been achieved in 92 to 100% of patients who have undergone repeated treatments.[45] Local anesthesia with antianxiety medication may be given but general anesthesia is often used.

Follow-up care and instructions after laser surgery should include the following:

- Advise the patient to use mild analgesics.
- Advise the patient to take nothing per vagina for approximately four weeks (no intercourse, baths, swimming, or douching).
- Vaginal dilator (or digital dilatation) may be used after extensive vaporization to prevent stenosis.[45]
- In postmenopausal women, vaginal application of estrogen cream two to three times/week (if not contraindicated) may promote healing.
- Have the patient make a follow-up appointment in two weeks to assess healing, and in four to eight weeks when healing is complete.[43]

Laser treatment of VIN can also be quite successful; less than 10% of patients have persistent disease within the first year following therapy.[45] Treating condyloma is more difficult, with persistence or recurrence found in about 20 to 34% of patients following laser vaporization. But with multiple treatments 90% of patients are cured.

Postoperative pain can be quite traumatic and thus requires sensitive and empathetic management. Follow-up care and instructions should include:

- Use of sitz baths with tepid saline water several times a day and following urination or defecation, followed by blow drying with a hair dryer on a cool setting. If urination causes burning in the treated area, pouring water over the vulva while voiding can minimize discomfort. Applying a hydrogel provides a moist wound environment, facilitating the healing process. The concept of leaving a wound dry to promote healing is unfounded; clinical science shows that neither dehydration nor toxic agents are good for humans or for open wounds. Moisture helps wounds heal because a moist wound/dressing environment facilitates recruitment of vital host defenses and the necessary cell population, such as macrophages, that help promote healing. And the acidification of wounds under hydrogels may inhibit bacterial growth.[46] But perhaps the most significant advantage of wound gels is their potential for relieving pain and discomfort.
- Application of viscous lidocaine jelly, 2% silver sulfadiazine ointment, or tannic acid compresses (i.e., tea bags) may be recommended as comfort measures.[45]
- Manual separation of the labia may be necessary to prevent coaptation. It can be more comfortably accomplished during sitz baths. In instructing the patient to perform her postlaser care, one must assess how comfortable the patient is with touching her genitalia as well as her knowledge of her own anatomy. A mirror and return demonstration may be helpful.
- Advise the patient to avoid intercourse or tight clothing for 4–6 weeks or until the vulva has completely healed.
- Follow-up in 2 weeks to assess healing, and again in 4–6 weeks. More frequent follow-up may be indicated after treatment of extensive lesions, to observe for coaptation and to provide satisfactory pain control and emotional support.

- Inform patients that male partners should also be evaluated for condyloma, although the presence of HPV infection in men is often subclinical. Penile or urethral lesions should be treated, and the couple should be encouraged to use condoms.

Excisional Therapies

LEEP. Conization of the cervix with loop electrosurgical procedure (LEEP) is a relatively new treatment option for women with CIN. It is also referred to as large loop excision of the transformation zone (LLETZ).[21] Developed in Great Britain, then introduced in the United States, LEEP equipment consists of a loop wire electrode and a generator that delivers a high-frequency, low-voltage–radio frequency current that vaporizes tissue faster than the laser. The loop wire electrodes come in various sizes, and selection is made according to the geometry of the lesion.[47] Selecting the proper loop is most important.

Nonsteroidal anti-inflammatory drugs (NSAID) are usually given 20–30 minutes prior to the LEEP to decrease prostaglandin release, and subsequent pelvic cramping, during the procedure. The patient is then placed in the lithotomy position and a grounding pad placed on the thigh. A nonconductive, insulated speculum is inserted, and the smoke evacuator tubing is attached via an adaptor. Next the cervix is viewed with a colposcope and acetic acid applied to dissolve mucus and mark abnormal areas. Intracervical anesthesia with 4–8cc of 1% xylocaine with epinephrine is given. The cervix is then painted with Lugol's solution to view or highlight the abnormal tissue, which will not stain. The wire loop is then positioned at 9 o'clock, passed horizontally through the transformation zone, and pulled out at 3 o'clock, using a sweeping motion (Figure 2.8). Multiple passages with different-sized electrodes are sometimes necessary. The actual procedure takes only about five to ten seconds. The specimen is then removed and sent to pathology. A ball-tip electrode is inserted into the probe, and

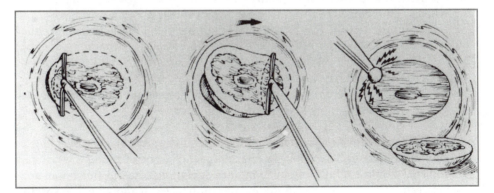

FIGURE 2.8. Procedure for the LEEP.

Source: Reproduced with permission from Nordquist, S.R.B. (1994). *Practice Protocol and Procedure.* Miami: Gynecologic Oncology Associates.

the generator is set on coagulation current to seal vessels for homeostasis. Finally, Monsel's solution, which acts as a chemical cautery, is applied.[43]

The LEEP as a form of excisional therapy has two distinct advantages: It is both a diagnostic and a treatment modality. As with a cold-knife excisional cone biopsy, the affected tissue is removed entirely with little thermal damage and sent for histopathologic analysis. Additional advantages of the LEEP are that:

1. It is performed in an office/clinic or outpatient setting, with minimal discomfort and in a short period of time.
2. It is cost-effective.[47]
3. The squamocolumnar junction has been found to be visible in 94% of patients after the LEEP.[48]

Postoperative complications are rare, with serious bleeding requiring intervention occurring 1 to 2% of the time and cervical stenosis less than 1% of the time.[48] Light bleeding usually occurs for a few days following the LEEP.

The LEEP has been well documented to be a safe and effective treatment of CIN. As women undergoing this procedure are commonly of reproductive age, the effects of treatment on subsequent fertility is a concern. Turlington, Wright, and Powell performed a retrospective, cohort study of women of reproductive age who were treated for CIN with the LEEP. Follow-up surveys revealed 11 of the 12 women who desired pregnancy became pregnant in the interval between treatment and completion of the survey.[49] These preliminary results are encouraging.

Conization of the Cervix.   Conization of the cervix is a minor outpatient surgical procedure usually performed under general anesthesia, although local anesthesia is sometimes used. Conization involves the removal of a portion of the cervix with a scalpel (cold knife) or laser, allowing serial histologic sectioning of the excised cervical tissue for review. Scalpel conization results in a cone-shaped defect (Figure 2.9), whereas laser conization results in a cylindrical defect.[1]

Conization of the cervix is performed to treat CIN in the following situations:

* If colposcopic examination is unsatisfactory
* If ECC results are positive
* If there is a discrepancy between cytology, colposcopy, and biopsy results
* To rule out microinvasive or invasive disease[4]

Bleeding is the major short-term complication of conization. The overall difference in complication rates between knife conization and laser conization is worth noting. Larson et al. report overall complication rates, including bleeding, infection, and stenosis, between laser conization and knife conization as 4.2% and 23.6%, respectively. Thus laser conization, although offering no therapeutic advantage over knife conization, is associated with less morbidity.[50]

FIGURE 2.9. Procedures for cone biopsy.

Source: Reproduced with permission from DiSaia, P.J., & Creasman, W.T. (1997). *Clinical Gynecologic Oncology* 4th ed. St. Louis, MO: Mosby Year Book, Inc.

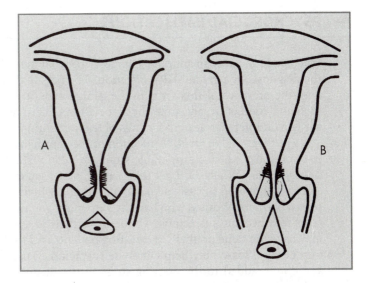

Adequate follow-up is essential to ensure treatment success. Even if the margins of the conization specimen are free of neoplasia, the patient still requires long-term follow-up since new lesions can develop. If the margins of the cone specimen are involved with neoplasia, the patient is considered for further treatment with hysterectomy. At the time of the five-year follow-up, Ahlgren et al. noted 98% cure rates if the margins were lesion-free, versus 70% if the margins were involved.[51] Data emphasize, however, that it is not always mandatory to perform hysterectomy if the margins of the cone are involved with CIN. Kolstad and Klein followed 1,128 patients for fifteen to twenty-five years and found that 21 of 25 patients with positive margins were free of disease for up to fifteen years.[52] These and other data support follow-up rather than immediate hysterectomy for patients with positive margins, especially for women who want to continue childbearing.[4]

Hysterectomy. Hysterectomy is an accepted method of management in a patient with CIN who has completed her childbearing, providing she is made aware of other more conservative treatment options.[1] If hysterectomy is planned for a HGSIL, it should always be preceded by a cone biopsy to rule out invasive disease.

In selecting the optimal treatment option, patient compliance to follow-up should be an important consideration. However, careful follow-up after hysterectomy is also required, as the patient is at increased risk of developing genital intraepithelial neoplasia at other sites.[1] Thus the need for patient education here cannot be understated. Many woman feel that gynecological follow-up is no longer necessary after hysterectomy. Therefore education in the immediate posthysterectomy period may be the only opportunity to emphasize the significance of the need for lifetime follow-up.

✳ PSYCHOSOCIAL IMPLICATIONS

Emotional trauma is an apt phrase to describe what many women experience following the diagnosis of a genital HPV infection. The personal and societal images associated with the presence of this virus in the genital area often lead to much emotional turmoil and conflict. In addition, the association of certain types of HPV with cancers of the genital tract may lead to feelings of fear and vulnerability.[53]

The diagnosis of an HPV infection or intraepithelial neoplasia of the lower genital tract may also cause considerable strain on relationships with sexual partners. Questions such as "When did I get this?" and "Who gave this to me?" are generally unanswerable, but tend to cast suspicion and doubt, which may lead to blaming the self or sexual partners. Women who have been in monogamous relationships for a number of years may become suspicious, wondering if their partners have been faithful. Partners may have the same doubts.[53] Educating patients and their partners on the natural history of the disease may help eliminate suspicions. Misinformation resulting in blame and doubt, added to the existing stress of the diagnosis, can have disastrous consequences for these patients' relationships. As is often the case in sexuality counseling, the nurse or physician must initiate the discussion. Most patients desire such education and counseling, yet they admittedly do not verbalize their concerns unless given the opportunity.

Gossfeld studied twenty patients with CIN to evaluate the impact of the diagnosis and treatment on self-esteem, body image, and sexual concepts.[54] The subjects completed four questionnaires throughout the diagnosis, treatment, and posttreatment process. Findings and recommendations included the following:

- Women with CIN are concerned about cancer and sexual functioning at all visits. However, sexual counseling is most effective if received at the time of diagnosis or postsurgery. Fear and anxiety are so high initially that patient education should focus on the disease process and treatment. Just as with invasive cancers, patients are more receptive to sexual information after the initial crisis of diagnosis is over.
- Far too often, the patients are hurried through the clinic or office with insufficient time and attention from the health care provider. All patients require information to be given in a caring, professional manner.[54]

Counseling for patients with genital HPV infections and intraepithelial neoplasia can provide the opportunity to voice concerns about sexuality, fertility, physical discomfort related to treatment, fears of recurrence, and risk of cancer. Women with long-term HPV, and their partners, require ongoing educational counseling and emotional support to effectively cope with the diagnosis. Support groups can be helpful in educating people, reducing the stigma and isolation, and sharing ways of coping with the virus and its ramifications.[54]

✻ Future Directions

What efforts may improve the early detection and treatment of women with HPV? Improvements in early detection could be made by increasing the use of the Pap smear (particularly in high-risk populations), decreasing the false-negative rate of the Pap smear, automating the screening process to lower the cost, and better defining which patients need to be referred for expensive colposcopy.[20] A promising development in

---

TABLE 2.7
Diagnostic Cluster

Screening and Prevention Period

NURSING DIAGNOSIS

1. Potential altered health maintenance related to insufficient knowledge of basic reproductive female anatomy, cancer prevention, and screening recommendations

2. Anxiety related to insufficient knowledge about screening techniques, uncertainty about outcomes, and possible cancer diagnosis

---

Diagnostic/Preoperative and Treatment Period

COLLABORATIVE PROBLEMS
Potential Complication: Bleeding/Hemorrhage
Potential Complication: Infection/Sepsis

NURSING DIAGNOSIS

1. Potential altered health maintenance related to insufficient knowledge of condition, diagnostic tests, prognosis, and treatment options

2. Decisional conflict related to insufficient knowledge of treatment options

3. Anxiety/fear related to impending surgery, and insufficient knowledge of preoperative routines, intraoperative activities, and postoperative self-care activities

4. Anxiety/fear related to insufficient knowledge of potential impact of condition and treatment on reproductive organs and sexuality

5. Grieving related to potential loss of fertility and perceived effects on lifestyle

6. Potential altered comfort related to effects of surgery, disease process, or immobility

7. Potential altered health maintenance related to insufficient knowledge of dietary restrictions, medications, activity restrictions, self-care activities, symptoms of complications, follow-up visits, and community resources

the management of HPV infections is the potential for a vaccination against genital strains of the disease. The goal of these studies is the production of an inexpensive and effective vaccination that can be used worldwide.[15]

The most promising areas of research will include those that focus on understanding the natural history and immunobiology of HPV infections as they progress to intraepithelial lesions, vaccine trials and their effects on the natural history of lesions, and understanding the process of cervical carcinogenesis and how it can be interrupted with chemopreventive agents.[20]

✖ REFERENCES

1. Nolte, S., & Hanjani, P. (1990). Intraepithelial neoplasia of the lower genital tract. *Semin Oncol Nurs,* 6(3), 181–189.
2. Disaia, P.J., & Creasman, W.T. (1997) *Clinical Gynecologic Oncology* 5th ed. (pp. 1–50). St. Louis, MO: Mosby.
3. Richart, R. M. (1973). Cervical intraepithelial neoplasia. *Pathol Ann,* 8, 301–328.
4. Herbst, A.L. (1992). The Bethesda System for cervical/vaginal diagnosis. *Clin Obstet Gynecol,* 35(1), 22–27.
5. Cytyc Corporation (1997). *Thinprep® Pap Test™ Quick Reference Guide, Endocervical Brush/Spatula Protocol.* Boxborough, MA.
6. National Cancer Institute Workshop (1989). The 1988 Bethesda System for reporting cervical/vaginal cytologic diagnosis. *JAMA,* 262(7), 931–934.
7. National Cancer Institute Workshop (1991). The revised Bethesda System for reporting cervical/vaginal cytologic diagnosis: Report of the 1991 Bethesda Wokshop. *JAMA,* 267(14), 1892.
8. Kurman, R., Malkasian, G.D. Jr., Sedalis, A., & Solomon, D. (1991). From Papanicolaou to Bethesda: The rationale for a new cervical cytologic classification. Reprinted with permission from the American College of Obstetrics & Gynecology. *Obstet Gynecol,* 77(5), 779–782.
9. Edwards, C.L., Tortolero-Luna, G., Linares, A.C., Malpica, A., Baker, V.V., Cook, E., Johnson, E., Mitchell, M.F. (1996). Vulvar intraepithelial neoplasia and vulvar cancer. *Obstet Gynecol Clin North Am,* 23(2), 295–324.
10. Abercrombie, P.D., Korn, A.P. (1998). Vulvar intraepithelial neoplasia in women with HIV. *AIDS Patient Care and STDs,* 12(4), 251–254.
11. National Cancer Institute (1986). Publication: *Questions and Answers about DES Exposure During Pregnancy and before Birth.* Washington, DC: National Cancer Institute.
12. Yoder, L., & Rubin, M. (1992). The epidemiology of cervical cancer and its precursors. *Oncol Nurs Forum,* 19(3), 485–493.
13. Nordqvist, S.R.B. (1981). DES exposure in utero: What are the effects? In S.C. Balloon, ed. *Controversies in Cancer Treatment* (pp. 113–122). Boston: Hall Medical.
14. Zurhausen, H. (1977). Human papilloma viruses and their possible role in squamous carcinomas. *Curr Top Microbiol Immunol,* 78(1), 1–28.
15. Daley, E.M. (1998). Clinical update on the role of HPV and cervical cancer. *Cancer Nurs,* 21(1), 31–35.
16. Reid, R. (1996). The management of genital condylomas, intraepithelial neoplasia, and vulvodynia. *Obstet Gynecol Clin North Am,* 23 (4), 917–991.
17. Turek, L.P., Smith, E.M. (1996). The genetic program of genital human papillomaviruses in infection and cancer. *Obstet Gynecol Clin North Am,* 23 (4), 735–758.
18. Kulski, J.K., Demeter, T., Rakocxy, P., Sterrett, G.F., & Pixley, E.C. (1989) Human papilloma virus coinfections of the vulva and uterine cervix. *J Med,* 27(3), 244–251.
19. Bosch, F.X., Manos, M.M., Munoz, N., Sherman, M., Jansen, A.M., Peto, J., et al. (1995) Prevalence of human papilloma virus in cervical cancer: a worldwide perspective. International biological study on cervical cancer (IBSCC) study group. *J Natl Cancer Inst,* 87, 796–802.
20. Mitchell, M.F., Tortolero-Luna, G., Wright, T., Sarkar, A., Richards-Kortum, R., Hong, W.K., Schottenfeld, D. (1996). Cervical human papillomavirus infection and intraepithelial neoplasia: a review. *J Natl Cancer Inst Monographs,* 21, 17–25.
21. Ferenczy, A., Jenson, A.B. (1996). Tissue effects and host response: the key to the rational triage of cervical neoplasia. *Obstet Gynecol Clin North Am,* 23(4), 759–782.
22. Kurman, R., Schiffman, M.H., Lancaster, W.E.D., et al. (1988). Analysis of individual human papilloma virus types in cervical neoplasia: A possible role for type 18 in rapid progression. *Am J Obstet Gynecol,* 159(2), 293.
23. Graham, C.A. (1993). Cervix cancer prevention

and detection update. *Seminars in Oncol Nurs,* 9(3), 155–162.

24. Lorincz, A.T., Reid, R., Jenson, B., et al. (1992). Human papilloma virus infections of the cervix: Relative risk associations of fifteen common anogenital types. *Obstet Gynecol,* 79(3), 328–337.

25. Cox, J.T. (1996). Clinical role of HPV testing. *Obstet Gynecol Clin North Am,* 23 (4), 811–851.

26. Lucas, V.A. (1990). Clinical implications of perinatal and childhood human papilloma virus infections. *Nurse Pract Forum,* 1(1), 40–46.

27. Kiguchi, K., Bibbo, M., Hasegawa, T., et al (1981). Dysplasia during pregnancy: A cytologic follow-up study. *J Reprod Med,* 266(1), 66.

28. Gemignani, M., Maiman, M., Fruchter, R.G., Arrastia, C.D., Gibbon, D., Ellison, T. (1995). CD4 lymphocytes in women with invasive and preinvasive cervical neoplasia. *Gynecol Oncol,* 59, 364–369.

29. Wright, T.C., Sun, X.W. (1996). Anogenital papillomavirus infection and neoplasia in immunodeficient women. *Obstet Gynecol Clin North Am,* 23(4), 861–893.

30. CDC: (1993) 1993 revised classification system for HIV infection and expanded surveillance case definition for AIDS among adolescents and adults. *MMWR* 41, 1.

31. CDC: (1998). Sexually transmitted disease guidelines. *MMWR* 47, RR-1.

32. Abercrombie, P.D., Korn, A. (1995). Vulvar intraepithelial neoplasia (VIN) in HIV-infected women {abstract FC-209}. In Program and abstracts of HIV Infections in Women: Setting a New Agenda Conference. Washington, D.C., pp. S59.

33. Carlone, J.P., Schenk, C.P. (1990). Genital HPV infection in the nonpregnant woman: Diagnosis and management options. *Nurse Pract Forum,* 1(1), 16–24.

34. Barter, J. (1984). *Gynecologic Oncology Review Notes.* Washington, DC: Division of Gynecologic Oncology, Georgetown University.

35. Fife, K.H. (1998). New treatments of genital warts less than ideal (abstract and commentary). *JAMA,* 279(24), 2003–2004.

36. CDC (1989). 1989 sexually transmitted disease guidelines. *MMWR,* 38(2), 18–21.

37. Kirby, H., Dunne, A., King, K.H., & Corey, L. (1990). Double-blind randomized clinical trial of self-administered podofilox solution verses vehicle in the treatment of genital warts. *Am J Med,* 88(5), 465–469.

38. Evans, R.M., & Wiley, D. (1997). External genital warts: diagnosis and treatment. *AMA Continuing Medical Education Program.* Chicago: American Medical Association.

39. Edwards, L., Ferenczy, A., Eron, L, et al, and the HPV Study Group. (1998). Self-administered topical 5% imiqimod cream for external anogenital warts. *Arch Dermatol,* 134, 25–30.

40. Gaydos, T.L., Lambe, H.A., Schwartz, K., Krall, J.M. (1998). Dimethylether treatment for condyloma acuminata in women. *J Lower Genital Tract Dis,* 2 (3), 148–50.

41. Reid, R. (1994). Preinvasive disease. In J.S. Berek & N.F. Hacker (Eds.), *Practical Gynecologic Oncology* (pp. 201–241). Baltimore: Williams and Wilkins.

42. Syrjanen, S., Syrjanen, K. (1986). HPV DNA sequences demonstrated by in situ hybridization in serial paraffin-embedded cervical biopsies. *Arch Obstet Gynecol,* 239(1), 39–48.

43. Nordqvist, S.R.B. (1994). *Practice Protocol and Procedure.* Miami: Gynecologic Oncology Associates.

44. Baggish, M.S., Dorsey, J.H., & Adlelson, M. (1989). A ten-year experience treating cervical intraepithelial neoplasia with the CO2 laser. *Am J Obstet Gynecol,* 161(1), 60.

45. Holloway, R., Barnes, W., & Barter, J. (1988). The CO2 laser: A guide to its use in lower genital tract disorders, part II: Vaginal and vulvar lesions and condyloma acuminata. *Female Patient,* 14(8), 14–19.

46. Kirstein, M. (1994). Overview of wound healing in moist environment. *Am J Surg,* 167(1A), 15–16.

47. Paniscotti, B.M. (1992). Introducing the LEEP. *J Gynecol Oncol Nurs.* Fort Worth, TX: Publication of the Society of Gynecologic Nurse Oncologists.

48. Wright, T.C., Gagnon, S., Richart, R.M. & Ferenczy, A. (1992). Treatment of cervical intraepithelial neoplasia using the loop electrosurgical excision procedure. *Obstet Gynecol,* 79(2), 173–178.

49. Turlington, W.T., Wright, B.D., Powell, J.L. (1996). Impact of the loop electrosurgical excision procedure on future fertility. *J Reprod Med,* 41(11), 815–818.

50. Larson, G., Gullberg, B.O., & Grundsell, H. (1983). A comparison of laser and cold-knife conization. *Obstet Gynecol,* 62(2), 213–217.

51. Ahlgren, M., Ingemarsson, I., & Lindberg, L.G., et al. (1975). Conization as treatment of carcinoma in situ of the uterine cervix. *Obstet Gynecol,* 46(2), 135.

52. Kolstad, P., & Klein, V. (1976). Long-term follow-up of 1121 cases of carcinoma in situ. *Obstet Gynecol,* 48(2), 125.

53. Lehr, S.T., & Lee, M.E. (1990). The psychosocial and sexual trauma of a genital HPV infection. *Nurse Pract Forum,* 1(1), 25–30.

54. Gossfeld, L. (1991). Evaluation of the impact of the diagnosis and treatment of cervical intraepithelial neoplasia (CIN): Patient's self-esteem, body image, and sexual concepts. *J Gynecol Oncol Nurs.* Fort Worth, TX: Publication of the Society of Gynecologic Nurse Oncologists.

CHAPTER 3

Invasive Cancer of the Cervix

Margaret Anne Lamb, PHD, RN

器 INTRODUCTION

Since the 1940s, with the initial study of screening for cervical cancer by Papanicolaou et al., use of the Pap smear has not only decreased the incidence of cervical cancer by half but also reversed the prognosis of this disease. In 1998, it was estimated that 13,700 new cases of invasive cancer of the cervix would be diagnosed in the United States.[1] Cervical cancer occurs more frequently in younger women (44% <45 years). However, women ≥65 years account for the most frequent deaths.[1] (See Figure 3.1.) Estimates were approximately 4,900 deaths from cervical cancer in the United States in 1998, with a mortality rate twice as high for black women as for white women.[1]

Anatomy

The cervix is one of the two major parts of the uterus (Figure 3.2). The body, or corpus, of the uterus is the section immediately above and adjacent to the cervix. The narrowest part of the corpus is the lower end, or isthmus, of the uterus and is just above the cervix. The cervix, or neck of the uterus, extends from the isthmus to the vagina. It is the narrow, cylindric segment of the uterus; it enters the vagina through the anterior vaginal wall and lies, in most instances, at right angles to it. In most women, it measures 2 to 4 centimeters in length. Anteriorly, the cervix is separated from the bladder by fatty tissue and is connected laterally by the broad ligaments and parametrium. The cervix receives its blood supply through the parametrium. The lower portion of the cervix projects into the vault of the vagina and is covered by a mucous membrane.

The endocervical canal is the passageway between the cervix's lower opening (the external os) and the upper opening (the internal os).[3] It is lined with columnar ep-

FIGURE 3.1. Cervical cancer by age, 1991–1995.

Source: SEER Cancer Statistics Review, 1973–1995 (NCI 1998); *Cancer Facts & Figures, 1998* (ACS 1998)

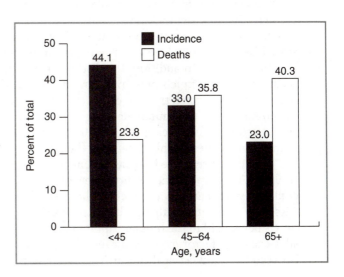

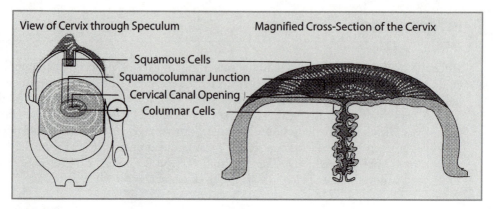

FIGURE 3.2. View of cervix through speculum.

Source: Reproduced with permission from Waye, R.D. (1990). *The Pap Smear and Your Cervix.* Chicago: Medfax-Sentinel.

ithelial cells. The ectocervix and the vagina are lined with squamous epithelial cells. The point at which these two types of epithelial cells meet is called the squamocolumnar junction, or transformation zone. The transformation zone is the usual site of cervical carcinoma.[3]

Etiology

As discussed in Chapter 2, and as with many cancers, the exact etiology of cervical cancer remains unknown. The progression to abnormality seems to be related to repeated injuries sustained by the cervix. Squamous cell carcinoma of the cervix is virtually nonexistent in celibate populations; only one case has been reported in the literature.[4] The risk factors known to be associated with squamous cell carcinoma of the cervix include sexual intercourse at an early age, multiple male sexual partners, male sexual partners who themselves have had multiple sexual partners, HPV infection, and smoking.[4,5,6] In addition, the disease in younger women (teens to age 40 years) seems to follow a much more rapid progression with an accompanying poorer prognosis.[7,8] It is projected that the occurrence of cervical cancer in the elderly will rise as the population in the United States ages.[9,10] There is no correlation with frequency of sexual activity. The disease is more prevalent in women of color in lower socioeconomic groups, presumably because of their poor access to health care and screening.[11]

Certain viruses have been studied as potential etiologic agents for cervical cancer. In the 1970s, herpes simplex virus type 2 (HSV-2) was implicated as oncogenic. Great controversy remains about whether the virus is oncogenic, carcinogenic, or simply a passenger associated with a multiplicity of sexual partners. And currently, great attention is being paid to the human papilloma virus (HPV) infection of the cervix as a possible causative factor to cervical cancer.[12,13,14] Most studies demonstrate a strong link between HPV and cervical cancer. The high-risk types of HPV, known to be associated with the development of cervical cancer, are types 16, 18, 31, 33, and 35. These high-risk types are seen in the majority of women diagnosed with cervical cancer.[6,7,8] HIV infection and AIDS have also been considered recently as a risk factor for the development of cervical cancer.[12,17,18] This is most likely the result of both opportunistic malignancies due to an immunosupressed state and the presence of concomitant infections such as HPV and HSV-2. In addition, a genetic variation raises the risk of cervical cancer sevenfold. Women with two copies of the variant of the gene for the tumor suppressor protein p53 are seven times more likely to have cervical cancer than are patients with one copy of the variant gene. And finally, the use of estrogen replacement therapy was examined to determine if a relationship between it and the development of cervical cancer existed. The findings suggested that exogenous estrogen use did not increase the risk of cervical cancer and may, in fact, decrease the risk.[18]

Pathology

Table 3.1 lists the types of cervical cancer. The nature of squamous cell cancer of the cervix is best described as a continuum, from normal cells, through degrees of dysplasia, to invasive disease (Figure 3.3). Invasive squamous cell carcinoma of the cervix spreads through direct invasion into adjacent tissues and metastasizes through lymphatic and vascular dissemination. Grossly, the tumors may be ulcerating, exophytic, or nodular. Ulcerating lesions are characterized by an absence of the superficial layers of the cervix, resulting in a concave defect. Exophytic lesions appear on the surface of the cervix and project into the vaginal or cervical canal. Nodular lesions are similar to exophytic lesions; however, they are more discrete and often better defined by palpation than visualization.

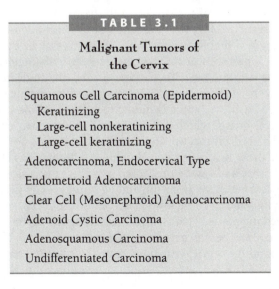

TABLE 3.1
Malignant Tumors of the Cervix

Squamous Cell Carcinoma (Epidermoid)
     Keratinizing
     Large-cell nonkeratinizing
     Large-cell keratinizing

Adenocarcinoma, Endocervical Type
Endometroid Adenocarcinoma
Clear Cell (Mesonephroid) Adenocarcinoma
Adenoid Cystic Carcinoma
Adenosquamous Carcinoma
Undifferentiated Carcinoma

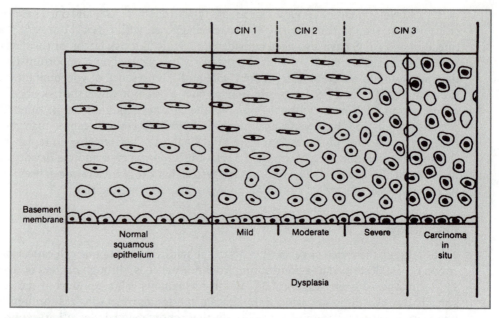

FIGURE 3.3. Cervical endothelium showing progressive degrees of cervical intraepithelial neoplasia (CIN).

Source: Reproduced with permission from Herbst, A. (1992). *Comprehensive Gynecology* 2nd ed. St. Louis, MO: Mosby Year Book, Inc.

Adenocarcinomas and mixed adenosquamous carcinomas range in incidence from 10 to 15% of all cancers of the cervix, with the remaining 85 to 90% being squamous carcinomas. An increase in the frequency of cervical adenocarcinomas has been reported in the recent literature.[4] Rather than a true rise in the actual numbers of adenocarcinomas, it has been postulated that the ratio of adenocarcinomas to squamous cell carcinomas is changing. This change may be due to decreased incidence of squamous cell cancers because of early detection and treatment of cervical dysplasia and CIS. It may also be due to better sampling techniques of the endocervix through use of the endocervical brush, which is far superior in detecting endocervical lesions than the previously used cotton-tip applicator. Risk factors for adenocarcinoma of the cervix include those associated with human papillomavirus (HPV). HPV is a sexually transmitted disease and can be prevented by safe sex practices.[4,5]

Adenocarcinoma arises from the endocervical mucus-producing gland cells (Figure 3.4). The location of these lesions within the endocervical canal is often what results in delayed diagnosis. That is, an adenocarcinoma of the cervix may be present for a considerable time before becoming clinically evident.[6] The lesions are typically bulky and expand the cervical canal to create the so-called barrel-shaped lesions of the

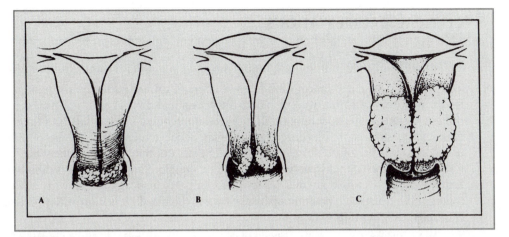

FIGURE 3.4. Gross appearance of cervical cancer. **A.** Carcinoma of the cervix may appear grossly to be extending from the cervix and filling the upper vaginal canal. This exophytic cancer is the most typical type. **B.** Squamous cell carcinoma of the cervix may also invade the cervical stroma with little exophytic component (endophytic lesion). **C.** Adeno-carcinoma of the endocervix often penetrates the cervical stroma and expands the cervix and lower uterine segment without an obvious lesion on the exocervix. This expanded lower uterine segment and cervix are designated a "barrel lesion."

Source: Reproduced with permission from Pearson, D., & Dawood, M. (1990). *Green's Gynecology* 4th ed. (p. 510). Boston: Little, Brown and Company.

cervix. The spread pattern of these lesions is similar to that of squamous cell cancer, with direct extension accompanied by metastases to regional pelvic lymph nodes as the primary routes of dissemination. Local recurrence is more common in these lesions, and this has resulted in the commonly held belief that they are more radioresistant than squamous cell lesions.[4] It may be, however, that the bulky, expansive nature accounts for the local recurrence. Hence, many oncologists recommend combined radiotherapy and surgery for these lesions. Survival statistics are comparable to squamous cell carcinoma stage for stage.[4]

Clear cell adenocarcinoma of the cervix and vagina has been associated with first-trimester exposure to a nonsteroidal synthetic estrogen. The most common synthetic estrogen associated with the occurrence of clear cell carcinoma is diethylstilbestrol (DES). Since DES is no longer prescribed during high-risk pregnancy, the incidence of this rare disease has decreased steadily since its peak in 1975. The age range for young women diagnosed with clear cell adenocarcinoma of the cervix/vagina is 7 to 34 years. Younger women (below age 15) have more aggressive tumors than older women (over 19 years).[4]

✖ CLINICAL MANIFESTATIONS

Symptoms

The symptoms of early cancer of the cervix often go unrecognized by the patient. The initial symptom is a thin, watery, blood-tinged vaginal discharge. It is painless and is often associated with douching or after sexual intercourse (postcoital).[4] As the malignancy progresses, more bleeding episodes may occur, which with time become heavier, more frequent, and of longer duration. The patient may also describe what seems to be an increase in menstruations. Ultimately, the bleeding becomes essentially continuous, with resulting anemia. A foul discharge is also associated with advanced stages of the disease. In postmenopausal women, the bleeding is more likely to prompt early medical attention.

All of these symptoms are associated with the tumor mass. Lesions are friable and bleed easily with trauma; hence, sexual activity or douching causes sloughing and bleeding of the lesion. Progressive bleeding and a foul discharge are associated with large, bulky necrotic tumors. These advanced lesions often bleed spontaneously and shed necrotic debris.

Late symptoms, indicators of more advanced disease, include the development of pain referred to the flank or leg. This is usually secondary to involvement of the uterus, pelvic wall, and/or sciatic nerve. Dysuria, hematuria, rectal bleeding, or constipation may signal bladder or rectal tumor invasion. Persistent edema of one or both lower extremities as a result of lymphatic and venous blockage by extensive pelvic wall disease are late manifestations of both primary disease and recurrent disease. Uremia may result from ureteral obstruction due to advanced lateral pelvic disease.[20]

Spread of Disease

The main routes of spread are (1) into the vaginal mucosa, extending microscopically down beyond visible or palpable disease; (2) into the myometrium of the lower uterine segment, especially with lesions that originate on the endocervix; (3) into the paracervical lymphocytes, and from there into regional and then distant lymph nodes—the internal, external, and common iliac lymph nodes and the obturator are common sites of lymphatic involvement; and (4) direct extension into adjacent structures or parametria. Extension of the disease to involve the bladder or rectum can occur with or without the occurrence of a vesicovaginal or rectovaginal fistula.

The cervix has a rich lymphatic network. Microscopic lymphatics lie beneath the cervical squamous mucosa and surround the endocervical glands. Interconnections exist between all the lymphatics from the various levels of the cervix with those of the uterus and upper vagina. The lateral collecting trunks are relatively large and leave the cervix with the uterine artery and veins (Figure 3.5). The prevalence of lymph node disease correlates with the stage and grade of the malignancy (Figures 3.6 and 3.7).

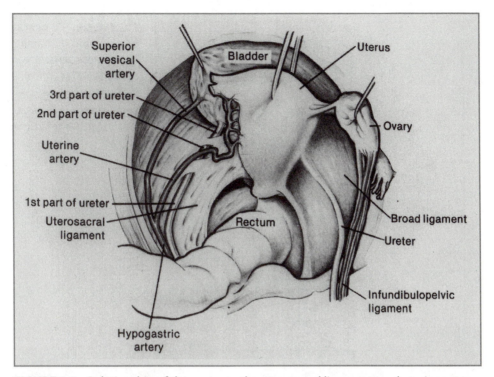

FIGURE 3.5. Relationship of the ureter to the uterosacral ligaments and uterine artery.

Source: Reproduced with permission from DiSaia, P.J., & Creasman, W.T. (1997). *Clinical Gynecologic Oncology* 5th ed. (p. 70). St. Louis, MO: Mosby Year Book, Inc.

Lymph node involvement in stage I is between 15 and 20%; in stage II, between 25 and 40%; and in stage III, it is assumed that at least 50% have positive nodes.[4]

Clinical Staging

The International Federation of Gynecology & Obstetrics (FIGO) staging system serves as a basis for comparing the results of therapy by various methods and in various centers throughout the world (Table 3.2). The FIGO staging system is also a useful guide in estimating prognosis, and furthermore provides general principles of therapy and specific details of treatment for patients with the same stage of disease. This staging system is based on palpable findings on abdominal, pelvic, and rectal examinations supplemented by information from imaging techniques.

The staging of cervical cancer is done clinically rather than surgically. Since staging is a means of communicating treatment results from one institution to another, it

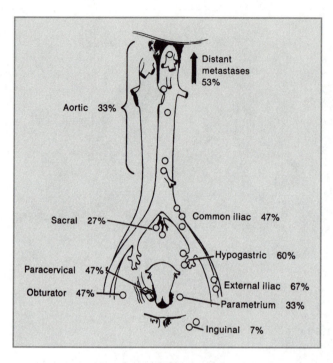

FIGURE 3.6. Percentage involvement of draining lymph nodes in untreated patients with cervical cancer.

Source: Reproduced with permission from Henriksen, E. (1949). *Am J Obstet & Gynecol, 58,* 924.

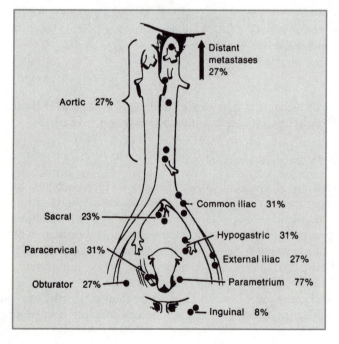

FIGURE 3.7. Percentage involvement of draining lymph nodes in treated patients with cervical cancer.

Source: Reproduced with permission from Henriksen, E. (1949). *Am J Obstet & Gynecol, 58,* 924.

TABLE 3.2

International Classification of Cancer of the Cervix by Stage

Stage	Description
0	Carcinoma in situ, intraepithelial carcinoma
I	Carcinoma strictly confined to the cervix (extension to the corpus should be disregarded)
Ia	Preclinical carcinomas of the cervix, that is, diagnosed only by microscopy
Ia1	Minimal microscopically evident stromal invasion
Ia2	Lesions detected microscopically that can be measured. The upper limit of the measurement should not show a depth of invasion of more than 5 mm taken from the base of the epithelium, either surface or glandular, from which it originates, and a second dimension, the horizontal spread, must not exceed 7 mm. Larger lesions should be staged as Ib.
Ib	Lesions of greater dimensions than stage Ia2, whether seen clinically or not. Preformed space involvement should not alter the staging but should be specifically recorded so as to determine whether it should affect treatment decisions in the future.
II	Involvement of the vagina but not the lower third, or infiltration of the parametria but not out to the sidewall
IIa	Involvement of the vagina but no evidence of parametrial involvement
IIb	Infiltration of the parametria but not out to the sidewall
III	Involvement of the lower third of the vagina, or extension to the pelvic sidewall All cases with a hydronephrosis or nonfunctioning kidney should be included, unless they are known to be attributable to other cause.
IIIa	Involvement of the lower third of the vagina but not out to the pelvic sidewall if the parametria are involved
IIIb	Extension onto the pelvic sidewall and/or hydronephrosis or nonfunctional kidney
IV	Extension outside the reproductive tract
IVa	Involvement of the mucosa of the bladder or rectum
IVb	Distant metastasis or disease outside the true pelvis

Source: Reproduced with permission from DiSaia, P.J., & Creasman, W.T. (1997). *Clinical Gynecologic Oncology* 5th ed. (p. 64). St. Louis, MO: Mosby Year Book, Inc.

is important to adhere to the standardized methods of staging. Staging determinations are based on physical examination, chest X-ray, colposcopy, cystoscopy, proctosigmoidoscopy, IVP, and contrast (barium) studies of the lower colon and rectum.[4] CT scans, MRI examinations, lymphangiograms (LAG), arteriography, and venography are not used to stage patients since these tests are not available in all institutions. Findings from MRI examinations and CT scans can influence treatment decisions; however, they should not influence initial staging determinations.[4] The detection of lymph node metastases from cervical cancer can be accomplished by LAG, CT, or MRI. However, since MRI and CT are less invasive and have the added benefit of assessing local tumor extent, they should be considered the preferred diagnostic tools when available.[21] As the population ages and more elderly women are diagnosed with this disease, certain imaging studies may be contraindicated, or the findings may be suboptimal due to preexisting conditions. For example, hip arthroplasty may reveal confounding lymphangiogram findings due to an alteration in the pelvic lymphatic drainage.[21]

The five-year survival rate for all cervical cancer patients is 66%. For patients diagnosed in the early invasive stages, however, the survival rate is 89%, and the survival rate for in situ cases is virtually 100 percent.

✖ TREATMENT

A strong causal relationship between HPV and cervical cancer has been established.[14,15,22] Primary prevention of HPV infection can be accomplished through (a) educating adolescents and health care providers regarding the strong association between HPV and cervical cancer, (b) encouraging delayed onset of sexual intercourse, (c) developing an effective vaccine, and (d) developing effective vaginal microbicides.[22]

Treatment decisions are based on the stage of the disease as determined by histopathogy, including grade of the tumor and radiologic findings; and the patient's general health and age. On completion of the initial work-up or pretreatment evaluation, the data are reviewed by a gynecologic oncologist, radiation oncologist, pathologist, and possibly diagnostic radiologist. Choice of treatment demands clinical judgment, but apart from the occasional patient for whom only symptomatic treatment may be best, the choice lies between surgery and radiotherapy.

The controversy between surgery and radiotherapy has existed for decades concerning the treatment of stage I and stage IIa cervical cancers. Currie[24] reported the results of 552 radical operations alone for cancer of the cervix, and Fletcher[25] reported on 2,000 patients treated with radiation therapy alone. In general, comparable survival rates are seen with both treatment methods for stages I and IIa (Table 3.3). All stages above I and IIa are treated with radiation therapy.

Surgery has noted advantages over radiation therapy in the treatment of early carcinoma of the cervix, particularly for younger patients. These advantages include shorter treatment time, preservation of ovarian function, higher patient acceptance, and limited sexual morbidity.[4] The more concrete-thinking patient often perceives surgical removal of the tumor as more effective in "getting the tumor out of her body." Additional reasons for the selection of surgery over radiation therapy include previous

	TABLE 3.3	
	Comparison of Five-Year Survival Rates by Treatment	
Stage of Disease	Surgery	Radiation Therapy
Stage I	86.3%	91.5%
Stage IIa	75	83.5
Stage IIb	58.9	66.5

Source: Adapted with permission from DiSaia, P.J., & Creasman, W.T. (1997). *Clinical Gynecologic Oncology* 5th ed. (p. 69). St. Louis, MO: Mosby Year Book, Inc.

pelvic irradiation therapy for other disease, concomitant inflammatory bowel disease or pelvic inflammatory disease, patient preference, and pregnancy.[4]

Cancer of the cervix in pregnancy is rare, accounting for only 0.01% of patients.[4] For cases of early invasion diagnosed at first trimester, traditional treatment (surgery or radiation) is indicated, and the pregnancy terminated.[26] In the second trimester, the therapy is similar, except that it may be necessary to evacuate the uterus first. After twenty-six weeks, in the third trimester, the treatment decision is more of a dilemma. Any decision to delay treatment should be made only after thorough deliberation with the patient and family. With the neonatal technologies currently available, fetuses can survive after thirty-two weeks' gestation. In this case, treatment would consist of Caesarean section followed by either surgery or radiation therapy. Prognosis for all stages of cervical cancer during pregnancy are considered to be consistent with nonpregnant patients with the same disease.[26]

Surgical Therapy

The radical nature of surgical treatment for patients with invasive cervical cancer depends on the risk of pelvic lymph node metastasis and the size of the tumor. There has been considerable debate in the literature about which parameters should be used to define patients who are not at risk for lymph node metastases or recurrence, as they may be treated with less radical approaches. This group of patients includes those with microscopic disease, the most common definition of which (originally put forward by the Society of Gynecologic Oncologists [SGO] in 1974) is a lesion in which neoplastic epithelium invades the stroma to a depth of less than or equal to 3 mm beneath the basement membrane and in which lymphatic or vascular involvement is not demonstrated.[27] These patients can be treated with either conization or a simple hysterectomy, that is, removal of the uterus and cervix but with no removal of intervening parametrial tissue or lymph nodes. Patients selected for simple hysterectomy over cone biopsy usually have completed their childbearing, or have associated pelvic pathology such as fibroids or dysfunctional bleeding.

Radical hysterectomy is the surgical treatment of choice for patients who have disease greater than 3 mm confined to the cervix, when probability of lymph node metastasis is less than 5%.[23,27] This procedure (Figure 3.8) involves removal of the uterus, upper third of the vagina, the entirety of the uterosacral uterovesical ligaments, and all of the parametrium on each side, along with pelvic node dissection encompassing the four major pelvic lymph node chains: urethral, obturator, hypogastric, and iliac.[4] The ovaries are preserved in young women since metastasis to the ovaries is rare.

Lateral ovarian transposition, or the surgical repositioning of the ovaries to a non-pelvic site, is performed at the time of surgery if postoperative radiation is likely and the patient is premenopausal. Deep invasion of the cervical stroma and metastatic disease to the lymph nodes both necessitate adjuvant radiation therapy, and shielding of the transposed ovaries during radiation therapy may prevent ovarian failure. But the success of ovarian transposition is unclear. Husseinzadeh[28] reported a 17% ovarian failure in women whose ovaries had been transposed and subsequently shielded dur-

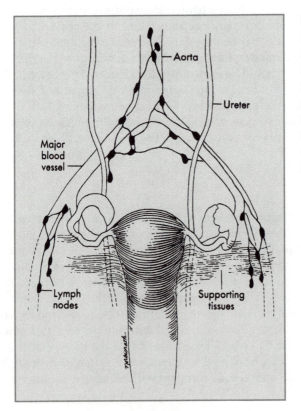

FIGURE 3.8. Radical hysterectomy: removal of uterus, nearby supporting tissues, uppermost part of vagina, and pelvic lymph nodes.

Source: Reproduced with permission from Phipps, W.J., Long, B.C., & Woods, N.F. (1995). *Medical Surgical Nursing: Concepts and Clinical Practice* 5th ed. St. Louis, MO: Mosby Year Book, Inc.

ing postoperative radiation. However, Feeney et al.[29] reported only a 50% preservation of ovarian function in similarly treated women.

Acute complications of radical hysterectomy, which occur in no more than 5% of cases, include infection, formation of ureteral fistulae, pulmonary embolus, and small-bowel obstruction.[27] The most common acute complication is febrile morbidity; however, the availability and prophylactic use of wide-spectrum antibiotics has reduced this problem. Fewer than 5% of patients experience wound infections, and this low incidence can be attributed greatly to provision of good nursing care.[30] Ureteral fistulae are even less frequent, 0 to 3%, and directly related to improvements in surgical techniques, such as avoiding intraoperative ureteral damage and assuring adequate collateral blood supply.[4]

Pulmonary embolism is the complication most commonly associated with mortality during the perioperative period. The intraoperative period is the most dangerous time for thrombus formation in the lower extremities or pelvic veins. Thus constriction of the leg veins should be vigilantly avoided. Prophylactic, preoperative, low-dose heparin or enoxaprin (Lovenox) reduces the incidence of this serious complication, without evidence of serious intraoperative bleeding. It is continued until the patient is ambulating on a regular basis. In addition, pneumatic compression stockings, worn during and after surgery for several days, have been shown to decrease the incidence of pulmonary embolism.[4]

Small-bowel obstruction is a very rare complication of radical hysterectomy, but Montz et al.[31] reported that small-bowel obstructions due to intraperitoneal adhesions are more common if concomitant radiotherapy is given. More specifically, 5% of those patients treated with radical hysterectomy alone developed a postoperative small-bowel obstruction, 20% of the women treated with adjuvant radiotherapy, and 22% who had also received preoperative radiotherapy.[31]

Subacute complications of radical hysterectomy include postoperative bladder dysfunction, formation of lymphocysts, and lymphedema of the lower extremities. The degree of bladder compliance is related to the width and extent of the surgical dissection. Typically, bladder volume is decreased and filling pressure increased for the first few days after surgery. The patient may also have a reduced sensitivity to filling and an inability to initiate voiding. Reports in the literature suggest that bladder dysfunction is a direct result of injury to the sensory and motor nerve supply to the detrusor muscle of the bladder.[32] This dysfunction is usually manifested in the patient by a loss of the sense of urgency to void and an inability to empty the bladder completely without a Crede maneuver. O'Laughlin[33] describes four major types of bladder dysfunction after radical hysterectomy: hypertonus of the bladder muscle, loss of sensation of bladder fullness, difficulty in initiating micturition, and bladder hypotonia. Long-term, or possibly permanent, bladder dysfunction can be avoided by preventing overdistention of the bladder. Once the indwelling urinary catheter is removed, the bladder should be emptied regularly, and this can be achieved by either micturition or intermittent catheterization every four hours. Residual urine volume should be maintained at or below 100cc, checked by either ultrasound or postvoid catheterization. Nocturnal overdistention can be avoided by decreasing fluids several hours before bedtime and voiding or self-catheterization immediately prior to retiring for the night. Although some patients learn to compensate and return to near normal function, patients frequently need to be taught intermittent self-catheterization. Thus discharge planning should include self-catheterization and care of the catheter to prevent urinary tract infection. Postoperative use of a suprapubic catheter and urethral catheter has helped decrease the incidence of long-term bladder dysfunction.

The formation of lymphocysts within the pelvis is reduced with the provision of adequate drainage of the retroperitoneal space postoperatively via continuous-suction catheters.[4] Lymphocysts rarely cause injury and generally resolve in time by reabsorption, but surgical management is necessary when the rare lymphocyst causes ureteral obstruction. Some women are discharged with a continuous-suction device in place to prevent accumulation of drainage and subsequent infection. These patients should be taught how to empty the device, record volumes, and assess for infection. Percutaneous aspiration increases the risk of subsequent infection.

Lymphedema of the lower extremities is a complication that rarely occurs after radical hysterectomy alone. However, the incidence increases with the addition of postoperative radiation therapy. Werngren-Elgstrom and Lidman[34] reported slight swelling (>5% volume increase) in 28% of women treated with surgery and radiotherapy for cancer of the cervix. Six percent had moderate swelling (>10% volume increase) and 7% had severe swelling (>15% volume increase). Twenty-two percent had lymphedema that was severe enough to cause symptoms.[34] Routine use of custom-made elastic support hose by patients at risk during the first year postoperatively reduces the risk of lymphedema. Patients at risk include those with extensive lymphatic dissection and adjuvant radiation therapy, though collateral pathways of lymph drainage develop within the first year after completion of therapy. Streptococcal lymphangitis, should it occur, dramatically increases the incidence of lymphedema,[4] so prophylactic use of low-dose antibiotic therapy to prevent this infection also may be used. Women who experience this rare complication should be instructed to avoid dependent edema through positioning to support optimal drainage (i.e., legs elevated above heart). Regular exercise to improve drainage and augment the development of collateral channels is also recommended. Injections in the affected extremity should be avoided.

Note that concomitant obesity has not been shown to adversely affect the survival rate or the incidence of serious complications in women undergoing radical hysterectomy for cervical cancer. But Soisson et al.[35] reported that, although serious complications were not seen in these cases, the operative technique was more difficult, operating time was longer, and a greater blood loss occurred.

Radiation Therapy

As mentioned above, radiation therapy is a common treatment modality for cervix cancer, and cure rates for early stages are equal to those obtained with surgery.[36,37] Cure rates for advanced disease treated with radiation are 60% for stage II, 30% for stage III, and only 10% for stage IV.[27] Postoperative radiation may improve survival for patients with more than three positive nodes,[4] but the use of radiation in this subset of patients is quite controversial.[38,39] Very recent advances have demonstrated a significant improvement in survival for patients with advanced disease by combining radiation therapy and platinum-based chemotherapy.[40] These dramatic results have demonstrated a significant improvement in survival rates for women with bulky stage Ib through advanced stages of the disease (II–IV) by adding cisplatinum-based chemotherapy during irradiation therapy. Rates of bowel and urinary tract complications may increase with postoperative radiation therapy.[32,39,44]

Radiation therapy for all stages of cancer of the cervix consists of a combination of high-energy megavoltage pelvic irradiation to treat regional lymph nodes and the central cervical disease, and intracavitary brachytherapy to treat the rest of the central tumor (one cGy = 1 rad of absorbed dose). Treatment is given in daily fractions for a period of four to six weeks, followed by one or two intracavitary applications of cesium using a tandem source to deliver 4,000 to 5,000 cGy internally. Interstitial therapy may be considered with carcinoma of the cervix when accurate placement of conventional intracavitary applications is not possible because of tumor obstruction or vaginal contracture.[4]

Extended-field irradiation therapy has been employed to increase survival rates for patients with advanced cervical cancer with periaortic lymph node metastases. This radiation consists of targeting en bloc periaortic and pelvic portals to the level of the dome of the diaphragm and down to the obturator foramen.[4] Overall, the value of extended-field radiation is clouded because patients with periaortic involvement often have such advanced disease that any therapy is likely to have little or no effect.[4] Again, new advances in combining radiation and cisplatinum have changed the standard treatment protocols for these patients.[10]

The role of pretreatment surgical staging in cervix cancer remains unclear. Several large institutions across the United States routinely perform such procedures as prospective protocols, and the Gynecologic Oncology Group (GOG) has used pretreatment laparotomy as an integral part of many of their advanced cervix cancer protocols.[4] Whether data being collected in these studies will show enough survival benefit to recommend the procedure routinely remains to be seen. Kim et al. recommend CT treatment planning to prevent geographic miss and subsequent local pelvic failure. The availability of CT scans, however, is not universal; therefore, anterio-posterior and posterio-anterior pelvic therapy is the most reliable if CT planning is not a feasible option.[45]

Large, bulky stage II and stage III tumors of the cervix pose additional radiotherapeutic challenges. These tumors are often hypoxic at the core, rendering them more radioresistant. In an effort to maximize the effectiveness of radiation therapy in these cases, several avenues of research are currently being explored, including the use of radiosensitizers and identification of radiobiologically hypoxic tumors. Garcia-Angulo and Kagiya have described promising results with the use of intratumor and parametrial infusion of the radiosensitizer 3-nitrotriazole (AK-2123). AK-2123 was intratumorly injected thirty minutes prior to radiotherapy. The short-term effects demonstrated a good response in exophytic types of lesions; endophytic lesions responded less dramatically. Treatment was well tolerated, and no neurological toxicity occurred.[46] A modified radiotherapeutic approach may be indicated in tumors that are deemed hypoxic. Hockel et al. have described a method for determining the pO_2 of tumors prior to initiation of therapy. Significantly shorter survival and recurrence-free survival were found in those tumors with low pO_2. This procedure, known as intratumor pO_2 histography, would enable pretherapeutic selection of tumors for modification of therapy.[47]

Complications of radiation can be classified as early (acute) or delayed effects. Acute complications are often related to ionizing effects on the bowel and bladder. Symptoms include cramping, diarrhea, tenesmus, dysuria and, occasionally, bleeding from the bowel or bladder. A diet low in lactose, glucose, and protein may help treat bowel symptoms, and the addition of antispasmodic agents may be helpful for both bowel and bladder symptoms. A week of rest from radiation therapy may be required if symptoms are severe. The incidence of severe hemorrhagic cystitis following radiation for stage Ib cancer of the cervix is low but can occur many years following treatment.[48] Episodes of hematuria can be managed with urine culture and sensitivity with subsequent antibiotic therapy. Persistent bleeding is an indication for cystoscopy to rule out clot retention or recurrent disease. Heavy bleeding is managed with clot evacuation and continuous bladder irrigation.[48]

Late complications are relatively rare (8–18%), but may include bowel obstruction, fistula formation, perforation, and vaginal stenosis.[4] The rate of complications increases as higher doses of radiation are used and may occur up to several years after the completion of radiation therapy. Bowel obstruction may be treated conservatively with bowel rest, NPO, and placement of an intestinal tube to decompress the bowel. Surgical correction of bowel obstruction due to radiation and surgically induced adhesions may be necessary. Appropriate surgery, such as internal bypass procedures, may be necessary in persistent cases.

Radiation necrosis resulting in fistula formation or perforation is often mistaken for recurrent disease and patients may die of these complications unless aggressively treated. Thus accurate diagnosis of the cause of a fistula is necessary and may require treatment with surgical bypass or repair for care or palliation. Small-bowel fistulae rarely heal spontaneously. Their management involves total resection of the affected portion of the bowel. The potential for late rectal complications may be reduced by adjusting the fraction dose or intracavitary radiation techniques.[48]

Strategies to prevent vaginal stenosis as a result of radiation therapy are also important. The vagina undergoes some predictable changes following radiation therapy: decreased vascular engorgement and reduced vaginal lubrication, dyspareunia, and significant sexual disruption as a result of trauma to the vaginal epithelium.[49] Sore spots and ulcers may form in the initial treatment period and may take months to heal after radiation is completed. As the natural scarring process of vaginal tissue begins, it becomes fibrous and tough, losing its ability to stretch during sexual excitement and intercourse.[49] Dilation regimens following radiation therapy vary with regard to dilator size and suggested frequency of use. It is important to encourage women to either be sexually active on a regular basis or to utilize a vaginal dilator regularly. A weekly gentle vaginal douche with salt water or vinegar may be substituted. In sexually active patients, a water-soluble lubricant is also recommended. Continuing psychological support is important. (See Chapters 13 and 14 for a more in-depth discussion of radiation therapy and sexuality.)

Severe, permanent vaginal stenosis can occur if patients do not use a dilator or have not been sexually active during the two-year period following radiation therapy. Sexual activity is only one factor in the need for a functional vagina. Even if the woman is not and never wishes to be sexually active, frequent examinations of the vaginal cuff to detect cancer recurrence dictate the need for a functional vagina. In some cases, surgical reconstruction of the vagina is needed, although there is a further risk of rectovaginal or vesicovaginal fistula formation with this procedure.[50]

Vaccine

The discovery that HPV is present in 93% of all cancer of the cervix has led to efforts to develop vaccines against HPV. These vaccines would be both prophylactic and therapeutic.[14,22,47] Since the HPV virus inserts itself into cervical cells, it escapes the body's immune response. The investigational vaccines consist of a viral protein that the immune system recognizes as foreign and sends to cell surfaces, triggering an immune response.[14,47] The efficacy of these vaccines has been proven in animal models. Human clinical trials are in progress.[47]

Chemotherapy

The role of chemotherapy as a treatment modality in the management of cervical cancer is limited. Investigations are under way throughout the world, looking for neoadjuvant therapy for advanced squamous cell carcinoma of the cervix. Most of the regimens are cisplatin-based, often including bleomycin and vincristine.[50,52–55] These trials are being conducted using patients presenting with large-volume disease, whereas in the past, chemotherapy was reserved for patients with metastasis or recurrence after radiation therapy. Clinical trials are evaluating the effectiveness of newer drugs such as ifosfamide, dibromodulcitol, and taxol in the treatment of advanced cervix cancer.[56] Etoposide and vinblastine require further investigation. Tumors that have not received prior irradiation seem more susceptible to chemotherapy, presumably related to tumor perfusion. Since cervical cancer is more sensitive to radiotherapy, however, the incidence of an unirradiated cervical lesion is and should be rare. There is no evidence to show that cervical cancer is sensitive to hormonal therapy.

※ RECURRENT AND ADVANCED DISEASE

Adequate follow-up is the key to the early detection of recurrence following therapy for invasive cervical cancer. The yield of examinations such as IVP and chest X-ray in patients with initial early disease is so low that many clinicians have discontinued their routine use. However, frequent internal examinations and Pap tests from the vaginal apex are recommended. The advanced-practice nurse is an appropriate care provider for these patients. DiSaia and Creasman[4] recommend seeing patients for pelvic examinations, Pap smears, and other tests as outlined in Table 3.4.

Caring for the patient with recurrent or advanced cancer of the cervix gives rise to special nursing challenges in the areas of active treatment and palliative care. Most patients are able to enjoy complete recovery following the treatment. However, some suffer great difficulties with side effects of treatment, surgery, or radiation, and some succumb to death from disseminated disease. Thus it is important to understand the psychological as well as the physical processes of recovery so that the ultimate goal of the health care team can be met: helping patients live as well as possible.

It is estimated that approximately 35% of patients with invasive cervical cancer will have recurrent or persistent disease after treatment. Over 75% of all recurrences are clinically evident within two years after completion of initial therapy.[4,27,50] The diagnosis, however, is often difficult to establish. The most common signs and symptoms of recurrent cervical cancer include unexplained weight loss; excessive unilateral leg edema; pelvic, thigh, or buttock pain; serosanguinous vaginal discharge; cough; hemoptysis; and chest pain[4] (Table 3.5). Histologic confirmation is essential since many of these symptoms can be due to side effects of therapy or other chronic conditions. Central recurrences at the vaginal cuff are quite accessible to biopsy, but other sites of recurrence may require radiologically directed needle biopsy.

Diagnostic evaluation at the time of suspected recurrence should include a chest X-ray, CT scan, and laboratory studies such as CBC, renal function, and liver function. The triad of symptoms of leg edema, pain, and weight loss is ominous. Leg edema is

---

TABLE 3.4

Frequency of Follow-up Examinations for the Asymptomatic Patient

Years	Frequency	Examination
1	3 mo.	Pelvic, Pap
	6 mo.	CXR, IVP
	1 yr	CBC, BUN, creatinine
2	4 mo.	Pelvic, Pap
		CXR, IVP
		CBC, BUN, creatinine
3–5	6 mo.	Pelvic, Pap

Source: Adapted with permission from DiSaia, P.J., & Creasman, W.T. (1997). *Clinical Gynecologic Oncology* 5th ed. (p. 85). St. Louis, MO: Mosby Year Book, Inc.

TABLE 3.5
Presenting Symptoms of Patients with Recurrent or Persistent Cervix Cancer

Weight Loss
Leg Edema
Pelvic, Thigh, or Buttock Pain
Vaginal Discharge
Progressive Ureteral Obstruction
Supraclavicular Lymphadenopathy
Persistent Cough/Hemoptysis

Source: Adapted with permission from DiSaia, P.J., & Creasman, W.T. (1997). *Clinical Gynecologic Oncology* 5th ed. (p. 86). St. Louis, MO: Mosby Year Book, Inc.

---

usually due to progressive lymphatic obstruction; however a thrombophlebitis should be ruled out. Some patients reporting pain describe it as radiating to the upper thigh or into the buttock; others describe pain in the groin.

Management

Persistent or recurrent disease is discouraging, with a one-year survival rate of between 10 and 15%. Treatment failures are more common with advanced initial stages of disease; therefore most patients are not candidates for a second curative approach. Most recurrences are suitable for palliative management only, though some gynecologic oncologists have suggested conservative surgery (radical hysterectomy) for recurrent cervical cancer after primary radiation therapy.[57,58] Unfortunately, the complication rate in these patients is often unacceptably high, including high fistula and operative mortality rates.[59]

Radiation Therapy

Women with recurrent disease who have been treated only surgically to date are candidates for radiation therapy in doses described earlier in this chapter. In addition, Monk et al.[60] describe some limited success with open interstitial brachytherapy for the treatment of cervical cancer recurrence after primary surgery.

When disease recurs outside of a previously irradiated field, local irradiation is frequently successful in providing local control and symptom relief. However, most patients who benefit from reirradiation are those who receive far less than optimal radiation during their initial treatment. But this circumstance has become rare in recent times, since sophisticated radiation therapy is available in most areas of the United

States. Therefore reirradiation for recurrent disease is usually not feasible. The potential for necrosis and fistulae formation with even moderate doses of reirradiation is unfavorable.

Chemotherapy

Management of disseminated cervical cancer has not improved despite the progress of modern chemotherapy. The Gynecologic Oncology Group has reported the most extensive experience with cisplatin in the treatment of cervix cancer. The size of this trial and the care with which it was conducted make it the definitive cisplatin study in cervix cancer. In this study, more than 300 patients were treated with cisplatin to define the optimal dose and schedule. Despite response rates of 17 to 18% for all dose rates, cisplatin alone remains as effective as any combination chemotherapy reported and confirmed in a large series.[4]

New combinations of chemotherapy are currently being researched, however. These include investigational protocols using dibromodulcitol and cisplatin[61] and cisplatin, 5-fluorouracil, and ifosamide.[62] Early results reveal promising response rates with tolerable toxicities.

Pelvic Exenteration

A small percentage of patients with recurrent or persistent central disease are eligible for a pelvic exenteration. Improved five-year survival after this ultraradical surgery allows some patients to rehabilitate and enjoy an acceptable quality of life, but presence of metastatic spread beyond the pelvis is a contraindication for continuing with plans for a pelvic exenteration. Such metastases may be found in the presurgical work-up or during initial stages of the laparotomy. Miller et al.[63] reported an aborted exenterative procedure rate of almost 33%. The reasons for aborting the procedure included the presence of peritoneal disease (44%), positive lymph nodes (40%), parametrial fixation (13%), and hepatic or bowel lesions (4.5%), all of which were found at the time of laparotomy despite extensive preoperative work-up. Hence, they concluded that disseminated disease can seldom be detected during the preoperative work-up; nonetheless a preoperative work-up should be performed on all prospective patients to decrease the likelihood of the devastating impact of an aborted exenterative procedure. This work-up includes chest X-ray, CT scan of the abdomen and pelvis with intravenous contrast, creatine clearance, liver and kidney function tests, and CBC with differential.[4]

Total pelvic exenteration includes removal of all pelvic viscera, including bladder and rectosigmoid colon, and is the treatment of choice for the patient with recurrent disease limited to the pelvis (Figure 3.9). In very carefully selected cases, either an anterior or posterior exenteration may be performed. An anterior exenteration entails removal of the bladder with preservation of the rectosigmoid (Figure 3.10). Posterior exenteration includes removal of the rectosigmoid with preservation of the bladder (Figure 3.11). Anterior and posterior exenterations alone are quite rare, since the risk

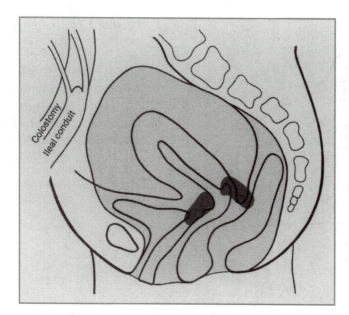

FIGURE 3.9. Total exenteration: removal of all pelvic viscera. Fecal stream is diverted via colostomy, and urinary diversion is via an ileal or sigmoid conduit or continent pouch.

Source: Reproduced with permission from DiSaia, P.J., & Morrow, C.P. (1973). *Calf Med, 118,* 13.

of remaining disease is quite high. In addition, the remaining organ often incurs multiple postoperative complications and malfunctions.

Thus the risk of such an extensive procedure can be justified only when there is a chance of long-term survival. The data from various studies indicate a 15 to 62% five-year survival rate.[4] The tumor needs to be totally resectable, and the patient should

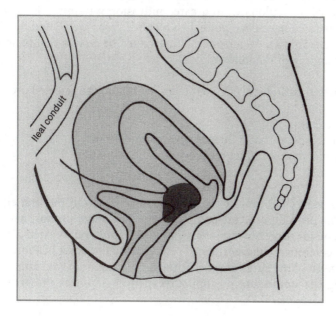

FIGURE 3.10. Anterior exenteration: removal of all pelvic viscera except rectosigmoid. Urinary stream is diverted into an ileal or sigmoid conduit or continent pouch.

Source: Reproduced with permission from DiSaia, P.J., & Morrow, C.P. (1973). *Calf Med, 118,* 13.

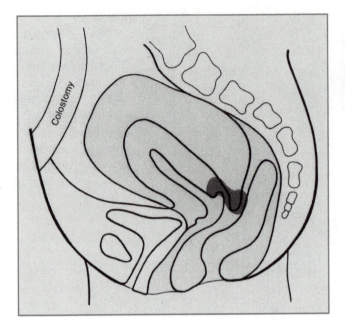

FIGURE 3.11. Posterior exenteration: removal of all pelvic viscera except bladder. Fecal stream is diverted via colostomy.

Source: Reproduced with permission from DiSaia, P.J., & Morrow, C.P. (1973). *Calf Med,* *118,* 13.

have physical and mental reserves adequate for recovery. Surgeons weigh many factors before exenteration, including the surgical risks, financial costs (hospital and convalescent), ability to learn ostomy care, emotional and social adjustment, pain control, and potential relief from palliative surgery.

The woman who undergoes pelvic exenteration requires monitoring of intravenous fluids, medications, meticulous wound care, and ostomy training. Excellent teaching plans for these women have been published by both Yarbrough[64] and the Patient Education Department at M.D. Anderson.[65] Nurses must be certain that patients have a thorough understanding of the following:

- Type of exenteration and pathologic circumstances leading to the selected procedure
- Criteria for patient selection
- Specific intraoperative aspects that influence postoperative care
- Patient and family concerns that affect recovery and rehabilitation
- Long-term patient needs

Complications, both acute and long-term, generally occur within the first eighteen months following the procedure. Acute complications are similar to those associated with other types of major surgery: pulmonary embolism, pulmonary edema, myocardial infarction, and cerebrovascular accidents.[4] Cardiovascular complications are directly related to the length of the surgical procedure and the extent of the intraoperative blood loss. During the immediate postoperative period, sepsis is the greatest threat. This can originate from either pelvic abscess or pelvic cellulitis. The occurrence of this complication diminishes after the first week postoperatively. Postoperative small-bowel obstruction is also a serious complication, but surgical techniques to prevent the small bowel from adhering to the denuded pelvic floor have decreased its incidence.[4]

Long-term complications are most commonly related to urinary diversion. Both urinary obstruction and infection pose the most serious long-term threat. Prophylactic, ongoing urinary antisepsis is often recommended to prevent pyelonephritis. Ureteral obstructive disorders can result from ureteral strictures and obstructions resulting in hydronephrosis. Should it occur, this requires immediate correction to prevent permanent renal damage.[4]

Sexual adjustment related to neovaginal reconstruction is an issue that must be addressed. This may be a concern for both the client and her sexual partner. Vaginal intercourse remains possible but the sensations during foreplay and intercourse are altered. The exterior female genitalia remains unchanged, therefore clitoral stimulation and orgasm remain unaltered. However, the sensation of a vaginal orgasm will be altered. The natural vaginal lubrication is also no longer present, and therefore a water-soluble lubricant should be used. Vaginal intercourse should be avoided until the neovagina is completely healed. A pelvic exam will determine the maturity of the reconstruction. Alternative ways of expressing physical love can be implemented until the neovagina has completely healed.

Pain Management in Advanced Disease

Pain is one of the most compelling problems that those with cancer and their caretakers will ever have to face. In fact, one of the greatest fears associated with the diagnosis of cancer is that it inevitably results in the occurrence of pain for which there is no relief. No other experiences we have as nurses have as significant an impact on our skills, our hearts, and our memories as those in which a person has suffered from pain that we have not been able to control. Certainly many of our most challenging clinical situations have focused on the dynamic interplay among patient, nurse, and physician that takes place as we struggle to find solutions to the problems of pain. But the crux of the cancer-pain management dilemma is not that methods to relieve pain are nonexistent, but rather that the pain is often not assessed properly or interventions are not utilized appropriately.

Pain assessment and management for women with advanced cervical cancer is a major nursing concern. Seventy to 75% of women with advanced cervical cancer experience unrelieved cancer pain. Barriers to pain relief are many, including systems issues, health care provider issues, and patient/family issues. Nurses need to try to discover what the particular barriers are for each patient and begin an education process to help overcome them.

To do so, nurses first assess the pain to determine its etiology and then try to make recommendations. Some common types of pain profiles found in women with cervix cancer include:

TABLE 3.6

Diagnostic Cluster

Diagnostic/Preoperative and Postoperative Period

COLLABORATIVE PROBLEMS
Potential Complication: Bleeding/hemorrhage
Potential Complication: Thromboembolic event
Potential Complication: Infection/sepsis
Potential Complication: Fluid/electrolyte imbalance
Potential Complication: Atelectasis/pneumonia
Potential Complication: Bowel dysfunction
Potential Complication: Urinary dysfunction

NURSING DIAGNOSIS
1. Potential altered health maintenance related to insufficient knowledge of condition, diagnostic tests, prognosis, and treatment options
2. Decisional conflict related to insufficient knowledge of treatment options
3. Anxiety/fear related to impending surgery, and insufficient knowledge of preoperative routines, intraoperative activities, and postoperative self-care activities
4. Anxiety/fear related to insufficient knowledge of potential impact of condition and treatment on reproductive organs and sexuality
5. Grieving related to potential loss of fertility and perceived effects on lifestyle
6. Potential altered respiratory function related to immobility secondary to imposed bedrest and pain
7. Potential fluid volume deficit related to losses secondary to surgical wound, or gastrointestinal dysfunction
8. Altered comfort related to effects of surgery, disease process, and immobility
9. Potential for infection related to susceptibility to bacteria secondary to wound, invasive vascular access, or urinary catheter
10. Potential altered nutrition: less than body requirements, related to disease process, wound healing, and decreased caloric intake
11. Impaired physical mobility related to surgical interruption of body structures, incisional site pain, and activity restriction
12. Potential bowel dysfunction related to decreased peristalsis secondary to surgical manipulation of bowel, effects of anesthesia and analgesia, and immobility
13. Potential urinary dysfunction related to loss of sensation of bladder distention secondary to surgical or pharmaceutical interventions
14. Potential impaired skin integrity related to surgical wound, decreased tissue perfusion, ostomy stomas, drain sites, or immobility
15. Potential impaired tissue integrity/infection related to lymphedema secondary to surgical removal of lymph nodes

TABLE 13.6 *(continued)*

16a. Potential sexual dysfunction related to disease process, surgical intervention, fatigue, and/or pain

16b. Potential moderate or possible permanent alterations in sexual activity related to disease process, surgical intervention, fatigue, and/or pain

16c. Severe or permanent inability to engage in genital intercourse

17. Alteration in coping related to infertility

18.c Potential altered health maintenance related to insufficient knowledge of dietary restrictions, medications, activity restrictions, self-care activities, symptoms of complications, follow-up visits, and community resources

Treatment Period

COLLABORATIVE PROBLEMS
Potential Complication: Preexisting medical conditions
Potential Complication: Anasarca
Potential Complication: Fluid/electrolyte imbalance

NURSING DIAGNOSIS
1. Anxiety/fear related to loss of feelings of control of life, unpredictability of nature of disease, and uncertain future
2. Anxiety/fear related to insufficient knowledge of prescribed radiation therapy and necessary self-care measures
3. Anxiety/fear related to insufficient knowledge of prescribed gynecologic radiation implant: conventional afterloading procedure
4. Anxiety/fear related to insufficient knowledge of prescribed gynecologic radiation implant: remote afterloading procedure
5. Potential for infection related to immunosuppression neutropenia secondary to chemotherapy and/or radiation therapy
6. Potential for bleeding related to immunosuppression thrombocytopenia secondary to chemotherapy and/or radiation therapy
7. Potential alteration in skin integrity related to treatment modality and/or disease process
8. Potential altered health maintenance due to insufficient knowledge of colostomy/ileostomy and/or ileal conduit
9. Potential for impaired elimination related to development of fistulae

1. Visceral abdominal pain, or pain from deep structures, tumor-related from distension or torsion, not well localized; "deep" and "aching" pain commonly reported
2. Sacral syndrome, aching pain in the low back, exacerbated by lying or sitting; may indicate bony infiltration
3. Lumbar plexopathy, pain that may reflect nerve infiltration in L1 to L3 radiating to anterior thigh or groin, or L5 to S1 radiating down leg to heel, with numbness
4. Sacral plexopathy, a dull, aching pain with sensory loss

5. Treatment-related pain. Radiation fibrosis chemotherapy induces peripheral neuropathies or postsurgical adhesions.
6. Tumor-related pain, or pressure or distention in the pelvic or abdominal area or bone; obstruction; or bowel or ureter fistula development

A nurse's role in medication selection is critical, as is assessing for the potential side effects of the medications. Common issues concerning side effects include occurrence with initial prescription or dose increase, the importance of ruling out other causes, and the physiologic adaptation that occurs over time. Treatment options for side effects include titrating down the dose, adding a coanalgesic, changing the opioid dose, and involving the patient in the prioritization of goals. Particularly challenging in cervix cancer are constipation,[66] nausea, and vomiting. Both disease and treatment may cause problems in these areas, requiring more detailed assessment and management plans.

Nonpharmocologic interventions for cancer pain management are varied and have been reported as successful by both patients and clinicians. Examples of nonpharmacologic pain-management methods include massage, applying alternating heat and cold, transcutaneous nerve stimulation, biofeedback acupuncture, and music therapy.[67–71]

Excellent work on cancer pain management has been done by such authors as Spross et al.[67,68,69] and Wilkie.[71] In addition, the entire issue of *Seminars in Oncology Nursing* (1985), vol. 1, no. 2, is devoted to cancer pain. Refer to these authors' works for a more comprehensive discussion of the physiology of pain. In addition, the Agency for Health Care Policy and Research (AHCPR) has published two valuable references for the clinician managing acute pain and cancer pain.[72,73] These free references from the DHHS outline specific pain management techniques, including pain prevention, assessment, and management options.

✳ NURSING MANAGEMENT

Nursing management of the woman with cervical cancer begins at the time of diagnosis. A diagnosis of cancer by itself has an impact that has been well described in the literature.[30,72–75] In addition, a diagnosis of cervical cancer sometimes causes an added stigma because of public awareness of the potential venereal causation factor.

Nursing care in the diagnosis and initial work-up phases revolves around patient teaching and support.[76] Those women who are eligible and opt to have a radical hysterectomy should have thorough preoperative teaching. Jusenius[76] wrote a comprehensive booklet for the woman undergoing radical hysterectomy, an outstanding teaching pamphlet that can be adapted by any gynecologic nurse oncologist for her/his particular setting. The teaching plan should include standard preoperative teaching (turning, coughing, deep breathing, early ambulation, etc.) but also an in-depth discussion of the possibility of postoperative voiding difficulties, including self-catheterization. Corney et al.[75] researched 105 patients who had undergone surgery for gynecologic malignancies. A high proportion of the women in the sample indicated that they wished they had received more information on the after-effects of the operation, including the long-term physical, sexual, and emotional effects of the surgery.

Nursing care issues for women who undergo radiation therapy also consist of thorough patient education and support, both before and throughout the course of treatment. Nursing care during radiation therapy revolves around reinforcement of teaching and the management of side effects. The most common side effects during treatment include diarrhea and fatigue. Long-term teaching needs include the use of water-soluble lubricants before sexual intercourse or vaginal dilator use for the sexually inactive woman. Nursing care related to the acute and long-term effects of radiation therapy are covered in Chapter 13.

Sexuality is an ongoing concern for everyone diagnosed with cancer but especially for the woman with cancer directly affecting her sexual and reproductive organs. Refer to Chapter 14 for an in-depth discussion of this aspect of nursing care.

Women who are diagnosed with recurrent, persistent, or advanced disease pose a special challenge to the gynecologic nurse oncologist. Few will be appropriate candidates for pelvic exenteration; the remainder will require long-term palliative care. Psychosocial and spiritual care become increasingly important aspects of nursing care in these cases.[77] Hospice care should be initiated early to optimize the transition from palliative to terminal care. Often difficult ethical issues arise during this phase of cancer care.[78] Euthanasia is one such issue that is becoming a more prevalent dilemma, and oncology nurses' attitudes regarding physician-assisted dying vary.[79] Gynecologic nurse oncologists should expect this and other ethical dilemmas to impact on their own practice. Continuing education, focus groups, and support networks can aid the clinician in coping with these ethical practice dilemmas. The emotional care of the patient with recurrent cancer of any type warrants careful nursing assessment to address coping and rehabilitative action.

✳ REFERENCES

1. ACS *Cancer Facts & Figures—1998.* American Cancer Society, Atlanta, GA.
2. JNCI (1998). Age distribution of cervical cancer. *J Natl Cancer Inst, 90*(20), 1510.
3. McCance, K.L., Huether, S.E. (1998). *Pathophysiology: The Biological Basis for Disease in Adults and Children* 3rd ed. St. Louis, MO: Mosby.
4. DiSaia, P.J., Creasman, W.T. (1997). *Clinical Gynecologic Oncology* 4th ed. St. Louis, MO: Mosby.
5. Richart, R.M., Masood, S., Syrjanen, K.J., Vassilakos, P., et al. (1998). Human papillomavirus. International Academy of Cytology Task Force summary. Diagnostic cytologu towards the 21st century: An international expert conference and tutorial. *Acta Cytol, 42*(1), 50–58.
6. Hording, U., Daugaard, S., & Visfeldt, J. (1997). Adenocarcinoma of the cervix and adenocarcinoma of the endometrium: Distinction with PCR-mediated detection of HPV DNA. *APMIS, 105*(4), 313–316.
7. Cannistra, S.A., Niloff, J.M. (1996) Cancer of the uterine cervix, *N Engl J Med, 334*(16), 1030–1038.
8. Bolli, J.A. & Maners, A. (1992). Age as a prognostic factor in cancer of the cervix: The UAMS experience. *J Ark Med Soc, 89*(2), 79–83.
9. Kaplan, M. (1989). Investigation of age as a prognostic factor in early stage invasive cancer of the cervix: Implications for nursing. *Cancer Nurs, 12*(3), 177–182.
10. Mandelblatt, J. (1993). Squamous cell cancer of the crevix: Immune senescence and HPV: Is cervical cancer an age-related neoplasm? *Adv Exp Med Biol, 330*, 13–26.
11. Mandelblatt, J., Andrews, H., Kerner, J., Zauber, A, & Burnett, W. (1991). Determinants of late stage diagnosis of breast cancer and cervical cancer: The

impact of age, race, social class, and hospital type. *Am J Public Health, 81*(5), 646–649.

12. Kelley, K.F., Galbraith, M.A., & Vermund, S.H. (1992). Genital human papilloma virus infection in women. *J Obstet Gynecol Neonatal Nurs, 21*(6), 503–515.

13. zur Hausen, H. (1994). Molecular patheogenesis of cancer of the cervix and its causation by specific human papilloma virus types. *Curr Top Microbiol Immunol, 186,*131–156.

14. zur Hausen, H. (1994). Disrupted dichotomous intracellular control of human papilloma virus infection in cancer of the cervix. *Lancet, 343*(8903), 955–957.

15. Lowy, D.R. & Schiller, J.T. (1998) Papillomaviruses and cervical cancer: Pathogenesis and vaccine development. *J Natl Cancer Inst, Supp. Monograph* (23), 27–30.

16. Storey, A., Thomas, M., Kalita, A., Harwood, C., Gardiol, D., Mantovani, F., Breuer, J., Leigh, I.M., Matlashewski, G., Banks, L. (1998) Role of p53 polymorphism in the development of human papilloma- virus-associated cancer. *Nature, 393,* 229–234.

17. AIDS Alert (1992). HIV-infected women threatened by cervical cancer. *AIDS Alert, 7*(2), 17–21.

18. Levine, A.M. (1993) AIDS-related malignancies: The emerging epidemic. *J Natl Cancer Inst, 85*(17), 1382–1397.

19. Parazzini, F., La Vecchia, C., Negri, E., Franceshi, S., Moroni, S., Chatenoud, L., Bolis, G. (1997) Case-controlled study of oestrogen replacement therapy and risk of cervical cancer. *Br Med J, 315*(7100), 85–88.

20. Hopkins, M.P., & Morley, G.W. (1993). Prognostic factors in advanced stage squamous cell cancer of the cervix. *Cancer, 72*(8),2389–2393.

21. Corn, B.W., Lanciano, R.M., King, S., & Cope, C. (1993). Lymphangiography as a staging tool for cervix cancer: Limited value after hip arthroplasty. *Clin Oncol, 5*(5),319–320.

22. Scheidler, J., Hricak, H., Yu, K.K., Subak, L., Segal, M.R. (1997) Radiologic evaluation of lymph node metastases in patients with cervical cancer: A meta-analysis. *JAMA, 278*(13), 1096–1101.

23. Cervical Cancer. NIH Consensus Development Conference Statement 1996 April 1–3; 14(1), 1–38.

24. Currie, D.W. (1971). Operative treatment of carcinoma of the cervix. *J Obstet Gynecol Br Commonw, 78*(5), 385–405.

25. Fletcher, G.H., & Rutledge, F.N. (1972). Extended field technique in the management of the cancers of the uterine cervix. *Am J Radiol, 114*(1), 116–122.

26. Hacker, N.F., Berek, J.S., & Lagase, L.D. (1982). Carcinoma of the cervix associated with pregnancy. *Obstet Gynecol, 59*(6), 735–746.

27. Hatch, K.D. (1989). Cervical cancer. In J.S. Berek & N.F. Hacker, eds. *Practical Gynecologic Oncology.* Baltimore: Williams & Wilkens.

28. Husseinzadeh, N., Nahhas, W.A., Velkley, D.E., Whitney, C.W., & Morrel, R. (1984). The preservation of ovarian function in young women undergoing pelvic radiation therapy. *Gynecol Oncol, 18*(3), 373–379.

29. Feeney, D.D., Moore, D.H., Look, K.Y., Stehman, F.B., & Sutton, G.P. (1995). The fate of the ovaries after radical hysterectomy and ovarian transposition. *Gynecol Oncol, 56*(1), 3–7.

30. Thompson L. (1990). Cancer of the cervix. *Semin Oncol Nurs, 6*(3), 190–197.

31. Montz, F.J., Holschnedier, C.H., Solh, S., Schuricht, L.C., & Monk, B.J. (1994). Small-bowel obstruction following radical hysterectomy: Risk factors, incidence, and operative findings. *Gynecol Oncol, 53*(1), 114–120.

32. Carenza, L., Nobili, F., & Giacobini, S. (1982). Voiding disorders after radical hysterectomy. *Gynecol Oncol, 13*(2), 213–219.

33. O'Laughlin, K.M. (1986). Changes in bladder function in the woman undergoing radical hysterectomy for cervical cancer. *J Obstet Gynecol Neonatal Nurs, 15*(5), 380–385.

34. Werngren-Elgstrom, M., & Lidman, D. (1994). Lymphedema of the lower extremities after surgery and radiotherapy for cancer of the cervix. *Scand L Plast Reconst Surg Hand Surg, 28*(4), 289–293.

35. Soisson, A.P., Soper, J.T., Berchuck, A., Dodge, R., & Clarke-Pearson, D. (1992). Radical hysterectomy in obsese women. *Obstet Gynecol, 80*(6), 940–943.

36. Perez, C.A. (1993). Radiation therapy in the management of cancer of the cervix. *Oncology, 7*(2), 89–96.

37. Russell, A.H. (1994). Contemporary radiation treatment planning for patients with cancer of the cervix *Semin Oncol, 21*(1), 30–41.

38. Morrow, C.P. (1980). Is pelvic radiation benefical in the postoperative management of stage Ib squamous cell carcinoma of the cervix with pelvic node metastasis treated by radical hysterectomy and pelvic lymphadenectomy? *Gynecol Oncol, 10*(1), 105–110.

39. Monk. B.J., Cha, D.S., Walker, J.L., & Burger, R.A. (1994). Extent of disease as an indication for pelvic radiation following radical hysterectomy and bilateral pelvic lymph node dissection in the treatment of stage Ib and IIa cervical carcinoma. *Gynecol Oncol, 54*(1), 4–9.

40. Johnston, C. (1998) Multiple therapies hit cervial cancer best. *Lancet, 352*(9103), 652.

41. Lanciano, R.M., Martz, K., Montana, G.S., & Hanks, G.E. (1992). Influence of age, prior abdominal surgery, fraction size, and dose on complications after radiation therapy for squamous cell cancer of the uterine cervix. *Cancer, 69*(8), 2124–2130.

42. Keys, H.M., Bundy, F.B., Stehman, F.B., Muderspach, L.I., Chafe, W.E., Suggs, C.L., Walker, J.L, Gersell, D. (1999) Cisplatin, radiation and adjuvant hysterectomy compared with radiation and adjuvant hysterectomy for bulky stage Ib cervical carcinoma. *N Engl J Med, 340*(15), 1154.

43. Rose, P.G., Bundy, B.N., Watkins, E.B., Thigpen, J.T., Deppe, G., Maiman, M.A., Clarke-Pearson, D.L., Insalaco, S. (1999) Concurrent cisplatin-based radiotherapy and chemotherapy for locally advanced cervical cancer. *N Engl J Med, 340*(15), 1144.

44. Morris, M., Eifel, P.J., Lu, J., Grigsby, P.W., Levenback, C., Stevens, R.E., Rotman, M., Gershenson, D.M., Mutch, D.G. (1999) Pelvic irradiation with concurrent chemotherapy compared with pelvic and para-aortic radiation for high-risk cervical cancer, *N Engl J Med, 340*(15), 1137.

45. Kim, R.Y., McGinnis, L.S., Spencer, S.A., & Meredith, R.F. (1995). Conventional four-field pelvic radiotherapy technique without computed tomography treatment planning in cancer of the cervix: Potential geographic miss and its impact on pelvic control. *Int J Radiat Oncol Biol Phys, 31*(1), 109-112.

46. Garcia-Angulo, A.H., & Kagiya, V.T. (1992). Intratumoral and parametrial infusion of 3-nitrotriazole (AK-2123) in the radiotherapy of the urerine cervix cancer, stage II-III: Preliminary positive results. *Int J Radiat Oncol Biol Phys, 22*(3), 589–591.

47. Hockel, M., Vorndran, B., Schlenger, K., Baussmann, E., & Knapstein, P.G. (1993). Tumor oxygenation: A new predictive parameter in locally advanced cancer of the uterine cervix. *Gynecol Oncol, 51*(2), 139–140.

48. Ogino, I., Kiramura, T., Okamoto, N., et al., (1995). Late rectal complication following high dose rate intracavitary brachytherapy in cancer of the cervix. *Int J Radiat Oncol Biol Phys, 31*(4), 725–734.

49. Andersen, B.L., & Turnquist, D.C. (1989). Psychological issues. In J.S. Berek and N. Hacker, eds. *Practical Gynecologic Oncology.* Baltimore: Williams & Wilkens.

50. Shingleton, H.M., & Orr, J.W. (1983). Cancer of the cervix: Diagnosis and treatment. New York: Churchill Livingstone.

51. McNeil, C. (1997) HPV vaccine treatment trials proliferate, diversify. *J Natl Cancer Inst, 89*(4), 280–1.

52. Stehman, F.C., Ballon, S.C., & Lagasse, L.D. (1979). Cisplatin in advanced gynecologic malignancy. *Gynecol Oncol, 7*(3), 349–360.

53. Omura, G.A. (1992). Current status of chemotherapy for cancer of the cervix. *Oncology, 6*(4), 27–32.

54. Dottino, P.R., & Segna, R.A. (1994) Neoadjuvant chemotherapy in cervix cancer. *Cancer Treat Res, 70,* 63–71.

55. Omura, G.A. (1994). Chemotherapy for cervix cancer. *Semin Oncol, 21*(1), 54–62.

56. McGuire, W.P., & Ball, H.(1990). *A Phase II Trial of Taxol in Patients with Advanced Cervical Carcinoma.* Philadelphia: Gynecologic Oncology Group.

57. Coleman, R.L., Keeney, E.D., Freedman, R.S., & Burke, T.W. (1994). Radical hysterectomy for recurrent carcinoma of the uterine cervix after radiotherapy. *Gynecol Oncol, 55*(1), 29–35.

58. Rutledge, S., Carey, M.S., Prichard, H., & Allen, H.H. (1994). Conservative surgery for persistent carcinoma of the cervix following irradiation: Is exenteration always necessary? *Gynecol Oncol, 52*(3), 353–359.

59. Magrina, J.F. (1993). Complications of irradiation and radical surgery for gynecologic malignancies. *Obstet Gynecol Surv, 48*(8), 571–575.

60. Monk, B.J., Walker, J.L., Tewari, K., & Ramsignhani, N.S. (1994). Open interstitial brachytherapy for the treatment of local-regional recurrences of uterine corpus and cervix cancer after primary surgery. *Gynecol Oncol, 52*(2), 222–228.

61. Omura, G.A., Hubbard, J.L., Harch, K.D., Schlaerth, J.B., & Blessing, J.A. (1992). Chemotherapy of cervix cancer with mitolactol (dibromodulcitol, NCS 104800) and cisplatin: A phase I study of the Gynecologic Oncology Group. *Am J Clin Oncol, 15*(3), 185–187.

62. Fanning, J., Ladd, C., & Hilgers, R.D. (1995). Cisplatin, s5-flourouracil, and ifosamide in the treatment of recurrent or advanced cervical cancer. *Gynecol Oncol, 56*(2), 235–238.

63. Miller, B., Morris, M., Rutledge, F., & Mitchell, M.F. (1993). Aborted exenterative procedures in recurrent cervical cancer. *Gynecol Oncol, 50*(1), 94–99.

64. Yarbrough, B. (1981) Teaching plan for patient undergoing total pelvic exenteration. *Onocol Nurs Forum, 8*(2), 36–40.

65. Anderson, M.D. (1981). Patient education series: Pelvic exenteration. *Oncol Nurs Forum, 8*(4), 54–56.

66. Canty, S.L. (1994). Constipation as a side effect of opioids. *Oncol Nurs Forum, 21*(4), 739–750.

67. Spross, J.A., McGuire, D.B., & Schmitt, R.M. (1990). Oncology Nursing Society position paper on cancer pain, part I. *Oncol Nurs Forum, 17*(4), 595–614.

68. Spross, J.A., McGuire, D.B., & Schmitt, R.M. (1990) Oncology Nursing Society paper on cancer pain, part II. *Oncol Nurs Forum, 17*(5), 751–760.

69. Spross, J.A., McGuire, D.B., & Schmitt, R.M. (1990). Oncology Nursing Society position paper on cancer pain, part III. *Oncol Nurs Forum, 17*(6), 943–955.

70. Beck, S.L. (1991). The theraprutic use of music for cancer-related pain. *Oncol Nurs Forum, 18*(8), 1327–1337.

71. Wilkie, D.J. (1990). Cancer pain management: State of the art nursing care. *Nurs Clin North Am, 25*(2), 331–343.

72. Agency for Health Care Policy and Research (1994). *Clinical Practice Guideline: Management of Cancer Pain* (no 9). Rockville, MD: US Department of Health and Human Services.

73. Agency for Health Care Policy and Research (1992). *Clinical Practice Guideline: Acute Pain Management: Operative or Medical Procedures and Trauma* (no 1). Rockville, MD: US Department of Health and Human Services.

74. McMullin, M. (1992). Holistic care of the patient with cervical cancer. *Nurs Clin North Am, 27*(4), 847–858.

75. Corney, R., Everett H., Howells, A., & Crowther, M. (1992). The care of patients undergoing surgery for gynecologic cancer: The need for information, emotional support and counseling. *J Adv Nurs, 17*(6), 667–671.

76. Jusenius, K. (1983). A reaching aid for the radical hysterectomy patient. *Oncol Nurs Forum, 10*(2), 71–75.

77. Mahon, S. (1991). Managing the psychosocial consequences of cancer recurrence: Implications for nurses. *Oncol Nurs Forum, 18*(3), 577–583.

78. Winters, G., Glass, E., & Sakurai, C. (1993). Ethical issues in oncology nursing practice: An overview of topics and strategies. *Oncol Nurs Forum, 20*(10) suppl., 21–34.

79. Young, A., Volker, D., Rieger, P.T., & Thorpe, D.M. (1993). Oncology nurses' attitudes regarding voluntary physician-assisted dying for competent terminally ill patients. *Oncol Nurs Forum, 20*(3), 445–454.

CHAPTER 4

Cancers of the Vulva and Vagina

Giselle J. Moore-Higgs, ARNP, MSN, AOCN

❈ INTRODUCTION

Overview

Malignancies of the vulva and vagina are relatively rare genital neoplasms, with the greatest frequency of occurrence in the seventh and eighth decades of life. Historically, malignancies of the vulva have accounted for approximately 3 to 5% of all female genital malignancies, and malignancies of the vagina have accounted for 1–2%.[1] In the 1997 FIGO annual report, 3–5% of female genital malignancies are found on the vulva.[2] Green also reported that, in his experience, malignancies of the vulva accounted for 5% of gynecologic malignancies seen from 1927 through 1961 but increased to 8% in the next twelve years.[3] This increase is probably reflective of two epidemiologic factors that may be significantly impacting the incidence of both malignancies. The first is the rapid growth of the population of women in their seventh and eighth decades of life. Since 1900, the percentage of people over the age of 65 has tripled, and the trend continues. It is estimated that by the year 2000, 13% of the population of the United States will be over 65 years of age, with women making up the majority.[4] The second factor is the increasing number of women under age 65 who are presenting with human papilloma viral infections, intraepithelial neoplasia, and subsequent invasive malignancies of the vaginal and vulvar epithelium (Table 4.1). This phenomenon, along with the extensive morbidity associated with treatment, continues to challenge the health care team in all facets of both diseases.

TABLE 4.1

Incidence of Cancer of the Vulva

Age Groups	Intraepithelial (%)	Invasive (%)
20–30	9.8	2.5
31–40	29.2	14.2
41–50	17.1	13.3
51–60	9.8	25.8
61–70	26.8	25.0
71–80	4.9	12.5
81–90	2.4	6.7
Total	100.0	100.0

Source: Reprinted with permission from Krupp, P.J. Jr. (1992). Invasive tumors of the vulva: Clinical features, staging, and management. In M. Coppleson, ed., *Gynecologic Oncology: Fundamental Principles and Clinical Practice* 2nd ed. (p. 480). New York: Churchill Livingstone.

Anatomy of the Vulva and Vagina

The vulva consists of those portions of the female genital tract that are externally visible in the perineal region, lying between the genitocrural folds laterally, the mons pubis anteriorly, and the anus posteriorly (Figure 4.1). Included are the vulvar vestibule, the clitoris, the labia minora, labia majora, and the mons pubis.

The vulvar vestibule is the portion of the vulva that extends from the exterior surface of the hymen to the frenulum of the clitoris anteriorly, fourchette posteriorly, and to Hart's line laterally.[5] Hart's line is a distinctive mark on the vulva where the nonkeratinized squamous epithelium of the vestibule joins the more papillated-appearing keratinized epithelium of the lateral labia minora. The vestibule is composed of stratified, nonkeratinized squamous epithelium. Structures within the vestibule include the urethral orifice, vaginal introitus, openings of the Bartholin's gland ducts, and openings of the minor vestibular glands.[5] The urethral orifice is a small (4–6 mm) opening situated about 2.5 cm below the clitoris. It is surrounded by the Skene's glands, which are homologous to the prostate in the male. The Bartholin's glands (also known as the greater vestibular glands) are a pair of pea-sized mucus-secreting glands that are visible on each side of the vestibule, between the hymen and the labia minora.

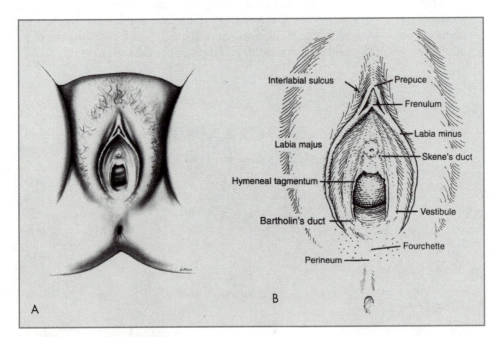

FIGURE 4.1. Anatomy of the vulva.

Source: Reproduced with permission from Wilkinson, E.J., & Stone, I.K. (1995). *Atlas of Vulvar Disease* (pp. 1–13). Baltimore, MD: Williams & Wilkins.

The hymen, a thin, vascularized membrane that separates the vagina from the vestibule, is usually not present after the onset of vaginal coitus. The clitoris is a small erectile organ, rich in sensory receptors, that is situated at the lower border of the symphysis and is homologous to the corpus cavernosum of the male penis. The clitoris consists of two cylindrical erectile bodies, called the corpora cavernosa, that terminate in the vulvar vestibule as the glans. The epithelium is primarily squamous mucosa without glands or dermal papillae.[5]

The labia minora lie between the labia majora and are separated laterally from the labia majora by the intralabial sulcus. Anteriorly, the labia minora split, then fuse beneath the clitoris as the frenulum and above the clitoris to form the prepuce. They are thin folds of redundant connective tissue, composed of highly vascular erectile tissue covered with stratified squamous epithelium, which is not keratinized on the vestibular surface and thinly keratinized on the lateral surface. The labia minora are relatively prominent in children since the labia majora are not well developed until puberty.

The labia majora are two longitudinal folds of skin that extend in an elliptical manner from the mons pubis posteriorly to enclose the vulvar cleft. The labia majora are covered with stratified squamous epithelium, which is hair-bearing in the lateral and midportions of the labial surface and hairless on the medial surfaces.[5] These hair shafts are associated with sebaceous glands and apocrine sweat glands. Both the sebaceous and apocrine glands are stimulated by sex hormones; however, the apocrine sweat glands are functional throughout life.[5] In some postmenopausal women, the labia majora tend to atrophy, and the labia minora again become prominent.

The mons pubis is the portion of the vulva presenting as the rounded, fleshy prominence over the symphysis pubis. The surface of the mons is composed of stratified squamous epithelium, similar to that of the labia majora, with hair and sebaceous glands distributed throughout its substance. The underlying tissue of the mons is composed primarily of adipose tissue.[5]

The vagina is a thin-walled, muscular, dilatable tube averaging 8 to 10 cm in length that passes obliquely upward and backward at an angle of approximately 45 degrees from the introitus in the vestibule to the uterus (Figure 4.2). It attaches circumferentially to the uterine cervix at a higher point on the posterior wall than on the anterior wall, forming a circular groove at the junction, called the *fornix*. The base of the bladder is in direct contact with the upper third of the anterior vaginal wall, the urethra is in contact with the lower two-thirds of the anterior vaginal wall, and the rectum lies directly below the posterior vaginal wall.

The vagina is composed of three layers of tissue. The lower part of the vagina is lined with a thick, nonkeratinizing, nonglandular, stratified squamous epithelium. The upper two-thirds is derived initially from glandular tissue, which usually undergoes a process of metaplasia in utero to form a "mucosa" of nonkeratinized, stratified squamous epithelium extending onto the ectocervix. This process is halted or modified in those pregnancies where maternal DES ingestion has occurred and, occasionally, without DES exposure.[6] The mucosa forms many transverse folds, called rugae, and is lubricated by mucus emanating from the cervix and, during intercourse, from

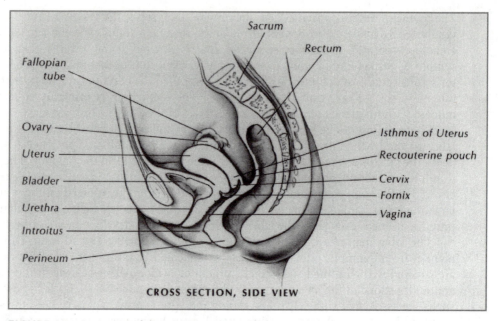

FIGURE 4.2. Anatomy of the vagina.

Source: Reproduced with permission from Bates, B. (1995). *A Guide to Physical Examination* 6th ed. (p. 378). Philadelphia: J.B. Lippincott.

the Bartholin's glands.[6] The muscularis layer is composed of smooth muscle fibers arranged circularly on the inner portion and longitudinally on the thicker outer portion. The adventitia is a thin, outer connective tissue layer that merges with that of adjacent organs.[7] The vaginal sphincter at the introitus is formed by skeletal muscle.

The blood supply to the vulva is abundant and comes from branches of the internal and external pudendal artery. The vagina is supplied with arterial blood from branches of the internal iliac and uterine arteries. The vulva, the lower third of the vagina, and the perineum are drained by a network of lymphatics that terminate in the inguinal and femoral lymph nodes (Figure 4.3). The lymphatic drainage of the upper vagina shares the lymphatic drainage of the cervix, namely, the ureteral, hypogastric, obturator, external iliac, lateral sacral, and promontory nodes in the pelvis (Figure 4.4).

The perineum is supplied by the pudendal nerve and its branches, as well as by direct fibers from the fourth sacral nerve. Autonomic nerves are conveyed to the lower vagina, to the erectile tissue of the vestibule, and to the clitoris by fibers from the inferior portion of the pelvic plexus, a continuation of the hypogastric plexus. The vaginal sympathetic nerve supply is derived from the hypogastric plexus, with parasympathetic fibers supplied from the second and third sacral nerves.

FIGURE 4.3. Lymphatic drainage of the vulva.

Source: Reproduced with permission from DiSaia, P.J., & Creasman, W.T. (1997). Invasive cancer of the vulva. *Clinical Gynecologic Oncology* 4th ed. (p. 244). St. Louis, MO: Mosby Year Book, Inc.

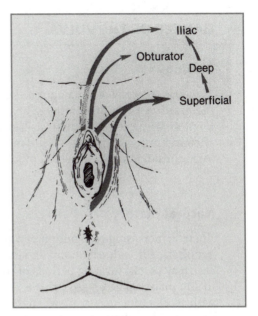

FIGURE 4.4. Lymphatic drainage of the vagina. Metastases from vaginal carinoma may spread to the pelvic (A) and inguinal lymph nodes (B). The pattern is contingent on the location of the cancer in the vagina. Disease in the lower two-thirds of the vagina can spread by way of the pelvic or inguinal lymph nodes. Upper vaginal disease is more likely to metastasize only to pelvic lymph nodes.

Source: Clarke-Pearson, D.L., & Darwood, M.Y. (1990). *Green's Gynecology: Essentials of Clinical Practice* 4th ed. (p. 560). Boston: Little, Brown and Company.

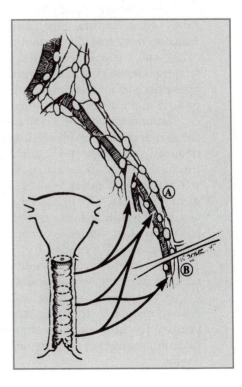

✠ CANCER OF THE VULVA

Etiology

The exact etiology of squamous cell carcinoma of the vulva is unknown, although it is theorized to be multifactorial. Debate continues regarding the role of human papilloma viral infections, genetic cofactors, other bacterial and viral infections, and/or chemical exposure in the development of this disease. Chapter 1 outlines these etiologic considerations as well as epidemiologic factors.

Natural History

There is increasing recognition of a progression of vulvar disease from intraepithelial neoplasia, through carcinoma in situ, to invasive carcinoma. The intraepithelial disease may persist for long periods of time; case data indicate ten years or longer for the in situ phases. The invasive disease tends to be slowly progressive in the early stages, with acceleration occurring when the disease penetrates the epithelial basement membrane and lymphatic dissemination occurs.[8]

Vulvar cancer spreads by three common routes: direct extension to adjacent organs (vagina, urethra, anus), lymphatic embolization to regional lymph nodes, and hematogenous spread to distant organs (liver, lungs, and bone).[9] Lymphatic drainage of the vulva is a progressive systematic mechanism, with the superficial inguinal lymph nodes serving as the primary, or sentinel, lymph nodes of the vulva; followed by the deep femoral lymph nodes; and finally, the pelvic lymphatics. The incidence of positive inguinal and pelvic lymph nodes varies considerably in the literature. The recent introduction of lymphatic mapping techniques used immediately prior to surgical resection may provide the necessary information to resolve this controversy. Most frequently, the ipsilateral inguinal group of lymph nodes is involved first, with contralateral metastases occurring rarely.[8] Lymphatic invasion increasingly occurs as the size of the lesion grows. With invasive lesions up to 3 cm in size, lymph node involvement is found in 9.7% of cases, increasing to 42.5 % in larger lesions.[10] The overall incidence of lymph node metastasis in cancer of the vulva is approximately 30%. Hacker has reported an incidence of nodal metastasis in terms of the FIGO stages (1969) as approximately 10% in stage I, 26% in stage II, 65% in stage III, and 90% in stage IV.[11] The incidence of pelvic lymph node involvement is approximately 5%, occurring rarely in the absence of clinically positive inguinal lymph nodes.[12]

As the primary invasive lesion progresses, other sites on the vulva may proceed to neoplasia, resulting in multifocal sites of disease. The progression of the primary lesion is often accompanied by increasing size, necrosis, and secondary infection producing an extremely foul odor. Hematogenous spread is late and uncommon.[8]

Clinical Manifestations

In 1854, Charles Meigs astutely observed that successful treatment of vulvar neoplasia was significantly impaired by delayed diagnosis resulting from patients' and physicians' attitudes.[13,14] Although 135 years have passed since Meigs's observation, numerous reports in the medical literature confirm that the two most significant obstacles to the successful evaluation and treatment of vulvar neoplasia continue to be delayed patient presentation (2–16 months) and delayed physician evaluation with biopsy for definitive diagnosis (up to 12 months or longer).[14]

There are a variety of presenting symptoms related to malignancies of the vulva. The most common symptoms are a mass or lump with associated pruritus (Table 4.2). Pruritus is present in up to 80% of patients with early invasive disease and may have been present for many years.[15] Bleeding, discharge, dysuria, dyspareunia, a lesion that does not heal, and vulvar pain are more common in advanced stage disease. Occasionally, urinary incontinence, due to fistulae or urethral obstruction, is present in extensive disease involving the anterior wall of the vagina. Metastatic disease to one or both groins, presenting as a mass or lump, may also be the first indication of a problem, although this is rare. The duration of symptoms does not appear to correlate with the size of the lesion, presence of metastatic disease in regional lymph nodes, or recurrence rates and may be an indication only of the duration of coexistent dystrophy.[16]

On physical examination, the lesion may also have a variety of manifestations (Figures 4.5 and 4.6). It may appear superficial or deep and ulcerated; raised and fleshy; leukoplakic; warty; or as a firm lump. Warty tumors have been reported to account for 20% of vulvar squamous lesions.[17] Most squamous cell malignancies arise as unilateral lesions on the labia majora (40%), more commonly on the right than the left.[18] Other primary sites, in descending order of frequency, are the labia minora (20%), the clitoris, prepuce and mons (10%), and the perineum and posterior

TABLE 4.2
Clinical Presentation of Cancer of the Vulva
Lump or Mass
Vulvar Pruritus
Bleeding
Discharge
Dysuria
Dyspareunia
Lesion that will not heal
Incontinence
Vulvar Pain

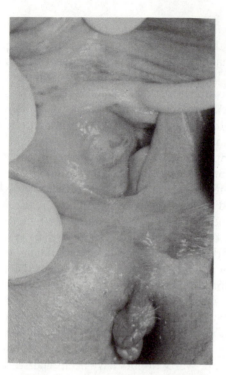

FIGURE 4.5. Early stage malignancy of the vulva.

Source: Courtesy of the Division of Gynecology Oncology, Department of Obstetrics and Gynecology at the University of Florida College of Medicine, Gainesville, FL.

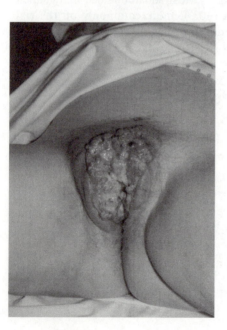

FIGURE 4.6. Late stage malignancy of the vulva.

Source: Courtesy of the Division of Gynecology Oncology, Department of Obstetrics and Gynecology at the University of Florida College of Medicine, Gainesville, FL.

fourchette (15%).[19] Multifocal lesions occur in 10 to 30% of cases.[16] Early-stage lesions are usually localized and well demarcated; however, in advanced-stage disease, the disease on the vulva may be so extensive that precise determination of the primary site may be difficult.

Diagnostic Method

During initial presentation, a detailed history and careful examination of the entire vulva, vagina, and cervix assist in defining symptoms and contributing factors. Figure 4.7 is an example of an assessment form used for vulvovaginal consultations. Such a form is helpful in the documentation of both symptoms and contributing factors for both benign and malignant lesions. In addition, a diagram and written description of the lesion should be included, and lesions should be distinguished primarily by their surface contour, size, color, and anatomy involved. Table 4.3 provides a useful descriptive classification of different types of lesions.

Using the colposcope to provide a magnified examination of the vagina and cervix, as well as obtaining a Pap smear of the cervix, is encouraged to evaluate for additional lesions. A tissue biopsy of the lesion is necessary to determine the histology, which will influence recommendations for treatment. DiSaia and Creasman recommend using the following indications for excisional biopsy of a vulvar nevus: a change in surface area of the nevus, a change in elevation, a change in color, a change in surface type (smooth to scaly to ulcerated) or a change in sensation (itching or tingling).[20] Usually these procedures can be performed without difficulty in an office setting (Figure 4.8). Shaving the vulva, or even the biopsy site, is not necessary, though clipping a portion of the pubic hair with scissors may be helpful. Biopsies of vulvar tissue should be performed under sterile conditions and after appropriate preparation of the skin with an antiseptic solution. Subcutaneous injections of the biopsy site with a small amount of local anesthetic solution (e.g., 1% lidocaine hydrochloride, with or without epinephrine) using a 25-gauge needle usually provides satisfactory relief from pain.[21] Occasionally, tender, inflamed lesions may benefit from a topical preanesthetic (e.g., 20% benzocaine spray) before infiltration with lidocaine.[5] A dermatologic punch is commonly used to obtain biopsies and is available as a disposable instrument. The punch is pushed against the area to be biopsied, and a circular area of skin or tissue is removed. Depending on the site of the biopsy, closure of the site is easily accomplished with absorbable suture; delayed absorbable suture material may also be used. If the biopsy is taken from the core of a large, erosive defect, closure may not be possible, in which case packing may be necessary to prevent hemorrhage or infection. Monsel's (ferrous subsulfate) solution may also be useful to stop bleeding from large tumor masses. Hematomas of the vulva have resulted from use of a punch biopsy pressed too deeply into the subcuticular tissue. These are painful and may increase the risk of a superficial infection.

Proper fixation, orientation, and labeling of specimens are critical for determining histology and depth of invasion. They should be received by the laboratory fixed in an

Vulvovaginal Consultation

Patient Name: _____ MR #: _____

Name: _____ Date: _____ Age: _____

Ht.: _____ Wt.: _____ Race: ☐ White ☐ Black ☐ Asian ☐ Hisp. ☐ Other _____

Marital Status: ☐ Married ☐ Single ☐ Widowed ☐ Divorced Parity: ☐ Term ☐ Prem ☐ AB ☐ Living

LMP: _____ Contraception: _____

Menstrual Hygiene: ☐ N/A ☐ Tampons ☐ Pads ☐ Both ☐ Deodorant Coital Frequency: _____

Occupation: _____ Sports/Exercise: _____

Present Illness: _____

Major Symptoms: _____

_____ Duration: _____

Changed by: ☐ Coitus ☐ Menses ☐ Clothing ☐ Position/Activity ☐ Diet ☐ Other _____

Similar Disease in Family/Partner: _____ On Other Body Sites: _____

Recent Therapy: _____

Relevant History: _____

Surgical: _____ Psychiatric: _____

Medical: _____ Medication: _____

Foreign Travel: _____

Spinal Injury, Surgery, or Symptoms: _____

Estrogen Replacement: _____ Allergies: _____ Diabetes: Family _____ Self _____

Prior Vaginitis: _____ HPV: _____ HSV: _____ Other STD: _____

Underwear Fabric: _____ Laundry Products Now Used: _____ Incontinence: _____

Vulvar Hygiene: _____ Douche Hx: _____

Hot Tub/Spa: _____ Ever Catheterized? _____

Description of Findings: _____

Vulva: _____

Attach Photo

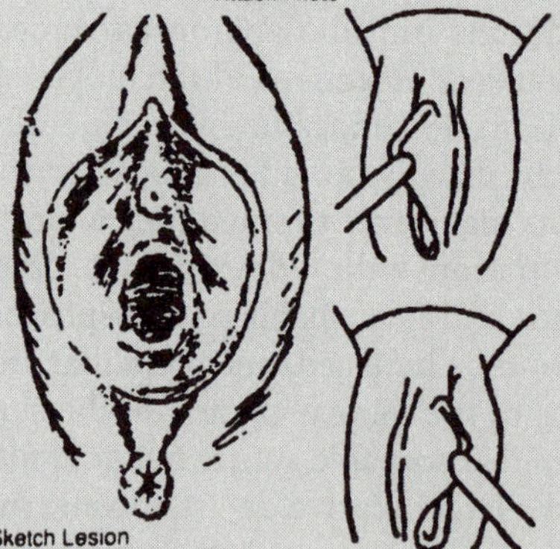

Vagina: Cells: ☐ Clue ☐ WBC

pH: _____ Flora: _____

Discharge: _____

Mucosa: _____

Cervix: _____

Bimanual: _____

Initial Impression: _____

_____

Plan: _____

_____

Sketch Lesion
Indicate Biopsy Site ⊗

_____ , MD
Director/Attending

FIGURE 4.7. Vulvovaginal consultation form.

Source: Reproduced with permission from Wilkinson, E.J., & Stone, I.K. (1995). *Atlas of Vulvar Disease* (pp. 1–13). Baltimore, MD: Williams & Wilkins.

TABLE 4.3

Classification of Vulvar Lesions by Visual Clinical Presentation

Type of Lesion	Definition
Macule	A flat lesion demonstrating no elevation above contiguous skin
Papule	A well-defined, elevated lesion with solid matrix
Plaque	An elevated, relatively flat area of skin
Verruca	An elevated lesion with a horny appearance
Erosion	A defect resulting from partial loss of the epithelium
Ulcer	A depressed defect in the skin that results from destruction or loss of the dermis and epidermis
Tumor	A neoplasm in the skin or subcuticular tissue

Source: Reprinted with permission from Wilkinson, E.J., & Stone, I.K. (1995). *Atlas of Vulvar Disease* (pp. 1–13). Baltimore, MD: Williams & Wilkins.

appropriate solution, placed on a piece of lens paper or some other adhesive, and oriented either on edge or on end. The specimens' orientation should be indicated so that the technician can appropriately reorient the tissue in the paraffin block. Some pathologists prefer solutions other than 10% formalin because they yield comparatively better cytologic characteristics, especially if fixation of the specimens is delayed.[22]

FIGURE 4.8. Outpatient vulva biopsy set.

Source: Reproduced with permission from Deppe, G., & Lawrence, W.D., Intraepithelial vulvar neoplasia, in S.B. Gusberg, H.M. Singleton, & G. Deppe, eds., *Female Genital Cancer,* Churchill Livingstone, New York, 1988, p. 226.

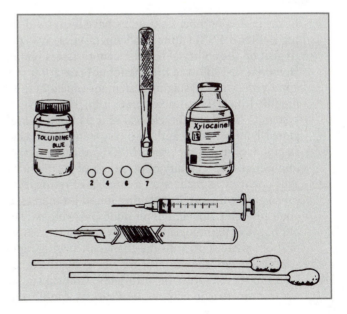

TABLE 4.4	
Diagnostic Studies for Vulva Cancer	
Radiologic Study	*Rationale*
Chest X-ray	Identify possible metastatic disease
IVP	Identify ureteral obstruction
Urethroscopy	Identify invasion of the urethra
Barium Enema	Identify invasion of the rectum
Colonoscopy	Identify invasion of the rectum
CT Scan or MRI (Abdomen/Pelvis)	Identify metastatic disease within the pelvis, retroperitoneum, and groin
Lymphangiography or lymphatic mapping	Identify involvement of lymphatics

Only histologic evaluation of the lymph nodes can determine metastatic involvement. This is obtained with a fine-needle aspiration or during lymphadenectomy. However, careful clinical examination of the regional lymph nodes that drain the vulva is vital in determining the probable extent of the disease. This includes palpation of the superficial inguinal lymph nodes and deep femoral lymph nodes. Additional studies that may be obtained to determine extent of disease and metastatic disease are listed in Table 4.4.

Staging

In the past, a number of systems have been used to stage cancer of the vulva, including a clinical TNM (tumor/node/metastasis) system, adopted in 1971, which was contingent on the ability of the clinician to assess lymph node involvement by palpation.[1] However, in 1989, the International Federation of Gynecology & Obstetrics (FIGO) approved a surgical staging system for cancer of the vulva (Table 4.5). This system was modified in 1995 to incorporate a microinvasive category into Stage I disease. This system is based on the clinical and pathologic evaluation of the primary lesion, regional lymph nodes, and sites of potential metastasis (TNM) classification. Surgical staging recognizes the prognostic significance of the status of the lymph nodes and acknowledges the inability of palpation of groin nodes to determine metastatic disease.[9] This change was made after a number of retrospective studies comparing initial clinical staging with surgical staging found an increased incidence of nodal metastasis in clinically nonpalpable lymph nodes, as well as overdiagnosis of clinically suspicious but negative pathologic inguinal lymph nodes.[1] It is important to remember that publications written prior to the change in staging report data utilize the original clinical staging system; therefore, it may be difficult to compare patient outcome with that found in the literature prior to 1989. Clinical staging may still be used in the woman who for any reason may not be a surgery candidate, however.

TABLE 4.5

Surgical Staging of Vulva Malignancies

Stage	Tumor (T)	Node (N)	Metastasis (M)	Clinical Findings
Stage 0	TIS	N0	M0	Carcinoma in situ; intraepithelial carcinoma
Stage I	T1	N0	M0	Tumor confined to the vulva and/or perineum; 2 cm or less in greatest dimension; no nodal metastasis
Stage Ia				Lesions 2 cm or less in size confined to the vulva or perineum and with stromal invasion no greater than 1.0 mm*; no nodal metastasis
Stage Ib				Lesions 2 cm or less in size confined to the vulva or perineum and with stromal invasion greater than 1.0 mm; no nodal metastasis
Stage II	T2	N0	M0	Tumor confined to the vulva or perineum; more than 2 cm in greatest dimension; no nodal metastasis
Stage III	T3	N0	M0	Tumor of any size with adjacent spread to the urethra, vagina, or the anus or with unilateral regional lymph node metastasis
	T3	N1	M0	
	T1	N1	M0	
	T2	N1	M0	
Stage IVa	T1	N2	M0	Tumor invading upper urethra, bladder mucosa, rectal mucosa, pelvic bone; or bilateral regional node metastases
	T2	N2	M0	
	T3	N2	M0	
	T4	Any	M0	
Stage IVb	Any T	Any N	M1	Any distant metastasis, including pelvic lymph nodes

* The depth of invasion is defined as the measurement of the tumor from the epithelial-stromal junction of the adjacent most superficial dermal papilla to the deepest point of invasion.

Source: Used with permission of the American Joint Committee on Cancer (AJCC®), Chicago, Illinois. The original source for this material is the *AJCC® Cancer Staging Manual,* 5th edition (1997) published by Lippincott-Raven Publishers, Philadelphia, Pennsylvania.

Histopathology

Most malignancies of the vulva arise within squamous epithelium already involved by an epithelial cell abnormality. Studies have reported that an estimated 85% of superficial invasive squamous cell carcinoma lesions and 60% of frankly invasive lesions have adjacent vulvar intraepithelial neoplasia.[23] In addition, lichen sclerosis, usually associated with squamous cell hyperplasia, can be found in 15 to 40% of cases.[9]

The pathologic features that must be evaluated in addition to tumor stage include the type of tumor, grade of tumor, depth of invasion, vascular space invasion, and the growth pattern of the tumor. The depth of invasion is defined as the measurement from the epithelial stromal junction of the most superficial adjacent dermal papilla to the deepest point of invasion. Tumor thickness is measured from the overlying surface epithelium, or the bottom of the granular layer if the surface is keratinized, to the deepest point of invasion, as specified by the International Society of Gynecologic Pathologists (ISGP) subcommittee. Vascular space involvement can be defined as the findings of tumor within an endothelial-lined vascular space; it is associated with a higher frequency of lymph node metastasis and an overall lower five-year survival rate in cancer of the vulva.[24,25] The description of the tumor growth pattern, such as confluent, compact, or fingerlike, may also influence the rate of lymph node metastasis and subsequent survival.[9]

Table 4.6 shows histologic classification of malignant tumors, and Table 4.7 lists the incidence of each classification.

Paget's disease of the vulva is rare. These lesions typically present as an eczematous, red, weeping area on the vulva, often localized to the labia majora, perineal body, clitoris, or other sites. In advanced disease, there may be spread to the mon pubis, thighs, vagina, and buttocks.[22] Paget's disease commonly occurs in older, postmenopausal white women. It is often misdiagnosed initially, since the presentation is similar to benign skin diseases; consequently, it may have been present for a long period of time. Approximately 15% of women with Paget's disease of the vulva have an underlying primary adenocarcinoma arising within the apocrine glands or the underlying Bartholin's glands.[9] Treatment and prognosis are dependent on the presence of adenocarcinoma, thus stressing the importance of adequate assessment by palpation and tissue biopsy during initial evaluation.

Squamous cell carcinomas are the most common malignant lesions found on the vulva. They vary from small pigmented flat lesions, to shallow, indurated ulcers with elevated, nodular margins, to large, fungating confluent neoplasms with necrotic, hemorrhagic, and infected surfaces. The surrounding vulvar skin may appear normal but commonly shows localized or generalized dystrophy.[16] The vast majority of squamous cell carcinomas of the vulva are well-differentiated (grade I) lesions.[22] There are some variants of vulvar squamous cell carcinoma, including adenoid squamous, squamous cell carcinoma with tumor giant cells, sebaceous cell carcinoma, and spindle cell–squamous cell carcinoma.[9]

Since squamous cell carcinoma is the most common malignancy found on the vulva, the majority of the data regarding staging, prognostic factors, natural history, and primary treatment of cancer of the vulva are based on this histology.

TABLE 4.6

Histologic Classification of Malignant Tumors of the Vulva

Primary Tumors	
Carcinomas	
Intraepithelial	Squamous cell neoplasia (VIN)
	Adenocarcinoma (Paget's disease)
Invasive	Squamous cell carcinoma
	Verrucous carcinoma
	Basal cell carcinoma
	Basaloid (cloacogenic) carcinoma
	Melanoma
	Neuroendocrine (Merkel cell)
	Adenocarcinoma and variants
Sarcomas	Rhabdomyosarcoma and other rare variants
Metastatic Tumors	
Carcinomas	Breast, lung, cervix, gastrointestinal
Sarcomas	

Source: Adapted with permission from Ferenczy, A. (1992). Pathology of malignant tumors of the vulva and vagina. In M. Coppleson, ed., *Gynecologic Oncology: Fundamental Principles and Clinical Practice* 2nd ed. (p. 419). New York: Churchill Livingstone.

TABLE 4.7

Incidence of Cancer of the Vulva by Histology

Histology	*Percentage*
Epidermoid	86.2
Melanoma	4.8
Sarcoma	2.2
Basal Cell	1.4
Bartholin's Gland	1.0
Adenocarcinoma	0.6
Undifferentiated	3.9

Source: Adapted with permission from Plentl, A.A., & Friedman, E.A. (1971). *Lymphatic System of the Female Genitalia* (p. 28). Philadelphia: W.B. Saunders.

Verrucous carcinoma is another variant of squamous cell carcinoma and presents as a florid, white, exophytic, cauliflowerlike papillary growth that may be locally destructive and include direct bone invasion.[26] Some of the larger lesions may present with superficial ulcerations and a prurulent drainage. These lesions usually occur in postmenopausal women who have a warty lesion that has been present for a long period of time and appears to be growing slowly. Metastasis to regional lymph nodes is rare. These lesions lend themselves to aggressive local excision and overall have a good prognosis. Radiotherapy is not advised, as there is a poor cure rate and a significant risk of malignant transformation of the tumor into an anaplastic carcinoma.[27]

Basal cell carcinoma is a relatively rare tumor of the vulva, comprising 2 to 4% of infiltrative neoplasms arising on the vulva.[9] The etiology of these lesions on the vulva is obscure, considering that most basal cell carcinomas appear to be related to sun exposure. They are commonly found on the labia majora of elderly women and are slow-growing malignancies arising from primordial basal cells of the epidermis. The two most common types are the superficial plaque, which has a rough, darkly pigmented or reddish crusted surface, and the rodent ulcer, which consists of a circumscribed, indurated nodule with elevated borders and central, superficial ulceration.[22] Presenting symptoms may include pruritus with occasional bleeding and interval periods of healing. These tumors tend to be locally invasive, with infiltrative margins and satellite nodules. Occasionally, they present as multicentric lesions. Lesions with positive margins after biopsy have a high rate of recurrence. Metastasis to regional lymph nodes is rare, lending to a good overall prognosis with adequate wide local excision of the lesion.

Basaloid (cloacogenic carcinoma) is a rare lesion of the vulva that appears as a firm, nodular growth deep in the labia majora, rectovaginal septum, or perineum.[22] The prognosis is generally poor due to early lymph node metastasis.

Neuroendocrine (Merkel cell) carcinomas are very aggressive neoplasms that histologically resemble small cell carcinomas of the neuroendocrine type in other body sites, such as lung and the head and neck region. These tumors frequently have both regional lymph node and distant metastasis and are associated with a poor prognosis.[9]

Adenocarcinoma and Bartholin's gland carcinoma. Most adenocarcinomas arise in the Bartholin's glands, although they may arise occasionally in the vestibular glands or rarely in the sweat gland. They are rare, representing 0.1% of all female genital tract neoplasms and 2 to 3% of all vulvar carcinomas.[19] Variants of vulvar adenocarcinoma include mucoepidermoid carcinoma, adenoacanthoma, adenosquamous, papillary, mesonephric adenocarcinoma, and endodermal sinus tumor in infants.[22]

Carcinoma of the Bartholin's gland generally occurs in older women. These tumors are often deeply invasive and difficult to detect in their early growth. Due to the location of the gland, dyspareunia is often the initial symptom noticed. Patients may give a lengthy history of inflammation of the gland. In general practice, if a woman over 50 years presents with an enlarged Bartholin's gland that does not resolve after attempt at aspiration, a biopsy should be performed.

Other malignancies of the vulva. A number of other rare malignancies can occur as either primary or metastatic lesions to the vulva. The other primary lesions include malignant melanoma, malignant schwannoma, yolk sac tumors, adenocarcinoma arising in ectopic breast tissue, transitional cell carcinomas, and adenoid cystic carcinoma.[9] An in-depth review of malignant melanoma of both the vulva and vagina is presented later in this chapter. Lesions metastatic to the vulva tend to arise in the labia majora and Bartholin's gland, with the primary sites including the lower genital tract, lower gastrointestinal tract, breast, kidney, stomach, and/or lung. Although these lesions are rare, the treatment options and prognosis are based on the accurate pathologic evaluation and the natural history of the primary malignancy.

Primary sarcomas of the vulva. A number of sarcomas may arise primarily in the vulva. These include leiomyosarcoma, malignant fibrous histiocytoma, epithelioid sarcoma, malignant rhabdoid tumor, angiosarcoma, Kaposi's sarcoma, hemangiopericytoma, rhabdomyosarcoma, alveolar soft part sarcoma, and liposarcoma.[9] Further discussion of these tumors is found in Chapter 9.

Treatment

Surgery

Radical vulvectomy, along with surgical excision of the bilateral regional lymph nodes, was described in 1912 by Basset as the standard approach to the treatment of carcinoma of the vulva.[28] Taussig[29] and Way[30] pioneered improvements to the procedure, with establishment of the en bloc radical vulvectomy and bilateral inguinal lymphadenectomy, with or without pelvic node dissection, as the treatment of choice for all patients with operable vulvar cancer. This radical surgery substantially improved overall cure rates, with corrected five-year survival rates for stages I and II reported by many authors as approximately 90%.[1] Unfortunately, this extensive procedure led to a significant postoperative morbidity, including a high rate of skin incision separation, wound breakdown, and infection, necessitating healing by secondary intention and prolonged hospitalization. In turn this led to subsequent devastating and disabling alterations in sexual function and body image due to both the disfiguring procedure and severe scar formation with concentric narrowing of the vagina, urethra, and/or anus.

Recently, the emphasis has been on individualization and the preservation of as much normal anatomy as possible through the use of new surgical approaches to both the primary lesion and regional lymphatics. These modifications to the en bloc principle for management of invasive squamous cell carcinoma of the vulva have resulted from a change in the demographics of the patient population presenting with vulvar lesions, as well as a series of prognostic observations reported during the past fifteen years.[31] The size, depth of invasion, and histologic subtype of the primary lesion, as well as degree of lymphatic and vascular invasion, have been found to closely correlate with the incidence of regional lymph node involvement and prognosis.[32,33,34] Demographic changes, including women of childbearing age and women living into their 80s and 90s, have promoted a need to decrease the overall morbidity of the treatment. These findings have supported the use of less radical resection of early invasive lesions, changes in regional lymph node management with respect to both the inguinal femoral nodes and deep pelvic nodes, and implementation of preoperative radiation therapy and/or chemotherapy to reduce tumor volume.

Choice of surgical methods depends on the site and extent of the primary lesion, the statistical risk of regional lymph node involvement, and importantly, patient preference when possible. The following is a brief discussion of the most common procedures and indications for their use:

Radical local excision, also referred to as wide *local excision* or *modified radical vulvectomy,* is a wide and deep resection of the primary lesion with a 2 cm margin and deep dissection to the level of the inferior fascia of the urogenital diaphragm or the aponeurosis over the pubic symphysis. The width of the margins may be influenced by the known lymphatic pathways and altered by the lateral crural folds, anus, and vagina.[31] This procedure is primarily used for early-stage disease, when the primary lesion is 2 cm or less in diameter. Depending on the site of the lesion, the procedure is usually clitoris-sparing, and with the use of small rhomboid flaps to fill tissue defects, it may provide the least disfiguring result.

Skinning vulvectomy removes the epidermal layer of vulvar skin, allowing a new growth of normal epidermis. It has been used primarily for noninvasive conditions such as vulvar intraepithelial neoplasia (VIN).

Regional lymphadenectomy is the removal of regional lymph nodes that may be at risk or clinically suspicious for metastatic disease. The procedure may be performed either through separate groin incisions or en bloc with the vulvectomy dissection. The procedure for separate incisions involves the removal of an ellipse of skin 1 cm below and parallel to the groin crease, through which the femoral and inguinal lymph nodes are removed.[9] This approach decreases the risk of wound complications due to the smaller volume of tissue removed. It also allows for unilateral lymphadenectomy in the patient who is a candidate for a hemivulvectomy or radical wide excision of an early stage lesion but who may also be at risk of regional lymph node involvement.

En bloc radical vulvectomy (Figure 4.9) is the dissection of the invasive primary lesion, contiguous skin, subcutaneous fat, regional inguinal and femoral lymph nodes, and vulva (labia minora, labia majora, clitoris, and perineal body).[35] This procedure is primarily used for stage II and III lesions, and may be tailored to the extent of disease when there is involvement of the urethra, vagina, and/or anus. The vulvectomy may also be performed with separate regional lymphadenectomy incisions (Figure 4.10).

Pelvic exenteration (discussed in Chapter 3) may be combined with a radical vulvectomy and lymphadenectomy in patients with locally advanced primary lesions that extensively involve the urethra, bladder, vagina, and/or rectum. These procedures are tailored to the extent of disease and may involve cystectomy, vaginectomy, and/or anoproctectomy. Recent use of preoperative radiotherapy to decrease the volume of tumor has reduced the need for such radical procedures.

Graft procedures may be used to close surgical defects after surgery of the vulva. Split thickness skin grafts are free skin grafts that are completely detached from

FIGURE 4.9. En bloc radical vulvectomy incision.

Source: Reproduced with permission from Hacker, N.F., Eifel, P., McGuire, W., & Wilkinson, E.J. (1992). Vulva. In W.J. Hoskins, C.A. Perez, & R.C. Young, eds., *Principles and Practice of Gynecologic Oncology* (p. 552). Philadelphia: J.B. Lippincott.

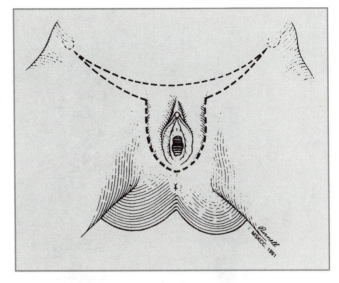

the donor site. They are used primarily to cover skin defects where there is little or no loss of subcutaneous tissue, such as after a skinning vulvectomy. Rotational or transposition flaps, such as rhomboid flaps (Figure 4.11), contain skin, underlying subcutaneous tissue, and occasionally the deep fascia. They may be derived from adjacent vulva, perineal, buttock, or thigh skin. Unfortunately, their limited size may prevent their use in large defects of the vulva.

Since the development of myocutaneous flaps in the early 1950s, a variety of musculocutaneous grafts have been described for the purpose of closing extensive defects of the vulva, including the gracilis, rectus abdominis, tensor fascia lata,

FIGURE 4.10. Vulvectomy with separate groin incisions.

Source: Reproduced with permission from Hacker, N. (1989). Vulvar cancer. In J.S. Berek & N.F. Hacker, eds., Practical *Gynecologic Oncology* (p. 404). Baltimore, MD: Williams & Wilkins.

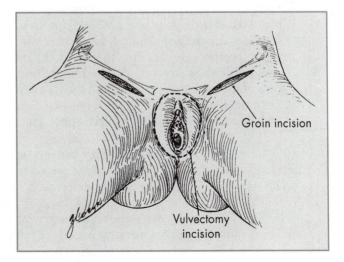

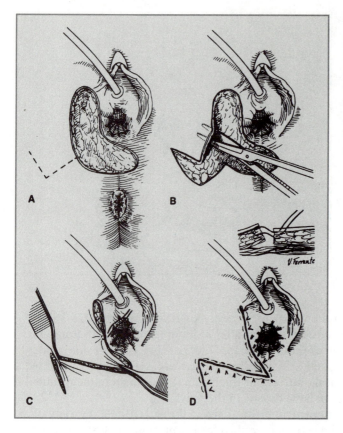

FIGURE 4.11. Technique for rhomboid flap repair.

Source: Reproduced with permission from Hacker, N.F., Eifel, P., McGuire, W., & Wilkinson, E.J. (1992). Vulva. In W.J. Hoskins, C.A. Perez, & R.C. Young, eds., *Principles and Practice of Gynecologic Oncology* (p. 553). Philadelphia: J.B. Lippincott.

gluteus maximus, and latissimus dorsi flaps (Figure 4.12). They are suitable because of a wide arc of rotation and transfer of an island of skin rather than a broad-based pedicle, as in rotational flaps. In addition, they bring a new blood supply to the recipient wound, which may have been devascularized by surgery and/or preoperative radiation therapy.[36] The circumstances influencing choice of graft include size, contour, depth of the deformity to the potential donor site, presence of necrosis and infection, and the requirement of a new blood supply.[37] In some situations, it may be necessary to use several reconstructive procedures, simultaneously or serially, to achieve optimal reconstruction.

Despite the advanced age of many patients with vulvar cancer, surgery is usually remarkably well tolerated, and age alone should never be a contraindication to appropriate surgery.[38] Underlying health issues, such as cardiovascular status, respiratory status, and presence of chronic illness that may increase the overall morbidity and mortality of the surgery, may impact management, however. Common complications during the immediate postoperative period are primarily related to the protracted sur-

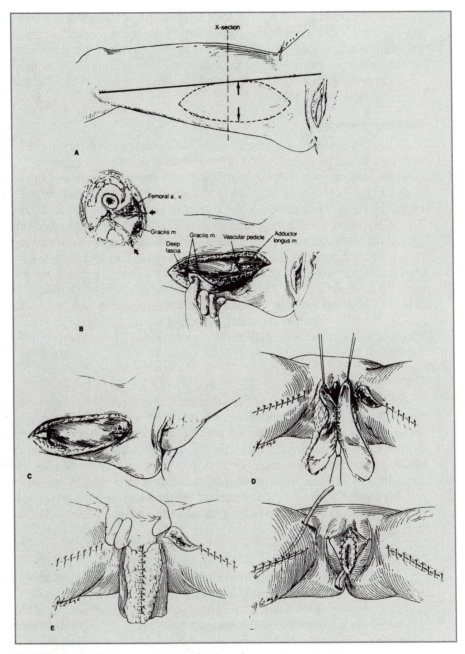

FIGURE 4.12. Myocutaneous graft procedure.

Source: Reprinted with permission from The American College of Obstetricians and Gynecologists. Berek, J.S., Hacker, N.F., & Lagassee, L.D. Vaginal reconstruction performed simultaneously with pelvic exenteration, in *Obstetrics and Gynecology* (1984), vol. 63, p. 318.

gical wound healing and may include infection/sepsis, deep-vein thrombosis, bleeding, seromas, and lymphocyst formation. Long-term complications may include chronic leg edema with subsequent recurrent episodes of lymphangitis or cellulitis, urinary stress incontinence, introital stenosis, and symptoms from pelvic floor prolapse. Recommendations for prevention and management of these complications are discussed later in this chapter.

Radiation Therapy

The role of radiation therapy in the management of vulvar cancer has been controversial in the past. Recent improvements in the methods of delivering treatment to both the primary site and regional lymphatics have led to a number of new studies evaluating the efficacy of radiation in the preoperative and postoperative settings. As surgical radicality has declined, the role of radiotherapy has consequently expanded. The preoperative radiotherapy studies have focused primarily on use of radiation therapy to decrease the volume of disease and subsequent decrease in the radicality of surgery. In addition, the use of radiotherapy versus lymphadenectomy is being evaluated in the management of at-risk or clinically positive regional lymphatics. In the postoperative setting, the use of radiation therapy has been studied in patients with extensive regional lymphatic involvement and/or close or positive surgical margins. Although some study data regarding the use of radiation therapy in these settings have been published, there is no consensus regarding overall morbidity and long-term outcomes.

Chemotherapy

The use of chemotherapy in malignancies of the vulva remains investigational. Generally this treatment modality has been used to enhance the response of radiation therapy, in an attempt to reduce tumor volume prior to surgery, or as salvage therapy. Agents such as bleomycin, methotrexate, 5-fluorouracil, vinblastine, and cisplatin have been used in either single- or multiple-agent protocols.[9] To date, the use of this modality alone or in combination with radiation and/or surgery has not shown a significant impact on the overall outcome of the disease. It is often poorly tolerated in the primarily elderly population who present with malignancies of the vulva. Further studies are needed.

Special Circumstances

The occurrence of a malignancy of the vulva during pregnancy, although rare, does present a challenge to the health care provider. Such lesions occur much more frequently in younger women in the intraepithelial form, presenting difficult diagnostic and management problems. Issues such as accuracy of diagnosis, staging, and treatment are compounded by the presence of the unborn fetus. Treatment of the malignancy must be highly individualized, with attention to several parameters such as stage, lesion size and location, and gestational age. Several factors may significantly impact surgical morbidity during pregnancy, including increasing genital vascularity and a greater likelihood of thromboembolic complications secondary to increased levels of fibrinogen, increased activity of serum coagulation factors, and decreased activity of antithrombin II and antifactor Xa. In the puerperium, the incidence of thromboembolic complications is increased three- to fourfold over that during pregnancy, although it rapidly reverts to the normal state during the first week after delivery.[39] Selection of an appropriate mode of delivery must also be individualized. Although successful vaginal delivery is possible after radical vulvectomy, a Caesarean section may be considered for obstetrical indications. If treatment is planned after delivery, issues such as hemorrhage and possible laceration of lesions on the vulva must be take into consideration. Lymphatic tumor embolization facilitated by vaginal birth is also of hypothetical concern.[40]

Prognosis

The overall prognosis for cancer of the vulva is good, primarily because most patients now present with relatively early disease.[9] Hacker reports an overall five-year survival rate of approximately 70% when patients are treated with curative intent.[11] The most important prognostic factor is presence of metastatic disease in regional lymph nodes at time of presentation. Factors influencing the presence of lymphatic involvement include clinical nodal status, tumor thickness, lesions larger than 2 cm, histologic spray patterns, lymphovascular space involvement and tumor grade. The introduction of flow cytometry in the evaluation of these tumors may provide further understanding of the tumor-related factors that influence prognosis and subsequently alter treatment approaches to improve outcome.[19] Patients with no evidence of metastatic disease in regional lymph nodes have a five-year survival rate of approximately 90%, but it drops to 50% when metastatic disease is present.

✖ CANCER OF THE VAGINA

Overview

Primary carcinoma of the vagina is one of the rarest malignancies in the female genital tract, representing 1 to 2% of all gynecologic malignancies.[1] It is defined as a malignancy that arises in the vaginal epithelium and does not involve the cervix or vulva. Metastatic lesions to the vagina, from either direct extension, lymphatic, or hematogenous spread, are much more frequent than primary lesions of the vagina. Spread by direct extension from either a cancer of the cervix or the vulva account for most metastatic lesions. Other primary malignancies that may present with lesions in the vagina include those of the endometrium, ovary, urethra, bladder, rectum, and gestational trophoblastic neoplasia.[1]

Etiology

The exact etiology of vaginal carcinoma remains unknown. The predominance of lesions in the upper third and on the posterior wall has led to speculation that an accumulation of irritating or macerating substances that pool in the posterior fornix produce a chronic irritation leading to a malignant degeneration. Additional predisposing factors, which have been postulated but not validated, include use of a vaginal pessary, prolapse of the vaginal wall, leukorrhea, and leukoplakia.[1] Use of radiation therapy to the pelvis for a previous bladder, cervical, endometrial, or rectal carcinoma also appears to increase the risk of the development of primary cancers of the vagina.

The proximity of the vagina to the cervix and the similarity of epithelium makes it logical to assume that risk factors may be similar. This has provoked a controversy regarding screening of the vagina with Pap smears and pelvic examination after hysterectomy for benign disease. Several studies have attempted to resolve this controversy, including Peters et al., who reported that 38% of the patients in their series treated for primary cancer of the vagina had undergone previous hysterectomy for benign disease.[41] DiSaia and Creasman recommend Pap smears of the vagina every two to three years for such women.[1]

Intrauterine exposure to diethylstilbestrol (DES) has been associated with clear cell adenocarcinomas of the vagina. This drug was used in the 1950s and early 1960s during early pregnancy in an attempt to prevent miscarriage. In 1970 Herbst and Scully reported an unusually high frequency of clear cell adenocarcinomas of the vagina in young women over a relatively short period of time in the Boston area. Their epidemiologic review found a close correlation between the annual incidence of clear cell adenocarcinoma of the vagina and cervix and the estimated use of DES for pregnancy support in the United States.[42] They have since maintained a registry of such cases, with more than 500 reported.[43] Study data indicated that the median age at diagnosis was nineteen years, and the risk was greatest for those exposed during the first sixteen weeks in utero. With discontinuation of the use of DES during pregnancy, incidence declined rapidly. However, research continues in regard to long-term effects of such exposure, particularly as "DES babies" reach their fourth and fifth decades of life.

Natural History

Cancer of the vagina spreads by local invasion and lymphatic permeation with embolization. The spread pattern is similar to that of cancers of the cervix and vulva. More than half of invasive lesions occur in the posterior wall of the upper third of the vagina, where they may displace the vaginal mucosa and invade the deep rectovaginal tissue.[6] The second most common primary site is the anterior wall of the lower third of the vagina, where the lesion may penetrate the vesicovaginal septum. In addition, lesions may invade the paracolpal and parametrial tissues, extending into the obturator fossa, cardinal ligaments, lateral pelvic walls, and uterosacral ligaments.[7] The lymphatics of the proximal one-third of the vagina drain to the lateral and posterior pelvic nodes, the central portion of the vagina drains to the lateral pelvic nodes, and the distal vagina drains to the inguinal lymph nodes (Figure 4.4). The incidence and extent of lymphatic involvement is dependent on the location and magnitude of disease at the primary site. It is not uncommon to find metastatic disease within lymph nodes that do not directly drain the primary site; that finding probably accounts for the overall poor prognosis of this disease.

Clinical Manifestations

The common presenting signs and symptoms of cancer of the vagina include painless, abnormal vaginal bleeding; a watery or discolored discharge; and dyspareunia. Approximately 50 to 75% of patients present with bleeding, either dysfunctional or postcoital.[44] Bladder or bowel symptoms, such as dysuria, hematuria, frequency of urination, and changes in consistency and form of stool, may be present in more advanced disease.

The lesion most frequently presents as either ulcerative or exophytic. Occasionally there may be only a thickened or firm nodule in the vagina as the lesion grows beneath the superficial vaginal mucosa. Early infiltration of the submucosa is a frequently observed feature, and local reaction and induration tend to give the impression of significant extension, even in small lesions.[6]

Diagnostic Method

A complete history and physical examination, including pelvic examination with speculum and palpation of the vagina, should be performed. The speculum should be rotated as it is withdrawn so that anterior and posterior wall lesions, which occur frequently, are not overlooked.[7] During visual inspection of the vagina, it is critical to assess for the presence of disease on the vulva and cervix. If disease is present on either of these adjacent organs, the staging protocols dictate that the vagina cannot be considered as the primary site. Exfoliative cytologic studies, including a Pap smear and tissue biopsies, are necessary to identify the histology of the lesion. Metastatic evaluation should include cystoscopy, proctosigmoidoscopy, chest X-ray, intravenous pyelogram, and where indicated, a barium enema, lymphangiogram, computed tomography, and magnetic resonance imaging. Careful examination of the inguinal and femoral lymph nodes is necessary, and any suspicious indurated lesions should be further evaluated.

Staging

Cancer of the vagina is staged clinically using the FIGO system (Table 4.8). It may be necessary to examine the patient under anesthesia in order to secure an accurate assessment of the extent of disease.

TABLE 4.8

Staging of Vaginal Cancer

TNM Category	FIGO Stage	Definitions
		Primary Tumor (T)
Tx		Primary tumor cannot be assessed
T0		No evidence of primary tumor
Tis	0	Carcinoma in situ
T1	I	Tumor confined to vagina
T2	II	Tumor invades paravaginal tissues but not to pelvic wall
T3	III	Tumor extends to pelvic wall
T4	IVA	Tumor invades mucosa of bladder or rectum and/or extends beyond the true pelvis (Bullous edema is not sufficient evidence to classify a tumor as T4)
M1	IVB	Distant metastasis
		Lymph Node (N)
NX		Regional lymph nodes cannot be assessed
N0		No regional lymph node metastasis
		Upper two-thirds of vagina:
N1		Pelvic lymph node metastasis
		Lower one-third of vagina:
N1		Unilateral inguinal lymph node metastasis
N2		Bilateral inguinal lymph node metastasis
		Distant Metastasis (M)
MX		Presence of distant metastatis cannot be assessed
M0		No distant metastasis
M1	IVB	Distant metastasis

Stage Grouping

	AJCC/UICC			FIGO
0	Tis	N0	M0	Stage 0
I	T1	N0	M0	Stage I
II	T2	N0	M0	Stage II
III	T1	N1	M0	Stage III
	T2	N1	M0	
	T3	N0	M0	
	T3	N1	M0	
IVA	T4	Any N	M0	
IVB	Any T	Any N	M1	Stage IVB

*Note: If the bladder mucosa is not involved, the tumor is Stage III.

Source: Used with permission of the American Joint Committee on Cancer (AJCC®), Chicago, Illinois. The original source for this material is the *AJCC® Cancer Staging Manual,* 5th edition (1997) published by Lippincott-Raven Publishers, Philadelphia, Pennsylvania.

Histopathology

Squamous cell carcinomas represent 80 to 90% of primary malignant vaginal neoplasms.[7] Variants that may be found in the vagina include verrucous carcinoma and small cell carcinoma. Malignant melanoma is the second most common cancer of the vagina and is discussed later in this chapter. There have also been rare reports of primary sarcomas involving the vagina, including endometrial stromal sarcoma, alveolar soft part sarcoma, malignant fibrous histiocytoma, synovial-like sarcoma, malignant mixed mesodermal tumor, angiosarcoma, and hemangiopericytoma. Embryonal rhabdomyosarcoma is the most common tumor of the vagina in infants and children, with 90% occurring in children younger than five years.[7] Adenocarcinomas, primarily clear cell adenocarcinoma, were discussed earlier in association with DES exposure in utero. Primary adenocarcinomas of the vagina are rare and occur predominantly in postmenopausal women.

Treatment

Radiation Therapy

Radiation therapy is the most frequently used treatment modality for primary malignancies of the vagina due to the excellent tumor control and good functional results obtained.[45] The radiation therapy is individualized but usually consists of a combination of external beam and brachytherapy with a paravaginal or parametrial interstitial implant.[7] Common complications associated with this therapy include proctitis, cystitis, fibrosis of the vagina, mucosal necrosis, and fistulae.

Surgery

Early-stage carcinoma of the vagina may be treated with surgery, depending on the exact site and extent of disease. Surgical procedures may consist of wide local excision or total vaginectomy, with or without reconstruction. These procedures provide the opportunity to preserve ovarian function, particularly in premenopausal women in whom childbearing is a consideration. If the early lesion is in the vaginal fornix, near the cervix, a radical hysterectomy with partial or complete vaginectomy may be indicated.[6]

Surgery may also be used in situations where an early vaginal recurrence has occurred after radiation. The procedure is individualized to the extent of the recurrence, and options include wide local excision, vaginectomy, radical hysterectomy, or pelvic exenteration.[6]

Reconstruction Procedures

Vaginal reconstruction is usually performed to revise or replace a vagina that has stenosed as a result of surgery or radiation or to create a neovagina when the vagina has been removed surgically.[46] Although it may offer a woman the opportunity to resume or maintain vaginal intercourse, it takes an extensive amount of education and support to assist her and her partner in adjusting to the physical changes. In addition, protracted healing periods and the need for active participation in maintaining patency can affect overall acceptance and success.

Vaginal stenosis may occur after surgery or radiation and is usually manifested by progressive dyspareunia. Nonsurgical approaches are often the first line of therapy offered, including use of vaginal dilators and topical estrogen cream. Sexual activity on a regular basis helps to maintain the patency and pliability of the vaginal tissues.[47] Surgery may be performed to remove small areas of scar tissue or stenosis, primarily using a procedure called *perineorrhaphy,* to correct the defect.

Vaginal obliteration occurs primarily after extensive surgery or radiation. The vaginal mucosa becomes scarred and stenotic, with subsequent loss of patency and pliability. Surgery may be used to remove the scar tissue or the stenotic vagina, and a skin graft is placed to form a neovagina. The most common donor sites for these tissue grafts are the buttocks and medial thigh. The skin graft is placed over a vaginal stent, which is then inserted into the pelvic defect created by removal of the stenotic tissue. The Heyer-Schulte stent (Figure 4.13) is preferred for this purpose, as it is inflatable and can be removed and replaced easily by the patient.[48]

Neovagina construction, with or without the reconstruction of the pelvic floor, may also be performed during pelvic exenteration. Both split-thickness skin grafts and myocutaneous grafts may be used. The myocutaneous gracilis graft, harvested from the inner aspect of the thigh, and the bulbocavernosus myocutaneous pedicle graft, from the vulva, have both been used for this purpose. These procedures may be performed at the time of initial surgery or in a delayed procedure several months later.

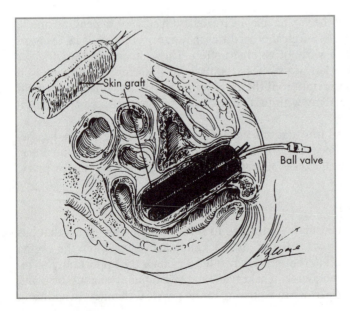

FIGURE 4.13. Heyer-Schulte vaginal stent.

Source: Reproduced with permission from Berek, J.S. (1989). General surgical operations. In J.S. Berek & N.F. Hacker, eds., *Practical Gynecologic Oncology* (p. 541). Baltimore, MD: Williams & Wilkins.

Chemotherapy

Several drugs used in combination with radiotherapy or surgery for treatment of squamous cell carcinomas of the vagina have been studied. These drugs include cisplatin, bleomycin, mitomycin-C, etoposide, mitoxantrone, doxorubicin, lomustine, and semustine.[6,7] Most of the data have not shown significant improvement in overall outcome over radiotherapy or surgery alone. However, chemotherapy may be used in the management of rare sarcomas of the vagina in combination with another modality.

Prognosis

Survival rates of patients with carcinoma of the vagina are comparable to those reported for carcinoma of the cervix, although local recurrences after radiotherapy remain a constant problem. Perez and Camel reported long-term (5-year) survival rates of patients treated with radiation therapy for invasive carcinoma of the vagina as follows: stage I, 90%; stage IIa, 58%; stage IIb, 32%; stage III, 40%; and stage IV, 0%.[49]

✳ MELANOMA OF THE VULVA AND VAGINA

Overview

Melanoma of the female genital tract is a rare disease that challenges the women diagnosed with it and the oncology teams who treat it. There have been some remarkable improvements in the understanding of malignant melanoma over the past twenty years, which have had a direct impact on the approach to screening, diagnosis, and management of the disease. The current ability to identify both low- and high-risk groups, based on clinical and histologic data, has kept surgery as the primary mode of treatment and has led to improved survival due to earlier diagnosis. Historically, melanoma of the genital tract has been a malignancy known for its potential to metastasize quickly, with a consequent poor prognosis. Although the overall prognosis has not significantly improved, approaches to treatment have broadened in an attempt to reduce the necessity for radical surgical procedures that affect the patient's body image and sexual function. Below is an overview of cutaneous melanoma in general, as well as vulvar and vaginal melanoma in particular.

Natural History

Cutaneous melanoma arises from melanocytes, which are cells specializing in the biosynthesis and transport of melanin. These pigment-producing cells migrate from the neural crest to the skin, uveal tract, meninges, and ectodermal mucosa. Melanocytes are found in the basal portion of the epidermis and are present in fetal tissue by eight weeks' gestation.[50] The exact origin of the melanocytes in the vulvar and vaginal mucosa has been extensively debated. In melanoma of the vulva, the lesion may arise from preexisting pigmented lesions containing a junctional or compound nevus, or from normal-appearing skin.[51] Melanoma lesions of the vagina tend to be located on the anterior wall of the lower third.[1] Melanoma spreads by both the lymphatic and hematologic routes and, although unpredictable, lesions do metastasize to other sites in the lower genital tract, including the cervix, urethra, and rectum. They may be aggressive and metastasize widely or lie dormant for a number of years and then reappear after minor stress to the local tissue, such as a surgical procedure.

Etiology/Epidemiology

Malignant melanoma of the skin accounts for 1% of all cancers in the United States.[51] An estimated 41,600 new cases were reported for 1998 and an estimated 7,300 deaths. It is the leading cause of death from diseases of the skin, with a mortality rate that is increasing faster, approximately 4% per year since 1973, than any other cancer with the exception of lung cancer in women.[52] Melanoma now occurs in 1 out of 150 adults and is estimated to occur in 1 out of 100 adults by the year 2000.[53]

Genital melanomas account for 1 to 5% of all cases.[51] Although rare, malignant melanoma of the vulva is the second most common malignant lesion found in this tissue, accounting for approximately 5 to 10% of all malignant lesions of the vulva.[54] Melanoma of the vaginal mucosa is an extremely rare malignancy, accounting for less than 0.3% of cutaneous melanomas and 0.5% of all vaginal malignancies.[1] Melanoma of the vulva and vagina are found primarily in postmenopausal Caucasian women.[51]

Factors that have been associated with the transformation of melanocytes to malignant melanoma are trauma, hormonal influences, and exposure to sunlight (ultraviolet light). Additional known factors include genetic influences and immunologic deficits. Potential factors, such as the role of hormones and chemical carcinogens, are under investigation.[55] The incidence of melanoma increases in areas of the world close to the equator, and in body sites exposed to the sun. Melanoma is rare in blacks, and when it does occur, it is generally limited to the nonpigmented areas of the body such as the palm of the hand and sole of the foot.

Personal risk factors for the development of melanoma (Table 4.9) include a family history of melanoma, poor or no tanning ability, sunburn in childhood or adolescence, light hair, and blue eyes. For these reasons, primary preventative measures include the use of sunscreen, limiting sun exposure during midday, and wearing protective clothing and headgear. Recommended secondary measures include careful skin self-examination and regular examination of all skin surfaces by a health care professional.

Clinical Manifestations

The clinical features associated with melanomas, regardless of site, are known by the acronym ABCD. A melanoma tends to have an asymmetrical (A), irregular border (B), variegated (tan, red, brown, black) color (C), and/or diameter (D) greater than the

TABLE 4.9

Factors Associated with Increased Risk of Developing Melanoma

Risk Factors	Relative Risk
1. Changing mole	Very high
2. Adulthood (Δ 15 yrs)	88
3. One or more large or irregular pigmented lesions	
a. Dysplastic, + familial	148
b. Dysplastic, – familial	27
c. Lentigo maligna	10
4. Congenital mole	21
5. Caucasian	12
6. Previous melanoma	9
7. Melanoma in parent, sibling, or child	8
8. Immunosuppression	4
9. Sun sensitivity	3
10. Excessive sun exposure	3

Source: Reproduced with permission from Rhodes, A.R., Weinstock, M.A., Fitzpatrick, T.B., Mihon, M.C., & Sober, A.J. (1987). Risk factors for cutaneous melanoma: A practical method of recognizing predisposing individuals. *JAMA,* 258, 3146–3154. Copyright 1987, American Medical Association.

size of a dime (6 mm).[56] As malignant melanoma progressess, its neoplastic cells eventually penetrate from the epidermis into the subjacent dermis.[55] The lesion continues to expand both horizontally and vertically and, in time, may appear as an enlarging pigmented macule with superimposed papules and/or nodules, a pigmented plaque, or rarely, as a single nodule.[56]

Lesions of the female genital tract may not be easily identified by the patient until symptoms occur. Vaginal bleeding, vaginal discharge, and presence of a polypoid mass are the most common symptoms reported by patients with vaginal melanoma. The lesions may be single or multiple and may show a variation in size, pigmentation, and growth pattern.[1] In melanoma of the vulva, the lesions are usually raised, nodular, and pigmented, although occasionally (10%) they present as an amelanotic lesion similar in appearance to squamous cell carcinoma lesions.[9] Melanomas may arise anywhere on the vulva; however, they commonly occur in non–hair-bearing areas, specifically, the labia minora and clitoris.[51]

The diganosis of malignant melanoma in its later stages is based on not only the primary lesion but also additional history and symptomatology such as neurologic, respiratory, or musculoskeletal, and confirming radiologic studies.

Histopathology

Vulvar malignant melanomas may be classified into three categories: superficially spreading melanoma (SMN), nodular melanoma (NM), and acral lentiginous melanoma (ALM).[57] Vaginal melanomas are similar to those of the vulva and other sites.

Superficial spreading melanomas generally arise in a preexisting nevus. They constitute approximately 70% of all melanomas. They are characterized by their large centrifugal growth phase that occurs after stromal invasion, followed by a rapid progression after the vertical growth begins. Nodular melanomas are more aggressive tumors that commonly arise without evidence of a preexisting lesion. They constitute 15 to 30% of all melanomas, show only vertical growth, and are generally more advanced at the time of diagnosis. Acral lentiginous melanomas occur on the palms of the hands, soles of the feet, or beneath the nail beds; they constitute approximately 2 to 8% of all melanoma lesions. But in non-Caucasians, they comprise 35 to 60% of melanoma lesions found and resemble tan or brown flat stains with very irregular borders. Ulceration is common in neglected ALM lesions and is often mistaken for a fungal infection.[58]

Diagnostic Method and Staging

Pigmented lesions that present on the vulva or in the vaginal mucosa should be biopsied to determine histology and presence of a melanoma. Additional studies, such as chest X-rays and CT scan of the chest, abdomen, and pelvis, assist in determining the presence of metastatic disease. If the patient presents with symptoms of headaches, visual disturbances, or gait change, a CT scan or MRI of the brain should also be performed. A bone scan with correlating skeletal films can identify bone metastasis and should be performed in patients who are experiencing musculoskeletal discomfort.

Level of invasion and tumor thickness are measurements used in the evaluation of malignant melanoma and directly impact overall prognosis.[9] Several classification systems have been used to describe melanoma. After biopsy, the pathologist measures the melanoma thickness (Breslow microstaging system) and determines the level of invasion (Clark system). Breslow's system[59] is the quantitative assessment of the maximum tumor thickness in millimeters as measured by an ocular micrometer. The Clark system[60] categorizes the five levels of invasion that reflect increasing depth of penetration into the underlying dermis or subcutaneous tissue.[58] Chung et al. have modified the Clark level definitions.[54] Table 4.10 illustrates the three systems. The Breslow and Clark classification systems, however, are not applicable for vaginal melanoma because the layers of submucosal connective tissue are poorly defined and skin appendages are absent, making accurate assessments impossible.

Treatment

The treatment of malignant melanoma is primarily surgical. Current recommendations for surgical therapy for melanoma of the vulva include:

TABLE 4.10

Microstaging Systems for Melanomas, Including Those of the Vulva

	Clark	*Chung*	*Breslow*
I	Intraepithelial	Intraepithelial	< 0.76 mm
II	Into papillary dermis	≤ 1 mm from granular layer	0.76–1.50 mm
III	Filling dermal papillae	1–2 mm from granular layer	1.51–2.25 mm
IV	Into reticular dermis	> 2 mm from granular layer	2.26–3.0 mm
V	Into subcutaneous fat	Into subcutaneous fat	> 3.0 mm

Source: Reprinted with permission from Hacker, N.F., Eifel, P., McGuire, W., & Wilkinson, E.J. (1992). Vulva. In W.J. Hoskins, C.A. Perez, & R.C. Young, eds., *Principles and Practice of Gynecologic Oncology* (p. 559). Philadelphia: J.B. Lippincott.

- Excise all junctional or compound nevi of the vulva
- Biopsy all pigmented lesions found on the vulva
- Excise only for in situ melanoma
- Consider wide local excision only for lesions <1 mm, obtaining a lateral margin of 1 cm, with or without superficial inguinal lymph node excision
- Perform radical vulvectomy or hemivulvectomy with inguinal/femoral lymphadenectomy for moderate- to high-risk lesions without distant metastasis
- Attempt to "microstage" lesions to help choose low-risk patients for conservative approach (wide local excision) using the Breslow and Clark staging systems.

Immunotherapy and hormonal therapy with tamoxifen citrate have also been employed.[7] Radiation therapy may be used to palliate bleeding or painful sites of disease, reduce tumor volume, or for patients who cannot tolerate surgery. No successful chemotherapeutic agent or combination of agents has consistently yielded results in metastatic melanoma.

As many as 80% of vulvar melanomas may involve the vagina at the mucocutaneous border, and this involvement can make it difficult to determine the primary site. Many of these tumors may actually arise at the vulvovaginal junction. Surgical management may involve a more radical procedure, including a partial or total vaginectomy, radical vulvectomy, pelvic exenteration, or any combination of these. The oncology team must carefully consider the advantage of local tumor control with these techniques against the possibility of prompt appearance of distant metastatic disease and the psychosocial implications of these procedures for the woman and her family.

Multiple therapies for melanoma of the vagina have been attempted during the past several decades, but radiation therapy and chemotherapy have not proven to be effective.[1] Surgical approach should be tailored to the location of the lesion and may include radical vulvectomy and regional lymphadenectomy, and/or exenteration.

Prognosis

Overall prognosis for malignant melanoma is poor. The mean five-year survival rate reported for melanoma of the vulva is 32%.[7] Prognosis for melanoma of the vagina is extremely poor, with an overall five-year survival rate of 5%.[1]

NURSING MANAGEMENT

The nursing care of women with malignancies of the vulva and vagina can be very challenging. From the process of initial diagnosis, through treatment and rehabilitation, and into long-term follow-up, a number of issues arise that nursing may have a direct impact on.

Education is a vital component of the process of diagnosis. With the emphasis on prevention and early detection of cancer, participation in community education concerning vulvar self-examination and early evaluation of symptoms is important. In addition, nurses need to encourage women who have had a hysterectomy to continue with scheduled gynecologic care. Gynecologic oncology nurses may provide education directly to women in their health care setting, or in their communities, through participation in screening programs and seminars. Education of health care peers in facilities caring for women, particularly elderly women, can improve the rate of early detection of these malignancies.

Once the diagnosis has been established, preparation of the patient for treatment becomes the primary focus. Extensive education is important regarding the disease, the treatment options, and potential complications. In addition, there should be steady emotional support as the patient and family adjust to the diagnosis, the issues surrounding treatment, and the psychosocial issues involved in a potentially disfiguring procedure, including those of self-esteem, body image, and sexuality. The preoperative care of a patient having a radical procedure involving the vulva and/or vagina requires the coordinated efforts of many members of the health care team, including the surgeon, nursing staff, and social worker. Additional team members may include the medical oncologist, enterostomal therapist, physical therapist, and nutrition specialist. Elderly patients tend to have multiple system disorders, with consequent direct or indirect effects on the process of treatment, and may require the involvement of physicians in other specialties such as cardiology or pulmonology.

Preoperative assessment is critical and may be performed in the outpatient or inpatient setting. A careful evaluation of the patient's preoperative functional status provides a baseline on which a realistic postoperative plan of care and rehabilitation can be built. In addition to medical history and medications, the assessment should include the patient's ability to perform the activities of daily living, mobility status, and use of assistive devices or oxygen therapy. If other services, such as physical therapy, enterostomal therapy, and nutrition specialists are available, they may value the opportunity to evaluate the patient at this time, in order to accurately plan for the postoperative period. The coordination of these evaluations can help to eliminate frustration and failure during the postoperative period, when the patient is unable to meet unrealistic expectations such as bed-to-chair transfers or walking. A complete nutrition assessment, including patient preferences for food, can identify potential deficiencies. Early nutritional interventions are necessary to promote wound healing and resolution of fatigue, decrease the risk of incapacitating constipation and/or bowel obstruction, and promote general well-being.

Preoperative assessment by enterostomal or wound care specialty nurses helps identify patients who are at risk for poor wound healing or nonsurgical skin integrity issues, such as pressure sores with prolonged bed rest. Early intervention and prevention may reduce the incidence of these problems, improving patient comfort and compliance with therapy and shortening the hospital stay. Patients who are scheduled to undergo an exenteration procedure benefit from early intervention and education regarding stoma placement and postoperative expectations.

Preoperative preparation usually begins a day or two prior to surgery. These procedures often include bowel preparation with clear-liquid diets, enemas, laxatives, and oral antibiotics. Additional focus should be placed on assessment of the patient's and family's knowledge and understanding of the disease, the proposed treatment, and expected postoperative experiences. Preoperative education should also include use of deep-breathing exercises and equipment, techniques for splinting the wound during coughing, and methods of access to pain medication, particularly if infusion pumps will be used. Foreknowledge helps in decreasing the potential for anxiety and frustration after surgery.

Early postoperative problems are those commonly associated with most radical surgery procedures, primarily hemorrhage, decreased intravascular fluid volumes, and respiratory compromise associated with anesthesia. Due to the advanced age of many of these patients, chronic diseases such as cardiovascular, respiratory, or renal disease may impact care within the first forty-eight hours. In addition to routine postoperative care, reduction of stress on the wound and prevention of deep-vein thrombosis (DVT) development is important in this patient population.

Bed rest for three to four days after surgery to immobilize wounds has been advocated, although some physicians have found that early mobilization with ambulation does not significantly impact wound healing and may decrease the risk of DVT. If bed rest is ordered, careful positioning to decrease tension on the wounds should be implemented. Log rolling may be used to assist patients in changing positions. Specialty beds or mattresses help to decrease the risk of skin breakdown if prolonged bed rest is necessary. Low-pressure suction drains are usually placed under the incisions, particularly lymphadenectomy or graph incisions, at the time of surgery in order to prevent collections of serosanguinous fluid and subsequent abscess formation or wound dehiscence. These should be closely monitored to ensure unobstructed, adequate suction and early identification of postoperative hemorrhage. Normal drainage is clear to slightly serosanguinous in color and odor-free. A sharp decrease in the amount of fluid drainage in the first forty-eight hours after surgery may indicate an obstruction. If the drain tubing is not kinked, then the drains should be evaluated for the possibility of clots; however, the drains should not be irrigated, in order to prevent infection or wound dehiscence. Pneumatic calf compression, elastic support hose, subcutaneous heparin sodium, and range-of-motion exercises may be employed to decrease the risk of DVT. The timing of oral intake is dependent on the extent of the surgery. In most vulvectomy patients, a return to a full diet occurs within the first few days. However, due to the extensive perineal resection, care should be taken to avoid constipation through adequate fluid intake and an appropriate diet.

Wound Healing

Once the patient has recovered from the initial effects of surgery, the most common postoperative complication is related to wound healing. Vulvectomy wounds, in particular, are under a tremendous amount of stress, and it is estimated that 50% of patients have some degree of wound breakdown.[1] Both groin and vulvar incisions are difficult to immobilize, thus subject to an undue amount of tension on them. In addition, the technique for removing lymph nodes involves undermining the skin, creating pockets of dead space in which fluid collection may occur. Despite the placement of drains within the wounds, the lack of tissue adherence to underlying tissue delays healing and increases the risk of infection. Last, the anatomy of the vulva does not lend itself to adequate dressings that protect the wound, particularly with the proximity to urine and stool. Finding an appropriate, cost-effective approach to supporting the wound healing process can be challenging.

Patients who receive radiation therapy are also at significant risk of wound complications. In the patient receiving radiation preoperatively, the extensive moist desquamation involving the primary tumor mass and surrounding tissue can be painful and difficult to manage. In the postoperative setting, moist desquamation may occur in the treatment fields, particularly if the surgical wound is within the field. These patients are primarily treated as outpatients, and therefore careful consideration in regard to daily traveling to and from treatment needs to be included in the plan of care. Availability of wound dressing supplies, ability to care for the wound, and careful management of pain associated with the moist desquamation should be considered.

Wound healing or repair is a fundamental response to tissue injury. The end product is a dense connective tissue consisting predominantly of collagen, but the process by which this end product is produced is very complex.[61] The basic theory of wound healing has changed dramatically over the past decade in response to new scientific data. In the past, all wounds were treated aggressively and maintained with dry, microbe-free environments. Recent research generally supports that topical agents, dressings, and treatment modalities do not make wounds heal faster, but that some do not hinder the repair process as much as others and are better at fostering the natural healing process.[62] All wounds are liable to be contaminated with a variety of microorganisms, yet the majority do not get infected. This supports the concept that healthy wounds are able to combat most infections via granulocytes and the immune response and heal without any major problems if the body is allowed to do what it is supposed to do. Wound treatments should be used to treat infection if present, to cleanse the wound, debride the wound, provide an optimal environment for healing, relieve pain and discomfort, and prevent complications.[62]

Radical gynecologic surgery most commonly involves dermal wounds. Dermal wounds involve the complete epidermis, dermis, and subcutaneous tissues of the skin; they may also involve muscles and bone.[63] The healing of dermal wounds is highly complex and goes through three phases before healing occurs: the inflammatory phase, the fibroblastic phase, and the remodeling phase. The inflammatory phase serves primarily to control bleeding and prevent bacterial invasion beyond the trauma site. Characteristics of this phase are localized edema, erythema, and tenderness. This process lasts approximately two to three days and eventually prepares the wound site for subsequent formation of granulation tissue. The fibroblastic phase, also called the proliferative phase, rebuilds the damaged structures and provides strength to the wound. This phase lasts approximately four to twenty days after the injury occurs. During this phase, macrophages arrive and replicate and there is production of fibro-blasts, secretion of collagen by the fibroblasts, and capillary budding and development. The changes that are visible, namely the presence of new granulation tissue, include a wound bed that is beefy red, moist, friable, and has a shiny, cobblestone appearance. Finally, the remodeling phase modifies the immature scar to a mature scar to fit the wound, providing the final form to the wound. This phase begins approximately twenty days after injury and extends beyond one year.[64] The three phases may overlap each other, with the end of one phase stimulating the beginning of the next phase.

There are several types of healing wounds. Primary closure, or healing by first in-tention, occurs when full-thickness surgical incisions or other acute wound edges with minimal skin loss are approximated and sutured together. Further healing takes place by reepithelialization only. This is the least complicated type of wound healing. Secondary closure, or healing by secondary intention, occurs in open, large, full-thickness wounds with soft-tissue loss. These wounds take longer to heal, and the process is much more extensive. The wounds undergo collagen deposition, wound contraction with subsequent scar formation, granulation, and finally epithelialization. Delayed primary closure or healing by third intention occurs in more extensive wounds, which are either heavily contaminated or at risk of developing an infection during the acute phase of healing. By delaying the closure, the team can monitor the healing progress, and if the wound becomes infected, therapeutic intervention can be initiated.[63]

A number of factors affect the normal healing of wounds. Both systemic and local factors have an adverse impact. These factors may cause inflammatory arrest, failure of contraction, failure of epithelialization, failure to produce and cross-link collagen, and failure to neovascularize. In the elderly patient, take into consideration a decrease in Langerhans cells and T-cell lymphocytes, which impact cellular immunity; a reduction in microvasculature; and a reduced perception of pain. The most common local and systemic factors are listed in Table 4.11.

When evaluating a patient with dermal wounds, a complete evaluation includes three components: history and subjective examination, review of laboratory tests and

TABLE 4.11

Local and Systemic Factors Affecting Wound Healing

Local Factors	Systemic Factors
Blood Supply	Age
Denervation	Anemia
Hematoma	Anti-inflammatory Drugs
Lack of Protection	Cytotoxic Drugs
Local Infection	Diabetes Mellitus
Mechanical Stress	Jaundice
Presence of Foreign Materials (drains)	Malignant Disease
Previous Radiation	Malnutrition
Surgical Technique	Obesity
Suture Material and Technique	Systemic Infection
Type of Tissue	Temperature
	Trauma
	Uremia
	Vitamin Deficiency
	Zinc Deficiency

Source: Adapted with permission from Harding, K. (1994). Wound management in general practice. *Fourth Coastal Wound Symposium.* Savannah, GA.

procedures, and objective examination. Performing an accurate wound assessment should include objective measurements that allow for serial monitoring of progress toward healing. Factors such as wound location, shape (length, width, depth, tunnels), and depth of tissue injury should be evaluated first. The presence and consistency of any drainage should be evaluated, including type (serous, prurulent, sanguineous), amount, color, and odor, and should be documented. Finally, the type of tissue involved, and existing structures within the wound as well as the status of the skin surrounding the wound, should be identified.

Once the evaluation is complete, formulation of short- and long-term goals that are specific and measurable should be made and an appropriate treatment plan devised to achieve the goals (Figure 4.14). Methods for protection of the wound from undue stress, friction, or trauma should be identified. These may include pressure-relief devices, patient positioning, and/or specific dressing ideas. A method of wound cleansing, debridement, and dressing, as follows, should be included.

Cleansing.   Wound cleansing and preparation is the most important step in reducing the risk of wound infection.[65] Effective cleansing removes loosened debris and toxic residue from topical agents and produces a moist environment for wound healing. This can be accomplished by mechanical cleansing, wound irrigation or lavage, or water agitation such as whirlpool therapy.

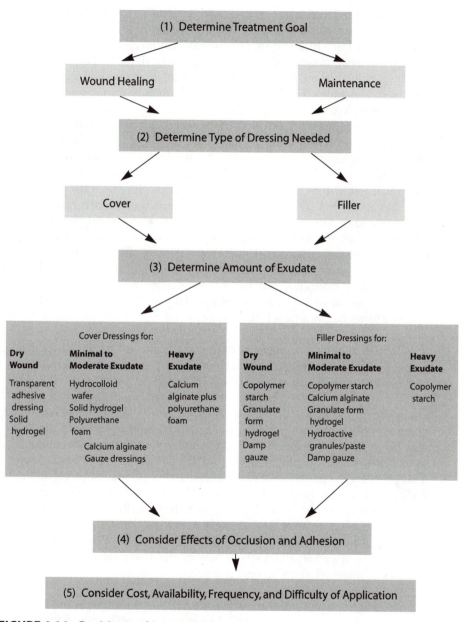

FIGURE 4.14. Decision-making model for wound healing.

Source: Reproduced with permission from Doughty, D. (1992). Topical therapy: From concepts to results. *The Symposium on Advanced Wound Care.*

Mechanical cleansing is the gentle removal of debris from the wound using moistened gauze. Isotonic saline is an effective cleanser in most cases. In 1993, a study was conducted in which sixteen commercial wound cleansers were evaluated to determine the relative toxicity of each on granulation tissue.[66] The toxicity index for the cleansers ranged from 10 to 100,000, indicating a one tenfold dilution to five tenfold dilutions. This index may provide useful information for making a decision of which cleanser to utilize in a specific wound.

Wound irrigation is an effective way to remove debris and contaminants in partially healed wounds or those without hard eschar. It is also the single most effective method of reducing bacterial counts on wound surfaces or in sinus tracts.[65] Irrigation may be performed via syringe or high-pressure lavage. Take care to use the minimum amount of force necessary, to avoid tissue trauma. Hydrotherapy or whirlpool therapy may also be utilized. This is a very effective method of cleansing for women who have undergone extensive resection of the perineum, as in radical vulvectomy. Hydrotherapy helps to soften and loosen debris and necrotic tissue, and consequently decreases the odor that is associated with the extensive wounds and moist healing process. In addition, various antimicrobial agents may be added to the water to kill bacteria present in infected wounds.[65] Sitz baths may also accomplish cleansing of the perineum and can be performed in either a commercially available bath that attaches to a toilet seat or a clean bathtub with wet towels or a foam pillow to provide comfort.

Debridement.   The presence of necrotic tissue or foreign matter in a wound may predispose it to infection. Thus early intervention with debridement decreases this risk and enhances the development of healthy granulation tissue. There are four basic methods of debridement: mechanical, sharp/surgical, enzymatic, and autolytic. Mechanical removal of necrotic tissue by means of wet to dry dressings may be used in some wounds. Although soft necrotic tissue may be removed with the dressings, there may be inadvertent removal of healthy tissue as well as trauma and pain. Sharp or surgical debridement may be necessary to remove extensive necrotic tissue or eschar. This procedure is painful and may necessitate local/regional or general anesthesia. In addition, there may be inadvertent removal of healthy tissue. Enzymatic debridement is accomplished by use of an agent to lyse fibrin, collagen, and elastin. It can be accomplished relatively quickly and is effective if used correctly. Autolytic debridement is nature's way of cleansing the wound by using the body's own enzymes. It is painless and selective, however, and may not be very effective if the necrotic tissue is thick and leathery or attached to the wound margins.[65]

Dressing.   Major changes are taking place in the types of dressing used for wounds. These changes began with the finding that occlusion of the wound, preventing dehydration of granulation tissue, has a stimulatory effect on the process of epithelialization.[67] (The major obstacle to the use of occlusive dressings used to be the assumption that maintaining hydration of the wound site would lead to increased incidence of infection.) In response to these and other findings, there are now over 2,000 dressing materials available commercially, making it impossible to remember trade names, actions, indications, and contraindications of all the products. To make the number more manageable, eight commonly used categories have been identified: gauze, nonadherent, hydrocolloid, semipermeable film, semipermeable hydrogels, semipermeable foams, exudate-absorbing, and biologic. Proper dressing selection requires accurate wound assessment and careful identification of the stage of healing.[68] Table 4.12 provides a list of principles that should be considered in making a decision regarding the appropriate type of dressing based on the characteristics of the wound.

In most vulvectomy wounds that break down, the wounds are usually clean and not infected. Most of these wounds have a moderate amount of clear exudate secondary to the lymphadenectomy. The plan of care should include a method of cleansing, removal of necrotic tissue, and a dressing that provides absorption of the exudate as well as a moist healing environment. In addition, care should be taken to avoid breakdown of surrounding tissue with tape products. Burn net can be cut to form panties that hold the dressings in place and reduce the need for tape. Some patients may prefer to use panty hose that have had the legs cut off; it also keeps dressings in place and allows air to the perineum to decrease moist accumulations.

TABLE 4.12

Principles of Topical Therapy

Principle	Rationale
1. Remove necrotic tissue.	Necrosis prolongs the inflammatory process, thus delaying wound healing.
2. Eliminate any infection.	Infection prolongs inflammation and causes additional tissue damage.
3. Obliterate dead space by packing wounds with sinus tracts.	Packing prevents premature closure and abscess formation.
4. Absorb excess exudate.	Large amounts of exudate may macerate the surrounding skin and may inhibit fibroblast activity as a result of the effects of bacterial toxins and breakdown products.
5. Maintain a clean and moist wound surface.	A moist wound surface promotes cellular function and cellular migration; drying delays the wound healing process.
6. Insulate the wound surface.	Insulation enhances blood flow and the rate of epidermal migration.
7. Protect the healing wound from trauma and bacterial invasion.	Trauma disrupts newly formed tissues, delaying wound healing. Open wounds are vulnerable to infection, which delays wound healing.

Source: Reproduced with permission from Doughty, D. (1990). The process of wound healing: A nursing perspective. *Progressions, 2*(1), 105.

TABLE 4.13

Diagnostic Cluster

Diagnostic/Preoperative and Postoperative Period

COLLABORATIVE PROBLEMS
Potential Complication: Bleeding/Hemorrhage
Potential Complication: Thromboembolic Event
Potential Complication: Infection/Sepsis
Potential Complication: Fluid/Electrolyte Imbalance
Potential Complication: Atelectasis/Pneumonia
Potential Complication: Bowel Dysfunction
Potential Complication: Urinary Dysfunction

NURSING DIAGNOSIS

1. Potential altered health maintenance related to insufficient knowledge of condition, diagnostic tests, prognosis, and treatment options

2. Decisional conflict related to insufficient knowledge of treatment options

3. Anxiety/fear related to impending surgery, and insufficient knowledge of preoperative routines, intraoperative activities, and postoperative self-care activities

4. Anxiety/fear related to insufficient knowledge of potential impact of condition and treatment on reproductive organs and sexuality

5. Grieving related to potential loss of fertility and perceived effects on lifestyle

6. Potential altered respiratory function related to immobility secondary to imposed bedrest and pain

7. Potential fluid volume deficit related to losses secondary to surgical wound or gastrointestinal dysfunction

8. Altered comfort related to effects of surgery, disease process, and immobility

9. Potential for infection related to susceptibility to bacteria secondary to wound, invasive vascular access, and/or urinary catheter

10. Potential altered nutrition: less than body requirements, related to disease process, wound healing, and decreased caloric intake

11. Impaired physical mobility related to surgical interruption of body structures, incisional site pain, and/or activity restriction

12. Potential bowel dysfunction related to decreased peristalsis secondary to surgical manipulation of bowel, effects of anesthesia and analgesia, and/or immobility

13. Potential urinary dysfunction related to loss of sensation of bladder distention secondary to surgical and/or pharmaceutical interventions

14. Potential impaired skin integrity related to surgical wound, decreased tissue perfusion, ostomy stomas, drain sites, and/or immobility

15. Potential impaired tissue integrity/infection related to lymphedema secondary to surgical removal of lymph nodes

TABLE 4.13 *(continued)*

16a. Potential sexual dysfunction related to disease process, surgical intervention, fatigue, and/or pain

16b. Potential moderate or possible permanent alterations in sexual activity related to disease process, surgical intervention, fatigue, and/or pain

16c. Severe or permanent inability to engage in genital intercourse

17. Potential altered health maintenance related to insufficient knowledge of dietary restrictions, medications, activity restrictions, self-care activities, symptoms of complications, follow-up visits, and community resources

Treatment Period

COLLABORATIVE PROBLEMS
Potential Complication: Preexisting medical conditions
Potential Complication: Anasarca
Potential Complication: Fluid/electrolyte imbalance

NURSING DIAGNOSIS

1. Anxiety/fear related to loss of feelings of control of life, unpredictability of nature of disease, and uncertain future

2. Anxiety/fear related to insufficient knowledge of prescribed radiation therapy and necessary self-care measures

3. Potential for infection related to immunosuppression neutropenia secondary to chemotherapy and/or radiation therapy

4. Potential for bleeding related to immunosuppression thrombocytopenia secondary to chemotherapy and/or radiation therapy

7. Potential alteration in skin integrity related to treatment modality and/or disease process

8. Potential altered health maintenance due to insufficient knowledge of colostomy/ileostomy and/or ileal conduit

9. Potential for impaired elimination related to development of fistulae

For patients who have developed extensive moist desquamation due to radiation therapy, cleansing at least twice a day can be performed with warm water soaks in a clean bathtub or shower, taking care not to remove the treatment field markings. A clear hydrogel or silver sulfadiazine cream or a combination of both may be applied to provide a moist environment for healing. It is important to remove the ointments at least one hour prior to treatment to avoid a bolus effect to the skin by the radiation. However, they can be replaced immediately afterward. Patients need to be instructed that healing will not take place until the completion of treatment, and that it may take two to three weeks before the moist desquamation resolves. Careful planning of treatment times and bathing helps to avoid lengthy periods of time without a moist covering on the wound.

In the patient who has undergone vaginal reconstruction with a skin graft, a vaginal stent is placed during surgery to maintain the neovagina. The patient must be instructed on how to remove, clean, and replace the stent daily. Once healing is complete, the patient and her partner should be instructed on the importance of vaginal intercourse in the prevention of vaginal stenosis.[48] If the patient does not have a partner, or is having difficulty with vaginal intercourse, she should be instructed on the use of vaginal dilators or continued use of the stent to maintain patency. Whatever method is selected should be used a minimum of twice a week.

Rehabilitation

All members of the health care team must continue to provide emotional support as the patient adjusts to the physical changes that have occurred, including the mourning of her loss of normal body function. Rehabilitation starts immediately after surgery and may continue for many months. It is the process of promotion of well-being and returning the patient to her pretreatment health status. This includes activities of daily living, mobility, skin integrity, sexual function, and decreasing the risk of long-term complications related to the disease and its treatment.

After vulvectomy, long-term complications may include lower extremity lymphedema, vaginal stenosis, and urinary incontinence secondary to pelvic relaxation (cystocele, rectocele, or uterine prolapse). In addition, patients may experience "urine spray" when voiding due to dissection of the urethral meatus. Simple techniques such as use of a plastic funnel to void into can alleviate frustration and promote well-being. Removal of a significant amount of tissue from the vulva, especially the clitoris, can result in decreased sexual satisfaction, as can a decrease in the range of motion of the legs due to removal of subcutaneous tissue. Counseling and appropriate referral should be included in the plan of care. Chapter 14 provides an overview of the sexuality issues that may arise in these women and recommendations for the management of these issues.

Lymphedema

Lymphedema of the lower extremities is a common complication of both surgery and radiation therapy. It occurs more frequently in women who have had regional lymph nodes removed or irradiated, particularly the inguinal and femoral nodes. Patients should be educated on methods to prevent lymphedema, including the wearing of loose-fitting clothes; avoidance of restrictive bands around ankle, knee, and groin; and use of range-of-motion or low-impact exercise to maintain muscle tone. Once lymphedema occurs, it becomes a chronic problem, and patients should be encouraged to participate in a diligent program of lymphedema compression and drainage. Custom-made elastic support stockings that provide support to the tissue of the lower extremities and encourage venous flow should be worn. Some patients may benefit from, or prefer the use of, sequential compression pumps, which are used for one to two hours per day. Manual lymphatic drainage using massage therapy is also an excellent option. However, it is important that the therapist has training in this special technique. A lymphedema compression program emphasizing lymphatic drainage should be maintained until adequate collateral pathways develop.

Patients with lymphedema are at risk of the development of cellulitis or lymphangitis. In patients who have significant risk because of poor venous flow in the lower extremities (e.g., those with diabetes, peripheral vascular disease, or obesity), low-dose prophylactic antibiotic therapy may be beneficial. Additional education should be provided regarding ways to avoid infection, including wearing appropriately fitting shoes; avoidance of walking in bare feet; protecting oneself from cuts, scratches, and insect bites; and having regular pedicures.

In sum, postoperatively it is important that patients who have had cancer of the vulva or vagina receive close follow-up. Recurrences may be local or distant, or both. Salvage therapy may be available if disease recurrence is small and conducive to therapy. Patients and their families need to receive continued education about the importance of recognition of new symptoms and immediate evaluation. In addition, they need continual emotional support to manage the long-term effects of both therapy and/or disease progression.

✵ REFERENCES

1. DiSaia, P.J., & Creasman, W.T. (1993). *Clinical Gynecologic Oncology* 4th ed. St. Louis, MO: Mosby.
2. Sheppard, J., Sideri, M., Benedet, J. et al (1998). Carcinoma of the vulva. *J Epidemiol Biostatistics, 3*(1), 111–27.
3. Green, T.H. (1978). Carcinoma of the vulva: A reassessment. *Obstet Gynecol, 52,* 462–468.
4. US Bureau of the Census, *Current Populations Reports* (series P-25, nos. 519–917). Washington, DC: US Bureau of the Census.
5. Wilkinson, E.J., & Stone, I.K. (1995). *Atlas of Vulvar Disease.* Baltimore: Williams & Wilkins.
6. Monoghan, J.M. (1992). Invasive tumors of the vagina: Clinical features and management. In M. Coppleson, ed., *Gynecologic Oncology: Fundamental Principles and Clinical Practice* 2nd ed. New York: Churchill Livingstone.
7. Perez, C.A., Gersell, D.J., Hoskins, W.J., & McGuire, W.P. (1992). Vagina. In W.J. Hoskins, C.A. Perez, & R.C. Young, eds., *Principles and Practice of Gynecologic Oncology.* Philadelphia: Lippincott.
8. Krupp, P.J. Jr. (1992). Invasive tumors of the vulva: Clinical features, staging, and management. In M. Coppleson, ed., *Gynecologic Oncology: Fundamental Principles and Clinical Practice* 2nd ed. New York: Churchill Livingstone.
9. Hacker, N.F., Eifel, P., McGuire, W., & Wilkinson, E.J. (1992). Vulva. In W.J. Hoskins, C.A. Perez, &

R.C. Young, eds., *Principles and Practice of Gynecologic Oncology.* Philadelphia: Lippincott.
10. Krupp, P.J., Lee, F.Y.L., Bohm, J.W., et al. (1975). Prognostic parameters and clinical staging criteria in epidermoid carcinoma of the vulva. *Obstet Gynecol, 46,* 84.
11. Hacker, N.F. (1989). Vulvar cancer. In J.S. Berek & N.F. Hacker, eds., *Practical Gynecologic Oncology.* Baltimore: Williams & Wilkins.
12. Curry, S.L., Wharton, J.T., & Rutledge, F. (1980). Positive pelvic nodes in vulvar squamous cell carcinoma. *Gynecol Oncol, 9,* 63.
13. Meigs, C.D. (1854). *Women: Her Diseases and Remedies* (pp. 35). Letter, Ill.
14. Lawhead, A.R., & Majmudar, B. (1990). Early diagnosis of vulvar neoplasia as a result of vulvar self-examination. *J Reprod Med, 35*(12), 1134–1137.
15. Buscema, J., Stern, J.L., & Woodruff, J.D. (1981). The significance of the histologic alterations adjacent to invasive vulvar carcinoma. *Am J Obstet Gynecol, 59,* 563.
16. Elliott, P.M. (1992). Early invasive carcinoma of the vulva: Definition, clinical features and management. In M. Coppleson, ed., *Gynecologic Oncology: Fundamental Principles and Clinical Practice* 2nd ed. New York: Churchill Livingstone.
17. Rastkar, G., Okagaka, T., Twiggs, L.B., & Clark, B.A. (1982). Early invasive and in situ warty carci-

noma of the vulva: Clinical, histologic, and electron microscopic study with particular reference to viral association. *Am J Obstet and Gynecol, 143,* 814.

18. Kunschner, A., Kanbour, A.I., & David, B. (1978). Early vulva carcinoma. *Am J Obstet Gynecol, 132,* 599.

19. Morrow, C.P., & Curtin, J.P. (1998). Tumors of the vulva. In C.P. Morrow & J.P. Curtin, eds, *Synopsis of Gynecologic Oncology,* 5th ed. Philadelphia: Churchill Livingstone.

20. DiSaia, P.J. & Creasman, W.T. (1997). Invasive cancer of the vulva. In P.J. DiSaia & W.T. Creasman, eds, *Clinical Gynecologic Oncology,* 5th ed. St. Louis: Mosby.

21. Hall, D.J., & Hurt, W.G. (1984). Lesions of the vulva. *J Fam Pract, 18*(1), 129.

22. Ferenczy, A. (1992). Pathology of malignant tumors of the vulva and vagina. In M. Coppleson, ed., *Gynecologic Oncology: Fundamental Principles and Clinical Practice* 2nd ed. New York: Churchill Livingstone.

23. Dvoretsky, P.M., Bonfiglio, T.A., Helmkamp, F. et al. (1984). The pathology of superficially invasive, thin vulvar squamous cell carcinoma. *Int J Gynecol Pathol, 3,* 331.

24. Wilkinson, E.J., Kneale, B., & Lynch, P.J. (1986). Report of the ISSVD Terminology Committee. *J Reprod Med, 31,* 973.

25. Wilkinson, E.J., Roco, M.J., & Pierson, K.K. (1982). Microinvasive carcinoma of the vulva. *Int J Gynecol Pathol, 1,* 29.

26. Buckley, C.H., & Fox, H. (1988). Epithelial tumors of the vulva. In C.M. Ridley, ed., *The Vulva* (pp. 261–333). New York: Churchill Livingstone.

27. Kraus, F.T., & Perez-Mesa, C. (1966). Verrucous carcinoma: Cervical and pathologic study of 105 cases involving oral cavity, larynx, and genitalia. *Cancer, 19,* 27.

28. Basset, A. (1912). Traitement chirurigical operatoire de l'epitheliome primitut du clitoris. *Rev Chir (Paris), 46,* 546.

29. Taussig, F.J. (1940). Cancer of the vulva: An analysis of 155 cases. *Am J Obstet Gynecol, 40,* 764.

30. Way, S. (1948). The anatomy of the lymphatic drainage of the vulva and its influence on the radical operation for carcinoma. *Ann R Coll Surg Engl, 3,* 187.

31. Greer, B.E., & Berek, J.S. (1991). Evolution of the primary treatment of invasive squamous cell carcinoma of the vulva. In *Current Topics in Obstetrics and Gynecology.* New York: Elsevier.

32. Donaldson, E.S., Powell, D.E., Hanson, M.B., et al. (1984). Prognostic parameters in invasive vulvar cancer. *Gynecol Oncol, 11,* 184.

33. Shimm, D.S., Fuller, A.F., Orlow, E.L., et al. (1986). Prognostic variables in the treatment of squamous cell carcinoma of the vulva. *Gynecol Oncol, 24,* 343.

34. Sedlis, A., Homesley, H., Bundy, B.N., et al. (1987). Positive groin lymph nodes in superficial squamous cell vulvar cancer. *Am J Obstet Gynecol, 156,* 1159.

35. Walczak, J.R., & Klemm, P.R. (1993). Gynecologic malignancies. In S.L. Groenwald, M.H. Frogge, M. Goodman, & C.H. Yasko, eds., *Cancer Nursing: Principles and Practice* 3rd ed. Boston: Jones and Bartlett.

36. Shepard, J.H., Van Dam, P.A., Jobling, T.W., & Breach, N. (1990). The use of rectus abdominous myocutaneous flaps following excision of vulvar cancer. *Br J Obstet Gynaecol, 97,* 1020.

37. Stern, J.F., & Lacey, C.G. (1987). Vulvovaginal reconstruction following radical surgery. *Bailliere's Clin Obstet Gynaecol, 1,* 287.

38. Lawton, F.G., & Hacker, N.F. (1990). Surgery for invasive gynecologic cancer in the elderly female population. *Obstet Gynecol, 76,* 287.

39. Hathaway, W.E., & Bonner, J. (1978). *Perinatal Coagulation.* New York: Grune & Stratton.

40. Moore, D.H., Fowler, W.C., Currie, J.L., & Walton, L.A. (1991). Squamous cell carcinoma of the vulva in pregnancy. *Gynecol Oncol, 41,* 74.

41. Peters, W.A., Juman, N.B., & Morley, G.W. (1985). Carcinoma of the vagina: Factors influencing treatment outcome. *Cancer, 55,* 892.

42. Herbst, A.L., & Scully, R.E. (1970). Adenocarcinoma of the vagina in adolescence: A report of seven cases including six clear cell carcinomas (so-called mesonephromas). *Cancer, 25,* 745.

43. Herbst, A.L., & Scully, R.E. (1983). Newsletter: *Registry for research on hormonal transplacental carcinogenesis.*

44. Herbst, A.L., Welder, H., & Poskanzer, D.C. (1971). Adenocarcinoma of the vagina: Association of maternal stilbestrol therapy with tumor appearance in young women. *N Engl J Med, 284,* 878.

45. Underwood, R.B., & Smith, R.T. (1971). Cancer of the vagina. *JAMA, 217,* 46.

46. Magrina, J.F., & Masterson, B.T. (1981). Vaginal reconstruction in gynecologic oncology: A review of techniques. *Obstet Gynecol Surg, 36,* 1.

47. Berek, J.S. (1989). General surgical operations. In J.S. Berek & N.F. Hacker, eds., *Practical Gynecologic Oncology.* Baltimore: Williams & Wilkins.

48. Berek, J.S., & Andersen, B.L. (1992). Sexual rehabilitation: Surgical and psychological approaches. In W.J. Hoskins, C.A. Perez, & R.C. Young, eds., *Principles and Practice of Gynecologic Oncology.* Philadelphia: Lippincott.

49. Perez, C.A., & Camel, H.A. (1982). Long term follow-up radiation therapy of carcinoma of the vagina. *Cancer, 49,* 1308.

50. Ketcham, M., & Loescher, L.J. (1994). Skin cancers. In S.L. Groenwald, M.H. Frogge, M. Goodman, C.H. Yarbro, eds., *Cancer Nursing: Principles and Practice* 3rd ed. (pp. 1238–1257). Boston: Jones and Bartlett.

51. Curtin, J.P., & Morrow, C.P. (1992). Melanoma of the female genital tract. In M. Coppelson, ed., *Gynecologic Oncology: Fundamental Principles and Clinical Practice* 2nd ed. New York: Churchill Livingstone.

52. Landis, S.H., Murray, T., Bolden, S., & Wingo, P.A. (1998). Cancer Statistics, 1998. *CA Cancer J Clin, 48*(1), 5–40.

53. Balch, C.M., Houghton, A., & Peters, L. (1989). Cutaneous melanoma. In V.T. DeVita, S. Hellman, & S.A. Rosenberg, eds., *Cancer: Principles and Practice of Oncology* 3rd ed. Philadelphia: Lippincott.

54. Chung, A.F., Woodruff, J.M., & Lewis, J.L. (1975). Malignant melanoma of the vulva. *Obstet Gynecol, 45,* 638.

55. Friedman, R.J., Rigel, D.S., Silverman, M.K., Kopf, A.W., & Vossaert, K.A. (1991). Malignant melanoma in the 1990s: The continued importance of early detection and the role of physician examination and self-examination of the skin. *CA Cancer J Clin, 41*(4), 201.

56. Friedman, R.J., Rigel, D.S., & Kopf, A.W. (1985). Early detection of malignant melanoma: The role of physician examination and self-examination of the skin. *Cancer, 35,* 130.

57. Benda, J.A., Platz, C.E., & Anderson, B. (1986). Malignant melanoma of the vulva: A clinical pathologic review of sixteen cases. *Int J Gynecol Pathol, 5,* 202.

58. Singeltary, S.E., & Balch, C.M. (1991). Malignant melanoma. In A.I. Holleb, D.J. Fink, & G.P. Murphy, eds., *American Cancer Society Textbook of Clinical Oncology* (pp. 263–270). Atlanta: American Cancer Society.

59. Breslow, A. (1970). Thickness, cross-sectional areas, and depth of invasion in the prognosis of cutaneous melanoma. *Ann Surg, 172,* 902–908.

60. Clark, W.H., from Bernardino, E.A., et al. (1969). The histogenesis and biologic behavior of primary human malignant melanomas of the skin. *Cancer Res, 29,* 705–727.

61. Jackson, D.S., & Rovee, D.T. (1988). Current concepts in wound healing: Research and theory. *J Enterostomal Ther, 15,* 133.

62. van Rijswijk, L. (1995). General principles of wound management. In P. Gogia, ed., *Clinical Wound Management.* Thorofare, NJ: Slack, Inc.

63. Gogia, P. (1995). Physiology of wound healing. *Clinical Wound Management.* Thorofare, NJ: Slack, Inc.

64. Bryant, R. (1987). Wound repair: A review. *Journal of Enterostomal Therapy, 14*(6), 262.

65. Marquez, R.R. (1995). Wound debridement and hydrotherapy. In P. Gogia, ed., *Clincial Wound Management.* Thorofare, NJ: Slack, Inc.

66. Foresman, P.A., Payne, D.S., Becker, D., Lewis, D., & Rodeheaver, G.T. (1993). A relative toxicity index for wound cleansers. *Wounds, 5*(5), 226.

67. Hinman, C.D., & Maibach, H.I. (1963). Effect of air exposure and occlusion on experimental human skin wounds. *Nature, 200,* 377.

68. Cuzzell, J., & Drasner, D. (1995). Wound dressings. In P. Gogia, ed., *Clinical Wound Management.* Thorofare, NJ: Slack, Inc.

Cancer of the Endometrium

Bridget M. Paniscotti, RN, BSN

❈ INTRODUCTION

Carcinoma of the endometrium is the most common pelvic malignancy in women in the United States. The American Cancer Society estimated that 37,400 new cases of corpus uterine cancer would be diagnosed in the United States in 1999. Of this number, 6,400 were estimated to die as a result of the disease, making it the seventh leading cause of death from malignancy among women.[1] Endometrial carcinoma is predominantly a disease of postmenopausal women, with an average age at diagnosis of 61 years. However, 25% of the cases occur in premenopausal women, and 5% occur in women younger than 40 years.[2,3] Survival rates for endometrial carcinoma are 76% for patients with stage I, 50% for those with stage II, 30% for those with stage III, and 9% for those with stage IV. The incidence rate of endometrial carcinoma increased by a third during the 1970s in the United States, followed by a near comparable decline during the 1980s. The increase in incidence may be attributed to increased use of exogenous estrogens during the 1960s, without knowledge of their full effects.[4] Other likely contributing factors include increased access to health care for women, increased clinical awareness, improved detection methods, and changes in histopathologic criteria for endometrial cancer. However, there has also been a rising incidence of endometrial carcinoma in Norway, Japan, and England, despite the fact that estrogens are rarely prescribed or unavailable in these countries, which suggests that environmental, dietary, and/or other unknown factors may influence its development.[5,6]

❈ ANATOMY

The uterus occupies the space between the bladder and the rectum, and is divided structurally and functionally into two parts, the corpus (or body) and the cervix, which are separated by a slight narrowing of the uterus known as the *isthmus*. This is the level of the internal os of the cervix. The cervix is divided into the supravaginal portion, which is closely approximated to the bladder, and the vaginal portion, which projects into the cavity of the vagina. The walls of the uterus are composed of muscular tissue called the *myometrium*. The epithelial membrane that lines the uterine corpus is called the *endometrium*. The endometrium is composed of glandular epithelium and endometrial stroma. The principal ligaments of support for the uterus are the broad ligaments, the round ligaments, the uterosacral ligaments, and the cardinal ligaments. Blood is supplied to the uterus by the uterine artery, which is a branch of the hypogastric or internal iliac artery, and enters the wall of the uterus at the isthmus. The lymphatics of the myometrium drain into the subserosal network of lymphatics, which coalesce into larger channels before leaving the uterus. Lymph flows from the fundus toward the adnexa and the infundibulopelvic ligaments. Lymph flow from the lower and middle thirds of the uterus tends to spread in the base of the broad ligaments toward the lateral pelvic sidewall.[7]

The endometrium is hormonally sensitive and changes throughout the menstrual cycle and during pregnancy.

✱ RISK FACTORS

Endometrial carcinoma occurs in both the reproductive and postmenopausal years. Obese women have an increased risk of developing it, with a threefold risk for those 30 pounds over ideal weight and a tenfold risk for those 50 pounds overweight (Table 5.1).[8] Hormonal abnormalities noted in women with upper body fat distribution (android obesity) appear to increase risk. Nulliparous women have a two times greater risk than primiparous women. Young women with a history of polycystic ovaries or Stein-Leventhal syndrome of infertility, menstrual irregularities, and anovulation are at risk for developing endometrial hyperplasia or carcinoma, which is attributed to the steady stimulation of estrogen to the endometrial lining without progestin influence. It is possible to reverse this process through progesterone therapy or by performing a wedge resection of the ovary.[9] Women with a history of hormone-secreting tumors, particularly of ovarian origin, are at risk for developing endometrial hyperplasia or

TABLE 5.1	
Risk Factors for Endometrial Cancer	
Risk Factors	*Increased Risk*
Obesity	
>30 lbs. over ideal weight	3x
>50 lbs. over ideal weight	10x
Nulliparous	2x
Late menopause	2.4x
"Bloody" menopause	4x
Diabetes mellitus	2.8x
Hypertension	1.5x
Unopposed estrogen	9.5x
Complex atypical hyperplasia	29x

Source: Reproduced with permission from Hoskins, W.J., Perez, C.A., & Young, R.C., eds. (1992). *Principles and Practice of Gynecologic Oncology* (pp. 663–693). Philadelphia: J.B. Lippincott.

carcinoma. Women with menopause occurring after age 52 have a 2.4 times greater risk for developing endometrial carcinoma than those who experience menopause before age 49.[10] Other medical conditions, specifically diabetes mellitus, hypothyroidism, and hypertension, are frequently present in women with endometrial cancer.[9] The associations are not clearly understood; however, these conditions are also common among obese females. Women who take tamoxifen for breast cancer are also thought to be at increased risk. Tamoxifen has the ability to trigger the proliferation of cells in the lining of the uterus. Studies support that the benefit from tamoxifen is substantially greater than the risk of endometrial cancer. Appropriate surveillance for this patient population must be available.[11]

Exogenous and Endogenous Estrogens

Women taking unopposed (without progestin) exogenous estrogen therapy are at high risk for developing carcinoma of the endometrium (Figure 5.1). Estrogens are taken to control or prevent the symptoms of menopause. The risk of endometrial cancer is reduced, but not eliminated, by adding progestin to the medicinal regimen when initiating hormone replacement therapy. Women with presumed estrogen-induced endometrial cancers typically have well-differentiated, superficially invasive tumors, although the increased risk is not limited to these favorable cases.[12]

There is also a correlation between endogenous estrogen and its effect on the endometrium. After menopause, most of the estrogens are normally derived from the

FIGURE 5.1. Natural history of endometrial neoplasia.

Source: Reproduced with permission from Moore, T.R., Reiter, R.C., Rebar, R.W., & Baker, V.V. *Gynecology and Obstetrics: A Longitudinal Approach.* Churchill Livingstone, New York, 1993, p. 702.

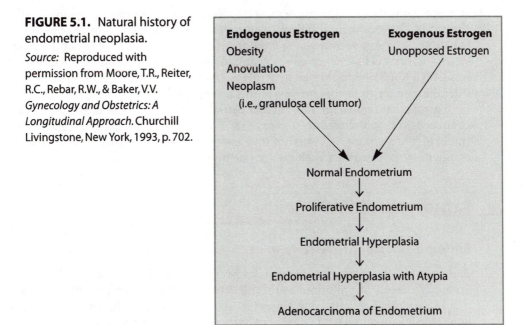

conversion of androgens of adrenal origin. The ovaries continue to secrete testosterone and androstenedione (androgen). Androstenedione is converted peripherally to estrone, a non–protein-bound estradiol that is considered carcinogenic in large amounts.[13,14] There appears to be a greater conversion of androstenedione to estrone in patients with endometrial cancer than in healthy menopausal women. There is also increased estrone production in obese females, which relates to the conversion of the precursor androgen, aromatase, from adipose tissue, causing higher amounts of estradiol to be in circulation.[15] In addition, android obesity is associated with significantly depressed levels of sex hormone–bound globulin (SHBG). This level is normally inversely proportional to the level of estradiol.[16] With lower SHBG, there is greater endogenous production of non–protein-bound estradiol.[14] Thus a state of hyperestrogenism is created, causing constant stimulation of the endometrium.

A hereditary pattern, referred to as the Lynch syndrome II, is associated with endometrial carcinoma. Lynch syndrome II features a significant genetic association between hereditary nonpolyposis colorectal cancer and the development of endometrial carcinoma.[17] Other cancers noted in the same families include carcinoma of the ovary, urologic system, stomach, small bowel, pancreas, and breast.[18] It is therefore imperative to obtain a complete family cancer history to determine the possibility of a Lynch syndrome II phenomenon.

❈ ETIOLOGY

Hormonal imbalance is the single most important causative factor for endometrial carcinoma.[19] The endometrial lining is controlled in a cyclic fashion by the predominant female sex hormones, estrogen and progesterone. The actual etiology of the progression of normal cells to carcinoma is unknown since the process can occur spontaneously in normal, atrophic, or hyperplastic tissue.[7] Therefore, it is necessary to consider the stated risk factors present in this disease process.

Factors that reduce the risk of endometrial cancer are the use of combination oral contraceptives, which reduces menstrual proliferation; weight loss; and cigarette smoking. But smoking is a cause of lung cancer and associated with the development of other diseases and clearly should not be promoted.[9]

❈ PATHOPHYSIOLOGY

Endometrial Hyperplasia

Endometrial hyperplasia is defined as an overgrowth of the endometrial lining of the uterus as a result of prolonged estrogenic stimulation of the endometrium. Endometrial hyperplasia may clinically present as abnormal bleeding. It can occur in progesterone-deficient young women who are infertile because of anovulation.

In addition, endometrial hyperplasia may precede endometrial carcinoma; it is considered a precursor state to endometrial carcinoma. It may also occur simultaneously with endometrial cancer.[9]

Classification of hyperplasia defines benign as well as premalignant conditions. The term *endometrial hyperplasia* refers to the histopathologic state of the endometrial glands and stroma. The histopathologic classification accepted by the International Society of Gynecological Pathologists consists of three categories: simple (cystic without atypia), complex (adenomatous without atypia), and atypical (simple cystic with atypia or complex adenomatous with atypia).

Hyperplasias with cellular atypia are considered to be premalignant, while those without atypia are benign. However, the endometrium continues to be predisposed to the development of carcinoma in the absence of cytologic atypia based on the underlying pathophysiologic state.[9] The progression of hyperplasia to carcinoma in patients with simple hyperplasia is 1%, and for complex hyperplasia, 3%. The progression rate to carcinoma is much higher when atypia accompanies hyperplasia: 8% with simple atypical hyperplasia and 29% with complex atypical hyperplasia.[7]

Adenocarcinoma of the Endometrium

Carcinoma of the endometrium arises from the glandular component of the endometrial mucosa. The disease may be locally confined to a polyp, or it may be diffuse disease commonly involving the upper portion of the uterine cavity.[20] Endometrial tumor growth tends to be slow, invading the myometrium and advancing toward the isthmus and cervix. Extrauterine spread occurs by direct extension of tumor cells through the fallopian tubes, resulting in peritoneal implants; lymphatic invasion, resulting in metastasis to the pelvic, aortic, and inguinal lymph nodes; and hematogenous spread, frequently involving the pulmonary system (Figure 5.2).[9]

The initial pathologic evaluation of endometrial tissue determines the cell type and histologic grade. Following surgery, depth of myometrial invasion and lymph node involvement are pathologically defined. The evaluation must also include a thorough microscopic evaluation of the cervix for evidence of tumor extension.[7] These factors determine prognosis and assist in developing an individualized treatment plan.

Grade 1 endometrial cancers are well differentiated and generally associated with a good prognosis. Grade 2 tumors are moderately differentiated and have an intermediate prognosis; and grade 3 reflects poorly differentiated lesions, which have a poor prognosis. As the tumor becomes less differentiated, the risk of deep myometrial invasion and lymph node metastases increases.[14,21,22,23]

Endometrioid adenocarcinoma is the most common histologic cell type found in endometrial carcinoma (Table 5.2), comprising 75 to 80% of all cases.[24] There are four main variants of adenocarcinoma: adenocanthomas, adenosquamous carcinomas, papillary adenocarcionomas, and secretory adenocarcinomas. Some tend to be more aggressive, but all are treated about the same. Adenoacanthomas are composed of benign squamous metaplasia and adenocarcinoma. These lesions tend to be well differentiated.[14] Adenosquamous carcinomas contain a malignant squamous compo-

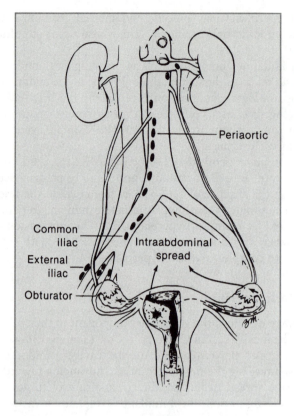

FIGURE 5.2. Spread pattern of endometrial cancer.

Source: Reproduced with permission from DiSaia, P.J., & Creasman, W.T. (1993). *Clinical Gynecologic Oncology* 4th ed. (p. 172). St. Louis, MO: Mosby Year Book, Inc.

nent, which is poorly differentiated and associated with extrauterine spread.[7] Papillary adenocarcinomas tend to have greater myometrial invasion and peritoneal surface involvement. This cell subtype is common in black women and older women.[14] Secretory adenocarcinoma is an uncommon cell subtype that is usually well differentiated and carries a favorable prognosis.

Other Endometrial Carcinomas

Mucinous carcinoma is a rare cell type and common in the endocervix. Serous carcinoma is a poor prognostic and aggressive tumor type associated with early lymphatic and myometrial spread.[7] Clear cell carcinoma cell type often occurs in older women and tends to be aggressive, with a poor prognosis.

Overall prognosis is dependent on both uterine and extrauterine factors. Uterine factors include histologic cell type, tumor grade, depth of myometrial invasion, occult extension to the cervix, and vascular space invasion. Extrauterine factors include intraperitoneal and adnexal spread, positive peritoneal cytology, pelvic lymph node

TABLE 5.2
Classification of Histologic Cell Types

Endometrioid adenocarcinoma	Serous carcinoma
Adenocanthoma	Clear cell carcinoma
Adenosquamous carcinoma	Squamous carcinoma
Papillary carcinoma	Undifferentiated carcinoma
Secretory carcinoma	Mixed types
Mucinous carcinoma	Metastatic carcinoma

metastases, and aortic lymph node involvement.[6] The uterus may or may not be enlarged; therefore, size is not a reliable indicator. To adequately evaluate prognostic factors and extent of disease, a surgical staging procedure is necessary. Surgical stage criteria were defined in 1988 by the International Federation of Gynecology & Obstetrics (FIGO), based on degree of myometrial invasion, endocervical involvement, nodal spread, and metastatic disease (Table 5.3, Figure 5.3).

❈ CLINICAL PRESENTATION

The cardinal symptom for both hyperplasia and endometrial carcinoma is abnormal vaginal bleeding. In younger patients, the development of endometrial carcinoma may be associated with obesity and a history of anovulation.[25] It is sometimes diagnosed during an evaluation for infertility, when symptoms include intermenstrual spotting or heavy abnormal menstrual bleeding (menometrorrhagia, oligomenorrhea). In postmenopausal women, vaginal bleeding is an indicator for malignancy and should be investigated to rule out atrophic vaginitis or medicinal withdrawal bleeding.[9] Any bleeding that occurs twelve months after menses have stopped is considered abnormal. A prurulent, sometimes blood-tinged vaginal discharge may also be a presenting symptom. Pelvic pressure, pain, ascites, and hemorrhage may indicate advanced disease.[9, 26]

❈ DIAGNOSIS

A thorough history and physical examination includes a bimanual pelvic and rectovaginal exam. The entire cervix and vagina are inspected and palpated. Bleeding may be visible at the external os. Particular attention should be given to the vagina and suburethral area since these are frequent sites for metastasis. A Pap smear may be

TABLE 5.3

Corpus Cancer Staging

TNM	FIGO	Definition
		Primary Tumor (T)
TX	—	Primary tumor cannot be assessed
T0	—	No evidence of primary tumor
Tis	—	Carcinoma in situ
T1	I	Tumor confined to the corpus uteri
T1a	IA	Tumor limited to the endometrium
T1b	IB	Tumor invades up to or less than one-half of the myometrium
T1c	IC	Tumor invades more than one-half of the myometrium
T2	II	Tumor invades the cervix but not extending beyond the uterus
T2a	IIA	Endocervical glandular involvement only
T2b	IIB	Cervical stromal invasion
T3 and/or N1	III	Local and/or regional spread as specified in T3a, b, N1 and FIGO IIIA, B, and C below
T3a	IIIA	Tumor involves the serosa and/or adnexa (direct extension or metastasis) and/or cancer cells in ascites or peritoneal washings
T3b	IIIB	Vaginal involvement (direct extension or metastasis)
N1	IIIC	Metastasis to the pelvic and/or paraaortic lymph nodes
T4*	IVA	Tumor invades the bladder mucosa or the rectum and/or the bowel mucosa
M1	IVB	Distant metastasis (*excluding* metastasis to the vagina, pelvic serosa, or adnexa; *including* metastasis to intra-abdominal lymph nodes other than paraaortic, and/or inguinal lymph nodes)
		Regional Lymph Nodes (N)
NX		Regional lymph nodes cannot be assessed
N0		No regional lymph node metastasis
N1		Regional lymph node metastasis
		Distant Metastasis (M)
MX	—	Presence of distant metastasis cannot be assessed
M0	—	No distant metastasis
M1	IVB	Distant metastasis

pTNM Pathologic Classification
The pT, pN, and pM categories correspond to the T, N, and M categories.

TABLE 5.3 *(continued)*				
Stage Grouping				
	AJCC/UICC			*FIGO*
Stage 0	Tis	N0	M0	
Stage IA	T1a	N0	M0	Stage IA
Stage IB	T1b	N0	M0	Stage IB
Stage IC	T1c	N0	M0	Stage IC
Stage IIA	T2a	N0	M0	Stage IIA
Stage IIB	T2b	N0	M0	Stage IIB
Stage IIIA	T3a	N0	M0	Stage IIIA
Stage IIIB	T3b	N0	M0	Stage IIIB
Stage IIIC	T1	N1	M0	Stage IIIC
	T2	N1	M0	
	T3a	N1	M0	
	T3b	N1	M0	
Stage IVA	T4	Any N	M0	Stage IVA
Stage IVB	Any T	Any N	M1	Stage IVB

Note: The presence of bullous edema is not sufficient evidence to classify a tumor as T4.

Source: Reproduced with permission from Beahrs, O.H., Henson, D.E., Hutter, R.V.P., & Kennedy, B.J. (1992). *Manual for Staging of Cancer* 4th ed. (p. 162). Philadelphia: W.B. Saunders.

taken, but it is not a reliable method of detecting endometrial cancer. Note that it is not unusual for the entire physical examination to be normal.[9]

The standard method for diagnosing abnormal bleeding is through histologic evaluation of endometrial and endocervical tissues. An accepted and reliable method for initial evaluation is an endometrial biopsy and endocervical curettage performed in the outpatient office setting. The endometrial biopsy is obtained with a suction catheter or curette, which is inserted through the cervical os into the uterus and rotated with multiple strokes to aspirate an adequate sample. The cervix should be cleansed with povidine-iodine solution prior to the procedure. A tenaculum may be necessary to hold the cervix, to facilitate insertion of the curette.

Nursing considerations include assessing for iodine allergy as well as explanation of the procedure and the cramplike discomfort associated with the biopsy. A non-narcotic analgesic, such as acetaminophen, ibuprofen, or aspirin (if not contraindicated), may be administered before the procedure to reduce discomfort. The procedure is usually tolerated well and does not require general anesthesia. Vaginal spotting or bleeding may occur following the biopsy, thus the use of peripads may be necessary for the first twenty-four to forty-eight hours afterward. The patient should be instructed to count the number of pads used in a twenty-four-hour period so that adequate assessment can be made in the event of heavy bleeding.

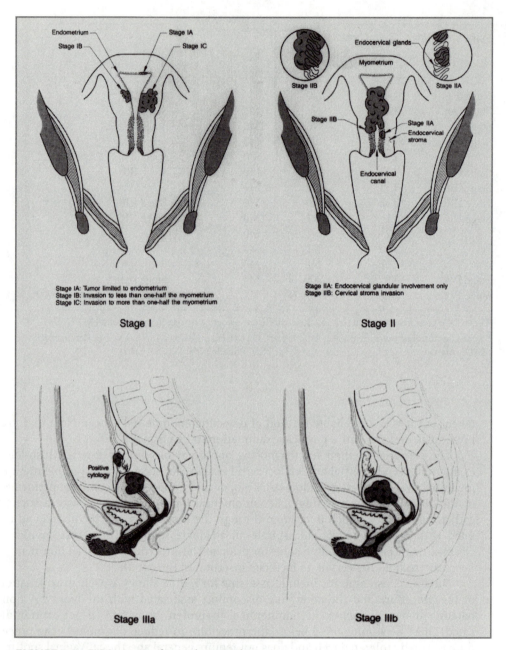

FIGURE 5.3. FIGO staging for endometrial cancer.

Source: Reproduced with permission from DiSaia, P.J., & Creasman, W.T. (1993). *Clinical Gynecologic Oncology* 4th ed. (pp. 161–162). St. Louis, MO: Mosby Year Book, Inc.

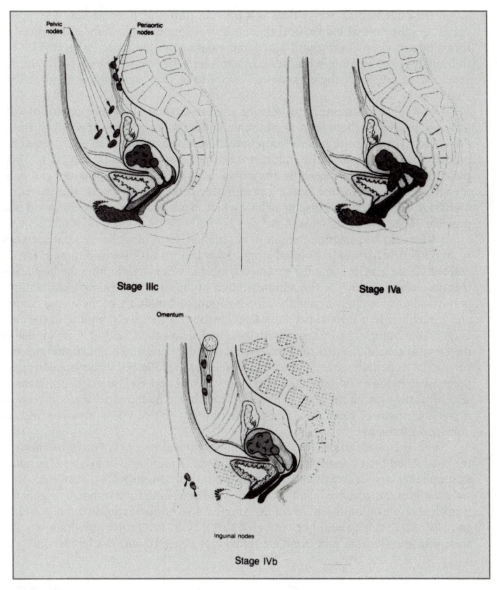

FIGURE 5.3. *(Continued)*

If the endometrial biopsy does not provide sufficient information, if symptoms persist despite normal biopsy, or if there is a strong suspicion of cancer, a formal fractional dilatation and curettage (D&C) and examination under anesthesia (EUA) are indicated. In conjunction with these, hysteroscopy may be indicated, to allow endoscopic visualization of the endometrial cavity to identify and biopsy abnormal mucosa.[14]

Transvaginal ultrasound can also be used to evaluate postmenopausal bleeding through measuring the thickness of the endometrial lining, or stripe. When the endometrial stripe is less than 3 to 5 mm in thickness, the incidence of endometrial neoplasia is low.[27] However, if the endometrial stripe is greater than 10 mm, 10 to 12% of patients will have hyperplasia or carcinoma. This additional information can define the advisability of a formal D&C, especially for patients who are an anesthesia risk. Transvaginal ultrasound is also beneficial when an adequate pelvic examination is not possible, especially in obese women.[9]

A D&C can be performed under mild sedation, local block, or general anesthesia in an outpatient setting or hospital surgical day facility. Risk status and need for general anesthesia are the two most common concerns when determining the location for this procedure. Following the administration of anesthesia, a pelvic examination is performed to adequately define the size, position, and mobility of the uterus, adnexa, and parametria in a relaxed pelvis. A D&C involves extensive sampling of the entire endometrial lining. The uterus is initially sounded and then, with the use of dilators, the cervical canal is dilated to allow insertion of the curette. The fractional curettage consists of a circumferential endocervical canal scrape followed by a systematic, comprehensive endometrial curettage. The endocervical and endometrial specimens are sent separately for pathologic evaluation. This classic fractionated method serves to detect the origin of carcinoma and to determine if the cervix is involved with endometrial carcinoma.[28]

Nursing considerations include providing written preoperative instructions for the patient and her partner. A brochure about D&C should also be given to the patient as supplementary information for informed consent. Questions are answered, financial arrangements reviewed, and the necessity of arranging for a responsible person to furnish transportation to and from the surgical site on the appointed day should be emphasized. Patients should be reassured that a D&C is a minor operation requiring short acting anesthesia, and complete recovery is expected within a few hours.

✼ TREATMENT

Hyperplasia

Reproductive-Aged Women

Progestin therapy creates a medical curettage that reverses hyperplasia by holding it in a regressive state.[29] For women diagnosed with hyperplasia without atypia who desire pregnancy, ovulation can be induced to stimulate production of endogenous progesterone. Cyclic progestins may also be administered to reduce estrogen stimulation of the endometrium. Follow-up includes periodic endometrial biopsy and transvaginal sonograms. For women diagnosed with hyperplasia with atypia, progestin therapy should be administered as a continuous regimen for six months. An endometrial biopsy should be obtained in three months to evaluate the response of the lesion, and a formal fractional D&C performed at completion of therapy. As long as a uterus is present, the need for progestin therapy remains because of the high risk of developing atypical hyperplasia, which can convert to carcinoma. Thus the endometrial cavity should continue to be periodically evaluated by endometrial sampling, transvaginal sonogram, or both.[9]

Postmenopausal Women

Endometrial hyperplasia carries a higher potential for malignancy in postmenopausal women.[30] It is therefore reasonable to consider surgical intervention for atypical hyperplasia in this age group. However, for those for whom surgery poses a risk, progestin therapy is an alternative intervention. For postmenopausal women who develop simple hyperplasia as a result of unopposed estrogen replacement therapy, adding progestin to the medical regimen is recommended.

Carcinoma of the Endometrium

After the diagnosis of endometrial carcinoma is histologically confirmed, the patient undergoes a complete evaluation to discover preexisting medical problems, suspicious lymph nodes, and areas of local and distal spread (Figure 5.4).

Hematologic studies should include routine preoperative blood work, clotting values, liver function tests, and measurement of CA-125 levels, as serum levels of the antigenic determinant CA-125 are elevated in most patients with advanced or metastatic endometrial cancers.[31,32] A chest X-ray is done to determine the cardiopulmonary status of the patient and to search for metastatic disease. If the lesion is poorly differentiated papillary, serous, clear cell, or sarcomatous, or if the patient has abnormal liver function tests, elevated serum CA-125, or parametrial or vaginal extension, a computed tomography (CT) scan of the abdomen and pelvis is indicated to evaluate the liver and retroperitoneal lymph nodes. Surgical staging according to the FIGO criteria then determines the need for adjuvant therapy.[7,33]

The therapeutic approach is individualized and based on prognostic factors, including stage, histologic cell type, degree of differentiation, degree of myometrial invasion, and nodal involvement. The grade of tumor and the degree of myometrial invasion can influence the risk for nodal metastases. Deep myometrial invasion is associated with a higher probability of extrauterine spread of disease, treatment failure, and recurrence.

Standard treatment for early stage endometrial carcinoma continues to be hysterectomy and bilateral salpingo-oophorectomy. Postoperative treatment is reserved

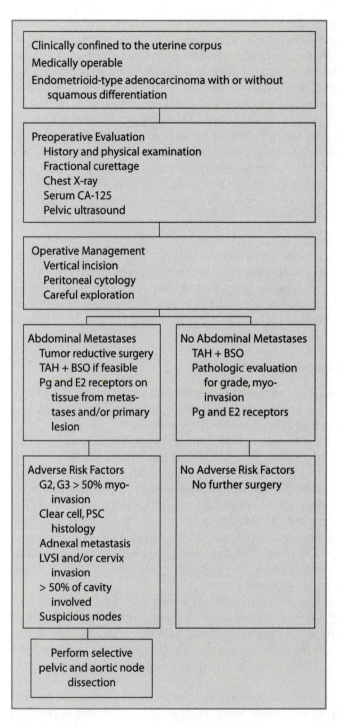

FIGURE 5.4. Schema for operative management of clinical stages I and II endometrial cancers.

Source: Reproduced with permission from Morrow, P.C., Curtin, J.P., & Townsend, D.E. *Synopsis of Gynecologic Oncology.* Churchill Livingstone, New York, 1993, p. 168.

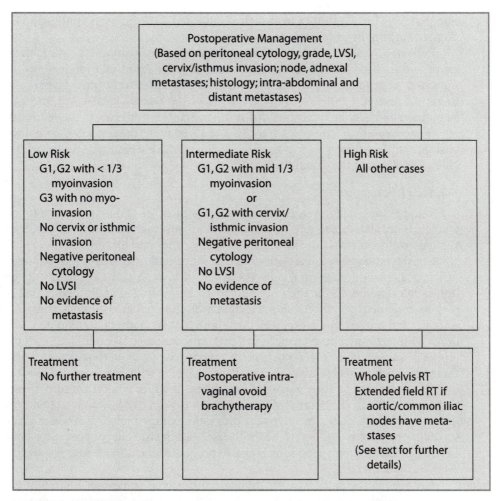

FIGURE 5.5. Endometrial carcinoma postoperative management schema.

Source: Reproduced with permission from Morrow, P.C., Curtin, J.P., & Townsend, D.E., *Synopsis of Gynecologic Oncology,* Churchill Livingstone, New York, 1993, p. 169.

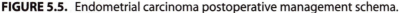

for those patients with poor prognostic factors as determined by pathologic staging based on FIGO criteria (Figure 5.5).

Surgical staging, as defined by FIGO criteria, involves an adequate abdominal incision, preferably vertical; sampling of peritoneal fluid for cytologic evaluation; and careful abdominal and pelvic exploration with biopsy or excision of any extrauterine lesions suspicious for tumor. For stage I disease, this procedure is followed by an extrafascial total abdominal hysterectomy and bilateral salpingo-oophorectomy. Suspicious lymph nodes should be removed, and routine sampling for pathologic evaluation performed.[23] No further treatment is indicated if the tumor is confined to the endometrium and the lesion is low grade.

For stage II endometrial carcinoma, with microscopic cervical invasion, the surgical procedure is the same as for stage I, at a minimum. A radical hysterectomy may be indicated, depending on cervical involvement. Postoperatively, intravaginal radiation therapy delivered to the vaginal vault reduces the risk of recurrence; and external beam radiation may be recommended if the margins or nodes are positive for cancer.

In most cases, treatment for stage III and IV endometrial cancers is combined and customized to the areas of metastasis. Treatments include surgery, radiation therapy, chemotherapy, and hormonal therapy.[9]

Adjuvant Treatments

Radiotherapy delivery methods in the treatment of endometrial cancer include whole pelvic, abdominal, and intravaginal. The intravaginal technique irradiates the vaginal vault to decrease the incidence of vaginal apex and local recurrence.

Considerable interest has been shown in the specific estrogen-progesterone receptors in malignant endometrial cells. Assays of these receptors have led to the collection of information on the presence and absence of estrogen and progesterone receptors in endometrial tumors, showing that well-differentiated tumors contain more estrogen and progesterone receptors than those that are poorly differentiated. Like patients with metastatic breast cancer, patients with endometrial carcinoma with progesterone-positive and estrogen-positive receptors have a high response to hormonal therapy.[14] Positive-receptor status has been associated with improved disease-free and overall survival rates. Thus progestational agents produce a good antitumor response and are valuable in the control of recurrent disease and can be administered orally or intramuscularly. Contraindications for progestin therapy include deep-vein thrombosis, pulmonary embolus, severe heart disease, and breast cancer. A receptor-poor status may predict not only a poor response to progestins but also a better response to cytotoxic chemotherapy.

The role of chemotherapy in endometrial cancer is somewhat limited; it is most commonly implemented as a palliative measure in advanced or recurrent disease. The most common agents used are doxirubicin, cisplatin, and paclitaxel.[34]

❋ FOLLOW-UP

Patients are advised on the routine follow-up schedule after the completion of treatment. For the first two to three years, the patient is examined every two to four months, depending on the risk for recurrence, then every six months. Each visit includes a physical exam, a speculum exam, a pelvic exam (vaginal and bimanual rectovaginal), peripheral lymph node examination, and a vaginal smear for cytology. Periodic chest X-rays and CT scans may also be beneficial in following this disease process.

Recurrence

Endometrial carcinoma usually recurs locally, within the vaginal vault or above the upper vagina. Treatment with surgery, radiation, or a combination of both is associated with good results. Recurrence beyond the vagina often requires hormonal therapy or chemotherapy. Tamoxifen will give a 20% response rate for patients who did not respond to standard progesterone therapy.[35]

If disease progresses while on progestins, chemotherapy should be also considered. Tamoxifen has been used as salvage therapy for endometrial cancer in an attempt to produce progesterone-receptor positivity.[36] Results vary; further research is needed.

Estrogen Replacement Therapy

After hysterectomy for endometrial carcinoma, many women suffer from the effects of estrogen deficiency, including vasomotor instability, dyspareunia, vaginal dryness, and the risks of osteoporosis, atherosclerotic heart disease, and Alzheimer's disease.[37] Osteoporosis may contribute to the risk of hip fractures in elderly women that is associated with a mortality of up to 24% within one year of the fracture.[38] Women with a history of endometrial carcinoma are usually denied estrogen replacement therapy, however, since adenocarcinoma of the endometrium is considered an estrogen-sensitive neoplasm, hormone replacement may stimulate residual tumor cells. This issue has been a long-standing controversy, since there are few scientific data to support or condemn its use.

Creasman et al. studied 221 patients with stage I adenocarcinoma of the endometrium; 17 patients received estrogen replacement after cancer therapy and 174 did not. Risk factors were similar for both groups. The group who received estrogen replacement had a longer disease-free survival rate, leading the researchers to conclude that hormone replacement does not appear to be contraindicated for patients with stage I endometrial cancer.[39]

In 1990, Lee et al. retrospectively studied 106 patients with stage I endometrial cancer where 44 patients were given estrogen replacement within the first postoperative year and 62 were not given estrogen. At five years, the estrogen-treated group did not have evidence of recurrent disease. One recurrence was documented in the non–estrogen-treated group.[40]

These significant data suggest that hormone replacement is safe for patients in the low-risk group. This finding will open the door for further research.

In 1990, the American College of Obstetricians & Gynecologists issued guidelines to identify appropriate candidates who are free of disease for estrogen replacement therapy, based on prognostic indicators and risk to the patient.[41] Patients should be encouraged to discuss these options with their physicians.

TABLE 5.4

Diagnostic Cluster

Diagnostic/Preoperative and Postoperative Period

COLLABORATIVE PROBLEMS
Potential Complication: Bleeding/hemorrhage
Potential Complication: Thromboembolic event
Potential Complication: Infection/sepsis
Potential Complication: Fluid/electrolyte imbalance
Potential Complication: Atelectasis/pneumonia
Potential Complication: Bowel dysfunction
Potential Complication: Urinary dysfunction

NURSING DIAGNOSIS
1. Potential altered health maintenance related to insufficient knowledge of condition, diagnostic tests, prognosis, and treatment options
2. Decisional conflict related to insufficient knowledge of treatment options
3. Anxiety/fear related to impending surgery, and insufficient knowledge of preoperative routines, intraoperative activities, and postoperative self-care activities
4. Anxiety/fear related to insufficient knowledge of potential impact of condition and treatment on reproductive organs and sexuality
5. Grieving related to potential loss of fertility and perceived effects on lifestyle
6. Potential altered respiratory function related to immobility secondary to imposed bed rest and pain
7. Potential fluid volume deficit related to losses secondary to surgical wound or gastrointestinal dysfunction
8. Altered comfort related to effects of surgery, disease process, and immobility
9. Potential for infection related to susceptibility to bacteria secondary to wound, invasive vascular access, and/or urinary catheter
10. Potential altered nutrition: less than body requirements related to disease process, wound healing, and decreased caloric intake
11. Impaired physical mobility related to surgical interruption of body structures, incisional site pain, and activity restriction
12. Potential bowel dysfunction related to decreased peristalsis secondary to surgical manipulation of bowel, effects of anesthesia and analgesia, and immobility
13. Potential urinary dysfunction related to loss of sensation of bladder distention secondary to surgical and/or pharmaceutical interventions
14. Potential impaired skin integrity related to surgical wound, decreased tissue perfusion, ostomy stomas, drain sites, and/or immobility
15. Potential impaired tissue integrity/infection related to lymphedema secondary to surgical removal of lymph nodes

TABLE 5.4 *(continued)*

16a. Potential sexual dysfunction related to disease process, surgical intervention, fatigue, and/or pain

16b. Potential moderate or possible permanent alterations in sexual activity related to disease process, surgical intervention, fatigue, and/or pain

16c. Severe or permanent inability to engage in genital intercourse

17. Alteration in coping related to infertility

18. Potential altered health maintenance related to insufficient knowledge of dietary restrictions, medications, activity restrictions, self-care activities, symptoms of complications, follow-up visits, and community resources

Treatment Period

COLLABORATIVE PROBLEMS
Potential Complication: Preexisting medical conditions
Potential Complication: Anasarca
Potential Complication: Fluid/electrolyte imbalance

NURSING DIAGNOSIS

1. Anxiety/fear related to loss of feelings of control of life, unpredictability of nature of disease, and uncertain future

2. Anxiety/fear related to insufficient knowledge of prescribed radiation therapy, and necessary self-care measures

3. Anxiety/fear related to insufficient knowledge of prescribed gynecologic radiation implant: conventional afterloading procedure

4. Anxiety/fear related to insufficient knowledge of prescribed gynecologic radiation implant: remote afterloading procedure

5. Potential for infection related to immunosuppression neutropenia secondary to chemotherapy and/or radiation therapy

6. Potential for bleeding related to immunosuppression thrombocytopenia secondary to chemotherapy and/or radiation therapy

7. Potential alteration in skin integrity related to treatment modality and/or disease process

8. Potential for alteration in elimination: diarrhea related to radiation-induced enteritis

9. Potential for impaired elimination related to development of fistulae

✖ NURSING MANAGEMENT

Formulating a plan of care poses a challenge to the nurse in managing the medical, surgical, and psychosocial components of patients with endometrial cancer. The diagnosis of cancer can be physically and psychosocially threatening to the patient, her partner, and her family. Nurses provide education, support, and therapeutic care in a comprehensive manner. Knowledge of the individual's physical and psychosocial needs are essential in formulating a realistic care plan and setting achievable goals.

It is not unusual to encounter multiple preexisting medical problems in this patient population. For example, obesity is a common risk factor in the development of endometrial cancer. Common medical and metabolic disorders associated with obesity are hypertension and diabetes mellitus. Nutritional status directly correlates with intraoperative success and postoperative recovery. As adipose tissue increases, so does the technical difficulty of surgery. Surgical incisions in obese patients are generally larger, and the tissue tends to be weak. This increases the risk of postoperative infection, incisional hernias, and wound dehiscence. Respiratory complications are also a concern because obesity decreases the efficiency of respiratory muscles, which inhibits effective coughing and deep breathing exercises postoperatively.

Diabetes mellitus predisposes a person to infection and inhibits healing. Standard glucose testing to determine if diabetes is controlled should be established before surgery. Blood glucose monitoring, with appropriate insulin coverage, needs to be carefully managed in the postoperative period.

The abdominal incision is at high risk for infection, hemorrhage, dehiscence, or evisceration, especially in the obese patient. These complications can occur at any time during the healing process. Observation of the incision for tension on suture sites, erythema, and increased serosanguineous drainage may indicate potential, partial, or complete dehiscence. Wound separations can be extremely distressing and frustrating to the patient and family. Wound dehiscence requires meticulous wound care to keep the site clean and free of exudate using aseptic techniques. Debridement may be indicated to remove necrotic tissue and allow for granulation. It is important to keep the patient informed about the progress of healing.

Cure for endometrial cancer is often achieved through surgical intervention alone, or in combination with postoperative external and/or intravaginal radiotherapy. These experiences can be overwhelming for the patient and her family from the time of diagnosis to the completion of therapy, though the treatment time span is relatively short compared with those of other gynecologic malignancies. A baseline psychosocial assessment to delineate the patient's role in and outside the family is helpful in providing appropriate intervention in the post-treatment period. Often, the patient may have difficulties in coping with the fact that a cancer was diagnosed and treated within a short time span. Allowing the patient to ventilate her feelings, fears, and concerns is encouraged. It is important for nurses to listen and validate patients' concerns and behaviors, in order to provide proper support. Referrals to support groups and/or cancer survivor groups may be offered so that the patient may share concerns with others in similar situations.

Menopause is induced by surgery for endometrial cancer in premenopausal women. But patients treated for endometrial cancer are not candidates for estrogen replacement therapy initially. Because of the lack of estrogen, the patient may report hot flashes, decreased vaginal lubrication, vaginal burning and pruritis, and dyspareunia. Nurses can advise on the use of a vaginal moisturizer to restore moisture to vaginal mucosa, and water-based lubricants to facilitate sexual relations. Patients may also report joint pain and backache as a result of osteoporosis. A calcium supplement and physical exercise are essential in protecting against bone loss. Accurate information regarding menopause and symptoms associated with a lack of estrogen can be helpful and reassuring to the patient with endometrial cancer.

✳ REFERENCES

1. American Cancer Society. (1999). *Cancer Facts and Figures 1999: Selected Cancers.* See http://www.cancer.org/statistics/cff99/ selectedcancers.html.
2. Gallup, D.G., & Stock, R.J. (1984). Adenocarcinoma of the endometrium in women 40 years of age or younger. *Obstet Gynecol, 64,* 417.
3. Whitaker, G.K., Lee, R.B., & Benson, W.L. (1986). Carcinoma of the endometrium in young women. *Mil Med, 151,* 25.
4. DeVesa, S.S., Silverman, D.T., & Young, J.L. Jr. (1987). Cancer incidence and mortality trends among whites in the United States: 1947–1984. *J Natl Cancer Inst, 79,* 701.
5. Lauritzen, C. (1977). Oestrogens and endometrial cancers: A point of review. *Clin Obstet Gynecol, 40,* 145.
6. Sutton, G.P. (1990). The significance of positive peritoneal cytology in endometrial cancer. *Oncology, 4,* 21.
7. Park, R.C., Grigsby, P.W., Muss, H.B., & Norris, H.J. (1992). Corpus: Epithelial tumors. In W.J. Hoskins, C.A. Perez, & R.C. Young, eds., *Principles and Practice of Gynecologic Oncology* (pp. 663–689). Philadelphia: Lippincott.
8. Wynder, E.L., Escher, G.C., & Mantel, N. (1966). An epidemiological investigation of cancer of the endometrium. *Cancer, 19,* 489.
9. Morrow, P.C., Curtin, J.P., & Townsend, D.E. (1993). *Synopsis of Gynecologic Oncology* 4th ed. New York: Churchill Livingstone.
10. Brinton, L.A., Berman, M.L., Mortel, R., et al. (1992). Reproductive, menstrual, and medical risk factors for endometrial cancer: Results from a case control study. *Am J Obstet Gynecol, 167,* 1317–1325.
11. Fisher, B., Constantino, J.P., Redmond, C.K. (1994). Endometrial cancer in tamoxifen treated breast cancer patients. Findings from the NSABP-B-14. *JNCI, 86(7)* 527–537.
12. Rubin, G.L. Peterson, H.B., & Lee, N.C. (1990). Estrogen replacement therapy and the risk of endometrial cancer: Remaining controversies. *Am J Obstet Gynecol, 162,* 148.
13. Barber, H.R.J.K. (1980). *Manual of Gynecologic Oncology* (p. 79). Philadelphia: Lippincott.
14. DiSaia, P.J., & Creasman, W.T. (1993). Adenocarcinoma of the uterus. In P.J. DiSaia & W.T. Creasman, eds., *Clinical Gynecologic Oncology* 4th ed. (pp. 156–193). St. Louis, MO: Mosby.
15. Schapira, D.V., Kumar, N.B., Lyman, G.H., et al. (1991). Upper-body fat distribution and endometrial cancer risk. *JAMA, 266,* 1808–1811.
16. Jasonni, V.M., Lodi, S., & Preti, S. (1981). Extraglandular estrogen production in postmenopausal women with and without endometrial cancer: Comparison between in vitro and in vivo results. *Cancer Detect Prev 4,* 469.
17. Lynch, H.T., Bardawil, W.A., & Harris, R.E. (1978). Multiple primary cancers and prolonged survival: Familial colonic and endometrial cancers. *Dis Colon Rectum, 21,* 165.
18. Lynch, H.T., Ens, J.A., & Lynch, J.F. (1990). Lynch Syndrome II and urological malignancies. *J Urol, 143,* 23.
19. Smith, D.B. (1986). Gynecologic cancers: Etiology and pathophysiology. *Semin Oncol Nurs, 2,* 270–274.
20. Huang, S.F., Berek, F.S., & Fu, Y.S. (1992). Pathology of endometrial carcinoma. In M.Coppelson, ed., *Gynecologic Oncology: Fundamental Principles and Clinical Practice* 2nd ed. (pp. 753–773). New York: Churchill Livingstone.
21. Cheon, H.K. (1969). Prognosis of endometrial carcinoma. *Obstet Gynecol, 34,* 680.
22. Creasman, T., Boronow, R.C., & Morrow, C.P. (1976). Adenocarcinoma of the endometrium: Its metastatic lymph node potential. *Gynecol Oncol, 4,* 239.

23. Piver, M.S., Lele, S.B., & Barlow, J.J. (1982). Para-aortic lymph node evaluation in stage I endometrial carcinoma. *Obstet Gynecol, 59,* 97.

24. Wilson, T.O., Podratz, K.C., & Gaffey, T.A. (1990). Evaluation of unfavorable histologic sybtypes in endometrial adenocarcinoma. *Am J Obstet Gynecol, 162,* 418.

25. Baird, S.B., McCorkle, R., & Grant, M. (1991). Gynecologic cancer. *Cancer Nursing: A Comprehensive Textbook* (pp. 514–519). Philadelphia: Saunders.

26. Haskell, C. (1985). *Cancer Treatment* 2nd ed. Philadelphia: Saunders.

27. Granberg, S., Wikland, M., & Karlsson, B. (1991). Endometrial thickness as measured by endovaginal ultrasonography for identifying endometrial abnormality. *Am J Obstet Gynecol, 164,* 47.

28. Creasman, W.T., & Weed, F.C. Jr. (1992). Carcinoma of the endometrium (FIGO stages I and II): Clinical features and management. In M. Coppleson, ed., *Gynecologic Oncology: Fundamental Principles and Clinical Practice* 2nd ed. (pp. 775–789). New York: Churchill Livingstone.

29. Kistner, R.W. (1970). The effects of progestational agents on hyperplasia and carcinoma in situ of the endometrium. *Int J Gynecol Obstet, 84,* 561.

30. Wentz, W.B. (1985). Progestin therapy in lesions of the endometrium. *Semin Oncol, 12,* 23.

31. Berchuck, A., Saisson, A.P., & Clarke-Pearson, D.L. (1989). Immunohistochemical expression of CA–125 in endometrial adenocarcinoma: Correlation of antigen expression with metastatic potential. *Cancer Res, 49,* 2091.

32. Olt, G., Berchuck, A., & Bast, R.C. Jr. (1990). The role of tumor markers in gyncologic oncology. *Obstet Gynecol Surv, 45,* 570.

33. Brinton, L.A., & Hoover, R.N. (1993). Estrogen replacement therapy and endometrial cancer risk: Unresolved issues. *Obstet Gynecol, 81(2),* 265–271.

34. Ball, H.G., Blessing, J.A., Lentz, S.S., et al. (1996). A phase II trial of paclitaxel in patients with advanced or recurrent adenocarcinoma of the endometrium: A Gynecological Group study. *Gynecol Oncol, 62(2),* 278–281.

35. Jick, S.S., Walker, A.M., Jick, H. (1993). Estrogens, progesterone, and endometrial cancer. *Epidemiology, 4(1),* 20–24.

36. Otte, D.M. (1990). Gynecologic cancers. In S.L. Groenwald, M. Frogge, M. Goodman, & C. Yarbro, eds., *Cancer Nursing: Principles and Practice* 2nd ed. (pp. 860–864). Boston: Jones and Bartlett.

37. Brinton, L.A., Schairer, C. (1997). Post menopausal hormone replacement therapy: time for a reappraisal? *N Engl J Med, 336(25),* 1821–1822.

38. Fisher, E.S., Baron, J.A., Malenka, D.J., et al. (1991). Hip fracture indidence and mortality in New England. *Epidemiology, 67(2),* 116–22.

39. Creasman, W.T., Henderson, D., Hinshaw, W., & Clarke-Pearson, D.L. (1986). Estrogen replacement therapy in the patient treated for endometrial cancer. *Obstet Gynecol, 67(3),* 326–330.

40. Lee, R.B., Burke, T.W., Park, R.C. (1990). Estrogen replacement therapy following treatment for stage I endometrial carcinoma. *Gynecol Oncol, 36,* 189–194.

41. American College of Obstetrics & Gynecology (1990, February). *Estrogen Replacement Therapy and Endometrial Cancer* (ACOG Committee Opinion, no. 80). Washington, DC: American College of Obstetrics & Gynecology.

CHAPTER 6

Epithelial Cancers of the Ovary and Fallopian Tube

JoAnn Huang Eriksson, RN, MS, AOCN
Sheryl Redlin Frazier, RN

❈ INTRODUCTION

It is estimated that 1 out of every 70 women will develop ovarian cancer, and 1 out of 100 women will die of this disease, in the United States.[1] Epithelial ovarian cancer is the leading cause of death from gynecologic malignancies. In 1999, 25,200 women were estimated to be diagnosed, with 13,342 dying from this disease.[2] Ovarian cancer is the fourth leading cause of cancer in women and accounts for 5% of all deaths from cancer.[2] With an insidious onset and often an advanced stage at time of diagnosis, ovarian cancer deaths exceed those of cervical and endometrial cancer combined.[1]

The treatment and care of the woman with ovarian cancer is complex and requires a thorough understanding of the disease.

❈ ANATOMY AND PHYSIOLOGY

The ovaries are pinkish grey, slightly nodular, solid, almond-shaped entities. The right ovary tends to be slightly larger than the left. They are located lateral to the uterus and slightly posterior and caudal to the fallopian tubes. The ovaries undergo significant changes in size, shape, position, and histology during a woman's lifetime and over the course of any given menstrual cycle. These changes are usually caused by various endocrine stimuli.[3]

The ovaries develop on the posterior wall, near the kidneys. They then descend into the true pelvis. They grow progressively larger and change shape and position between birth and puberty. During pregnancy they are lifted out of the true pelvis due to uterine enlargement. In the premenopausal state, ovaries measure approximately 3.5 × 2.0 × 1.5 cm.[3,4] Postmenopausal ovaries shrink and atrophy when the graafian follicles and ova disappear and become an inert residue consisting of white connective tissue. These may become as small as newborn ovaries and should not be palpable on pelvic examination.[3]

The blood supply to the ovary is from the ovarian artery, which branches off the abdominal aorta immediately below the renal artery. The right ovarian vein enters the inferior vena cava below the renal vein; the left ovarian vein drains into the left renal vein.[3,4]

The nerve supply of the ovaries comes from the level of the tenth thoracic vertebra.

Lymphatic drainage is into the para-aortic lymph nodes near the kidney. There are three primary routes of lymphatic drainage into the retroperitoneal lymph nodes. One route of drainage consists of a group of vessels that ascend bilaterally along the ovarian blood vessels to the nodes between the renal arteries and the aortic bifurcation. A second route consists of vessels that travel laterally toward the lateral and posterior pelvic wall and end in the high external and hypogastric nodes. From there, lymphatic drainage goes along the common iliac vessels into the para-aortic lymph nodes. A third route is along the round ligament into the external iliac and inguinal lymph nodes.[3,4] These drainage systems provide the routes for dissemination of ovarian cancer into the lymphatic system.

Epithelial ovarian tumors account for 90 to 95% of ovarian tumors.[5] They arise from the germinal epithelium or mesothelium on the surface of the ovary.[3,6] Germinal epithelium is thought to form invaginations into the ovarian stroma during adulthood, and these invaginations are the earliest developmental stage of the serous tumors. The common epithelial tumors arise where the surface epithelium has penetrated into underlying stroma, forming inclusion glands, or cysts. Repeated or incessant ovulation is thought to be an important etiologic factor in the development of an ovarian cancer.[7,8] Recent reports indicating that infertile women who have had hyperstimulation of the ovaries to induce ovulation have a higher risk of developing ovarian cancer seem to substantiate this theory.[9]

Low malignant potential (LMP) tumors, or tumors of borderline malignancy, are one subclass in the histologic classification of the epithelial tumors. No matter how anaplastic the epithelium may appear, these tumors are classified as LMP because there is no invasion of the stroma. But low malignant potential tumors may metastasize to the peritoneum or lymph nodes. Prognosis is dependent on the stage of the disease.[3,10]

The histologic classification of ovarian tumors is based primarily on morphology and histogenesis (Table 6.1). Although it is not perfect, it provides a standardized nomenclature for comparative studies. Low malignant potential tumors can be found in each of the different histologic subgroups.

The fallopian tube averages 12 cm in length and has an external diameter of 2 mm proximally and 1.5 cm distally. It is located on the edge of the mesosalpinx and extends from the uterus to the side of the pelvis. The lumen communicates proximally with the endometrial cavity and distally with the peritoneal cavity.[11]

TABLE 6.1

Neoplasms Derived from Coelomic Epithelium

Serous tumors

Mucinous tumors

Endometrioid tumors

Clear cell tumors

Transitional cell tumors

Mixed epithelial tumors

Undifferentiated carcinoma

Unclassified epithelial tumors

The fallopian tube has an external serosal layer, a middle muscular layer, and an internal mucosal layer. The mesothelial cells that cover the visceral peritoneum of the uterus also cover the serosal layer of the fallopian tube. The muscular layer has an external longitudinal and an inner circular layer. The mucosal layer is composed of fibrovascular stroma in a papillary pattern. This layer is covered by columnar epithelium.[11] It is the epithelial layer that is the origin of the majority of primary fallopian tube malignancies.[12] But no specific morphologic, ultrastructural, or immunohistochemical parameters to identify malignant epithelium as originating from the fallopian tube are available yet.[11] However, in an effort to define primary versus metastatic cancer of the fallopian tube, the following criteria have been recommended:[13]

1. The tumor is located in the fallopian tube and arises from the endosalpinx.
2. The histologic pattern is that of the epithelial mucosa, that is, revealing a papillary pattern.
3. The transition between benign and malignant tubal epithelium should be demonstrable if the wall of the fallopian tube is involved.
4. The ovaries and the endometrium are normal or contain less tumor than the fallopian tube(s).

Fallopian tube cancers are almost all adenocarcinomas. Papillary serous adenocarcinoma is the most common cancer of the fallopian tube, accounting for 90% of the adenocarcinomas. Adenoacanthomas and adenosquamous carcinomas have also been reported. Squamous, endometrial, and clear cell types are rare. Fallopian tube cancer appears to affect both tubes equally. Bilaterality is seen in 5 to 30% of patients.[11]

✹ EPIDEMIOLOGY/ETIOLOGY

Ovarian cancer occurs primarily in women in the 40 to 70 year age range.[14] The incidence rises steadily to the eighth decade, then drops off slightly. Peak incidence is in the 55 to 59 year age group, and the median age at time of diagnosis is 61 years.[3] The overall five-year survival rate is 35 to 40%,[15] with the survival rate for patients with early stage disease 81%, and 21% for those with advanced disease.[1]

Epidemiologic studies to evaluate risk factors for epithelial ovarian cancer indicate a higher incidence in nulliparous women or women with low parity. The risk of ovarian cancer is correlated with the length of time a woman has ovulated. Suppression of ovulation by pregnancy, lactation, and oral contraceptives seems to decrease the risk.[15,16] Preliminary reports indicate that infertile women who have had stimulation of ovulation by various gonadotropins are at higher risk of developing ovarian cancer.[9] These observations support the theory that the chronic irritation or damage to the ovarian epithelial surface occurs as a result of "incessant ovulation." That is, the rupture and repair process allows the possibility of aberrant repair. With increased number of ovulation cycles, the probability of developing ovarian cancer also increases.[17,18] Women who have never been pregnant and women who have used oral contraceptives have a 30 to 60% lower risk of developing ovarian cancer than nulliparous women and women without a history of contraceptive use.[1,16,19]

The theory of hormonal influence as a predisposing factor in ovarian cancer is also substantiated by several findings. There is an increased risk of developing ovarian cancer in women with a history of breast cancer. Conversely, women with a history of ovarian cancer have a two- to fourfold increased risk of developing breast cancer.[1] Whittemore et al.[7] have also identified a risk for epithelial ovarian cancer in women with abnormalities of ovulation that reduce fertility. However, exogenous use of estrogens alone has not been associated with an increased risk of ovarian cancer.[5,20]

Genetic Factors

Like all cancers, ovarian cancer is a genetic disease. It occurs in one of three forms: sporadic, familial, or hereditary. It is estimated that between 5 and 10% of all ovarian cancers are hereditary or familial.[21,22] In other words, in hereditary or familial cancer, the genetic alterations that contributed to the development of cancer can be attributed to the inheritance, from one generation to the next, of an abnormal copy of a predisposition gene. Inheritance of hereditary or familial cancer genes does not imply that the disease will occur in the individual during her lifetime, but does indicate an increased risk for disease occurrence.[21,22] Human beings have two copies of each gene. When one of those copies is ineffective, either through inheritance of an abnormal gene or through mutation or loss, a backup or second gene is placed into action; this is often referred to as the "spare tire" effect. Hereditary and familial cancers occur in individuals who have inherited an abnormal gene copy and through mutation or "loss" lose the second gene copy. Losing a gene copy is referred to as loss of heterozygosity, or LOH, and loss of genes occurs fairly commonly as cells divide. It is believed that in sporadic cancers, the first malfunction of a gene occurs as a mutation, and the second is a loss of chromosomal DNA from the gene thus permitting the development of cancer.

In inherited ovarian cancer, there are two major categories of dominant inheritance.[21] One includes cancer syndromes such as Peutz-Jegher (colon, ovary), Gardner (colon, brain, ovary), or Cowden (breast, colon, ovary).[21] In these disorders, cancer occurs as a secondary diagnosis.[21] The other category includes inherited cancer family syndromes such as Lynch syndrome II (colon, endometrium, ovary), site-specific ovarian cancer (ovary), and breast/ovarian cancer syndrome (breast, ovary).[21]

On the average, women with inherited ovarian cancer are usually diagnosed at an earlier age (average age at diagnosis is 59) than women with sporadic ovarian cancer.[1, 21] Prophylactic oophorectomy has been recommended by some physicians for women with a history of inherited ovarian cancer.[23] However, prophylactic oophorectomies are not a guarantee against ovarian cancer; there is still approximately a 15 to 20% risk of developing peritoneal carcinomatosis.[1] Hatcher[24] recommends the continuous use of birth control pills to suppress ovulation in women with a family history of ovarian cancer until the month before they desire to conceive. When the women have completed childbearing, preferably by age 35, then prophylactic bilateral oophorectomies are recommended. Barber[25] also recommends the use of birth control pills and prophylactic oophorectomies to prevent ovarian cancer in high-risk women.

As molecular geneticists move closer to discovering the causes of tumorogenesis, more information about which specific chromosomes can be implicated in contributing to the cause of ovarian cancer becomes evident. Currently it appears that chromosomes 1, 3, 6, 11, and 17 are involved in this cascade of events which drives the development of ovarian cancer. [22]

One gene associated with the hereditary breast ovarian cancer families that has been identified is the BRCA1 located at the 17q12-23 locus.[26] The BRCA1 is a tumor suppressor gene, and its mutation may contribute to the development of ovarian cancer.[26] BRCA2 and p53 are examples of other gene mutations implicated in ovarian cancer tumorogenesis. The p53 gene has been shown to be mutated or lost in as many as 75% of ovarian cancers.[26] Oncogenes, genes that regulate cell growth and proliferation, that are currently associated with ovarian cancer, are EGF (epidermal growth factor) and TGF-α which are thought to contribute to unrestrained proliferation of ovarian cancer cells.[26] TGF-β is thought to be a growth inhibitor of normal epithelial ovarian tissue, and its loss in ovarian cancer cell lines may contribute to some types of ovarian cancers.[26] Another EGF receptor under investigation in ovarian cancer is HER-2/*neu*.[26] HER-2/*neu* gene is *erb*B-2 and is found on chromosome 17q.[26] Studies have shown that the aggressive biologic behavior of some advanced ovarian cancers overexpresses HER-2/*neu*.[26] These findings are similar to studies in breast cancer which have shown an association between overexpression of HER-2/*neu* and poor survival.[26] Clearly the study of genes in ovarian cancers is an evolving science. It has become apparent that it takes more than one biologic event to develop ovarian cancer and these events differ from woman to woman. The use of the identified genes and the ones not yet implicated is also under investigation. It is certain that treatment of ovarian cancer in the future will include some kind of gene therapy.

Environmental Factors

Environmental factors have been investigated as risk factors for ovarian cancer, since the highest incidence occurs in industrialized countries, with the exception of Japan. Over time Japanese immigrants to the United States develop an increased risk of ovarian cancer that approaches the rate of native-born American women. However, it does not reach the level observed in Caucasian women.[1]

Studies on diets high in meat and animal fat as well as alcohol consumption as risk factors for ovarian cancer have been contradictory.[27,28] Obesity is associated with a slight increase in risk,[29] but cigarette and coffee consumption show no association.[16]

Cramer et al.[27] investigated the relationship between dietary factors and genetically determined levels of erythrocyte galactose-1-phosphate uridyl transferase and the risk of developing ovarian cancer. This study was based on the hypothesis that high levels of gonadotropins are secreted due to ovarian failure and faulty feedback control mechanisms in the pituitary gland (hypergonadotropic hypogonadism). It was also based on the observation that dietary galactose consumption and decreased levels of transferase are associated with hypergonadotropic hypogonadism. This study found that the mean transferase activity was significantly lower in women with ovarian cancer than in controls. The finding that the increase in ovarian cancer risk correlated with an increased lactose:transferase ratio was highly significant.

Exposure to industrial by-products and radiation has not been proved to be related to ovarian cancer. Migration of chemicals to the peritoneal cavity via the vagina and reproductive organs may account for exposure of the ovaries to carcinogens. Talc and asbestos exposure as a cause of ovarian cancer is controversial.[16,30]

Primary carcinoma of the fallopian tube is the least common of the gynecologic malignancies. It accounts for only 0.3 to 1.1% of all gynecologic cancers,[31,32] with an estimated 3.6 fallopian tube cancers per million women diagnosed annually. Only 15% of fallopian tube malignancies are of primary origin; the rest are metastatic from other sites, such as the ovary, endometrium, and gastrointestinal tract. Age at diagnosis ranges from 18 to 80 years, with the peak range at 60 to 64 years. Chronic infection has been implicated, but does not appear to play a role as a cause of fallopian tube cancer. Thus the etiology of primary carcinoma of the fallopian tube is as yet unknown.[11]

✖ DIAGNOSTIC EVALUATION

History and Physical Assessment: Clinical Manifestations

The initial spread of ovarian cancer is clinically occult. Approximately 75 to 85% of women have advanced disease at the time of diagnosis.[1] A significant proportion (10%) of women with tumor seemingly confined to the ovaries have microscopic spread at the time of diagnosis.[1]

The most common presenting symptoms of ovarian cancer are abdominal distention, discomfort, or pain. But ovarian cancer has an insidious onset, and symptoms are usually not thought to occur until advanced stages. However, close questioning of patients often reveals a multiple-month history of vague abdominal discomfort, dyspepsia, *urinary frequency*, increasing flatulence, a sense of bloating, gastrointestinal disturbances, vague pelvic symptoms, and *weight changes* which may also be indicative of advanced disease.[1]

Like epithelial ovarian cancer, women with fallopian tube malignancies can be asymptomatic, but more frequently they have symptoms that lead to earlier detection.[11] The most common symptom, presenting in greater than 50% of patients, is vaginal bleeding.[3] Colicky pelvic pain is a frequent symptom. It is often accompanied by a profuse, watery vaginal discharge called *hydrops tubae profluens*. The classic triad of pain, menorrhagia, and leukorrhea is considered pathognomonic for tubal malignancies; however, it occurs in less than 15% of patients.[33] Ascites and abdominal or pelvic mass (in 80% of patients) and a positive cervical cytology are other signs that can alert a practitioner to the presence of malignancy.[11,32]

Psychosocial Assessment

With the diagnosis of ovarian cancer, there are myriad initial responses, such as shock or fear of pain and death.[34] These responses are common with any cancer diagnosis. In addition, patients have sometimes spent an inordinate amount of time with physicians, undergoing various diagnostic tests to no avail. So persistent symptoms have frustrated the women, their families, and their physicians. Due to the time of life in which the disease frequently occurs, the women may be dismissed as having unmet psychologic needs. Some women may even have begun to doubt themselves. But with the progression of symptoms and development of ascites, the disease then manifests itself. With a diagnosis, some women are relieved that there truly is a cause for their symptoms. With the identification of a problem, then appropriate treatment may be sought.

Patients sometimes also express anger at their physicians, the medical profession as a whole, themselves, and their families. To them, the symptoms of their disease were obvious. They forget that hindsight is extremely clear, and that as the disease progressed it manifested itself more obviously. Sadly, time, more than anything else, was what helped confirm the diagnosis. Anger can often be an extreme impediment to the trust needed in relationships between patients and health professionals. It is very important to allow and help patients express their pain, anger, and frustration as a part of providing total care. However, the women must also be guided to move beyond the anger and focus on regrouping their resources to cope with the treatments now facing them.

Other important aspects of psychosocial assessment are:[34,35,36]

1. The patient's status in the life cycle and developmental issues for that particular stage of life
2. The patient's worldview, or her approach and attitude toward life
3. Coping mechanisms, or lack of effective coping mechanisms
4. The patient's available physical and psychological support systems
5. The basis of the patient's self-image, self-worth, and sexual identity
6. The patient's spiritual state
7. The financial situation, in particular insurance coverage

Physical Assessment

Diagnosis of ovarian cancer often occurs late in the disease process. The primary method of improving survival is earlier diagnosis, and different methods have been studied in an effort to accomplish this goal. However, at this time early diagnosis still remains elusive.

Pelvic Examination

A routine pelvic examination can detect an asymptomatic ovarian cancer, but this is rare. It is estimated that examination of only 1 of 10,000 asymptomatic women will reveal an ovarian cancer.[3,7] Most palpable adnexal masses in premenopausal women are not malignant. The enlargements are usually due to follicular or corpus luteum cysts, which regress in one to three menstrual cycles. Thus the management of a premenopausal woman with a palpable adnexal mass less than 8 cm consists of observation and a repeat of the pelvic exam in 1–2 months. However, an adnexal mass that is equal to or greater than 10 cm, enlarges beyond 5 cm while under observation, and/or appears to persist while a woman is on a contraceptive pill regimen needs to be evaluated surgically. A pelvic mass that cannot be definitely diagnosed as a uterine myoma in a postmenopausal woman also warrants surgical exploration.[1,37]

Other pelvic findings that may raise the index of suspicion for a malignancy include a mass in the ovary that is relatively immobile and painless; irregular mass; solid or mixed solid and cystic components; bilateral ovarian involvement; and presence of other masses on the exam. Though a pelvic examination is limited, it can provide important information for diagnosis.[15,37]

Cytology

A Pap smear is usually performed as part of the routine pelvic examination; however, detection of ovarian cancer by a Pap smear is rare. More often detection of malignant cells indicates the presence of exfoliated cells and possibly advanced disease.

Cytologic examination through culdocentesis or paracentesis is usually not warranted. The patient with suspicious pelvic and adnexal masses needs surgical exploration regardless of the results of these exams. There is a slight chance of cystic rupture and seeding of the tumor along the needle tract, which both increases the stage of the disease and affects survival.[3]

Paracentesis may be useful in patients for whom surgical exploration is contraindicated. Obtaining fluid for cytology could provide a presumptive diagnosis of ovarian cancer and allow medical treatment to begin. However, this test cannot accurately determine the primary tumor site.[3]

Imaging Techniques

Radiologic imaging is very useful in evaluation of a patient with an adnexal mass or symptoms of ovarian cancer. For example, although abdominal ultrasound cannot provide a definitive diagnosis, it can provide information on the characteristics of a mass. Bilateral ovarian involvement, irregular borders, presence of solid components with papillary projections, and multiple dense irregular septae are characteristics that are highly suggestive of a malignancy. Ultrasound can also provide information on the presence of ascites and involvement of other organs.[38]

The use of transvaginal sonography (TVS) for ovarian cancer screening was first started in 1986.[39] It is an improvement over abdominal sonography in terms of better visualization of the ovaries regardless of body habitus, greater patient comfort and acceptance, and increased efficiency. Commonly used in screening, TVS is also used to evaluate adnexal masses.

A morphology index has been developed in an attempt to improve the diagnostic accuracy of benign versus malignant masses. Though there is currently no standard morphology index, several scales have been proposed. Some features included in these scales are wall thickness, inner wall structure, characteristics of septae, and echogenicity.[40]

Vascular endothelial cell growth is stimulated during malignant transformation. Tumor angiogenesis can result in irregular blood vessels without a progressive decrease in the caliber of the vessels. Thus transvaginal color flow ultrasound is used to measure the flow patterns in ovarian vessels.[39,40,41] A high impedance to blood flow, as reflected by a pulsatility index greater than 1.0, is often used.[40] A resistance index of <0.6 revealed a sensitivity of 66% and a specificity of 81% in Bromley and colleagues' study of postmenopausal women.[42] Though neither TVS nor color flow Doppler imaging are completely accurate in differentiating benign from malignant lesions, together with CA-125 these tests proved the most sensitive available.

A barium enema or colonoscopy is sometimes used in the work-up of a patient suspected of having an ovarian malignancy. Their primary use is to rule out a colonic malignancy as the cause of an adnexal mass, especially in postmenopausal women. They are also helpful in defining extrinsic versus intrinsic causes of obstructive bowel symptoms.[43]

A chest X-ray is routinely used in the evaluation of the woman with suspected ovarian cancer. It is often required prior to surgery, but it is also needed to identify pulmonary involvement. Parenchymal pulmonary metastases are not common, but pleural effusions are frequently detected by chest X-ray. Chest X-rays may also be used to assess response to treatment when effusions are present.[38,40]

A mammogram may be ordered to rule out a primary breast malignancy. Since breast cancer can metastasize to the ovary and cause peritoneal carcinomatosis or ascites, it is important to know the origin of the cancer. A mammogram may also be used to rule out a second primary malignancy.[3,38]

Intravenous pyelogram (IVP) is helpful in identifying the relationship of the ureters to the tumor and other pelvic structures. However, it is not routinely used in the evaluation of an ovarian tumor.[38]

Computed tomography (CT) scans are frequently used in the diagnosis or preoperative evaluation of an ovarian malignancy. Magnetic resonance imaging (MRI) scans are not as commonly used. CT and MRI can be useful in identifying liver or lung nodules, and these scans are often used to monitor pelvic and abdominal masses for response to therapy.[43]

Immunoscintigraphy is the use of radiolabeled antibodies to detect intra-abdominal spread of ovarian cancer. The goal is to detect miliary spread or other tumor masses that may not be large enough to be visualized on an ultrasound, CT scan, or MRI scan. Discovering occult disease may contribute favorably to patient care by altering treatment. However, use of monoclonal antibodies can lead to the development of human antimouse antibodies (HAMA), which can make a second administration of the radiolabeled antibody potentially dangerous or of poor imaging quality. Nevertheless, there is some evidence that the test may still be performed despite the presence of HAMA.[44]

Use of other radiologic tests for diagnosis and preoperative evaluation of a suspected ovarian malignancy is usually not indicated. But additional tests may be employed on the basis of the physical exam and the index of suspicion.

Tumor Markers

Tumor-associated markers, or antigens, have been investigated in the detection and treatment of epithelial ovarian cancer in an attempt at early diagnosis. CA-125 has proven to be the most useful marker currently available.[45] The 125th monoclonal antibody studied was called *OC 125*. Its antigenic determinant was named CA-125. An assay developed to detect serum levels of CA-125 found that only 1% of 888 healthy individuals and 6% of 143 individuals with benign diseases had values above 35U/ml. However, in the presence of minimal disease, serum antigen levels are often undetectable.[46] Use of multiple markers has been found to be somewhat useful as a screening tool, but they are not cost-effective for this purpose. Thus there is no single good marker that is both sensitive and specific. The use of CA-125, transvaginal ultrasound with color flow Doppler, and pelvic exam together has been found to be somewhat useful in screening, but again, the cost of these multiple tests for general population screening is prohibitive.

The CA-125 assay has been found to be more useful in monitoring for response, progression, or recurrence of disease in patients in whom CA-125 was initially elevated because there is a correlation between the stage and amount of residual disease. CA-125 levels correlated well with disease progression or regression in 93% of patients originally studied. The CA-125 assay had an 88% sensitivity for detecting non-mucinous ovarian carcinomas after treatment. CA-125 was found to not correlate well, however, in patients with low malignant potential tumors or those with mucinous adenocarcinomas.[46]

Patients in whom CA-125 levels have fallen to normal within three months of chemotherapy are likely to have a negative second-look surgery. However, if it takes longer than three months for CA-125 to fall to normal range, persistent disease is usually found at second-look laparotomy.[46] Gard and Houghton[45] recommend using a lower level, 15U/ml, as a more useful predictive cutoff value in following patients with ovarian cancer. The patients that fell in the intermediate range (15–30U/ml) inevitably developed recurrent disease.

A variety of tests may be used to detect a fallopian tube malignancy. Cervical cytology is positive in 10 to 25% of patients.[11,31] Pelvic examination, ultrasound, or CT scan may be used to delineate the mass, but often it is indistinguishable from an ovarian or uterine process. Surgery is needed to establish a diagnosis.

STAGING

Ovarian cancer staging is based on surgical pathologic findings. An exploratory laparotomy, peritoneal washings, total abdominal hysterectomy, bilateral salpingo-oophorectomy (TAH-BSO), omentectomy, multiple peritoneal biopsies, and pelvic and para-aortic lymph node sampling are necessary for adequate staging.

In 1971, the International Federation of Gynecology & Obstetrics (FIGO) provided the first classification system for staging ovarian cancer. This system allowed more appropriate treatment, more accurate evaluation of treatments, and comparison of statistics on a worldwide basis. The classification system was revised in 1974 and 1987, reflecting the new information available.

The American Joint Committee on Cancer (AJCC) and the TNM committee of the International Union Against Cancer (UICC) developed a separate staging system. The FIGO system is most commonly used by gynecologic oncologists, but the TNM system is also used by some organizations. Both systems are shown in Table 6.2.

Fallopian tube cancer, like ovarian cancer, has the tendency to spread intra-abdominally. Therefore, the FIGO ovarian cancer staging system was adapted for use with fallopian tube malignancies (see Table 6.3). The majority of patients with fallopian tube malignancies are diagnosed at an earlier stage than are ovarian cancer patients. In a review of several articles, Markman et al.[11] found that 33% of 558 patients were found to have stage I disease, 33% stage II, and 34% were stage III or IV.

SURGICAL TREATMENT

Treatment of women with ovarian cancer requires multidisciplinary and multimodal approaches. Since women commonly present with advanced disease and many are older and have other medical problems, it is very important to address the goals of therapy and include the patient in the decision-making process.[1] If a woman is a poor surgical candidate, treatment may be aimed at palliation of symptoms once a presumptive diagnosis of ovarian cancer is made. But most of the women with epithelial ovarian cancer are between the ages of 40 and 60 years, and aggressive treatment is indicated in these women. Approximately 8% of the common epithelial ovarian malignancies occur in women younger than 35 years and this number appears to be rising.[1] As increasing numbers of women seek infertility treatment, there may also be more younger women diagnosed with ovarian cancer at an earlier stage

TABLE 6.2
FIGO and TNM Staging of Ovarian Cancer

FIGO	TNM	Definitions
TX		Primary tumor cannot be assessed
T0		No evidence of primary tumor
I		Tumor limited to the ovaries
Ia	T1a	Tumor limited to one ovary; capsule intact, no tumor on ovarian surface. No malignant cells in ascites or peritoneal washings*
Ib	T1b	Tumor limited to both ovaries; capsule intact, no tumor on ovarian surface. No malignant cells in ascites or peritoneal washings*
Ic	T1c	Tumor limited to one or both ovaries with any of the following: capsule ruptured, tumor on ovarian surface, malignant cells in ascites or peritoneal washings
II	T2	Tumor involves one or both ovaries with pelvic extension
IIa	T2a	Extension and/or implants on uterus and/or tube(s). No malignant cells in ascites or peritoneal washings.
IIb	T2b	Extension to other pelvic tissues. No malignant cells in ascites or peritoneal washings.
IIc	T2c	Pelvic extension (2a or 2b) with malignant cells in ascites or peritoneal washings
III	T3 &/or N1	Tumor involves one or both ovaries with microscopically confirmed peritoneal metastasis outside the pelvis and/or regional lymph node metastases
IIIa	T3a	Microscopic peritoneal metastasis beyond pelvis
IIIb	T3b	Macroscopic peritoneal metastasis beyond pelvis 2 cm or less in greatest dimension
IIIc	T3c &/or N1	Peritoneal metastasis beyond pelvis more than 2 cm in greatest dimension and/or regional lymph node metastasis
IV	M1	Distant metastasis (exclude peritoneal metastasis)

*The presence of nonmalignant ascites is not classified. The presence of ascites does not affect staging unless malignant cells are present.

Liver capsule metastasis is T3/Stage III, liver parenchymal metastasis M1/Stage IV. Pleural effusion must have positive cytology for M1/Stage IV.

Used with permission of the American Joint Committee on Cancer (AJCCA®), Chicago, Illinois. The original source for this material is the AJCC® Cancer Staging Manual, 5th edition (1997) published by Lippincott-Raven Publisher, Philadelphia, Pennsylvania.

TABLE 6.3	
Operative Staging of Fallopian Tube Carcinoma	
Stage I	Growth limited to the tubes
Ia	Growth limited to one tube; no ascites
Ib	Growth limited to both tubes; no ascites
Ic	Tumor either Ia or Ib with malignant ascites or positive peritoneal washings
Stage II	Growth involving one or both tubes with pelvic extension
IIa	Extension and/or metastases to the ovaries and/or uterus
IIb	Extension to other pelvic tissues
IIc	Tumor either stage IIa or IIb with malignant ascites or positive peritoneal washings
Stage III	Tumor involving one or both tubes with peritoneal implants outside the pelvis and/or positive retroperitoneal or inguinal nodes; tumor is limited to the true pelvis, but with histologically verified malignant extension to the small bowel or omentum
IIIa	Tumor involves one or both tubes with microscopic confirmed peritoneal metastases outside the pelvis and/or regional lymph node involvement
IIIb	Tumor of one or both tubes with histologically confirmed implants on abdominal peritoneal surfaces, none exceeding 2 cm in diameter; nodes negative
IIIc	Abdominal implants greater than 2 cm in diameter and/or positive retroperitoneal or inguinal nodes
Stage IV	Growth involving one or both tubes with distant metastasis; if pleural effusion is present, positive cytologic confirmation must be made; parenchymal liver metastasis equals stage IV

Source: Reproduced with permission from Hoskins, W.J., Perez, C.A., & Young, R.C., eds. (1997). *Principles and Practice of Gynecologic Oncology,* 2nd ed. (p. 1034). Philadelphia: J.B. Lippincott.

due to the close monitoring of the ovaries and the increased use of hormonal stimulation for hyperovulation. But this is a relatively new phenomenon and an area for further study.

Surgical Staging

Surgical staging and cytoreductive surgery provide the basis of treatment for ovarian malignancies. The staging laparotomy (Table 6.4) is performed to diagnose the malig-

TABLE 6.4

Staging Laparotomy Procedure

Purpose and Definition	A surgical procedure performed for the purpose of exploring the abdominal cavity to maximally resect the cancer, to determine the stage of the disease, and to allow selection of optimal postoperative therapy
Contraindications	Poor surgical risk
Content of the Procedure	1. Adequate incision; vertical recommended

2. Estimation of the volume of the free peritoneal fluid. Fluid should be sent for cytology. If no free fluid is present, washings should be obtained from the pelvis, pericolic gutters, and infradiaphragmatic area.
3. Inspection and palpation of all peritoneal surfaces for evidence of metastatic disease
4. Inspection of the omentum, removal of at least the infracolic omentum
5. Extrafascial total abdominal hysterectomy and bilateral salpingo-oophorectomy (in selected situations, unilateral salpingo-oophorectomy)
6. Removal of all gross disease
7. If initially there is no evidence of disease beyond the ovary or pelvis, and all gross tumor subsequently is resected, the following must be done:
   a. peritoneal biopsies
      1. cul-de-sac
      2. right and left pelvic sidewalls
      3. right and left pericolic gutters
   b. biopsy or scraping of the right diaphragm
   c. selective pelvic and periaortic lymph node sampling
8. Selective pelvic and periaortic lymph node sampling must be done on all of the following:
   a. all patients with no gross residual disease regardless of stage
   b. gross residual disease only in the pelvis
   c. gross residual disease outside the pelvis equal to or less than 1 cm in largest diameter
9. Histologically confirmed metastatic nodal disease makes further node sampling necessary.

Source: Reproduced with permission from Hoskins, W.J., Perez, C.A., & Young, R.C., eds. (1992). *Principles and Practice of Gynecologic Oncology* (p. 747). Philadelphia: J.B. Lippincott.

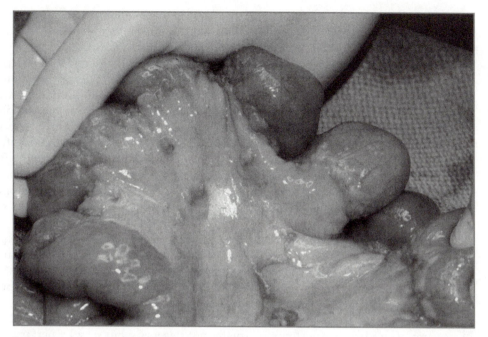

FIGURE 6.1. Peritoneal studding of ovarian cancer.

nancy and to accurately determine the extent of disease. This procedure provides a systematic approach for exploring the peritoneal surfaces of the abdominal cavity to determine the volume and distribution of disease (see Figures 6.1 and 6.2). The goal of cytoreductive surgery is to remove as much tumor as possible without undue surgical morbidity.

FIGURE 6.2. Peritoneal studding of ovarian cancer, which can lead to edematous bowl and carcinomatosis ileus.

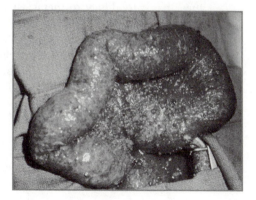

Cytoreduction can result in mechanical and metabolic improvements in the patient. A decreased tumor burden allows for improved tumor cell kinetics. Debulking surgery also allows for improved blood supply to the involved tissues.[47,48]

The surgical procedure is quite involved, requiring peritoneal and retroperitoneal exposure. A vertical midline incision from the symphysis pubis to above the umbilicus is needed for adequate exposure. If ascites is present, fluid is obtained for cytopathology. If no fluid is present, peritoneal washings are obtained and sent for cytopathology. The diaphragm, paracolic gutters, mesentery and serosa of the bowel, pelvic side walls, cul-de-sac, and omentum are all examined for disease. Biopsies are taken of suspicious lesions or of adhesions. Multiple selective biopsies of the peritoneal surfaces are also taken. The ovaries are inspected for excrescences, rupture, adhesions, and the presence of bilateral involvement. A total abdominal hysterectomy, bilateral salpingo-oophorectomy, omentectomy, and selective pelvic and para-aortic lymph node sampling are performed when possible.[47,48]

Cytoreduction of the tumor is attempted since it can convert a patient from a poor prognostic group to a more favorable prognostic group. The size of remaining tumor at the end of the operation is the most important prognostic indicator in patients with advanced ovarian cancer. Patients with remaining tumors ≤1 cm had a better prognosis than patients with more gross residual disease.[47,48]

Debulking surgery may include extensive dissection of pelvic masses and bowel resection if needed. A colostomy is usually not necessary but may be performed to prevent impending obstruction. Again, the goal is tumor reduction without excessive surgical morbidity.[47,48]

The young woman with stage I cancer or a tumor of low malignant potential may wish to preserve fertility. In this case, the contralateral ovary is evaluated and often sampled. A thorough examination of the abdominal cavity and lymph nodes is performed, and if possible the reproductive organs are preserved.[49]

The surgical treatment of primary fallopian tube cancer is identical to that of ovarian cancer. Staging, too, is based on the surgical/pathologic findings (Table 6.4). Diagnosis is rarely established preoperatively, so when confronted intraoperatively, the surgeon must be prepared to perform the required staging procedure. Fallopian tube cancer has a tendency to metastasize to the lymph nodes, especially the para-aortic lymph nodes; a 35 to 53% incidence of lymph node metastasis has been reported. As in ovarian cancer, patients with ≤1 cm residual tumor mass after surgery enjoyed a higher survival rate than those with larger residual disease. These findings underscore the necessity of performing a thorough ovarian cancer type staging and debulking procedure.[11]

Second-Look Surgery

A so-called second-look laparotomy is defined as an exploratory laparotomy performed on patients who have achieved a complete clinical response after primary therapy. The usefulness of this surgery is controversial in the medical community. Increasingly a second-look surgery, with its associated morbidity and seen and unseen costs, is viewed as unnecessary as it does not affect survival. A second-look operation is advocated only within the clinical trial setting. Others believe another laparotomy surgery is necessary to accurately evaluate response to treatment, determine the need for further treatment, and possibly perform further tumor debulking.[50,51]

It is further advocated by some to perform a secondary cytoreduction of tumor to improve the response to treatment. This is not a second-look laparotomy, but is referred to as a secondary cytoreductive surgery. In this case, a patient whose tumor was not completely resected at the original surgery, for various reasons, undergoes another laparotomy after short-term initial chemotherapy. This surgery is an attempt to further debulk the tumor. It is hoped that the subsequent resection of tumor to optimal size <1 cm) will result in improved response to adjuvant treatment.[52]

The secondary surgical procedure is similar to the initial staging laparotomy. A vertical abdominal incision is required for adequate visualization. Sampling of peritoneal fluid or pelvic washings are needed for cytopathologic examination. A systematic evaluation of all peritoneal surfaces and multiple biopsies of the peritoneal surfaces, suspicious lesions, and adhesions are done. Sampling of the pelvic and para-aortic lymph nodes is also done if tumor was present at staging laparotomy or if they were not sampled at the time of initial surgery.[52]

Second-look laparotomy has been used in the management of fallopian tube cancer. Its role is not clearly defined, though Barakat et al.[53] believe it provides useful prognostic information. The theoretical basis for the procedure is similar to the rationale for ovarian cancer—to evaluate the disease status and determine response to treatment in patients with clinically undetectable disease. In a review of the literature, Rose et al.[31] found 31 of 45 second-look laparotomies to be negative; however, 8 of the 31 patients (26%) later relapsed. Barakat et al.[53] found that approximately 80% of patients who had a negative second-look laparotomy after platinum-based chemotherapy remained disease-free.

Laparoscopy

Laparoscopy has historically been viewed as inadequate for fully evaluating an ovarian cancer. With the advent of improved instrumentation and surgical technique, however, it is increasingly being used in an effort to evaluate disease and minimize surgical morbidity.[54,55]

Laparoscopy is sometimes used as a second-look procedure. The ability to visualize the diaphragm, liver, and retroperitoneal spaces has allowed laparoscopy to replace laparotomy as the surgical procedure of choice at some institutions. Some surgeons schedule patients for second-look laparoscopy but are prepared to do an immediate laparotomy, if needed. If disease is found, documented, and evaluated, the laparotomy can be abandoned. However, if no residual disease can be documented or adequate visualization of all peritoneal surfaces is not possible, the surgeon then proceeds with the second-look laparotomy.[54,55]

✸ CHEMOTHERAPY

Conventional Treatment

Surgical staging, exploration, and cytoreduction provide the basis for systemic treatment of ovarian cancer. Single alkylating agents, such as melphalan, were considered standard treatment until 1978,[56] when several combinations of chemotherapeutic agents such as hexa-CAF (hexamethylmelamine, cyclophosphamide, methotrexate, and 5-fluorouracil) were tested against melphalan alone. Significant improvement in overall response rates, complete remissions, and significantly longer median survival were reported.[56]

In 1976, cisplatin was found to have a response rate of 26% in previously treated patients.[57] With the reports of platinum's activity in ovarian cancer, numerous prospective randomized trials containing platinum were performed. Multiple studies showing platinum-based regimens' superiority over non–platinum-containing multi-agent chemotherapy provided the basis for using cisplatin-based combination chemotherapy as the primary treatment.[58,59,60] Retrospective studies have indicated that the dose intensity of cisplatin is the most significant factor in achieving optimal responses.[1] However, dose escalation by a factor of 2 has not proved to affect response or survival.[61] Trials are under way to look at the concept of dose intensity with doses requiring hematologic support from stem cell transplantation.[62]

In the United States, cisplatin and cyclophosphamide became the standard regimen for treating primary advanced ovarian cancer. Median survival ranged from twenty-one to thirty-six months in patients receiving cisplatin in doses ranging from 50 mg/m^2 to 200 mg/m^2.[1]

Carboplatin was later developed in an attempt to find a platinum analogue with a better toxicity profile; the dose-limiting neurologic and nephrotoxicities have made administering dose-intense cisplatin regimens difficult. But several prospective randomized trials and meta-analyses comparing carboplatin with cisplatin as single agents and in combination showed no significant differences in the progression-free interval or survival rate between the two agents.[63,64,65]

The effectiveness of doxorubicin has also been studied in detail. The Gynecologic Oncology Group (GOG) reported no significant difference in progression-free interval or response in patients with advanced disease treated with cisplatin, doxorubicin, and cyclophosphamide (PAC) versus cyclophosphamide and cisplatin (CP).[66] But Conte et al.[67] and Bruzonne et al.[68] reported that the addition of doxorubicin to the PAC versus PC regimen provided a significantly higher pathologically complete response rate and a ten-month increase in median survival. A meta-analysis of four randomized trials comparing PAC and CP regimens reveals that the addition of doxorubicin had an increased survival benefit of between 5 and 7% in the two to six years following treatment.[69,70]

The optimal length of therapy has yet to be determined. A prospective randomized trial comparing five versus ten cycles of the PAC regimen in patients with advanced ovarian cancer showed no significant difference in medial survival rates, but the toxicity experienced with five cycles was significantly lower.[71]

McGuire et al.[72] first reported a 32% response rate with single-agent taxol for patients with refractory ovarian cancer. The GOG, in a prospective randomized trial of 394 suboptimal advanced ovarian cancer patients, showed the superiority of platinum and taxol (PT) over platinum and cyclophosphamide (PC), with improved clinical response rates, pathologically complete response rates, and progression-free intervals. However, the toxicity profile demonstrated that PT was significantly more toxic than cisplatin and cyclophosphamide in causing neutropenia, fever, and alopecia. There was no increase in sepsis. A greater number of cardiac events occurred in patients receiving cisplatin and taxol, but they were not clinically significant. The difference in response rates was significant enough that PT has become first-line treatment for patients with advanced ovarian cancer.[73]

Taxol originally was administered over twenty-four hours; however, Swenerton et al.[74] reported that taxol can be safely administered over one and three hours with premedication, to allow outpatient use of the drug. Taxol needs to precede a platinum-based compound for optimum effect.[75] Ninety-six hour intravenous taxol infusions as well as intraperitoneal administration of taxol are under investigation.

Second-line treatment with non–cross-resistant agents such as Altretamine (hexamethylmelamine) and ifosfamide have shown significant responses.[76,77] If paclitaxol has not been used previously, it should be the first agent used for salvage therapy.[78]

Response to second-line chemotherapy depends on several factors. These factors include prior exposure to chemotherapy, the interval between the last chemotherapy regimen and tumor recurrence, tumor response to prior chemotherapy regimen, and the amount of residual disease present at the start of second-line chemotherapy.[79] A platinum-free interval of ≥6 months indicates that response to retreatment with a platinum-containing regimen is likely,[77] whereas a disease-free interval of less than 6 months indicates a refractory response to retreatment with the same agent is likely.[77]

Agents such as topotecan, gemcitabine, liposomal doxorubicin, oral VP-16, navelbine, and docetaxel have been used as second-line treatment. The choice of treatment is dependent on prior response to treatment, quality of life desired, oral versus intravenous medications, and the toxicity profiles of the agents.[77]

New agents, different combinations of chemotherapeutic agents, dose-intense regimens, intraperitoneal administration routes, different administration schedules for taxol, combinations of different routes of chemotherapy administration within one regimen, use of growth factors, and agents to decrease drug resistance are among the different treatments being investigated.[80–83]

Intraperitoneal Chemotherapy

Since the 1950s, intraperitoneal chemotherapy has been used to control accumulation of malignant ascites. In the late 1970s, pharmacologic studies suggested that intraperitoneal administration may have a greater therapeutic index over intravenous therapy, due to several mechanisms. These mechanisms include (1) the ability to achieve a higher drug concentration within the peritoneal cavity, (2) bypassing the peritoneal barrier, and (3) detoxifying chemotherapy by the portal system, thereby allowing lower systemic toxicity.[84,85] Higher doses of drugs are associated with a greater tumor response. There is a significant difference between the peritoneal and plasma concentrations following intraperitoneal administration. This difference is considered the therapeutic ratio or pharmacologic advantage.

Cisplatin has been the primary drug studied in intraperitoneal chemotherapy. It has a large peritoneal/plasma concentration gradient. It has a fairly steep dose-response curve and does not cause local peritoneal toxicity. Studies have shown that there is a penetration of drug into tumors of only approximately six to eight cell layers, or 1 to 2 mm deep. Since most tumors are more than six to eight cell layers deep, it is necessary for chemotherapy agents to reach the tumors via capillary flow as well as direct peritoneal exposure to achieve maximum cell kill.[86,87] For this reason, patients with microscopic or minimal macroscopic disease are ideal candidates for intraperitoneal therapy. It is not recommended for patients with gross residual tumors.

Further studies are being made into intraperitoneal therapy with single agents such as taxol. Combinations of drugs for intraperitoneal administration and sequential intravenous/intraperitoneal chemotherapy are also being explored.

High-Dose Chemotherapy

Because of ovarian cancer's sensitivity to chemotherapy, high-dose chemotherapy with autologous bone marrow transplantation has been investigated. High-dose chemotherapy can be safely used in patients with ovarian cancer, especially those with disease previously responsive to chemotherapy and those with minimal residual disease.[62] Alkylating agents, etoposide, carboplatin, and ifosfamide, as single agents and in combination regimens, are among the agents used in pilot studies. Intravenous as well as intraperitoneal administration of the high-dose agents have been tested. It appears that the dose-limiting toxicities are nonhematologic, such as hepatotoxicity, neurotoxicity, and nephrotoxicity.[62,88] These studies show that responses can be achieved in heavily pretreated patients with just one course of treatment. However, the complication and mortality rates can be quite high.[1]

The introduction of growth factors has changed the field of high-dose chemotherapy with bone marrow rescue. Such hematologic support can decrease toxicities or their duration significantly. Hospital stays have decreased from an average of six to eight weeks to three to four weeks. However, the dose-limiting nonhematologic toxicities are not affected.

Peripheral stem cell transplantation, alone or with bone marrow transplantation, may allow multiple courses of high-dose chemotherapy to be given. This may ultimately have an impact on patients with large-volume disease and is currently an area under investigation. (For further information on high-dose chemotherapy, dose intensity/dose response relationships, and drug resistance, see Chapter 11.)

Neoadjuvant Chemotherapy

Neoadjuvant chemotherapy is the use of chemotherapy to decrease tumor burden prior to surgical resection. By decreasing tumor burden, it is believed that surgical resection can be made technically feasible and more patients can be optimally debulked, paving the way for further therapy.[89] Lim and Green[90] suggest that neoadjuvant chemotherapy may render debulking surgery feasible in a proportion of patients presenting with unresectable disease and can result in improved median survival. But Schwartz et al.[91] found that the progression-free survival for eleven women receiving neoadjuvant chemotherapy was not statistically different from eighteen women receiving the standard primary cytoreductive surgery and postoperative chemotherapy. However, the neoadjuvant chemotherapy was better tolerated. Further studies are in progress to better elucidate the role of neoadjuvant chemotherapy in ovarian cancer.

The development of chemotherapy in the treatment of fallopian tube cancer parallels that of ovarian cancer. Single agents that have shown activity include melphalan, chlorambucil, cyclophosphamide, thiotepa, doxorubicin, and cisplatin.[11] Use of single agents in advanced disease has primarily shown a response of short duration. Occasional long-term remissions (>2 years) have been reported. Combination chemotherapy consisting of cyclophosphamide and doxorubicin has been tried. And multiagent chemotherapy without cisplatin has shown a 29% response rate. Remissions lasting more than two years have been reported with the use of multiagent therapy in advanced disease.[11]

When cisplatin was determined to be the most active agent in the treatment of ovarian cancer, it was then incorporated into chemotherapy regimens in the treatment of fallopian tube malignancies. No doubt taxol is being used in fallopian tube cancers by some practitioners, but no data yet substantiate its use.

The addition of cisplatin into multiagent regimens has shown response rates of 81%.[92] The overall response survival rates have been reported to parallel those seen in patients with advanced ovarian cancer.[11] Barakat et al.,[93] however, found that patients with advanced disease who achieved a negative second look after platinum-based combination chemotherapy had a better possibility of remaining disease-free than patients with similar stage ovarian cancer.

✻ HORMONAL THERAPY

Hormonal therapy has been studied as a means for controlling ovarian cancer. Antiestrogens, antiandrogens, progestational agents, and gonadotropin-releasing hormone analogues have been used, with response rates of 4 to 15%.[94,95,96] There has been no correlation noted between hormone receptors and the response to various hormones. Since hormone therapy offers similar response rates to any second- or third-line chemotherapeutic agent, it is a viable treatment option for patients who have failed cytotoxic chemotherapy. Hormone therapy with an agent such as tamoxifen is a good option when considering quality of life, due to its minimal toxicity.[1]

The fallopian tube undergoes monthly cyclical change similar to that of the endometrium. Since it responds to hormonal influences, it logically follows that progestational agents have been tested in the treatment of fallopian tube carcinomas.[11] However, the data are insufficient to support this form of treatment at this time.

✖ IMMUNOTHERAPY

Nonspecific immunotherapy enhances cell-mediated immune function and antibody production, so it may also be effective in partially reversing the immunosuppression caused by cancer or cancer treatment. Nonspecific immunotherapy is the most extensively studied form of immunotherapy in women with ovarian cancer. BCG, with or without combination chemotherapy, did not affect survival in a GOG study.[97] *Corynebacterium parvum,* with or without melphalan, did not affect survival when administered intravenously. However, intraperitoneal administration of *C. parvum* has demonstrated tumor regression in some patients.[98] Interferon, given systemically or by the intraperitoneal route, has demonstrated response in patients with ovarian cancer.[99,100]

Adoptive immunotherapy in phase I/II trials using intraperitoneal interleuken-2 (Il–2) and lymphokine activated killer (LAK) cells has demonstrated activity. However, local peritoneal toxicity is increased when these two agents are given together.[1,101] Monoclonal antibodies have been used to detect as well as treat ovarian cancer. Gold-labeled monoclonal antibody, TC5, is being studied in the detection of serous and endometrioid types of adenocarcinomas of the ovary. Radioisotopes ^{125}I, [111]I, and ^{123}I or toxins such as recombinant ricin A chain and pseudomonas endotoxins have been used in phase I/II trials in the treatment of ovarian cancer,[102,103] but with significant pancytopenia, and central nervous system and peripheral neurotoxicities reported in the early phase I/II trials. Recent phase I/II studies using monoclonal antibodies have also reported substantial, but manageable, toxicities.[102,103,104] The use of cytokines continues to be researched in ovarian cancer. Intraperitoneal interferon and interleukin-12 are among clinical trials presently being conducted by the Gynecologic Oncology Group.

✖ GENE THERAPY

Growing scientific evidence supports the notion that gene therapy, classified as biologic cancer therapy, is a reasonable, potentially therapeutic cancer treatment. Therapeutic approaches can include "altering cells at the gene level, modifying the immune system, targeting cancer cell death with suicide genes, using foreign genes to mark a population of cells for further study, and promoting molecular alterations to augment traditional conventional chemotherapy."[105] Currently under investigation in ovarian cancer treatment is the insertion of genetic material (such as p53 or BRCA1) into cells using vectors (substances such as viruses used to "infect" or introduce material into a cancer cell). The therapy includes a type of vector, a route for delivery, the genetic material, the target tissue, and the desired response of the targeted tissue.[105] Ovarian cancer as a disease process provides a unique opportunity for the study of the therapeutic use of gene therapy because ovarian cancer is typically confined to the peritoneal cavity. The peritoneal cavity is an ideal setting in which to instill a vector containing genetic material, and using the same principles of intraperitoneal chemotherapy, the peritoneal surfaces and organs of the abdomen are exposed to the gene therapy.[106] It will be many years before the role of gene therapy in ovarian cancer management will be clearly defined, but it appears that at least two major areas of clinical research will be conducted. One approach is the use of gene therapy as an adjunct to chemotherapy. Second, gene therapy will likely be used for the purpose of disease prevention in women who are identified as at risk for development of ovarian cancer because of inherited genetic aberrations. Normally functioning genetic material will be given to at-risk women to prevent the development of ovarian cancer.

✳ RADIOTHERAPY

Radioactive Isotopes

Radioactive isotopes were first used in the treatment of ovarian cancer in 1945. Radioactive zinc (^{63}Zn), gold (^{198}Au), phosphate (^{32}P), and yttrium (^{90}Y) have all been studied, but currently only radioactive phosphate is used.[3] Radioactive phosphorus (^{32}P) has been used primarily to treat stage I and II ovarian cancers. It has also been used to treat patients with stage III disease after a negative second-look laparotomy.

Barber[3] summarizes his experience regarding the use of radioisotopes in the following way:

1. Malignant ascites can be controlled in up to 80% of patients.
2. Radioisotopes are not effective in treating malignant ascites when bulky disease is present.
3. Radioisotopes can improve survival rates, especially in stage I patients. (This point is not universally accepted.)
4. Patients with multiple adhesions have an unacceptable complication rate when radioisotopes are given.
5. The use of radioisotopes in patients who also receive external beam radiotherapy increases the rate of complications, especially gastrointestinal complications.

External Beam Radiotherapy

The use of external beam radiotherapy in the treatment of common epithelial ovarian cancer remains controversial. The natural history of ovarian cancer, with its transperitoneal spread, would make whole-abdominal radiation therapy seem like a viable option; however, the dose of radiation that can be given to the upper abdomen is less than the dose needed to eradicate macroscopic disease. Clinical trials have found that survival is better in patients treated with whole-abdominal radiation when there is only small macroscopic or microscopic disease. These trials have also found that abdominal and pelvic, not just pelvic, radiation therapy is required to adequately treat ovarian cancer, even in patients with early stage disease.[107,108]

Abdominopelvic radiotherapy has been given using two different methods: a moving strip technique and an open field technique. The two methods were compared in two randomized clinical trials, with no difference in survival or acute toxicity.[109,110] The open field technique has become standard because it is simpler and has a shorter length of treatment and less long-term toxicity. The para-aortic lymph nodes and the medial domes of the diaphragm are sometimes boosted to provide higher doses to areas of higher risk. The liver and kidneys require shielding during treatment.

Abdominopelvic radiation therapy has significant toxicities. The primary symptom is fatigue, and this increases with the duration of treatment. Nausea, abdominal cramping, and diarrhea are reported in approximately 75% of patients. Hematologic toxicity, especially thrombocytopenia (<50,000 platelets/mm^2), is also a common problem. Treatment delays are not uncommon in patients who have received prior chemotherapy.[107,108]

Acute adverse effects resolve a few weeks after treatment. However, late adverse effects can be persistent and severe. Liver toxicities, as evidenced by changes in liver function tests, can occur if the liver is not adequately shielded. Asymptomatic basal pneumonitis or fibrosis can be detected in 15 to 20% of patients when radiotherapy is given above the diaphragm.[107,108]

Gastrointestinal effects are the most common category of adverse effects. These present as diarrhea or persistent bloating in 10 to 15% of patients, but alterations in diet can usually control these side effects. Intermittent bowel obstruction and bowel obstruction requiring surgical intervention are the most serious side effects. The total dose of radiation, the dose per fraction, and the extent of previous surgery correlate with the frequency and severity of late gastrointestinal complications. If patients have undergone prior lymph node sampling, there is a greater risk for late complications.[107,108]

Abdominopelvic radiotherapy may also be used as adjuvant therapy in patients with stage I to III cancer with microscopic or small macroscopic (<5 mm) disease who have had initial staging laparotomies. Patients with stage Ia or Ib, grade 1 or 2 disease have a 90% cure rate and do not need postoperative radiotherapy.[107]

Whole-abdomen radiation therapy has been compared with chemotherapy in patients with ovarian cancer in several trials.[111,112,113] However, none of the studies included cisplatin in the treatment regimens, and the studies had technical weaknesses as well. Cooperative groups have been unsuccessful in comparing abdominopelvic radiation therapy with cisplatin-based combination chemotherapy due to investigator bias.[1]

The sequential use of whole-abdomen and pelvic radiotherapy after initial laparotomy along with cisplatin-based combination chemotherapy and secondary cytoreduction has been proposed. Some investigators have reported improved responses compared to the use of chemotherapy or radiotherapy alone; others have reported either increased or no difference in toxicity, without any improvement in tumor response.[114,115,116]

An increased complication rate is reported when whole-abdomen and pelvic radiation therapy is given after chemotherapy as salvage therapy. Patients who have had second-look laparotomies are at higher risk for late complications than patients with only one prior laparotomy. Any prior abdominal surgery can increase the risk of complications from external beam radiotherapy. Also, hematologic reserves are more depleted, leading to greater toxicities and the need for breaks between treatments. Hyperfractionation techniques have been studied in an attempt to decrease toxicity.[117]

Radiation therapy can be used for palliation in ovarian cancer, but it is rarely useful in treating ascites or painful hepatomegaly.[1] (See Chapter 13.)

Radiation therapy has been used to treat fallopian tube cancer after surgical intervention. However, the role of radiotherapy here is unclear. Since fallopian tube cancer is rare, no institution has had sufficient experience with it to produce reliable data. All the reports are retrospective over a long period of time concerning patients with a variety of stages and treatments.[11] Therefore, even the optimal technique to be used has not been clearly defined. The types of radiation therapy used include external beam therapy, brachytherapy, intraperitoneal radioisotopes, and radiation therapy concomitantly with chemotherapy. After reviewing the literature, Markman et al.[11] made the following generalizations:

1. Based on nonrandomized retrospective studies, patients treated with surgery plus postoperative radiotherapy have a survival advantage over patients treated with surgery alone.
2. Pelvic and whole-abdominal radiation therapy is superior to pelvic radiation therapy alone, even in early stage disease (stages I and II).
3. High-energy (megavoltage) radiation therapy gives significantly better results than orthovoltage radiation therapy. The pelvis should receive at least 50 Gy.

Intraperitoneal radioisotopes have been used in the treatment of patients with microscopic fallopian tube cancer. However, the experience with this form of therapy is too limited to draw any firm conclusions regarding its efficacy.[11,32]

Experience with concomitant use of radiotherapy and chemotherapy in the treatment of fallopian tube carcinoma is very limited. It is considered investigational.

✳ TREATMENT OF OVARIAN TUMORS OF LOW MALIGNANT POTENTIAL

Surgical intervention is the primary mode of treatment for ovarian tumors of low malignant potential (borderline malignancy). It should include a total abdominal hysterectomy, bilateral salpingo-oophorectomy (TAH-BSO), pelvic and para-aortic lymph node biopsies, peritoneal washings, and tumor debulking. In stage I disease, which frequently occurs during the childbearing years, women who have had conservative surgery (unilateral oophorectomy) have had equivalent survival rates as those who have undergone a TAH-BSO, that is, 95% versus 94%.[1] However, unilateral oophorectomy patients have had a higher recurrence rate, 15% versus 5%. The recurrent disease was effectively treated with surgery, and survival rates were the same.[1] Adjuvant therapy for early stage disease is not warranted.[10,118]

For patients with advanced disease, the surgical procedure is the same as that used for patients with invasive ovarian cancers. The benefit of postoperative therapy in advanced disease is not well established;[10] however, Benjamin and colleagues'[119] study found that platinum-based chemotherapy was effective for achieving surgically proven partial and complete responses in advanced stage ovarian serous carcinoma of low malignant potential. Platinum-based chemotherapy was also found to be effective as a salvage regimen in controlling persistent disease.[120]

✳ NURSING MANAGEMENT

As has been described, women with ovarian cancer often present with histories of long-standing gastrointestinal complaints that directly correspond with the metastatic status of the disease. It may be helpful to visualize the microscopic spread of neoplastic cells throughout the abdominal cavity as similar to the way in which the wind disperses the seeds of a mature dandelion. Many times symptoms of the disease are indicative of the organs on which the tumor grows, impairing normal function and causing pain and discomfort. There are many manifestations of this disease, so nurses should be aware that ovarian cancer can cause multisystem dysfunction. Metastases can appear in any organ or site. The four most common complications of metastatic disease are ascites, bowel obstruction, pleural effusions, and malnutrition. It is important to remember that nurses can identify and implement interventions to relieve symptoms and associated discomforts that are inherent in this disease—if we tune in to its signs and symptoms.

Ascites

Ascites is a common manifestation of ovarian cancer. Its presence is often indicative of advanced disease and has been associated with a poorer prognosis.[1,121] The development of abdominal ascites is thought to occur when tumor implants block or impede normal peritoneal lymph flow and when peritoneal surfaces produce an increased amount of fluid.[20,57,122] Under normal conditions, fluid flows freely in a state of equilibrium between the semipermeable membranes of the parietal and visceral peritoneum and the abdominal cavity.[122,123] Protein-rich serous fluid begins to accumulate when the ability to reabsorb is impaired. Often increasing abdominal girth is the symptom that compels the patient to seek a physician for an evaluation.[57]

Initially, ascites is most commonly relieved during the first laparotomy.[57,120] However, initiation of chemotherapy soon after surgery is necessary to prevent its reaccumulation.[1] A relatively small percentage of patients have ascites that is refractory to systemic chemotherapy when first diagnosed.[1,124]

Recurrent ascites presents a complicated management task for the medical team, as well as an emotional and physiologic burden for the patient. Often these patients have symptoms of early satiety, anorexia, indigestion, decreased bowel motility, constipation, and decreased bladder capacity.[122,125] As ascitic volume increases, there is a proportionate decrease in the space available for the organs of the abdomen. Abdominal skin becomes taut and shiny, the umbilicus may evert, and the flanks may begin to bulge.[122]

Assessment of ascites includes measurement of abdominal girth, percussion of the abdomen, detection of a fluid wave, and a review of the patient's symptoms.[122] Percussion of the abdomen can be achieved by asking the patient to recline on her back so the examiner may percuss her flanks. In the presence of ascites, dullness is heard in the flanks and tympany resonates from the mid-abdomen. Further assessment can be made by having the patient lie on one side, then the other, and repeating the procedure. The ascitic fluid shifts to the dependent side, so dullness can be heard from the dependent flank and tympany resonates from the upper flank.[125]

Detection of an abdominal fluid wave is performed, with the assistance of another clinician, by placing the ulnar side of one examiner's hand in the midline of the patient's abdomen and applying light pressure. The second examiner places each hand, palm down, on the patient's flanks. A positive fluid wave is felt by gently exerting a quick push on one flank; it is felt by the hand on the opposite flank.[125] Usually the presence of 500cc of ascitic fluid creates a positive fluid wave.

As the volume of fluid increases and the patient's symptoms worsen, paracentesis is considered. The patient is informed of the risks of the procedure, which include potential for injury to abdominal organs such as the bladder and intestine, pain, weakness and lowering of blood pressure, and peritonitis. Thus informed consent should be obtained prior to the procedure. It is useful to set up the drainage system before the procedure, with a three-way stopcock to obtain fluid for cytology, if desired. The patient should completely empty her bladder before beginning, to prevent bladder injury.[122] If the patient can tolerate it, she should be seated upright with her feet and legs supported; this allows the intestines to float away from the tap site.[126] Ultrasound guidance is helpful, if available. After the site is prepared aseptically, the abdominal wall is punctured with a needle or trochar and the fluid is drained, usually into a vacuum container.

The patient should be observed closely for the appearance of pallor, increased pulse rate, or decreased blood pressure. At the conclusion of the procedure, the patient should rest for a short time and be instructed to observe the site for signs of localized infection, an increase in abdominal pain, and a rise in body temperature.

The removal of large amounts of the plasma-rich ascitic fluid causes volume depletion and loss of valuable proteins and electrolytes in an already compromised patient.[57] Thus replacement fluids should be considered to maintain hemodynamic stability.

Repetitive paracenteses are not beneficial because of potential loculation of fluid, iatrogenic injury to the abdominal viscera, and risk of peritonitis. Removal of ascites is a temporary alleviation of symptoms, however, and to maximize the benefit of paracentesis, local or systemic measures such as intraperitoneal or intravenous chemotherapy should be undertaken. Other methods of treating recurrent ascites have been placement of a permanent peritoneovenous shunt,[120] use of peritoneovenous autotransfusion,[125] or intraperitoneal modalities.[122] The autotransfusion and shunt procedures have low success rates and some serious complications and are quite expensive.[1,127] Intraperitoneal chemotherapy, radioactive colloids, or biologic response modifiers have offered beneficial effects, but as with the other therapies, they are of short duration.[121]

For patients who have recurrent ascites, measures to promote comfort are the main goal. As the adverse effects of the ascitic fluid volume in the abdomen worsen, many patients experience bowel obstruction, malnutrition, anasarca, dyspnea, and lymphedema. In this case, noninvasive interventions should be considered (Table 6.5).[57] Although there are many possibilities, consideration must be given at this point to quality of life and what expectations the patient and her family have, with full knowledge of the course of disease.

Intestinal Obstruction

As many as half of all women with ovarian cancer develop intermittent or actual bowel obstruction during the disease course.[124,128] Indeed it is often the symptoms of bowel obstruction that first alert the clinician that the patient may have recurrent disease.[121] For the majority of these women, it is the progressive growth of tumor on or near the bowel that causes the symptoms.[124]

The presenting symptoms of bowel obstructions are nausea, vomiting, abdominal pain and cramping, diarrhea, or constipation.[121,129] The symptoms often progress slowly, and allow for nonemergent work-up. After a clinical assessment of symptoms and bowel sounds, which can be high-pitched or tinkling, an upright and flat-plate abdominal film should be obtained. In the presence of obstruction, the intestines appear on radiographic film as multiple, dilated loops with an appearance of air fluid levels.[129] Further diagnostic studies might include an upper GI with small bowel follow-through and a barium enema. Intestinal obstruction is not always confined to the small bowel; there can be carcinomatous involvement of any portion or the entire length of bowel (Table 6.6).[121,131]

TABLE 6.5	
Noninvasive Treatment for Ascites	
Diet	Patient should be encouraged to eat frequent, small meals that have high protein and low sodium content. In some cases, it may be beneficial to decrease total fluid volume intake in an attempt to minimize ascitic fluid production.
Diuretics	Use of diuretics that are electrolyte-sparing may be of some benefit at low doses. Patient should be closely observed for depletion of electrolytes and hypovolemia.
Rest	In most cases, the patient with ascites suffers from debilitating fatigue. She should be encouraged to rest frequently, particularly on her left side, with her feet elevated, to alleviate pressure on internal organs, improve vascular return from lower extremities, facilitate lymphatic flow, and improve diuresis.

Source: Adapted with permission from Kehoe, C. (1991). Malignant ascites: Etiology, diagnosis, and treatment. *Oncology Nursing Forum, 18*(3), 524.

Immediate management of the symptoms of bowel obstruction should be restriction of oral intake, or nothing by mouth until the symptoms abate. For the patient who desires to stay home and for whom a conservative management approach is considered appropriate, oral intake can slowly resume after several hours without symptoms. This should consist of fluid intake of clear liquids in small amounts, and when this is tolerated for several hours, then slow progress to full liquids. When full liquids are tolerated for several additional hours, then it is possible to begin soft foods in small amounts. This gradual dietary progression allows the bowel to resume peristaltic activity slowly and, in some situations, may temporarily delay invasive or surgical approaches to relieve the obstruction.

For the patient who is admitted to the hospital with symptoms of bowel obstruction, it is possible to conservatively manage the obstruction by withdrawing oral intake, decompressing the bowel with nasogastric intubation, and administering intravenous fluid or nutritional support.[129] Nevertheless, complete obstruction can occur, in which case palliative surgical intervention such as a bowel resection, diverting colostomy, and/or drainage gastrostomy tube is necessary.[121,130]

There is little supportive data in favor of long-term survival in patients with bowel obstruction who undergo palliative surgery.[124] However, the quality of life a patient can experience afterward often influences the medical team to attempt surgical alleviation of intestinal obstruction.[128] But there are prognostic factors that must be taken into consideration before surgery, including nutritional status, ascites, tumor burden, age, prior radiotherapy, and the tolerability of postoperative chemotherapy to allay recurrence of symptoms.[1,121]

TABLE 6.6

A Comparison of Clinical Manifestations of Large and Small Bowel Obstructions

Problem	Small Bowel	Large Bowel
Onset	Rapid	Insidious
Abdominal pain	Severe, crampy, intermittent attacks	Generally less severe; usually crampy
Vomiting	Occurs early; frequent and profuse	Occurs late; sometimes never
Bowel movement	Often presents as normal	Diarrhea; narrowing of stools, eventual obstipation
Abdominal distention	Early; life-threatening	Pronounced
Dehydration	Common	Late
Electrolyte and acid/base imbalances	Common	Rare

Source: Davis, L.S. Bowel obstruction. In J. Gross & B.L. Johnson, eds., *Handbook of Oncology Nursing* (p. 450). © 1992. Boston: Jones and Bartlett Publishers. Reprinted with permission.

For the patient in whom intestinal resection is not possible or has been unsuccessful, an alternative intervention can be the placement of a percutaneous endoscopic gastrostomy (PEG) tube.[1,131] This procedure has a low rate of morbidity, particularly when compared to surgical exploration. The PEG tube can be placed in the stomach or jejunum under light anesthesia, in a surgical suite or outpatient care facility. Its success is measured by alleviation of the symptoms of bowel obstruction and enhancement of the patient's quality of life. The PEG tube may allow the patient to resume drinking full liquids and eating small amounts of soft foods, which, although of no significant nutritional benefit, may be of great psychological benefit. Detailed instruction should be given to both the patient and her care givers in the care of the PEG tube site, to prevent wound breakdown from gastric contents or obstruction of the tube, which causes nausea and vomiting and necessitates medical intervention.

When there are no other alternatives, the medical team may elect to use total parenteral nutrition, either to temporarily nourish the patient during an obstructive event or to provide permanent nutrition. It is important to remember that intestinal obstruction developing as a result of recurrent disease predicts short-term survival; however, palliation of this feature of the disease is justified to improve the quality of life that remains.[130,132]

Pleural Effusion

The presence of pleural effusion(s) at the initial presentation of the woman diagnosed with ovarian cancer should be confirmed for malignancy by thoracentesis. If the fluid obtained is cytologically positive, she is given a diagnosis of stage IV disease (see Table 6.2). Most patients who present with pleural effusion(s) as a manifestation of stage IV disease and who receive systemic platinum-based chemotherapy will have resolution of the effusion(s) without sclerotherapy.[124]

It has been found in studies of patients with advanced stages of ovarian cancer that 25 to 30% develop pleural effusions, most commonly as a sign of recurrent or refractory disease.[121] The treatment of malignant pleural effusions in these patients can be difficult, requiring direct treatment of the pleural space.[121]

Physiologically, effusions develop when the flow of pleural fluid from the parietal pleura to the visceral pleura is impaired. Approximately 90% of pleural fluid flows between these two surfaces; the remaining 10% is absorbed by the lymphatics.[134] In the presence of carcinomatous involvement of the parietal and/or visceral pleura, these membranes suffer an inflammatory response and injury, with resulting increased output and accumulation of fluid in the pleural space.[122]

When such accumulation of fluid occurs, patients often present with symptoms of shortness of breath, hypoxia, pleuritic chest pain, and cough.[122] Many of these symptoms are related to the rate of accumulation of the pleural fluid rather than the total volume of fluid present.[121,122] On physical examination, the nurse finds markedly decreased breath sound, most frequently in the lung base(s).[122] A chest X-ray with both AP and lateral views should be obtained for confirmation.[122]

Once the diagnosis of a pleural effusion is made, the nurse should begin to prepare the patient for thoracentesis. In addition to a thoracentesis tray and vacuum bottles, there should be a source of oxygen at hand in case of an adverse event. An informed consent should be obtained and witnessed. Although thoracentesis is a relatively simple procedure, the patient should be well informed of possible complications, which include pain, infection, pneumothorax, and a reaccumulation of the effusion and/or pulmonary edema.

The patient should be placed in a comfortable, upright position over a pillow or tray table. If the patient's condition does not allow this optimal position, she can lie on her unaffected side. The physician chooses the site at which the thoracentesis is to be performed. The skin of the chest wall should be prepared aseptically, and a mild analgesic should be given at least fifteen minutes before the procedure. A local anesthetic is injected into the costal space prior to the thoracentesis. When adequate anesthetizing is achieved, the thoracentesis needle is inserted and the cavity is drained. During the procedure, the nurse should observe for increasing pleuritic or chest pain, increased respiratory rate, use of accessory muscles, dyspnea, uncontrollable cough, faintness or vertigo, or increased pulse rate. The rate at which the cavity is drained can have an effect on the patient's ability to tolerate the procedure. The adverse symptoms mentioned can sometimes be alleviated by slowing down the rate of flow or decreasing the pressure exerted by the vacuum.

When the procedure is complete, the needle is withdrawn, pressure is applied to the puncture site, and a sterile dressing is placed. The patient is observed for any adverse events for several minutes. In some cases, a chest X-ray is performed to evaluate the success of the procedure or to rule out incidental trauma such as a pneumothorax.

Despite the rapid relief of symptoms achieved by thoracentesis, it is usually temporary.[122] A high percentage of malignant pleural effusions reaccumulate in four to five days without initiation of systemic therapy.[122,124]

Those patients who have recurrent pleural effusions are considered for a thoracostomy, or placement of a chest tube with a drainage system (Figure 6.3). The procedure is similar to thoracentesis, with the exception that an incision is made; the pleural cavity is dissected; and a large-bore chest tube is inserted, sutured into place, and taped securely to the patient's chest wall.[133] The chest tube is connected to a chest drainage unit, most frequently using a wet suction system.[133] A sterile occlusive dressing is applied to the site of the chest tube to prevent air leaks. A chest X-ray is obtained to confirm placement and to rule out pneumothorax.[122]

The time frame for the duration of thoracostomy varies, but as the drainage slows, the decision for sclerosing the pleural cavity, or pleurodesis, is made. The goal of this therapy is to obliterate the pleural space through fibrosing (scarring) the tissues, thus preventing reaccumulation of fluid. Several agents have been tested in an attempt to

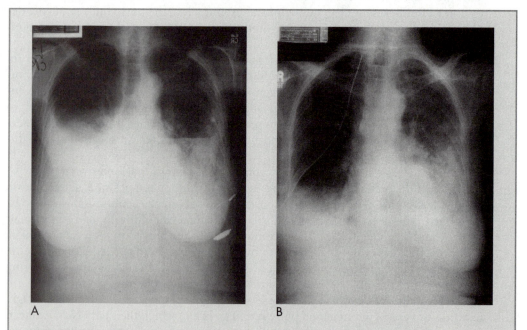

A   B

FIGURE 6.3. A. Bilateral pleural effusions. **B.** Resolution of pleural effusion in right lung with chest tube in place.

Source: Courtesy Vanderbilt University Medical Center, Nashville, TN.

achieve maximum benefit; talc, bleomycin, and doxycycline are the most commonly used agents.[122,134] While the agents are instilled, the nurse assists the patient to rotate into a variety of positions (i.e., right side, left side, Trendelenberg, reverse Trendelenberg, and combinations of each) so as to adequately distribute the sclerosing agent in the pleural cavity.[122] After the selected time frame, when the drainage has subsided after sclerosing, the chest tube is removed and a sterile dressing applied. The wound should be monitored closely for signs of infection.

Following pleurodesis, patients may be given additional systemic chemotherapy to prevent or allay further development of pleural effusions. In patients for whom pleurodesis is not successful, some institutions are achieving relief of symptoms by placing pigtail catheters or catheters with one-way valves to allow for constant or intermittent drainage, respectively.[135] This alternative to a chest tube allows for discharge to home with minimal intervention that can be easily managed by the patient's care givers.

Malnutrition

Virtually all cancer patients suffer from malnourishment during the course of their disease. In fact, it is estimated that as many as 40% of patients hospitalized for treatment of cancer suffer from obvious malnutrition.[136] The rapid growth of tumor cells illustrates the potential metabolic demands of cancer, although the exact mechanism is still unknown.[137] Regardless, the patient with cancer has a constant physiologic demand that can alter basal metabolic rate and diminish fat and protein stores.

In general, there is an alteration in carbohydrate, protein, and fat metabolism. Physiologically, the mechanisms for energy production, glycolysis, and oxidation of glucose into ATP are impaired.[138] To compensate for this inefficiency, the body uses accelerated gluconeogenesis to provide additional energy production, which in turn contributes to protein-calorie malnutrition.[139]

Protein loss is exhibited by the utilization of the proteins in muscle tissue for glucose and creation of a negative nitrogen balance related to a decrease in protein synthesis. Patients who suffer from a negative nitrogen balance may exhibit signs of anemia, muscle wasting, weakness, alteration in immunologic function, impairment of healing mechanisms, and skin breakdown.[138]

Many patients with cancer also experience an alteration in insulin utilization, with an associated increase in lipolysis, or mobilization and catabolism of fatty acids. This mechanism prevents the storage of fat and furthers the depletion of body fat.[137]

In addition to ineffective nutritional metabolism, the woman with ovarian cancer, in particular, faces a mechanical type of cachexia that is related to bowel obstruction and/or dysfunction, either intrinsic or extrinsic; excessive fluid or protein losses from the bowel; complications of chemotherapy; and pain.[136] Loss of fluids through the bowel and by other mechanisms leads to fluid and electrolyte imbalances manifested as hypoalbuminemia, hypercalcemia, hypokalemia, hypomagnesemia, and hyponatremia.

All of these system failures or malfunctions when added to the psychologic effects of an ovarian cancer diagnosis, such as anxiety, depression, feelings of loss of control, altered body image, and the impact of chronic pain, contribute to anorexia.[140] Anorexia is defined as a "diminished appetite; aversion to food."[141] Chronic anorexia induces cachexia, which is characterized by the wasting of tissues such as muscle and fat as well as profound weight loss.[142]

Appropriate nutritional support and intervention should begin after the diagnosis of ovarian cancer is made. By making an early assessment of nutritional status (Table 6.7), the nurse, with or without the assistance of a dietician, can identify:

1. Patterns of nutritional intake prior to diagnosis
2. Potential socioeconomic or religious barriers
3. Assessment of physiologic and/or psychologic impairments that may/will affect nutrition
4. Patients who are at higher than usual risk for nutritional deficits and malnutrition[139]

It is helpful to obtain a diet diary or calorie counts over three days to determine actual intake values. The baseline evaluation should include body weight prior to illness as well as current weight.[137] In so doing, the nurse may be able to delay the strong likelihood that the ovarian cancer patient will develop malnutrition by using carefully implemented interventions. Appropriate nutritional intake must be instituted to prevent potentially life-threatening protein-calorie malnutrition. After identification of certain factors that place the ovarian cancer patient at risk for malnutrition, the nurse, with the patient, should establish goals and interventions to delay or prevent nutritional deficit (Table 6.8).[139]

Some ovarian cancer patients simply cannot tolerate oral food intake. Sometimes it is the newly diagnosed patient, who is weakened by factors of the disease process in-

TABLE 6.7

Physical Evidence of Malnutrition

Focus of Assessment	Indications
Skin	Dry, flaky, taut, easily bruised, eruptions and/or dermatitis
Hair	Fine, dull, brittle, thin
Lips	Dry, swollen, cheilosis
Gums	Ulcerative, bleeding, swollen, reddened
Nails	Brittle, ridged
Eyes	Dull, dark, sunken areas below orbits, temporal wasting
Muscles	Wasted appearance
Mental Status	Irritability, confusion, diminished concentration

Source: Adapted with permission from Nunnally, C., Donoghue, M., & Yasko, J.M. (1982). Nutritional needs of cancer patients. *Nursing Clinics of North America, 17*(4), 557.

TABLE 6.8
Guidelines for Patients with Inadequate Nutritional Intake

Dietary	High-protein, high-calorie foods
Suggestions	Small, frequent meals
	Beer or wine (with physician's approval) may help to stimulate appetite
	Add herbs and spices (as tolerated)
	Avoid spicy or acidic foods
	Avoid foods high in fat or grease, or that are gas-producing
	Low fiber content
	Avoid milk products
	Avoid fluid intake during meals
	Moisten foods with gravies, broths, or sauces
Additional	Try Popsicles for mouth moisturizing
Suggestions	Try artificial saliva
	Try relaxation techniques
	Create meals that are attractive and stimulating
	Use antiemetics before meals
	Avoid stress at mealtime
	Exercise before meals
	Ambiance; dine with friends
	Eat slowly
	Play quiet music during meals

cluding surgical manipulation of the bowel, treatment complications, and age; other times it is the patient with recurrent disease, who is debilitated by harsh therapies, mechanical obstruction of the bowel, or a variety of other complications. Hyperalimentation may be the only alternative for such patients, and it may extend their lives.[130] Protein-calorie malnutrition is frequently the cause of death in ovarian cancer patients.[139]

Hyperalimentation may be given in either enteral or parenteral form. Enteral hyperalimentation for ovarian cancer patients commonly involves use of the gastrostomy tube. By using supplemental tube feedings, it is possible for the patient to take in small palate-pleasing meals and meet total protein and caloric requirements simultaneously.[143] Recommendations of appropriate supplemental formulas can easily be made by a dietician.[137]

Although the use of parenteral hyperalimentation, or TPN, is quite expensive, it quickly restores a positive nitrogen balance and thus may enable a severely nutritionally compromised patient to endure aggressive antineoplastic therapy.[144] In addition to its high cost, there is considerable risk of infection in an immunocompromised patient and the concern, although controversial, that TPN might increase tumor growth.[144] The administration of TPN requires constant vigilance by a trained nutritionalist and/or pharmacist. "The nurse should focus on prevention of complications and careful assessment to assure maximum benefits from therapy."[139]

Both forms of hyperalimentation are effective in maintaining nutrition, but determining appropriate candidates for this therapy can be difficult. It must be the consensus of the medical team that this intervention is ethical and appropriate for a given patient and will provide improvement in quality of life.[143,145]

Malnutrition is by definition a chronic process. Cachexia, as it relates to ovarian cancer, is caused by several factors, which include anorexia, malabsorption, and mechanical obstruction. Anorexia can be due to depression, which manifests as a lack of desire for food, sexual activity, and life itself.[137,146] It can also be influenced by fear and anxiety. For the ovarian cancer patient, who may already have had experiences with treatment-induced nausea and vomiting or a mechanical obstruction, the very act of eating a meal can be a source of stress and frustration.[57] Thus, after careful assessment of the patient's nutritional state, nursing intervention must focus on those issues that are supportive of the physiologic and psychologic factors influencing the development or perpetuation of malnutrition.[57]

Discharge Planning

It is an oncology nursing standard of care that the patient and her support system person(s) "manage stress within their individual physical, psychological, and spiritual capacities and their value systems."[147] For most patients, an assessment of coping mechanisms as well as the support system was established in the first-line treatment phase. Nevertheless, at those times when the patient's disease is in an acute phase, the family unit's ability to cope may be compromised and require frequent interventions.

Certainly as the patient's disease progresses, the level of stress she feels escalates, and does so proportionately in the family as well. It is important for both the patient and family to be well informed of the disease state and included in the decision making.[147] It may be necessary to locate support groups that are independent of the gynecologic oncology practice.

One resource available for continuity of care is the home health agency. Many gynecologic oncology practices have large referral bases that cover radiuses of a few hundred miles. It is important for nurses to develop working relationships with community-based home health agencies, especially considering the current trend toward delivery of care outside the hospital. Hospital-based nurses, staff, and clinical nurse specialists, outpatient facility–based nurses, and home health care–based nurses should have a symbiotic connection. There should be a continuous flow of up-to-date information and data to maintain continuity of care. This team of nurses must develop a plan of care with realistic expected patient outcomes and nursing strategies.

❋ QUALITY OF LIFE

Since Nightingale founded the nursing profession, nurses have centered delivery of care around improvement of quality of life for patients.[148] But recently there has been increased interest in quality of life as an outcome variable for the treatments of malignancies. For oncologic health care professionals in the evolving managed care environment, evaluation of quality of life may ultimately influence treatment plans. It is incumbent on professionals who are responsible for delivery of care to address the issues of treatment or outcomes of treatment that affect the patient's quality of life. As noted by Jones, "Length of survival is but one measure of successful treatment. The toxicity of the treatment must be weighed against the potential benefits."[120]

To determine quality of life, it must be defined. However, quality of life is subjective as it pertains to each individual.[149] For example, one woman's perspective of the impact of the diagnosis of ovarian cancer on her life is different from another's. The variety of complex manifestations of the disease are variables influencing each woman's ability to psychologically evaluate her quality of life.[132]

Quality of life is also multidimensional.[149,150] These dimensions are fundamental components of a person's well-being and include the physiologic, psychologic, sociologic, and spiritual domains.[150,151]

Certainly, in the initial phase of ovarian cancer, the central effect on a woman's quality of life is within the physical domain, impacting physical well-being with the consequences of primary surgery and therapy. Examples are the way in which cytoreductive ovarian cancer surgery can be disfiguring by creation of a colostomy, or the manner in which a bowel resection might cause chronic diarrhea. Initial therapy often causes alopecia, nausea with vomiting, or other difficult-to-manage side effects.[152] In the later course of the disease, women who have a recurrence experience physical symptoms of advanced disease, such as impairment of mobility, respiratory function, and skin integrity and/or alteration of nutritional status, all of which affect physical well-being.[153,154] Measurement of these dysfunctions typically is made using performance status measurements such as the Karnofsky[155] scale, WHO or Zubrod[156] scales, and the (Spitzer) Quality of Life Index.[157] However, these measurement tools evaluate only the medical functional abilities of the patient.[158] Personal aspects of quality of life should be obtained through the use of a patient-completed assessment.[149,154]

The second domain of quality-of-life assessment is psychological well-being.[150,151] Remember that many of the physiologic symptoms described above adversely affect the psychologic health of the woman. A variety of quality-of-life assessment factors can be evaluated, such as anxiety and depression, normalcy, self-esteem and body-image changes, loss of control as it relates to the administration of treatment, and fear of treatment outcome or recurrence.[149,159] These emotional issues are salient throughout the course of the disease and are worthy of assessment and strategic intervention.[160]

The sociologic domain pertains to the impact of the diagnosis on the woman's social relationships. Ovarian cancer alters relationships with her partner and her children and her role within the family unit, as well as her role as a provider. In turn, as her ability to work changes, her insurability may also change, consequently affecting the financial status of her family. As with other aspects of quality of life, the sociologic domain is interdependent with the other domains. As a woman's sexual function, for

TABLE 6.9
Diagnostic Cluster

Diagnostic/Preoperative and Postoperative Period

COLLABORATIVE PROBLEMS
Potential Complication: Bleeding/hemorrhage
Potential Complication: Thromboembolic event
Potential Complication: Infection/sepsis
Potential Complication: Fluid/electrolyte imbalance
Potential Complication: Atelectasis/pneumonia
Potential Complication: Bowel dysfunction
Potential Complication: Urinary dysfunction

NURSING DIAGNOSIS

1. Potential altered health maintenance related to insufficient knowledge of condition, diagnostic tests, prognosis, and treatment options

2. Decisional conflict related to insufficient knowledge of treatment options

3. Anxiety/fear related to impending surgery, and insufficient knowledge of preoperative routines, intraoperative activities, and postoperative self-care activities

4. Anxiety/fear related to insufficient knowledge of potential impact of condition and treatment on reproductive organs and sexuality

5. Grieving related to potential loss of fertility and perceived effects on lifestyle

6. Potential altered respiratory function related to immobility secondary to imposed bed rest and pain

7. Potential fluid volume deficit related to losses secondary to surgical wound or gastrointestinal dysfunction

8. Altered comfort related to effects of surgery, disease process, and immobility

9. Potential for infection related to susceptibility to bacteria secondary to wound, invasive vascular access, and/or urinary catheter

10. Potential altered nutrition: less than body requirements related to disease process, wound healing, and decreased caloric intake

11. Impaired physical mobility related to surgical interruption of body structures, incisional site pain, and activity restriction

12. Potential bowel dysfunction related to decreased peristalsis secondary to surgical manipulation of bowel, effects of anesthesia and analgesia, and immobility

13. Potential urinary dysfunction related to loss of sensation of bladder distention secondary to surgical and/or pharmaceutical interventions

14. Potential impaired skin integrity related to surgical wound, decreased tissue perfusion, ostomy stomas, drain sites, and/or immobility

15. Potential impaired tissue integrity/infection related to lymphedema secondary to surgical removal of lymph nodes

TABLE 6.9 *(continued)*

16a. Potential sexual dysfunction related to disease process, surgical intervention, fatigue, and/or pain

16b. Potential moderate or possible permanent alterations in sexual activity related to disease process, surgical intervention, fatigue, and/or pain

16c. Severe or permanent inability to engage in genital intercourse

17. Alteration in coping related to infertility

18. Potential altered health maintenance related to insufficient knowledge of dietary restrictions, medications, activity restrictions, self-care activities, symptoms of complications, follow-up visits, and community resources

Treatment Period

COLLABORATIVE PROBLEM
Potential Complication: Preexisting medical conditions
Potential Complication: Anasarca
Potential Complication: Fluid/electrolyte imbalance
Potential Complication: Ascites

NURSING DIAGNOSIS

1. Anxiety/fear related to loss of feelings of control of life, unpredictability of nature of disease, and uncertain future

2. Anxiety/fear related to insufficient knowledge of prescribed chemotherapy (including clinical trials) and necessary self-care measures

3. Anxiety/fear related to insufficient knowledge of prescribed intraperitoneal chemotherapy and necessary self-care measures

4. Anxiety/fear related to insufficient knowledge of prescribed radiation therapy and necessary self-care measures

5. Potential for infection related to immunosuppression neutropenia secondary to chemotherapy and/or radiation therapy

6. Anxiety/fear related to insufficient knowledge of prescribed biotherapy and necessary self-care measures

7. Potential for bleeding related to immunosuppression thrombocytopenia secondary to chemotherapy and/or radiation therapy

8. Potential alteration in skin integrity related to treatment modality and/or disease process

9. Potential alteration in respiratory function related to abdominal distention, decreased lung capacity, and/or lung metastasis

10. Potential altered health maintenance due to insufficient knowledge of colostomy/ileostomy and/or ileal conduit

example, is physiologically impaired by her disease, this in turn causes psychologic distress, which in turn affects her interpersonal relationships. Her need to be loved and supported is increased by the critical impact of the disease on the other domains of her quality of life.[151,161]

The fourth domain is spirituality, that is, the impact of the disease on the spiritual well-being of the woman with ovarian cancer. This aspect of quality of life, although certainly no less important than the others, is commonly the least explored.[153] Although unsubstantiated by research, health care providers (physicians, nurses) are thought to avoid spiritual assessment unless it manifests in some way as a physiologic or psychologic symptom.[162] Typically, when a spiritual problem is discovered, a referral is made to the chaplain or spiritual leader of the patient's choice. The difficulty of assessment of quality of life as it pertains to spirituality is the lack of standards or tools to define or assign a statistically significant meaning to patient responses. Too, spirituality is both highly individual and geographically regional. However, measures to assess the spiritual dimension of quality of life do exist, such as those used by Izsak and Medalie (1971),[163] Irwin (1982),[162] Danoff (1983),[162] and Cella et al. (1989).[149,164] Certainly, if there were a way to individualize spiritual assessment of quality of life, and if health care providers were better prepared to identify and implement strategies to facilitate improvement in a patient's spiritual well-being, then nurses would be better able to qualify the value of meeting the spiritual needs of patients.[165]

Regardless of the tool(s) used to assess quality of life, there must be an evolving or ongoing evaluation of coping strategies used by the patient in each of the four domains. The outcome of the assessment should indicate where nursing interventions are best implemented.[152] And as evidenced by the recent development of quality-of-life committees by oncology cooperative groups such as the GOG, ultimately the evaluations of quality-of-life measurements will influence both the types and radicality of medical treatment.

✽ REFERENCES

1. Ozols, R.F., Rubin, S.C., Dembo, A.J., & Robboy, S. (1993). Epithelial ovarian cancer. In W.J. Hoskins, C.A. Perez, & R.C. Young, eds., *Principles and Practice of Gynecologic Oncology* (pp. 731–782). Philadelphia: Lippincott.

2. Parker, S.L., Tong, T., Bolden, S., & Wingo, P.A. (1996). Cancer Statistics, 1996. *CA Cancer J Clin.* Atlanta, GA: American Cancer Society.

3. Barber, H.R.K. (1993). *Ovarian Carcinoma: Etiology, Diagnosis, and Treatment* 3rd ed. (p. 25). New York: Springer-Verlag.

4. Sadler, T.W. (1990). *Langman's Medical Embryology* 6th ed. (p. 260). Baltimore: Williams & Wilkins.

5. Harlap, S. (1993). The epidemiology of ovarian cancer. In M. Markman and W.J. Hoskins, *Cancer of the Ovary* (p. 79). New York: Raven Press.

6. Barber, H.R.K. (1988). Embryology of the gonad with reference to special tumors of the ovary and testis. *J Pediatr Surg, 23*(10), 967.

7. Whittemore, A.S., Wu, M.L., Paffenbarger, R.S. Jr., et al. (1989). Epithelial ovarian cancer and the ability to conceive. *Cancer Res, 49*(14), 4047–4052.

8. Dietl, J. (1991). Ovulation and ovarian cancer. *Lancet, 338*(8764), 445.

9. Rossing, M.A., Daling, J.R., Weiss, N.E., et al. (1994). Ovarian tumors in a cohort of infertile women. *N Engl J Med, 331*, 771–776.

10. Trimble, C.L., & Trimble, E.L. (1994). Management of epithelial ovarian tumors of low malignant potential. *Gynecol Oncol, 55*(3), S52–S61.

11. Markman, M., Zaino, R.J., Busowski, J.D., & Barakat, R.R. (1992). Carcinoma of the fallopian tube. In W.J. Hoskins, C.A. Perez, & R.C. Young, eds., *Principles and Practice of Gynecologic Oncology*, (pp. 783). Philadelphia: Lippincott.

12. Donnez, J., Casanas-Roux, F., Caprasse, J., Ferin, J., & Thomas, K. (1985). Cyclic changes in ovulation, cell height, and mitotic activity in human tubal epithelium during reproductive life. *Fertil Steril, 43*(4), 554–559.

13. Hu, C.Y., Taymor, M.L., & Hertig, A.T. (1950). Primary carcinoma of the fallopian tube. *Am J Obstet Gynecol, 59,* 58–67.

14. McGuire, W.P. (1993). Primary treatment of epithelial ovarian malignancies. *Cancer, Suppl 71*(4), 1541–1550.

15. Look, K.Y. (1993). Clinical aspects of ovarian cancer. In S.C. Rubin & G.P. Sutton, eds., *Ovarian Cancer* (p. 175). New York: McGraw-Hill.

16. Whittemore, A.S. (1994). Characteristics relating to ovarian cancer risk: Implications for prevention and detection. *Gynecol Oncol, 55*(3), S15–S19.

17. Casagrande, J.T., Louie, E.W., Pike, M.C., et al. (1979). Incessant ovulation and ovarian cancer. *Lancet, 2*(8135), 170–173.

18. Fathalla, M.F. (1971). Incessant ovulation: A factor in ovarian neoplasia? *Lancet, 2*(716), 163.

19. The WHO Collaborative Study of Neoplasia and Steroid Contraceptives (1989). Epithelial ovarian cancer and combined oral contraceptives. *Int J Epidemiol, 18*(3), 538–545.

20. Kaufman, D.W., Kelly, J.P., Welch, W.R., et al. (1989). Noncontraceptive estrogen use and epithelial ovarian cancer. *Am J Epidemiol, 130*(6), 1142–1151.

21. Lynch, H.T., Lynch, J.F., & Conway, T.A. (1993). Hereditary ovarian cancer. In S.C. Rubin & G.P Sutton, eds., *Ovarian Cancer* (pp. 189–217). New York: McGraw-Hill.

22. Gilbert, F. (1993). Genetics and Ovarian Cancer. In S.C. Rubin & G.P. Sutton, eds., *Ovarian Cancer* (pp. 3–19). New York, McGraw-Hill.

23. Averette, H.E., & Nguyen, H.N. (1994). The role of prophylactic oophorectomy in cancer prevention. *Gynecol Oncol, 55*(3), S38–S41.

24. Hatcher, R.A., Stewart, F.H., Trussel, J., et al. (1990). *Contraceptive Technology 1990–1992* (p. 246). New York: Irvington.

25. Barber, H.R.K. (1993). Prophylaxis in ovarian cancer. *Cancer, Suppl.* 71(4), 1529–1533.

26. Berchuck, A., Bast, Jr., R.C., (1993). Oncogenes and Tumor-Suppressor Genes. In S.C. Rubin & G.P. Sutton, eds., *Ovarian Cancer* (pp. 3–19). New York: McGraw-Hill.

27. Cramer, D.W., Welch, W.R., Hutchinson, G.D., Willett, W., & Scully, R.E. (1984). Dietary animal fat in relation to ovarian cancer risk. *Obstet Gynecol, 63*(6), 833–838.

28. Byers, T., Marshall, J., Graham, E., et. al. (1983). A case control study of dietary and nondietary factors in ovarian cancer. *J Natl Cancer Inst, 71*(4), 681–686.

29. Farrow, D.C., Weiss, N.S., Lyon, J.L., & Daling, J.R. (1989). Association of obesity and ovarian cancer in a case control study. *Am J Epidemiol, 129*(6), 1300–1304.

30. Cramer, D.W., Welch, W.R., Scully, R.E., et al. (1982). Ovarian cancer and talc: A case control study. *Cancer, 50*(2), 372–376.

31. Rose, P.G., Piver, M.S., & Tsukada, Y. (1990). Fallopian tube cancer: The Roswell Park experience. *Cancer, 66*(2), 2661–2667.

32. Podczaski, E., & Herbst, A.L. (1993). Cancer of the vagina and fallopian tubes. In R.C. Knapp & R.S. Berkowitz, eds., *Gynecologic Oncology*, (p. 308). New York: McGraw-Hill.

33. DiSaia, P.J., & Creasman, W.T. (1993). *Clinical Gynecologic Oncology*, 4th ed. St Louis, MO: Mosby.

34. Anderson, B.L. (1993). Predicting sexual and psychologic morbidity and improving the quality of life for women with gynecologic cancer. *Cancer, Suppl 71*(4), 1678–1690.

35. Eriksson, J.H. (1994). *Oncologic Nursing* 2nd ed. Springfield, PA: Springhouse Corp.

36. Lamb, M. A. (1995). Effects of cancer on the sexuality and fertility of women. *Semin Oncol Nurs, 11*(2), 120–127.

37. Curtin, J.P. (1994). Management of the adnexal mass. *Gynecol Oncol, 55*(3), S42–S46.

38. Dershaw, D.D., & Panicek, D.M. (1993). Radiologic evaluation of ovarian cancer. In M. Markman & W.J. Hoskins, eds., *Cancer of the Ovary* (p. 133). New York: Raven Press.

39. van Nagell, J.R., DePriest, P.D., Gallion, H.H., & Pavlik, E.J. (1993). Ovarian cancer screening. *Cancer, Suppl 71*(4), 1523–1528.

40. Brooks, S.E. (1994). Preoperative evaluation of patients with suspected ovarian cancer. *Gynecol Oncol, 55*(3), S80–S90.

41. Karlan, B.Y., & Platt, L.D. (1994). The current status of ultrasound and color Doppler imaging in screening for ovarian cancer. *Gynecol Oncol, 55*(3), S28–S33.

42. Bromley, B., Goodman, H., & Benacerraf, B.R. (1994). Comparison between sonographic morphology and Doppler waveform for the diagnosis of ovarian malignancy. *Obstet Gynecol, 83,* 434–437.

43. Bragg, D.G., & Hricak, H. (1993). Imaging in gynecologic malignancies. *Cancer, Suppl. 15*(4), 1648–1651.

44. Halpern, S.E. (1992). An overview of radioimmunoimaging. In R.T. McGuire & D. van Nostrand, eds., *Diagnosis of Colorectal and Ovarian Carcinoma* (pp. 1–22). New York: Marcel Decker.

45. Gard, G.B., & Houghton, R.S. (1994). An assessment of the value of serum CA-125 measurements in the management of epithelial ovarian carcinoma. *Gynecol Oncol, 53*, 283–289.

46. Bast, R.C., Klug, T.L., St. John, E., et al. (1983). A radioimmunoassay using a monoclonal antibody to monitor the course of epithelial ovarian cancer. *N Engl J Med, 309*(15), 883–887.

47. Hoskins, W.J. (1993). Primary cytoreduction. In M. Markman & W. J. Hoskins, eds., *Cancer of the Ovary* (p. 163). New York: Raven Press.

48. Hoskins, W.J. (1993). Surgical staging and cytoreductive surgery of epithelial ovarian cancer. *Cancer, Suppl. 15*(4), 1534–1540.

49. Colombo, N.C., Chiari, S., Maggioni, A., Bocciolone, L., Torri, V., & Mangioni, C. (1994). Controversial issues in managment of early epithelial ovarian carcinoma: Conservative surgery and the role of adjuvant therapy. *Gynecol Oncol, 55*(3), S47–S51.

50. Rubin, S.C. (1993). Second look laparotomy in ovarian cancer. In M. Markman & W. J. Hoskins, eds., *Cancer of the Ovary* (p. 175). New York: Raven Press.

51. Creasman, W.T. (1994). Second look laparotomy in ovarian cancer. *Gynecol Oncol, 55*(3), S122–S127.

52. Williams, L.L. (1993). Secondary cytoreduction in ovarian malignancies. In M. Markman, & W.J. Hoskins, eds., *Cancer of the Ovary* (pp. 187–204). New York: Raven Press.

53. Barakat, R.R., Rubin, S.C., Saigo, P.E., Lewis, J.L., Jones, W.B., & Curtin, J.P. (1993). Second look laparotomy in carcinoma of the fallopian tube. *Obstet Gynecol, 82*(5), 748–751.

54. Nezhat, C., Nezhat, F., Teng, N.N., Edraki, B., Nezhat, C.H., Burrell, M.O., Benigno, B.B., & Ramirez, C.E. (1994). The role of laparoscopy in the management of gynecologic malignancy (Review). *Semin Surg Oncol, 10*(6), 431–439.

55. Childers, J.M., & Surwit, E.A. (1993). Current status of operative laparoscopy in gynecologic oncology. *Oncology, 7*(11), 47–51.

56. Young, R., Chabner, B., Hubbard, S., et al. (1978). Advanced ovarian adenocarcinoma: A prospective clinical trial of melphalan (L-PAM) versus combination chemotherapy. *N Engl J Med, 299*(23), 1261–1266.

57. Eriksson, J.H., & Walczak, J.R. (1990). Ovarian cancer. *Semin Oncol Nurs, 6*(3), 214–227.

58. Omura, G., Blessing, J.A., Ehrlich, C.E., et al. (1987). A randomized trial of cyclophosphamide and doxorubicin, with or without cisplatin, in advanced ovarian carcinoma. *Cancer, 56*, 1725.

59. Neijt, J.P., ten Bokkel Huinink, W.W., van der Burg, M.E., et al. (1987). Randomized trial comparing combination chemotherapy regimens CHAP-5 versus CP in advanced ovarian carcinoma. *J Clin Oncol, 5*(8), 1157–1168.

60. Decker, D.G., Fleming, T.R., Malkasian, G.D., et al. (1982). Cyclophosphamide plus cis-platinum in combination: Treatment program for stage II or IV ovarian carcinoma. *Obstet Gynecol, 60*(4), 481–487.

61. McGuire, W.P., Hoskins, W.J., Brady, M.F., Homesley, H., & Clarke-Pearson, D.L. (1992). A phase III trial of dose-intense versus standard dose cisplatin and cytoxan in advanced ovarian cancer. *Proc ASCO, 11*, 226.

62. Shpall, E.J., Stemmer, S.M., Bearman, S.I., et al. (1993). High dose chemotherapy with autologous bone marrow support for the treatment of epithelial ovarian cancer. In M. Markman & W. J. Hoskins, eds., *Cancer of the Ovary* (p. 327). New York: Raven Press.

63. Rozencweig, M., Martin, A., Beltansody, M., et al. (1990). Randomized trial of carboplatin versus cisplatin in advanced ovarian cancer. In P.A. Bunn, R.F. Ozols, R. Canetta, & M. Rozencweig, eds., *Carboplatin: Current Perspectives and Future Directions* (pp. 195–196). Philadelphia: Saunders.

64. ten Bokkel Huinink, W.W., van der Burg, M.E.L., van Oosterom, A.T., et al. (1988). Carboplatin in combination therapy for ovarian cancer. *Cancer Treatment Rev, 15*(Suppl B), 9–15.

65. Wiltshaw, E., Evans, B., & Harland, S. (1985). Phase III randomized trial of cisplatin versus JM8 (carboplatin) in 112 ovarian cancer patients, stages III and IV. *Proc ASCO, 4*, 121.

66. Omura, G., Bundy, B.N., Berek, J.S., et al. (1989). Randomized trial of cyclophosphamide plus cisplatin, with or without doxorubicin, in ovarian carcinoma: A Gynecologic Oncology Group study. *J Clin Oncol, 7*(4), 457–465.

67. Conte, P.D., Bruzzone, M., Chiara, S., et al. (1986). A randomized trial comparing cisplatin plus cyclophosphamide versus cisplatin, doxorubicin, and cyclophosphamide in advanced ovarian cancer. *J Clin Oncol, 4*(6), 965–971.

68. Bruzzone, M., Repetto, L., Chiara, S., et al. (1990). A randomized trial comparing PC versus PAC chemotherapy in epithelial ovarian cancer: Seven years follow-up. *Proc ASCO, 9*, 610.

69. Ovarian cancer meta-analysis project. (1991). Cyclophosphamide plus cisplatin versus cyclophosphamide, doxorubicin and cisplatin chemotherapy of

ovarian carcinoma: A meta-analysis. *J Clin Oncol, 9*(9), 1668–1674.

70. Bertelsen, K., Jakobsen, A., Andersen, J.E., et al. (1987). A randomized study of cyclophosphamide and cisplatinum, with or without doxorubicin, in advanced ovarian carcinoma. *Gynecol Oncol, 28*(2), 161–169.

71. Hakes, T., Hoskins, W., Jones, W., et al. (1990). Randomized prospective trial of 5 versus 10 cycles of cyclophosphamide, doxorubicin, and cisplatin (CAP) in stage III and IV ovarian cancer. *Proc ASCO, 9*, 156.

72. McGuire, W.P., Rowinsky, E.K., Rosenshein, N.B., et al. (1989). Taxol: A unique antineoplastic agent with significant activity in advanced ovarian epithelial neoplasms. *Ann Int Med, 111*(4), 273–279.

73. McGuire, W.P., Hoskins, W.J., Brady, M.F., et al. (1993). A phase III trial comparing cisplatin/cytoxan (PC) and cisplatin/taxol (PT) in advanced ovarian cancer (AOC). *Proc ASCO, 12*, 808.

74. Swenerton, K., Eisenhauer, E., ten Bokkel Huinink, W., et al. (1993). Taxol in relapsed ovarian cancer: High versus low dose and short versus long infusion. *Proc ASCO, 12*, 810.

75. Rowinsky, E.K., Gilbert, M.R., McGuire, W.P., et. al., (1991). Sequences of taxol and cisplatin: A phase I and pharmacologic study. *J Clin Oncol, 9*, 1692–1703.

76. Moore, D.H., Valea, F., Crumpler, L.S., & Fowler, W.C. Jr. (1993). Hexamethylmelamine/altretamine as second line therapy for epithelial ovarian carcinoma. *Gynecol Oncol, 51*(1), 109–112.

77. Thigpen, J.T., Vance, R.B., & Khansur, T. (1993). Second line chemotherapy for recurrent carcinoma of the ovary. *Cancer, Suppl. 71*(4), 1559–1564.

78. Qazi, F., & McGuire, W.P. (1995). The treatment of epithelial ovarian cancer. *CA Cancer J Clin, 45*(2), 88–101.

79. Gore, M.E., Fryatt, I., Wiltshaw, E., & Dawson, T. (1990). Treatment of relapsed carcinoma of the ovary with cisplatin or carboplatin following initial treatment with these compounds. *Gynecol Oncol, 36*(2), 207–211.

80. Kavanagh, J.J., Kudelka, A.P., Freedman, R.S., et al. (1993). A phase II trial of taxotere (RP5696) in ovarian cancer patients refractory to cisplatin/carboplatin therapy. *Proc ASCO, 12*, 823.

81. Hansen, H.H., & Lund, B. (1992). Gemcitabine (2,2-difluorodeoxycitidine): A novel antineoplastic agent with activity in both lung and ovarian cancer. *Ann Oncol, 3*, 161.

82. Thigpen, T., Vance, R., Puneky, L., & Khansur, T. (1994). Chemotherapy in advanced ovarian carcinoma: Current standards of care based on randomized trials. *Gynecol Oncol, 55*(3), S97–S107.

83. Perez, R.P., Hamilton, T.C., Ozols, R.F., & Young, R.C. (1993). Mechanisms and modulation of resistance to chemotherapy in ovarian cancer. *Cancer, Suppl. 15*(4), 1571–1580.

84. Swenson, K.K., & Eriksson, J.H. (1986). Nursing management of intraperitoneal therapy. *Oncol Nurs Forum, 13*(5), 33–39.

85. Markman, M, Reichman, B., Hakes, T., et al. (1993). Intraperitoneal chemotherapy in the management of ovarian cancer. *Cancer, Suppl. 15*(4), 1565–1570.

86. Los, G., Mutsaers, P.H., Lenglet, W.J., et al. (1990). Platinum distribution in intraperitoneal tumors after intraperitoneal cisplatin treatment. *Cancer Chemother Pharmacol, 25*(6), 389–394.

87. Ozols, R.F., Young, R.C., & Speyer, J.L. (1982). Phase I and pharmacological studies of adriamycin administered intraperitoneally to patients with ovarian cancer. *Cancer Res, 42*(10), 4265.

88. Dauplat, J., Legros, M., Condat, P., et al. (1989). High dose melphalan and autologous bone marrow support for treatment of ovarian carcinoma with positive second look operation. *Gynecol Oncol, 34*(3), 294–298.

89. Surwit, E., Childers, J., Hallum A., et al. (1995). Neoadjuvant chemotherapy in advanced ovarian cancer. *Proc Soc of Gynecol Oncol* (abs. 23), 64.

90. Lim, J.T., & Green, J.A. (1993). Neoadjuvant carboplatin and ifosfamide chemotherapy for inoperable FIGO stage III and IV ovarian carcinoma. *Clin Oncol, 5*(4), 198–202.

91. Schwartz, P.E., Chamber, J.T., & Makuch, R. (1994). Neoadjuvant chemotherapy for advanced ovarian cancer. *Gynecol Oncol, 53*(1), 33–37.

92. Peters, W.A., et al. (1989). Results of chemotherapy in advanced carcinoma of the fallopian tube. *Cancer, 63*(5), 836–838.

93. Barakat, R.R., Rubin, S.C., Saigo, P.E., et al. (1991). Cisplatin-based combination chemotherapy in carcinoma of the fallopian tube. *Gynecol Oncol, 42*, 156–160.

94. Kavanagh, J.J., Roberts, W., Townsend, P., & Hewitt, S. (1989). Leuprolide acetate in the treatment of refractory or persistent epithelial ovarian cancer. *J Clin Oncol, 7*(1), 115–118.

95. Myers, A.M., Moore, G.E., & Major, F.J. (1981). Advanced ovarian carcinoma: Response to antiestrogen therapy. *Cancer, 48*(11), 2368–2370.

96. Hamilton, R.C., Davies, P., & Griffiths, K. (1981). Androgen and oestrogen binding in cytosols of human ovarian tumors. *J Endocrinol, 90*(3), 421–431.

97. Creasman, W.T., Omura, G.A., Brady, M.F., et al. (1990). A randomized trial of cyclophosphamide, doxorubicin, and cisplatin, with or without Bacillus Calmette-Guerin, in patients with suboptimal stage III and IV ovarian cancer: A Gynecologic Oncology Group study. *Gynecol Oncol, 39*(3), 239–243.

98. Bast, R.C., Berek, J.S., Obrist, E., et al. (1983). Intraperitoneal immunotherapy of human ovarian carcinoma with *Corynebacterium parvum. Cancer Res, 43*(3), 1395–1401.

99. Berek, J.S., Hacker, N.F., Lichtenstein, A., et al. (1985). Intraperitoneal recombinant alpha interferon for salvage immunotherapy in stage III epithelial ovarian cancer: A GOG study. *Cancer Res, 45*(9), 4447–4453.

100. Pujade-Lauraine, E., Colombo, N., Namer, N., et al. (1990). Intraperitoneal human r-IFN gamma in patients with residual ovarian carcinoma (OC) at second look laparotomy (SLL). *Proc ASCO, 9,* 156.

101. Steis, R.G., Urba, W.J., VanderMolen, L.A., et al. (1990). Intraperitoneal lymphokine-activated killer cell and interleukin-2 therapy for malignancies limited to the peritoneal cavity. *J Clin Oncol, 8*(10), 1618–1629.

102. Epenetos, A.A., Hooker, G., Krausz, T., et al. (1987). Antibody-guided irradiation of advanced ovarian cancer with intraperitoneally administered radiolabeled monoclonal antibodies. *J Clin Oncol, 5*(12), 1890–1899.

103. Freedman, R., Edwards, C., Kavanagh, J., et al. (1993). Intraperitoneal (IP) adoptive immunotherapy of epithelial ovarian carcinoma (EOC) with recombinant interleukin-2 (RIL-2)-expanded tumor infiltrating lymphocytes (TIL) plus low dose RIL-2. *Proc ASCO, 12,* 840.

104. Bookman, M.A., Caron, D.A., Hogan, W.M., et al. (1993). Phase I evaluation of dose-intense chemotherapy with interleukin-1a (IL-1a) for gynecologic malignancies. *Proc ASCO, 12,* 868.

105. von Gruenigen, V.E., Muller, C.Y., Miller, D.S., Mathis, J.M. (1997). Applying gene therapy to ovarian cancer. *Contemp OB/GYN,* (February), 113–114.

106. Tait, D.L., Obermiller, P.S., Redlin-Frazier, S., Jensen, R.A., Welsch, P., Dann J., King, M.-C., Johnson, D.H. Holt, J.T. (1997). A Phase I Trial of Retroviral BRCA1sv Gene Therapy in Ovarian Cancer. *Clin Cancer Res, 3,* 1–10.

107. Dembo, A.J. (1985). Abdominopelvic radiotherapy in ovarian cancer: A ten-year experience. *Cancer, 55*(9 suppl), 2285–2290.

108. Mychalczak, B.R., & Fuks, Z. (1993). The role of radiotherapy in the management of epithelial ovarian cancer. In M. Markman & W. J. Hoskins, eds., *Cancer of the Ovary* (p. 229). New York: Raven Press.

109. Fazekas, J.T., & Maier, J.G. (1974). Irradiation of ovarian carcinomas: A prospective comparison of the open field and moving strip techniques. *Am J Roentgenol, 120*(1), 118.

110. Dembo, A.J., Bush, R.S., Beale, F.A., et al. (1983). A randomized clinical trial of moving strip versus open field whole abdominal irradiation in patients with invasive epithelial cancer of the ovary. *Int J Radiobiol Related Stud Phys Chem 9*(52, suppl. 1), 97.

111. Smith, J.P., Rutledge, F., & Delclos, L. (1975). Postoperative treatment of early cancer of the ovary: A random trial between postoperative irradiation and chemotherapy. *National Cancer Institute Monograph, 42* 149–153.

112. Klaassen, D., Shelley, W., Starreveld, A., et al. (1988). Early stage ovarian cancer: A randomized clinical trial comparing whole abdominal radiotherapy, melphalan, and intraperitoneal chromic phosphate: A National Cancer Institute of Canada Clinical Trial Group report. *J Clin Oncol, 6*(8), 1254–1263.

113. Sell, A., Bertelsen, K., Anderson, J.E., et al. (1990). Randomized study of whole abdomen irradiation versus pelvic irradiation plus cyclophosphamide in treatment of early ovarian cancer. *Gynecol Oncol, 37*(3), 367–373.

114. Kersh, C.R., Randall, M.E., Constable, W.C., et al. (1988). Whole abdominal radiotherapy following cytoreductive surgery and chemotherapy in ovarian carcinoma. *Gynecol Oncol, 31*(1), 113–121.

115. Cain, J.M., Russell, A.H., Greer, B.E., et al. (1988). Whole abdomen radiation for minimal residual epithelial ovarian carcinoma after surgical resection and maximal first line chemotherapy. *Gynecol Oncol, 29*(2), 168–175.

116. Fuks, Z., Rizel, S., & Biran, S. (1988). Chemotherapeutic and surgical induction of pathological complete remission and whole abdominal irradiation for consolidation does not enhance the cure of stage III ovarian carcinoma. *J Clin Oncol, 6*(3), 509–516.

117. Morgan, L., Chafe, W., Mendenhall, W., & Marcus, R. (1988). Hyperfractionation of whole abdominal radiation therapy: Salvage of persistent ovarian cancer following chemotherapy. *Gynecol Oncol, 31,* 122.

118. Fort, M.G., Pierce, V.K., Saigo, P.E., et al. (1989). Evidence for the efficacy of adjuvant therapy in epithelial ovarian tumors of low malignant potential. *Gynecol Oncol, 32*(3), 269–272.

119. Benjamin, I., Barakat, R., Hakes, T., et al. (1995). Platinum-based chemotherapy for advanced stage ovarian serous carcinoma of low malignant potential. *Gynecol Oncol, 59*(3), 390–393.

120. Jones, H.W. (1988). Epithelial ovarian cancer. In H.W. Jones, A.C. Wentz, & L.S. Burnett, eds., *Novak's Textbook of Gynecology* 11th ed. (pp. 792–830). Baltimore: Williams & Wilkins.

121. Clarke-Pearson, D.C., Rodriguez, G.C., Boente, M., (1993). Palliative surgery for epithelial ovarian cancer. In S.C. Rubin & G.P. Sutton, eds., *Ovarian Cancer* (pp. 351–373). New York: McGraw-Hill.

122. Zehner, L.C., & Hoogstraten, B. (1985). Malignant effusions and their management. *Semin Oncol Nurs, 1*(4), 259.

123. Bender, M.D. (1992). Diseases of the peritoneum, mesentery, and omentum. In J. B. Wyngaarden, L.H. Smith, & J.C. Bennett, eds., *Cecil Textbook of Medicine* 19th ed. (p. 790). Philadelphia: Saunders.

124. Markham, M., & Hoskins, W.J. (1993). *Cancer of the Ovary* (pp. 217–228). New York: Raven Press.

125. Kehoe, C. (1991). Malignant ascites: Etiology, diagnosis, and treatment. *Oncol Nurs Forum, 18*(3), 523–530.

126. Brunner, L.S., & Suddarth, D.S. (1980). Assessment and management of patients with hepatic and biliary disorders—Paracentesis. In L.S. Brunner & D.S. Suddarth, eds., *Textbook of Medical-Surgical Nursing* 4th ed. (p. 810). Philadelphia: Lippincott.

127. Souter, R.G., Wells, C., Tarin, D., & Kettlewell, M.G. (1985). Surgical and pathologic complications associated with peritoneovenous shunts in the management of malignant ascites. *Cancer, 55*(9), 1973–1978.

128. Rubin, S.C., Hoskins, W.J., Benjamin, I., & Lewis, J.L. (1989). Palliative surgery for intestinal obstruction in advanced ovarian cancer. *Gynecol Oncol, 34*(1), 16–19.

129. Davis, L.S. (1992). Bowel obstruction. In B.L. Johnson & J. Gross, eds., *Handbook of Oncology Nursing* (pp. 446–458). Boston: Jones and Bartlett.

130. Abu-Rustum, N.R., Barakat, R.R., Venkatraman, E., Spriggs, D., (1997). Chemotherapy and total parenteral nutrition for advanced ovarian cancer with bowel obstruction. *Gynecol Oncol, 64*(3), 493–495.

131. Vasquez, B.M. (1993). Percutaneous endoscopic gastrostomy for palliation of small bowel obstruction in progressive ovarian carcinoma. In R. Cook & E.A. Hager, eds., *Gynecologic Oncology Nursing: Proceedings of the Tenth Annual Symposium in Gynecologic Oncology Nursing, 31,* 30–32. New York: SGNO.

132. Ersek, M., Ferrell, B.R., Dow, K.H., Melancon, C.H., (1997). Quality of life in women with ovarian cancer. *West J Nurs Res, 19*(3), 334–350.

133. Carroll, P. (1991). What's new in chest tube management. *RN, 54*(5), 34–40.

134. Windsor, P.G., Como, J.A., & Windsor, K.S. (1994). Sclerotherapy for malignant pleural effusions: Alternatives to tetracycline. *South Med J, 87*(7), 709–714.

135. Van Le, L., Parker, L.A., DeMars, L.R. MacKoul, P., Fowler, W.C., (1994). Pleural Effusions: Outpatient management with pigtail catheter chest tubes. *Gynecol Oncol, 54*(2), 215–217, Aug.

136. Smith, T.J., Kelly, K.G., & Blackburn, G.L. (1986). Nutrition and the cancer patient. In American Cancer Society, *Cancer Manual* (pp. 391–399). Boston: ACS.

137. Grant, M.M. (1986). Nutritional interventions: Increasing oral intake. *Semin Oncol Nurs, 2*(1), 36–43.

138. Gordon, A. (1987). Nutrition. In C.R. Ziegfeld, ed., *Core Curriculum for Oncology Nursing* (pp. 245–256). Philadelphia: Saunders.

139. Nunnally, C., Donoghue, M., & Yasko, J.M. (1982). Nutritional needs of cancer patients. *Nurs Clin North Am, 17*(4), 557.

140. Cushman, K.E. (1986). Symptom management: A comprehensive approach to increasing nutritional status in the cancer patient. *Semin Oncol Nurs, 2*(1), 30–35.

141. Hensyl, W.R. & Oldham, J.O., eds. (1982). *Stedman's Medical Dictionary* 24th ed. Baltimore: Williams & Wilkins.

142. Lindsey, A.M. (1986). Cancer cachexia: Effects of the disease and its treatment. *Semin Oncol Nurs, 2*(1), 19–29.

143. Irwin, M.M. (1986). Enteral and parenteral nutrition support. *Semin Oncol Nurs, 2*(1), 44–54.

144. Brennan, M.F. (1981). Total parenteral nutrition in the cancer patient. *N Engl J Med, 305*(7), 375–382.

145. Fry, S.T. (1986). Ethical aspects of decision making in the feeding of cancer patients. *Semin Oncol Nurs, 2*(1), 59–62.

146. Gastineau, C.F., DeWys, W., Martin, M.J., & Moxness, K. (1976). The patient who won't eat. *Dialogues in Nutrition, 1*(1), 1–8.

147. Davis, D.S. (1992). Coping. In B.L. Johnson & J.Gross, eds., *Handbook of Oncology Nursing* (pp. 129–144). New York: Wiley Medical.

148. Nightingale, F. (1858). *Notes on Nursing: What It Is, and What It Is Not.* Birmingham, AL: Classics of Medicine Library (1982).

149. Cella, D.F. (1991). Functional status and quality of life: Current views on measurement and intervention. *Cancer Nursing: Functional Status and Quality of Life in Persons with Cancer. Selected Papers from First National Conference on Cancer Nursing Research* (pp. 1–12). Atlanta: American Cancer Society.

150. Cella, D.F., & Tulsky, D.S. (1990). Measuring quality of life today: Methodological aspects. *Oncology, 4*(5), 29–38.

151. Ferrell, B.R. (1992). Overview of breast cancer: Quality of life. *Frontiers in Breast Cancer Symposium: 17th Annual Congress of the Oncology Nursing Society* (pp. 7–8).

152. Belcher, A.E. (1990). Nursing aspects of quality of life enhancement in cancer patients. *Oncology, 4*(5), 197–199.

153. Donovan, K., Sanson-Fisher, R.W., & Redman, S. (1989). Measuring quality of life in cancer patients. *J Clin Oncol, 7*(7), 959–968.

154. Anderson, B. (1994). Quality of life in progressive ovarian cancer. *Gynecol Oncol, 55,* S151–S155.

155. Karnofsky, D.A., Abelmann, W.H., Carver, L.F., & Burchenal, J.H. (1948). The use of the nitrogen mustards in the palliative treatment of carcinoma. *Cancer, 1,* 634–656.

156. Zubrod, C.G., Schneiderman, M., Frei, E., et al. (1960). Appraisal of methods of the study of chemotherapy of cancer in man: A comparative therapeutic trial of nitrogen mustard and triethylene thiophophramide. *J Chronic Dis, 11*(Jan.), 7–33.

157. Spitzer, W.O., Dobson, A.J., Hall, J., et al. (1981). Measuring the quality of life of cancer patients: A concise QL index for use by physicians. *J Chronic Dis, 34*(12), 585–597.

158. Schipper, H., Clinch, J., McMurray, A., & Levitt, M. (1984). Measuring the quality of life of cancer patients: The functional living index—cancer: Development and validation. *J Clin Oncol, 2*(5), 472–483.

159. Grant, M., Padilla, G.V., Ferrell, B.R., & Rhiner, M. (1990). Assessment of quality of life with a single instrument. *Semin Oncol Nurs, 6*(4), 260–270.

160. Kornblith, A.B., Thaler, H.T., Wong, G., Vlamis, V., Lepore, J.M., Loseth, D.B., Hakes, T., Hoskins, W.J., Portenoy, R.K. (1994). Quality of life of women with ovarian cancer. *Gynecol Oncol, 59,* 231–242.

161. Mankin, D. (1990). Impact of cancer on quality of life: A partner's perspective. *Oncology, 4*(5), 202–203.

162. Danoff, B., Kramer, S., Irwin, P., & Gottlieb, A. (1983). Assessment of the quality of life in long term survivors after definitive radiotherapy. *Am J Clin Oncol, 6*(3), 339–345.

163. Iszak, F.C., & Medalie, J.H. (1971). Comprehensive follow-up of carcinoma patients. *J Chronic Dis, 24,* 179–191.

164. Cella, D.F., Tulsky, D.S., Gray, G., et al. (1993). The functional assessment of cancer therapy scale: Development and validation of the general measure. *J Clin Oncol, 11*(3), 570–579.

165. Highfield, M.F., & Cason, C. (1983). Spiritual needs of patients: Are they recognized? *Cancer Nurs, 6*(3), 187–192.

Nonepithelial Cancers of the Ovary

Lois A. Winkelman, RN, MS

Connie L. Birk, RN, BSN, OCN

✻ INTRODUCTION

Nonepithelial ovarian cancer is a family of cancers that consists of two main categories: malignant germ cell tumors and ovarian stromal cancers. These tumors are similar in their presentation, diagnostic evaluation, and primary surgery, but different from one another in their histopathology, pathophysiology, natural history, adjuvant treatment, and prognosis. The incidence of these tumors is rare: malignant germ cell tumors account for 2 to 3% and stromal tumors account for 2% of all ovarian malignancies.[1] Because of their rarity, research in this area is difficult. However, information learned from testicular cancers has contributed enormously to the study of ovarian germ cell tumors and their recommended treatments.

The ovary consists of germ cells, gonadal stromal cells, and cells of mesenchymal tissue. Each tissue has the potential to form a tumor. During embryologic development, the ovary in its early phases is an indifferent organ with the potential to become either an ovary or a testis. During these phases, alterations can occur that may provide the setting for later cellular malfunction producing endocrine imbalances or malignancies.[1]

✻ GONADAL DEVELOPMENT

The sex of the embryo is predetermined at the time of fertilization, depending on the presence of an X or Y chromosome carried by the sperm. However, it is not until the seventh week of embryologic development that the gonads take on characteristics of male or female. The urogenital system consists of (1) the urinary system which excretes waste products and excess water, and (2) the genital system which produces germ cells and has endocrine functions. During development, the systems are closely related anatomically and embryologically. Both develop from the same mesodermal ridge along the posterior wall of the abdominal cavity, and the excretory ducts of both systems initially enter the same cavity, the cloaca.[2] The urogenital fold, or mesonephric ridge, is the ridge formed by both organs. It occupies the posterior portion of the primitive peritoneal cavity and runs the entire length of the fetus (Figure 7.1).[2] From this fold, the ovaries, kidneys, fallopian tubes, uterus, and parts of the vagina arise. The urogenital fold explains the interrelationship between these structures. Mesoderm is the major component in the development of the urogenital system. Endoderm, which develops into the gastrointestinal tract, and the ectoderm also make important contributions.[2]

Initially, the gonads appear as a pair of longitudinal ridges located on each side of the midline along the posterior wall of the embryo between the mesonephros and dorsal mesentery. They are formed by a proliferation of the coelomic epithelium and a condensation of the underlying mesenchyme. Primitive germ cells appear at about three weeks among the endodermal cells in the wall of the yolk sac close to the allantois (Figure 7.2).[2] It is not until the sixth week that the germ cells appear in the geni-

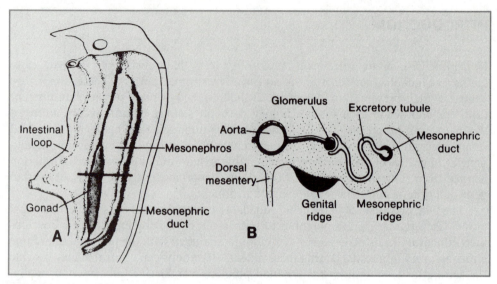

FIGURE 7.1. **A.** The relationship of the genital ridge and the mesonephros. Note the location of the mesonephric duct. **B.** Transverse section through the mesonephros and genital ridge at a level indicated in **A.**

Source: Reproduced with permission from Langman, J., & Sadlier, T.W. (1985). Urogenital system. *Langman's Medical Embryology* 5th ed. (p. 258). Baltimore, MD: Williams & Wilkins.

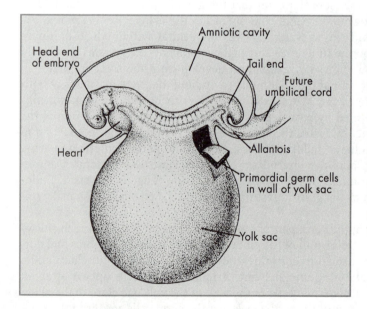

FIGURE 7.2. A three-week-old embryo showing the position of the primordial germ cells in the wall of the yolk sac, close to the attachment of the future umbilical cord.

Source: Reproduced with permission from Langman, J., & Sadlier, T.W. (1985). Urogenital system. *Langman's Medical Embryology* 5th ed. (p. 9). Baltimore, MD: Williams & Wilkins.

FIGURE 7.3. Migrational path of primordial germ cells along the wall of the hindgut and the dorsal mesentary into the genital ridge.

Source: Reproduced with permission from Langman, J., & Sadlier, T.W. (1985). Urogenital system. *Langman's Medical Embryology* 5th ed. (p. 259). Baltimore, MD: Williams & Wilkins.

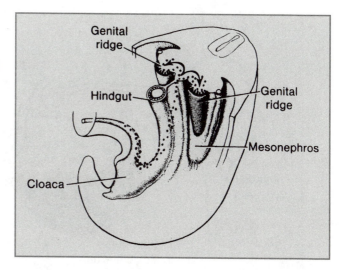

tal ridge, having migrated along the dorsal mesentery of the hindgut (Figure 7.3).[2] Primitive germ cells have an inductive influence on the further development of the gonad into a testis or ovary. The failure of the primitive germ cells to reach the gonadal ridge results in lack of gonadal development. Germ cells do not exist outside the genital ridge.[3]

Indifferent Gonad

Next, the coelomic epithelium of the genital ridge undergoes marked proliferation and some cells penetrate the underlying stroma. Continued growth produces a series of irregularly shaped cords, which are the primitive sex cords (Figure 7.4).[2] Before the arrival of the primitive germ cells in the gonadal ridges, though, the connection of the primitive sex cords and the surface epithelium produces a gonad that cannot be identified as male or female. This stage is referred to as the *indifferent gonad.*[2] Dysgerminomas and seminomas probably arise from cells at this level of development.[3]

Testis

The Y chromosome influences the development of the primitive sex cords into the male gonads. In the testis, primitive testis cords are separated from the coelomic epithelium by a layer of mesenchyme. A dense layer of connective tissue, called the *tunica albuginea*, completes the separation, and the epithelium on the surface of the testis flattens and disappears (Figure 7.5).[2] This distinguishes the testis from the ovary and explains why common epithelial carcinomas are not found in the testis. The tunica albuginea develops into the capsule of the testis. Further development of the gonad into testis occurs in the presence of sustentacular cells of Sertoli, derived from

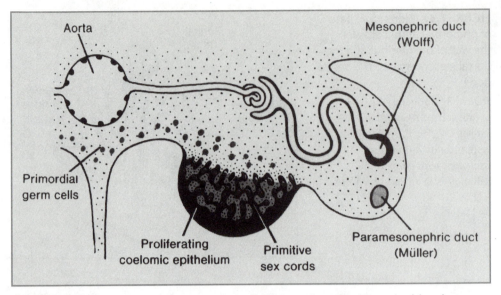

FIGURE 7.4. Transverse section through the lumbar region of a six-week-old embryo showing the indifferent gonad with the primitive sex cords. Some of the primordial germ cells are surrounded by cells of the primitive sex cords.

Source: Reproduced with permission from Langman, J., & Sadlier, T.W. (1985). Urogenital system. *Langman's Medical Embryology* 5th ed. (p. 259). Baltimore, MD: Williams & Wilkins.

surface epithelium, and interstitial cells of Leydig, derived from the original mesenchyme. At this point, testosterone produced by the Leydig cells begins, and the testis is now able to influence the sexual differentiation of the internal and external genitalia.[2]

Ovary

In the female, the primitive sex cords are broken up into cell clusters. These irregular clusters are located mainly in the medulla and contain groups of primitive germ cells (Figure 7.6A).[2] Later they disappear and are replaced by a vascular stroma that forms the ovarian medulla.[2]

The surface epithelium continues to proliferate. During the seventh week of development, a second set of cords, the cortical cords, penetrate the underlying mesenchyme while remaining close to the surface (Figure 7.6A).[2] At the fourth month, the cords split into isolated cell clusters, each surrounding one or more primitive germ cells (Figure 7.6B).[2] The germ cells develop into oogonia, and the surrounding epithelial cells form the follicular cells.[2]

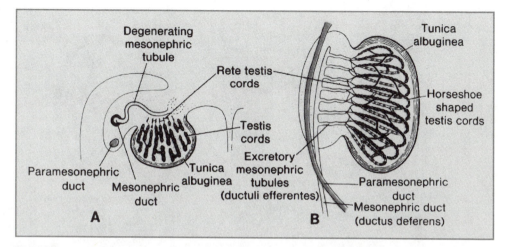

FIGURE 7.5. A. Transverse section through the testis in the eighth week of development. Note the tunica albuginea, the testis cords, the rete testis, and the primordial germ cells. The glomerulus and Bowman's capsule of the mesonephric excretory tubule are in regression. **B.** The testis and the genital duct in the fourth month of development. The horseshoe-shaped testis cords are continuous with the rete testis cords. Note the ductuli efferentes (excretory mesonephric tubules), which enter the mesonephric duct.

Source: Reproduced with permission from Langman, J., & Sadlier, T.W. (1985). Urogenital system. *Langman's Medical Embryology* 5th ed. (p. 261). Baltimore, MD: Williams & Wilkins.

The oogonia undergo multiple mitotic divisions. By the third month, some oogonia differentiate into primary oocytes. They increase in size, and the chromatin arrangement changes in preparation for the first mitotic division. The first oocytes can be identified at eight weeks and number about four million. The primary oocytes replicate their DNA and enter the prophase of the first mitotic division. During the fifth and sixth months of fetal life, many of the oogonia and primary oocytes degenerate. By the seventh month, the remaining primary oocytes are surrounded by flat epithelial cells forming follicles. At birth, no oogonia exist and the oocytes have reduced in number to two million. At age 7 years, only 300,000 oocytes remain.[4]

Primary oocytes remain in prophase; they do not finish their first meiotic division until puberty. At that time, under the influence of hormonal stimulation from the pituitary gland, many follicles start to mature each month, but only one reaches full maturity. The meiotic division of primary oocytes, which began during the third month of fetal life, is finally complete a few hours before ovulation.[1] This leads to the formation of two daughter cells of unequal size: a large secondary oocyte and a small, first polar body, both of which are haploid. The secondary oocyte immediately undergoes a

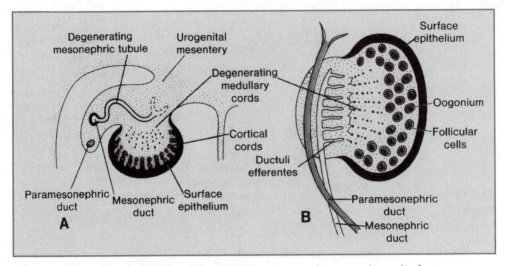

FIGURE 7.6. A. Transverse section through the ovary at the seventh week of development showing degeneration of the primitive (medullary) sex cords and the formation of the cortical cords. **B.** The ovary and genital ducts in the fifth month of development. Note the degeneration of the medullary cords. The excretory mesonephric tubules (ductuli efferentes) do not communicate with the rest. The cortical zone of the ovary contains groups of oogonia surrounded by follicular cells.

Source: Reproduced with permission from Langman, J., & Sadlier, T.W. (1985). Urogenital system. *Langman's Medical Embryology* 5th ed. (p. 262). Baltimore, MD: Williams & Wilkins.

second meiotic division, forming a mature ovum and a small secondary polar body. This occurs in the uterine tube, but only if fertilization takes place.[4]

Thus most oocytes remain in a prolonged prophase of first meiotic division lasting from fetal life to adulthood. Some germ cells may be suspended in prophase for as long as forty-five years. Prolonged exposure to adverse environmental factors can account for the relatively high incidence of chromosomal abnormalities in late-age pregnancies.[3]

To summarize, the presence of an X or Y chromosome at fertilization determines the sex of the embryo. In an XX sex chromosome, the medullary cords of the gonad regress and cortical cords develop. In an XY sex chromosome, the medullary cords develop into testis cords, and there is no second set of cortical cords. In males, the Wolffian system dominates during genital system development and the Muellerian system atrophies. In females, the opposite is true.[1]

Hormonal Control of the Ovarian and Endometrial Cycles

The female reproductive system undergoes a series of complex changes monthly. These changes may be described as the menstrual cycle and the ovarian cycle. The

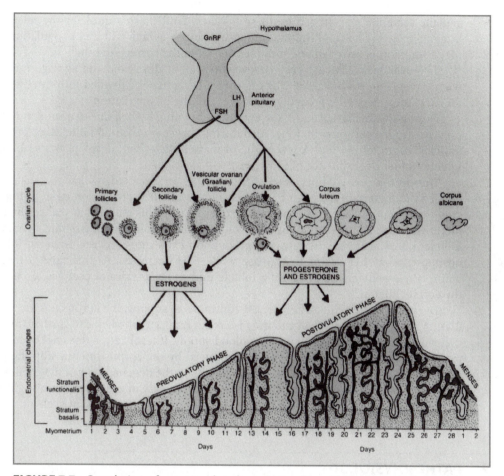

FIGURE 7.7. Correlation of menstrual and ovarian cycles with the hypothalmic and anterior pituitary gland hormones. In the cycle shown, fertilization and implantation have not occurred.

Source: Figure on p. 724 from *Principles of Anatomy and Physiology*, 6th ed., by Gerard Tortora and Nicholas Anagnostakos. Copyright © 1990 by Biological Sciences Textbooks, Inc., A & P Textbooks, Inc. & Elia-Sparta, Inc. Reprinted by permission of HarperCollins Publishers, Inc.

menstrual cycle allows the endometrium to thicken in preparation for a fertilized ovum. The ovarian cycle is the series of events that leads to the development of a mature ovum that may undergo fertilization.[5]

Both the menstrual cycle and the ovarian cycle are under hormonal control. They are regulated by the secretion of gonadotropic releasing factor (GnRF) by the hypothalamus (Figure 7.7).[6] GnRF stimulates the release of follicle-stimulating factor (FSH) from the anterior pituitary, which initiates the development of ovarian follicles and the secretion of estrogen by these follicles. GnRF also stimulates the release of luteinizing hormone (LH) from the anterior pituitary, which will lead to ovulation and the production of estrogen and progesterone from the corpus luteum.[5]

The average menstrual cycle lasts twenty-eight days, and the average range is twenty-five to thirty-five days. The menstrual cycle may be divided into three stages: the menstrual stage, the preovulation stage, and the postovulation stage.

During the menstrual stage, the endometrial lining is shed due to a sudden reduction of estrogen and progesterone. Also during this stage, ovarian follicles, or primary follicles, begin to develop. A few of the primary follicles will develop into secondary follicles under the influence of FSH.

During the preovulatory stage, FSH and LH are secreted, which stimulates increased production of estrogen by the secondary follicles. The endometrial lining begins to thicken in response to this release of estrogen. This may also be called the proliferative phase. At the end of this stage, one secondary follicle matures into a Graafian follicle, which increases its estrogen production even more. As the Graafian follicle nears ovulation, LH begins to increase while FSH decreases. At this time, a mature ovum is released and the remaining follicle undergoes a series of changes to become the corpus luteum.[6]

During the postovulatory stage, LH continues to support the corpus luteum, stimulating it to produce estrogen and progesterone. Progesterone helps to further thicken the endometrial lining and increase its blood supply. If fertilization does not occur, the rising estrogen and progesterone levels produced by the corpus luteum stop the production of LH by negative feedback. This results in the degeneration of the corpus luteum, leading to a sudden decrease of estrogen, a decrease of progesterone, a slight rise in FSH, and endometrial shedding and the beginning of a new ovarian cycle occur.[6]

❊ PATHOPHYSIOLOGY

Because of Teilum's extensive work on the comparative pathology of tumors of the ovary and testes, classification of identical tumors in male and female has evolved (Table 7.1).[7] This classification is based on their histogenetic basis and defines their pathology (Figure 7.8).[8] Because of the higher incidence of testicular cancers, data obtained from these diseases have provided a wealth of information for the management of nonepithelial ovarian cancers.

Germ Cell Tumors

Germ cell tumors may be derived from any or all of the three embryonic layers: ectoderm, mesoderm, and endoderm. In some, extraembryonic structures predominate, whereas in others immature or mature structures may be derived from any or all embryonic layers.[1]

TABLE 7.1

World Health Organization Classification of Nonepithelial Tumors of the Ovary

Germ Cell Tumors	Dysgerminoma
	Endodermal sinus tumor
	Embryonal carcinoma
	Polyembryoma
	Choriocarcinoma
	Teratoma
	Immature
	Mature (dermoid cyst)
	Monodermal (struma ovarii, carcinoid)
	Mixed Forms
	Gonadoblastoma
Sex Cord– Stromal Tumors	Granulosa-Stromal Cell Tumors
	Granulosa cell tumor
	Juvenile
	Adult
	Thecoma-fibroma
	Sertoli Stromal Cell Tumors
	Androblastomas
	Well differentiated
	Intermediate differentiation
	Poorly differentiated
	Sex Cord Tumor with Annular Tubules
	Gynandroblastoma
	Steroid (Lipid) Cell Tumors

Source: Reproduced with permission from Serov, S.F., Scully, R.E., & Sobin, I.H. (1973). Histological typing of ovarian tumors. *International Histological Classification of Tumors* (No.9). Geneva: World Health Organization.

Primitive germ cells, which are present in the adult, represent the oogonia and oocytes and give rise to embryonic tumors. The most common malignant embryonic tumor is the dysgerminoma, which arises at the indifferent stage of ovarian development. Hughesdon and Bennett reported that the origin of this tumor is probably linked to continuing proliferation of unencapsulated germ cells and the associated stimulation of surrounding ovarian mesenchymal cells.[9] Immature cells give rise to the embryonic carcinomas known as immature teratomas, and mature cells give rise to teratomas, which are either cystic or dermoid.[3]

The germ cell tumor classification also includes the extraembryonic mesoderm

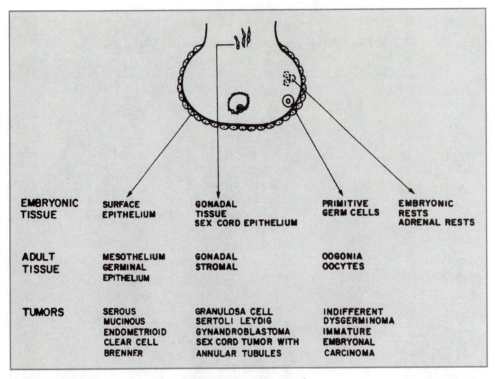

FIGURE 7.8. The histogenesis of primary ovarian neoplasms.

Source: Reproduced with permission from Barber, H.R.K. (1988). Embryology of the gonad with reference to special tumors of the ovary and testis. *Journal of Pediatric Surgery, 23*(10), 967–972.

tumors. This mesoderm seems to be derived, at least in part, from the inner surface of the trophoblast and differentiates before the endoderm has had time to spread around the anterior of the blastocysts. As a result, the primitive yolk sac has endoderm on its roof only. The remainder of the blastocyst cavity becomes lined with a thin layer of flattened mesothelial cells, representing the inner limiting layer of the extraembryonic mesoderm. This is in continuity with the primitive endoderm around its margins, which then closes the yolk sac. The primitive yolk sac is eventually converted into a smaller sac resembling an hourglass (Figure 7.9).[8] Part of the mesoderm covering the yolk sac is called the extraembryonic splanchnopleuric mesoderm. So-called yolk sac tumors of the human ovary reproduce these transient stages in the embryonic development of the yolk sac.[8]

The extraembryonal cells associated with the yolk sac give rise to endodermal sinus tumors as well as the trophoblastic cells. The trophoblastic cells consist of cytotrophoblasts and syncytial trophoblasts. Choriocarcinoma is derived from this

FIGURE 7.9. Primitive yolk sac.

Source: Reproduced with permission from Barber, H.R.K. (1988). Embryology of the gonad with reference to special tumors of the ovary and testis. *Journal of Pediatric Surgery,* 23(10), 967–972.

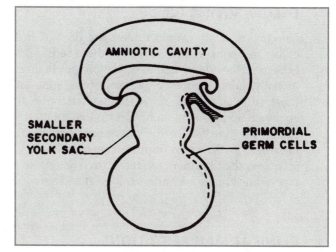

trophoblastic tissue. These tumors are highly malignant and have a counterpart in the testis.[1] Figure 7.10 illustrates the origins of germ cell tumors.

Gonadoblastoma is a tumor consisting of a mixture of germ cells and gonadal stromal cells. In most cases, it has been reported in intersex individuals and called *dysgenetic gonadoma.* Patients with gonadoblastoma have a genotype of 46, XY or XO/XY, and a phenotypic female habitus, amenorrhea, and possibly virilization.[1]

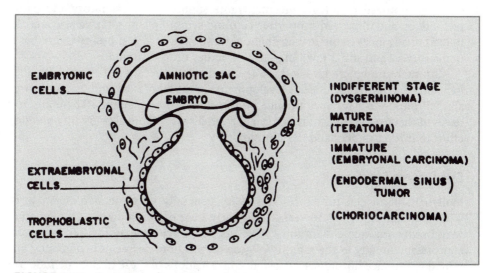

FIGURE 7.10. An extraembryonic ovarian tumor.

Source: Reproduced with permission from Barber, H.R.K. (1988). Embryology of the gonad with reference to special tumors of the ovary and testis. *Journal of Pediatric Surgery,* 23(10), 967–972.

Ovarian Stromal Tumors

One to 3% of all ovarian tumors are derived from the gonadal stroma and contain collagen-producing cells as well as theca cells, granulosa cells, Sertoli cells, and Leydig cells in various stages of differentiation (see Figure 7.8).[8] Most of these tumors are hormonally active, producing estrogens, progestins, androgens, and some corticosteroids.[3] Most stromal tumors show differentiation in an ovarian direction. Ovarian mesenchyme is capable of ambivalent differentiation.[8] Because of this ambiguity, stromal tumors are classified by their hormonal effects rather than histologic type. Gynandroblastoma, as the name implies, consists of male and female elements. Granulosa or granulosa-thecal tumors are categorized as female types; Sertoli-Leydig are of the male type. Some tumors are hormonally inert and are considered unclassified stromal tumors.[3]

✴ CLINICAL MANIFESTATIONS

Patients with germ cell tumors or stromal tumors of the ovary have similar presenting symptoms, surgical recommendations, and follow-up. (Adjunctive treatment depends on the unique histological characteristics of a particular tumor type and the individual medical needs of the patient.) On the whole, the treatment for malignant germ cell tumors has been one of the success stories in gyn-oncology.[10] More effective chemotherapy regimens that have evolved over the last twenty years and research data from testicular cancer studies have made the greatest contribution. More precise surgical staging, improved radiologic imaging, more sophisticated laboratory and pathology techniques, and improved supportive care and symptom control have also contributed to further advances in the management of these tumors.[11] A substantial number of patients survive and suffer few long-term toxicities from treatment.

Stromal tumors are rare and are less understood because of their rarity, indolent behavior, and late recurrences. Developments in the laboratory and patient care arenas are continuing to have an influence on the care of these patients. There are no standards of therapy yet for advanced or recurrent disease. Clinical trials are ongoing in an effort to further understand these tumors.[12]

Subjective Findings

Malignant germ cell tumors of the ovary generally occur in adolescent girls and women under the age of 30 years. In its early stage of development, an ovarian tumor may produce minimal symptoms. The degree of symptomatology and the physical signs relate directly to the rapidity of growth, position, degree of malignancy, and potential to produce hormones.[1] Possible complications of these tumors include torsion, hemorrhage, rupture, and infection.[1]

These tumors tend to occur most commonly at puberty, leading one to believe that some control mechanism may be activated, or that pituitary stimulation of a latent ovarian factor may be the triggering mechanism.[1] Until puberty, the ovary is an abdominal organ originating from the level of T10; after puberty, the ovaries descend into the pelvis. Therefore, ovarian tumors in adolescence are abdominal and thus highly susceptible to torsion because of a longer ovarian suspensory ligament.[1] Abdominal pain is the most common presenting symptom. The pain may be related to the relatively small pelvic and abdominal cavity, causing the tumor to stretch the peritoneum and produce pressure on adjacent organs. Other presenting symptoms may include abnormal vaginal bleeding, amenorrhea, or abdominal distention.[10]

In adult women, abdominal pain and symptoms similar to those of epithelial ovarian cancer (gastrointestinal discomfort, ascites) are common. Germ cell tumors are known to be associated with pregnancy in a small number of cases. That is, 15 to 20% of dysgerminomas are diagnosed during pregnancy or in the immediate postpartum period.[3]

Objective Findings

A general physical examination, including pelvic, rectal, and rectovaginal exam, should be performed and a health history taken. In children, it is impossible to palpate normal ovaries because they are abdominal organs. Thus if an ovary is enlarged on palpation, it can be assumed to be abnormal. Tumor size determines whether it can be felt abdominally or by rectoabdominal palpation.[1] In adult women, most ovarian masses can be detected on vaginal and rectovaginal exam.

If the tumor produces hormones, the clinical picture is related to the type of hormone secreted and its corresponding symptoms, which may include vaginal bleeding, isosexual precocity, virilism, or amenorrhea.[3]

Many malignant germ cell tumors possess the ability to produce biologic markers that can be measured in serum. The development of radioimmunoassay techniques for measuring human chorionic gonadotropin (hCG) and alpha fetal protein (AFP) have led to dramatic advances in monitoring patients.[10] Serial measurements of these tumor markers assist in diagnosis, monitoring response to treatment, and subsequent surveillance for tumor recurrence.[1] Table 7.2 lists the serum markers for various histologic tumor types.[10]

Another serologic marker that has been recently identified is the glycolytic enzyme lactic dehydrogenase (LDH). Certain LDH isoenzymes have been reported to be elevated in patients with testicular cancer as well as patients with ovarian dysgerminomas.[10] Further evaluation of LDH as a possible marker is warranted. Other tumor markers that may be elevated in malignant germ cell tumors include CA-125 and neuron-specific enolase.[12]

Progress is being made in identifying a circulating tumor marker for stromal tumors.[13] Most recent research has been done on inhibin, a peptide hormone that is produced by normal granulosa cells of the ovary in premenopausal women. Inhibin works by inhibiting the release of FSH from the pituitary gland. When inhibin is elevated in premenopausal women, infertility may result. After menopause, inhibin lev-

TABLE 7.2		
Serum Tumor Markers in Malignant Germ Cell Tumors of the Ovary		
Histology	AFP	BhCG
Dysgerminoma	−	±
Endodermal Sinus Tumor	+	−
Immature Teratoma	±	−
Mixed Germ Cell Tumors	±	±
Choriocarcinoma	−	+
Embryonal carcinoma	±	+

Source: Reproduced with permission from Gershenson, D. (1993). Update on malignant ovarian germ cell tumors. *Cancer, 71*(suppl. 4), 1582.

els are normally undetectable in the blood. But women who have a granulosa cell tumor of the ovary have increased levels, possibly due to inhibin being produced autonomously in the tumors themselves. Inhibin may be a good tumor marker for granulosa cell tumors, as its level is abnormally elevated prior to any clinical manifestation of disease. Also, it may be used to diagnose both primary and recurrent granulosa cell tumors. This is particularly important, as recombinant chemotherapy has improved prognosis and long-term remission in early stage tumors and tumors with small volume recurrences.[14,15]

When a patient has a suspicious pelvic mass, a diagnostic work-up is performed. This work-up should include blood count, blood chemistries, serum tumor markers, urinalysis, chest X-ray, intravenous pyelogram to rule out ureteral obstruction, and if indicated, gastrointestinal radiologic studies to rule out bowel involvement or other bowel disorders.[1] CT scan of the abdomen and pelvis is an alternative that can provide more information about the primary tumor and metastatic sites.[11] Ultrasound is optional, and the role of laparoscopy remains to be seen.[10] In patients suspected of having a hormone-producing tumor, hormone assays may be helpful.[12]

❈ GENERAL PRINCIPLES OF TREATMENT

Staging Laparotomy

For a patient suspected of having an ovarian mass, surgery establishes the diagnosis and is the primary therapy. An exploratory laparotomy as defined by the International Federation of Obstetrics & Gynecology (FIGO) is performed (see Table 6.3).[16] If the disease appears to be confined to one or both ovaries, it is imperative that appropriate staging biopsies be obtained.[1] Gynecologic oncology specialists are knowledgeable in the natural history of ovarian cancer spread, which is critical in order to perform the necessary staging laparotomy. Staging information is necessary to determine the extent of the disease, provide prognostic information, and guide postoperative treatment.[10] A meticulous approach is important for every patient, but it is of critical importance for a patient with presumed early stage disease in order to identify any occult or microscopic disease that may affect postoperative treatment recommendations.[1]

The type of primary surgery is dependent on the operative findings. Bilateral ovarian involvement is rare except in cases of pure dysgerminomas. Bilateral involvement may also be found in cases of advanced germ cell tumors in which metastasis from one ovary to the opposite one has occurred and in cases of mixed germ cell tumors with a dysgerminoma component. Stromal tumors are rarely bilateral.[16]

Role of Cytoreductive Surgery

Although there is very little information in the literature about the benefit of cytoreductive surgery in germ cell and stromal tumors, it is still recommended that the principles of tumor debulking applied in the surgical management of epithelial cancers be adhered to.[10] As long as it is technically feasible and safe, all visible tumor should be removed. Patients with completely resected disease at primary surgery have responded better to chemotherapy and had improvement in overall prognosis than those with incompletely resected disease.[10,11] In germ cell tumors, especially dysgerminomas, which are the most chemosensitive, the advisability of aggressive resection, especially of retroperitoneal lymph nodes, remains unclear. The morbidity due to the surgical procedure must be carefully weighed against the benefits.[11]

Conservative Surgery

A unilateral salpingo-oophorectomy (USO) with preservation of the contralateral ovary and uterus can be performed in most patients with early stage malignant germ cell tumors and stromal tumors, thus preserving fertility potential.[11] These tumors rarely involve both ovaries. Thus if the opposite ovary appears grossly normal, it should be left undisturbed. Unnecessary biopsy may result in future infertility because of peritoneal adhesions or ovarian failure. In cases of pure dysgerminoma, a biopsy of the opposite ovary may be considered, because occult or microscopic tumor does occur in 10 to 15% of patients. If the contralateral ovary appears enlarged or abnormal, a biopsy or ovarian cystectomy should be carried out. If frozen section analysis reveals malignant disease or a dysgenetic gonad, which is a nonfunctioning gonad that has a high risk of malignancy, a bilateral salpingo-oophorectomy is necessary. If a benign cystic teratoma (occurring in 5–10% of patients) is found, ovarian cystectomy with preservation of normal ovarian tissue is advised.[11] Even in the face of extensive metastatic disease, it is not uncommon for the surgeon to be able to preserve a normal contralateral ovary.

Historically, if a patient required bilateral salpingo-oophorectomy, a hysterectomy was also performed.[10] However, with the advent of in vitro fertilization technology, which involves donor oocyte and hormonal support, a woman wishing to sustain an intrauterine pregnancy may do so. If one ovary and the uterus are resected because of tumor involvement, modern techniques can provide the opportunity for oocyte retrieval from the remaining ovary. The oocyte can then be fertilized in vitro with sperm from her partner and implanted into a surrogate uterus.[11] Because of these advances, traditional guidelines for surgical treatment of patients with a gynecologic tumor are being reviewed, especially for young patients with germ cell tumors and stromal tumors. There is no substitute for surgical experience and a clear understanding of the biology of these tumors. The surgeon must use thoughtful and mature surgical judgment when encountering such situations, carefully weighing the risks and benefits.[11]

Because many of these patients receive initial surgical treatment at community hospitals, the incidence of inadequate surgical staging is widespread.[10] When the pathologic diagnosis reveals a malignant germ cell tumor or an ovarian stromal tumor, these inadequately staged patients are then referred to a gynecologic oncology specialist. In these cases, the question of reexploration for appropriate staging versus beginning adjunctive therapy arises. Postoperative studies that include CT scan of the abdomen and pelvis (if possible, lymphangiogram) and chest X-ray are performed to evaluate residual disease status. Unless bulky residual disease is present, it probably is not advisable to consider reexploration for adequate staging, but to begin therapy to these chemosensitive tumors as soon as possible.[11] In stromal tumors, secondary cytoreduction is believed to be beneficial, but there are differing opinions as to how much.[12]

Pathologic Review

Review of surgical pathology by an expert in the field of gynecologic oncology pathology is paramount. Because of the rarity and histological similarities of these tumors, misdiagnosis can easily occur. Thus many times surgical slides are reviewed by more than one pathology specialist to ensure accurate diagnosis. Only then can appropriate treatment recommendations and prognosis be determined.[1]

Role of Second-Look Surgery

Second-look laparotomy/laparoscopy has been part of the management of ovarian cancers for several years. Now the goal of second-look surgery is being reevaluated, however, especially in germ cell tumors and stromal tumors. Characteristics of nonepithelial ovarian cancers that have led to this reevaluation include the shorter natural history of germ cell tumors, the late recurrence of stromal tumors, the likelihood of negative findings, the benefits of early diagnosis of persistent disease, and the usefulness of tumor markers. It is not clear how successful salvage treatment would be at the time of a positive second look versus at the time of clinical progression. Therefore, it is believed that the number of patients that would benefit from reexploration would be small.[11] Further research in this area is ongoing.

❋ CLASSIFICATION

In 1973 the World Health Organization provided the classifications for ovarian germ cell and stromal tumors (see Table 7.1).[17] Staging of nonepithelial ovarian cancers is the same as that used for epithelial ovarian cancer (see Table 6.3).[16]

Germ Cell Tumors

Germ cell tumors can be divided into three major categories. The first is benign tumors, most of which are dermoid cysts and account for one-quarter to one-third of all ovarian tumors. These occur in young women most frequently, but can also occur in children and occasionally in the elderly. The second category, malignant tumors arising from constituents of dermoid cysts, accounts for 1% of all ovarian cancers and occurs in the same age group as surface epithelial ovarian cancer (median age 55).[10] The third category, primitive malignant germ cell tumors which recapitulate normal embryonic and extraembryonic cells and structures, almost always occurs in young women and accounts for 2 to 3% of ovarian cancers. This category includes the dysgerminoma, endodermal sinus tumor, immature teratoma, and mixed germ cell tumors.[16]

Dysgerminoma

Dysgerminoma is the most common ovarian malignant germ cell tumor, accounting for about half of the germ cell tumors of the ovary, although it is by no means common, representing 1 to 2% of all ovarian cancers.[16] Its homologue in testis cancer is seminoma.[1] It occurs predominantly in adolescent girls and women under the age of 30, although reports have included patients from age 7 months to 70 years.[16] The majority occur in normally developed phenotypic and genotypic females; 5 to 10% occur in maldeveloped patients.[11] Sixty-six percent of patients are diagnosed with stage I disease, and about 10% have bilateral involvement. The tumor is generally asymptomatic, being found on routine exam, especially when it has reached palpable size or when it has extended beyond the original site. Twenty-five percent have metastatic disease at primary surgery, occurring by extension through the capsule, by peritoneal spread, and by lymphatic and vascular routes.[12] Acute pain may occur if the capsule is ruptured or in the presence of torsion of the ovarian pedicle. Early stage disease can involve the opposite ovary. Involvement of mediastinal and supraclavicular nodes can occur in advanced stages and may also include bone, brain, liver, and lung metastasis.[3]

Primary surgery involves a staging laparotomy, discussed above, with removal of all visible tumor and the involved ovary, careful inspection of the contralateral ovary, retroperitoneal lymph nodes, and the entire peritoneal cavity, as well as biopsy of any suspicious findings.[10] If fertility is not an issue and the disease is early stage, a total abdominal hysterectomy with bilateral salpingo-oophorectomy (TAH-BSO) should be performed. If the disease is in stage I and fertility is a concern, conservative surgery, that is, removal of only the involved ovary, may be performed. Patients with stage Ia pure dysgerminoma are cured with surgery alone. In patients with greater than stage Ia, a high degree of differentiation, or mixed pathologic components, postoperative radiation therapy, and/or chemotherapy is indicated.[12] Because the tumor is chemotherapy and radiation sensitive, survival rates today are high.

For several decades, postoperative radiation therapy was used for patients with metastatic disease, unfortunately resulting in loss of fertility. Recurrent disease was treated with chemotherapy. Advances made in testicular cancer using chemotherapy documented the chemosensitivity of dysgerminomas.[10] Efforts to develop treatment strategies that would achieve equal efficacy, acceptable toxicity, and also preserve fertility began in the early 1970s, using chemotherapy agents such as vincristine, actinomycin, and cyclophosphamide (VAC). Even though this regimen had the potential for cure, only 50% were long-term survivors at that time.[18] However, by 1985, under the auspices of the Gynecologic Oncology Group (GOG), fourteen of fourteen patients with dysgerminoma (nine with advanced or recurrent disease) were without evidence of disease following VAC treatment.[19]

In the late 1970s, when cisplatin became available, treatment with testicular germ cell tumors using cisplatin-based regimens began to be studied. Using PVB (platinum, vinblastine, bleomycin), 66% long-term survivors were reported by the GOG. In addition, in testicular cancer, etoposide was substituted for vinblastine and found to have equal, if not superior, results with less toxicity. In a study by the GOG, nineteen of twenty patients with germ cell tumors who had had incomplete resection were treated with either PVB or BEP (bleomycin, etoposide, and cisplatin) and found to be disease-free for a median interval of twenty-six months.[20] BEP has also been used as adjunctive therapy for patients with inadequate surgical staging for pure dysgerminoma, who have an approximate recurrence rate of 20%. As of 1989, five of five were without evidence of disease.[21] Thus BEP has become the standard of therapy for both male and female dysgerminomas.

Conservative surgery in all stages, involving unilateral salpingo-oophorectomy in combination with postoperative chemotherapy, has raised hopes of equally impressive survival rates.[11] Chemotherapy is replacing radiation therapy as the standard of treatment for dysgerminomas in patients in whom fertility is a concern. In fact, in light of recent data proving its efficacy and decreased morbidity, chemotherapy (Table 7.3) is the clear choice, even if fertility is not an issue.[12, 22]

Microscopic evaluation of dysgerminomas requires thorough sectioning to rule out the presence of other malignant germ cell components, which are frequently found in association with these tumors.[10] It is imperative to distinguish pure dysgerminoma from mixed germ cell tumors, because treatment and prognosis can be dramatically different. Kurman and Norris[23] reviewed a series of thirty cases and found that the most common combination was dysgerminoma and endodermal sinus tumor. Early reports on the prognosis of dysgerminomas were poor because the distinct prognostic differences between dysgerminomas and nondysgerminomas were not appreciated.[23] But with development of assays for beta human chorionic gonadatropin (BhCG) and AFP, tumor markers produced by nondysgerminomatous elements, a clearer distinction in screening for pure dysgerminomas can be made. Pure dysgerminomas are not associated with hormonal activity. Once mixed germ cell tumors could be excluded, survival rates of pure dysgerminomas proved to be excellent when

TABLE 7.3			
Chemotherapy Regimens for Pure Dysgerminomas			
GOG Protocol 45:*	Cisplatin	20 mg/m^2	days 1–5
3–4 courses given	Vinblastine	12 mg/m^2	day 1
every 3 weeks	Bleomycin	20 U/m^2	each week
GOG Protocol 90:*	Cisplatin	20 mg/m^2	days 1–5
3 courses of BEP at	Etoposide	100 mg/m^2	days 1–5
3-week intervals,	Bleomycin	20 U/m^2	each week
followed by 3 courses		then	
of VAC at 4-week	Vincristine	1.5 mg/m^2	(max 2.0 mg)
intervals	Dactinomycin	350 ug/m^2	days 1–5
	Cytoxan	150 mg/m^2	days 1–5

*Doses of myelosuppressive drugs reduced 20% for prior radiotherapy, granulocytopenic fever, or thrombocytopenic bleeding.

Source: Reproduced with permission from Williams S.D., Blessing J.A., Hatch K.D., & Homesley, H.D. (1991). Chemotherapy of advanced dysgerminoma: Trials of the GOG. *Journal of Clinical Oncology, 9*(11), 1991.

surgery and radiation therapy were used, approximating 83%. This is because dysgerminomas are highly radiosensitive, but tumors possessing mixed elements are not.[22]

In summary, dysgerminoma has the best prognosis of all the malignant germ cell tumors. Even in advanced stages or in recurrence, if adequate treatment is given, the prognosis is still very good.[24]

Endodermal Sinus Tumors

Endodermal sinus tumors (ESTs), or yolk sac tumors, account for 20% of the primitive germ cell tumors, making them the second most common.[16] They are bilateral in less than 5% of cases.[10] ESTs are highly malignant and are characterized by overgrowth of extraembryonic mesoblast associated with yolk sac endoderm. They occur in adolescents and young adult women, most under the age of 30. Cure rates with radical surgery alone versus conservative surgery alone do not differ; only an occasional five-year survivor is reported. These tumors are not radiosensitive and are very rapidly growing tumors. The most frequent presenting symptom, abdominal pain, occurs within one week prior to presentation to the physician.[12]

This tumor metastasizes early via lymphatics to regional lymph nodes and hematogenously to the lungs, liver, and other organs. Extensive intra-abdominal disease is often found at presentation. Prior to the development of chemotherapy, most patients with stage Ia disease died.[11]

These tumors are chemosensitive (80% five-year survival rate) using agents that include the triple therapy of methotrexate, dactinomycin, and chlorambucil; or cyclophosphamide, actinomycin, vincristine, and doxorubicin. Recent studies using bleomycin, vincristine, and cisplatin have begun, but difficulty in accumulating a large series makes evaluation difficult. Chemotherapy is most effective when EST can be totally resected.[24] Poor prognostic factors include tumor greater than 10 cm, liver metastasis, bone marrow metastasis, poor performance status, and presence of ascites in the amount of 100 ml or greater.[24]

Most EST patients have significantly elevated serum levels of AFP, which is of great importance in monitoring the results of treatment and ruling out recurrences. However, normal AFP does not exclude the possibility of disease, since the parietal variant of EST does not produce AFP.[1]

Embryonal Carcinoma

Embryonal carcinoma is rare in ovarian germ cell tumors but has a high incidence in testicular tumors. These tumors are unilateral and typically encapsulated, ranging in size from 10 to 25 cm in one study.[23] They occur in girls and young women between the ages of 4 and 28. Most commonly, patients present with an abdominal mass, with 50% also presenting with abdominal pain, with the duration of symptoms being about three weeks. Embryonal carcinomas can be hormonally active; 60% manifest hormonal stimulation in the form of vaginal bleeding or precocious pseudopuberty (in adolescents) or amenorrhea (in older women).[16]

Histologically, embryonal carcinoma can be distinguished from other germ cell tumors based on distinctive microscopic characteristics. It differs from choriocarcinoma by the absence of well-defined syncytiotrophoblasts and cytotrophoblasts, though isolated syncytiotrophoblastic gland cells may be present. Both endodermal sinus tumors and embryonal carcinoma have mucinous glands and the presence of AFP. BhCG levels can also be elevated in both.[3]

Treatment includes conservative surgery (USO) followed by combination chemotherapy utilizing VAC, BEP, or PVB. These tumors are radioresistant.[16]

Choriocarcinoma

Pure nongestational choriocarcinoma is one of the rarest ovarian malignancies (40 cases in the literature) and is usually found combined with other elements in malignant germ cell tumors. It is found in girls, adolescents, and young adult women.[3] The tumor is unilateral, grows rapidly, and is highly malignant, with early metastasis, especially to the lungs.

Choriocarcinoma may produce BhCG, resulting in endocrine changes in the patient manifesting as sexual precocity and irregular bleeding.[8] This syndrome is in part triggered by ovarian estrogen production induced by chorionic gonadotropin produced by the tumor. Estrogen and chorionic gonadotropin levels may be markedly elevated at the time of diagnosis, decrease when tumor is excised, and rise if the tumor recurs.[1]

Radical surgery (TAH-BSO) has no advantage over conservative surgery if the tumor is unilateral and encapsulated. If it has spread outside the ovary, TAH-BSO and omentectomy should be performed. The tumor is not sensitive to radiation or chemotherapy. Unlike its gestational counterpart (GTN), choriocarcinoma is not folic acid–dependent and must be clearly distinguished from gestational choriocarcinoma because it has a worse prognosis and thus requires more aggressive, multiagent chemotherapy.[12] The lower sensitivity to chemotherapy may be related to the presence of other germ cell elements in the tumor.[1]

Teratomas

Teratomas are neoplasms consisting of tissues that are derived from two or three embryonic layers. They are subclassified according to whether tumor elements are immature, mature, or monodermal and highly specialized.[1] Immature teratomas are rare, representing less than 1% of all ovarian teratomas. They can occur in pure form or as part of a mixed malignant germ cell tumor. This type occurs in women aged 14 to 40 years. Patients present with pelvic or abdominal mass or pain.[3] Immature teratomas are almost all unilateral but can metastasize to the contralateral ovary. They can be associated with a synchronous or metachronous mature teratoma in the opposite ovary. Grossly, these tumors are large and mostly solid but may contain cystic areas. Microscopically, they consist of a variety of mature and immature elements from all three germ cell layers, but primitive neuroepithelium is the most abundant tissue. Adequate sampling and thorough examination for areas of immaturity are essential to distinguish an immature teratoma from a mature teratoma. A correlation exists between prognosis and degree of immaturity, which is thought to reflect metastatic capability.[25]

Norris et al.[25] devised the grading system for this tumor. Mature components are classified as grade 1, are present to a lesser degree in grade 2, and may be absent in grade 3. It is imperative that grade 1 tumors be distinguished from higher grades, because grades 2 and 3 require chemotherapy, even in patients with stage I disease. In their review of 58 cases of immature teratoma, Norris et al. found that the likelihood of metastatic spread was related to the grade of the primary tumor.

Immature teratomas invade adjacent adnexal structures and seed to the peritoneum. Metastasis can occur to the retroperitoneal and para-aortic lymph nodes and to distant sites. In patients whose tumor has spread outside the ovary, the grade of the tumor metastases is more important in determining treatment and prognosis. Mature implants (Grade 0–1) do not require additional treatment.[10] Grades 2 and 3 tumors and patients with malignant ascites require chemotherapy following conservative surgery. The chemotherapy agents used include vincristine, actinomycin, and cyclophosphamide (VAC), and methotrexate, actinomycin, and cyclophosphamide (MAC).[3] Chemotherapy is most effective when disease can be completely resected. Radiation has little value in treating immature teratomas.[10]

Mature solid teratoma (grade 0) is very rare, with the few (4) reports occurring in young women. Solid teratomas must be thoroughly sampled to rule out any immature elements which may alter treatment and prognosis.[26]

Mature cystic teratomas (or dermoid cysts) are benign tumors. They are bilateral in 12% of patients and account for 95% of all ovarian teratomas. They occur most commonly in the 20- to 30-year-old age group and can occur in pregnancy. Mature elements reflecting differentiation from all three embryonic germ layers (ectoderm, endoderm, and mesoderm) are present in 66% of cases.[26] It is common to find gastrointestinal squamous epithelium, sebaceous glands, cartilage, nerve, and respiratory elements on microscopic evaluation. A true dermoid cyst, however, consists of tissue from the ectodermal layer only. Surgery to remove the tumor is sufficient treatment for this benign tumor.[3]

Occasionally an overgrowth of thyroid tissue in a teratoma occurs, resulting in a struma ovarii.[1] To be designated a struma ovarii, thyroid tissue must be the major or sole component of the dermoid. Ten percent of the patients manifest thyrotoxicosis. Only a few of these tumors are malignant.[1]

Any of the constituents of a dermoid cyst has the potential to undergo benign or malignant changes, forming a tumor within a tumor. This occurs in 1 to 2% of cases and is usually confined to one ovary.[1] Tumors arising from dermoid cysts include squamous cell carcinomas, basal cell carcinomas, sebaceous tumors, malignant melanoma, adenocarcinoma, sarcoma, and neuroectodermal tumors.[8] Patients with squamous carcinomas have a better survival rate than patients with other forms.[1]

Mixed Germ Cell Tumors

Malignant mixed germ cell tumors contain at least two malignant elements. Kurman and Norris[23] found in a series of thirty patients that dysgerminoma was the most common constituent (80%), then endodermal sinus tumor (70%), immature teratoma (53%), choriocarcinoma (20%), and embryonal carcinoma (16%). Dysgerminoma and endodermal sinus tumor was the most frequent combination. Age for mixed types ranged between 5 and 33 years, and they caused abdominal pain, fever, vaginal bleeding, and precocious puberty in four out of twelve prepubertal patients. The composition and size of the tumor were the most important prognostic factors. The prognosis was poor if the tumor consisted of more than one-third of endodermal sinus tumor, choriocarcinoma, or grade 3 immature teratoma. But in patients with tumors less than 10 cm in diameter, all survived regardless of tumor composition. Overall survival of stage I tumor patients was 50%.[3]

Following resection of all tumors, patients receive postoperative chemotherapy. The regimen of VAC and PVB has been used most frequently. BEP is also being utilized.[10]

Gonadoblastoma

Gonadoblastoma is a rare tumor with a mixture of sex cord and germ cell elements first described in 1953 by Scully.[27] Because it had been reported previously in intersexual patients, it used to be called *dysgenetic gonadoma*. Gonadoblastoma is found exclusively in patients with androgen-insensitive tumors (testicular feminizing syndrome), Turner syndrome, pure gonadal dysgenesis, mixed gonadal dysgenesis, or hermaphroditism. This tumor occurs in young patients but most commonly in patients in their twenties. The tumor is bilateral in 33% of cases.[1]

Gonadoblastoma is the most common malignancy occurring in dysgenetic gonads and arises almost exclusively in them. Eighty percent are phenotypically female who are virilized, and 20% are phenotypic males with cryptorchidism, hypospadias, and female internal secondary sex organs. The most common karyotypes are 46, XY and 45 XO/46, XY (mosaic). Ninety percent of all patients have a Y chromosome. Patients present most often with primary amenorrhea, virilization, or developmental abnormalities of the genitalia. Patients may also present with gonadal tumors.[9]

Half of gonadoblastomas are associated with dysgerminomas, and another 10% are associated with other malignant germ cell tumors, including embryonal carcinoma, endodermal sinus tumors, teratoma, and choriocarcinoma.[1]

The malignant potential of gonadoblastoma has not been established. Aggressiveness may depend on the germ cell components present. Because these patients often reveal eunuchoidal features, sterility, or signs of Turner syndrome, and because the tumor may have a potential for malignancy, removal of both gonads is indicated.[27]

Ovarian Stromal Tumors

Ovarian stromal tumors are derived from primitive sex cords and gonadal stroma. They contain collagen-producing stromal cells as well as theca cells, granulosa cells, Sertoli cells, and Leydig cells in various stages of differentiation.[3] They account for only about 6% of all ovarian tumors, but they are the most common hormonally active ones.[28] Some gonadal stromal tumors have the potential to produce either an estrogenizing or a masculinizing effect. Although rare, they are of special interest because of their distinct histologic features and production of estrogens, androgens, progestins, and certain corticosteroids. These tumors most often affect children and young women.[27]

A clear understanding of these tumors is hampered by their rarity, indolent behavior, and tendency to recur after several years.[28] Early stage disease is treated with surgery alone, but some patients will develop recurrence and require additional treatment. However, the role of adjuvant chemotherapy or radiation is not well defined.[3] Patients with stage Ia do not require additional therapy unless rupture of the tumor occurs or a germ cell component is found in the pathology.[1] Tumor rupture results in significantly worse prognosis than tumors that are removed intact.[28] Radiation therapy has also been used in the past in this situation, but there are no clear guidelines for selecting patients with early stage disease who might benefit from adjuvant therapy.

For patients with advanced disease (primary or recurrent), there is no unequivocal recommendation for treatment. Radiation therapy, single-agent chemotherapy, and combination chemotherapy have all been reported, with varying degrees of success.[11] Postoperative chemotherapy is still controversial because of the small number of patients in any given report. Regimens that have been used include VAC, PVB, and BEP. There is little evidence for adjuvant radiation therapy, but it has been used in stromal tumors with small volume residual disease.[28]

Gonadal stromal tumors can be divided into (1) the female cell types, granulosa or granulosa-thecoma; (2) the male cell types, Sertoli-Leydig cell (arrhenoblastoma), Sertoli, and Leydig cell tumors; and (3) mixed cell type, gynandroblastoma.[1] These tumors are neither as common nor as malignant as germ cell tumors.

Granulosa Cell Tumors

Granulosa cells in the normal ovary are concerned primarily with the production and secretion of progesterone after ovulation has occurred.[3] Therefore categorization of granulosa cell tumors as a female cell type is no surprise. These tumors can also be found in combination with theca cell tumors.[29]

Granulosa cell tumors occur most frequently in women between the ages of 60 and 74. Only 5% appear in children before the age of 12; these are associated with iso-sexual pseudoprecocity caused by the estrogen secretion from the tumor.[28] The tumors have the capacity to produce estrogen from androstenedione, dehydroepiandrosterone, progesterone, and testosterone.[1] Endometrial hyperplasia has been frequently reported in association with granulosa cell tumors because of stimulation of the unopposed estrogen secreted by the tumor. As many as 13% of these patients will develop well-differentiated adenocarcinoma of the endometrium.[30] Other symptoms associated with the unopposed estrogen of granulosa tumors include breast swelling, tenderness, and pain. Increased incidence of infertility with granulosa cell tumors has not been reported, but Ohel et al.[31] report a fourfold increased incidence of breast cancer in Israeli patients.

The most common presenting symptoms of granulosa cell tumors are abnormal uterine bleeding and pain. In premenopausal women, amenorrhea may occur. Postmenopausal women may present with vaginal bleeding as well as symptoms that mimic epithelial ovarian cancer, such as vague abdominal complaints, increasing abdominal girth, and weight loss.[21]

In the juvenile variant of granulosa cell tumors, the patients are prepubertal. Approximately 90% of granulosa cell tumors found in prepubertal patients and women under age 30 are juvenile granulosa cell tumors. Microscopic features of this tumor distinguish it from the adult granulosa cell tumor.[31]

Granulosa cell tumors are unilateral in 95% of cases. Young et al.[32] reviewed a series of 124 patients and found that 121 had stage I disease and three had stage II. Rupture of the tumor has been reported in between 10 and 35% of cases. Torsion can produce acute abdominal pain, but even huge hemorrhagic tumors can be relatively asymptomatic.[28] If these tumors spread, it is by local, direct extension and intraperitoneal seeding. They rarely spread hematogenously or lymphatically.[28] Histologic grade and mitotic index are important prognostic factors.[30]

The tumor has a good prognosis, with malignancy rate of 25% in adults but only 3 to 6% in children. Recurrences are usually local; distant metastases are rare. Recurrences may take many years to appear but can happen at any time. These tumors are the most classic late-recurring malignancies in gyn-oncology,[28] ranging to more than five years, with the longest reported recurrence being thirty-three years. Schwartz and Smith[28] reported recurrences within three years in fourteen out of nineteen patients in their series, however.

Treatment for unilateral, encapsulated tumor is a unilateral oophorectomy with wedge resection of the opposite ovary if fertility is a concern. In the older patient who no longer desires childbearing or in advanced disease, a TAH-BSO should be performed. Use of adjuvant radiation therapy or chemotherapy is left to the discretion of the treating physician. These tumors are sensitive to radiation therapy as well as to multiple-agent chemotherapy.[1]

It is imperative that children with granulosa cell tumors be followed for life. A premenarchal child may show a vaginal cytology that reveals estrogen stimulation, which in turn may indicate recurrence. After childbearing, the remaining ovary should be removed.[1]

Theca Cell Tumors

Theca cell tumors, or theca-fibromas, constitute 1% of all ovarian tumors. Most are benign, and 66% occur in postmenopausal women. These tumors occur in association with granulosa cell tumors in 25% of cases and have similar presenting signs and symptoms because of their estrogen secretion.[1]

Benign thecomas are treated with surgery alone. Malignant thecomas are surgically staged and patients receive postoperative chemotherapy.[13]

Sertoli-Leydig Cell Tumors

Sertoli-Leydig cell tumors, or androblastomas, are rare sex cord–stromal tumors of the ovary, containing cells that are similar to Sertoli cells, Leydig cells, and indifferent stromal cells of the testes in cytological features and growth pattern.[13] The old name, arrhenoblastoma, has been replaced with the name of Sertoli-Leydig because the older term connotated masculinization, which is not a constant feature of this tumor. Many tumors are indeed associated with virilization, but some are inactive and others are estrogenic. If the predominant functioning cells of the tumor are Sertoli, the tumor may have a feminizing effect[1] and can be associated with isosexual precocity, menometrorrhagia, or postmenopausal bleeding. If Leydig cells predominate, the patient is first defeminized (e.g., breast atrophy, loss of female contours, amenorrhea) and then masculinized (e.g., hirsutism, clitoral hypertrophy, voice changes). The cause of these changes is androgens suppressing normal ovarian function, with resultant high levels of testosterone mediating masculinization. Defeminization and virilization occur in 70% of all differentiated Sertoli-Leydig cell tumors and 90% of less well-differentiated tumors.[1]

Sertoli-Leydig tumors affect women of childbearing age and are rare in children. The tumor is bilateral in only 5% of the cases and almost always has a benign course.[13] But 3 to 20% of these tumors manifest malignant behavior, as evidenced by intra-abdominal spread rather than by distant metastasis.[1]

Treatment for Sertoli-Leydig tumors involves conservative surgery. Most of the signs of masculinization regress after tumor excision; however, patients may be left with permanent hirsutism and voice changes. These tumors have a history of late recurrence, so the question of removal of reproductive organs after a patient has completed childbearing has been debated, with no definitive recommendation at this time.[12]

Gynandroblastoma

Gynandroblastoma (mixed type tumor) is extremely rare. It contains substantial elements of both granulosa-stromal and Sertoli-Leydig cell tumors. It is common for stromal tumors to have cells that are normally associated with gonads of the opposite sex.[28] Thus granulosa-stromal cell tumors may have Sertoli-Leydig cell elements and vice versa. To be categorized as a gynandoblastoma, the tumor must have at least 10% of the minor element. The presence of both male and female elements in the same tumor suggests a common origin of these tumors.[1] There are no reports of children having this type.

Unclassified Sex Cord–Stromal Tumors

Approximately 5 to 10% of sex cord–stromal tumors cannot be classified as either Sertoli-Leydig or granulosa cell because of features that are suggestive but not characteristic of either tumor. That is, the cells are not differentiated clearly into male or female elements. These tumors are usually poorly differentiated overall. They are also presumed to be more malignant than granulosa or Sertoli-Leydig tumors.[1]

✠ SALVAGE THERAPY

Little information can be found in the literature regarding salvage therapy for patients with malignant ovarian germ cell tumors with persistent, progressive, or recurrent tumor after primary chemotherapy.[9,10] Failures of the PVB regimen have been reported to have successful salvage with regimens consisting of etoposide and cisplatin or VAC.[11,33,34] Other drug regimens used include EMA-CO (etoposide, methotrexate, dactinomycin, cyclophosamide, and vincristine); etoposide, doxorubicin, and cyclophosphamide; and vincristine, dactinomycin, and ifosfamide.[10]

For patients whose first-line treatment containing cisplatin has failed, it is important to distinguish between platinum-resistant and platinum-sensitive tumors. Platinum resistance is defined as occurring in patients who have progressive disease while on therapy or within six to eight weeks of stopping it. Platinum-sensitive tumors recur more than six to eight weeks after first-line therapy has been discontinued. For patients who are platinum sensitive, a salvage regimen utilizing cisplatin, ifosfamide, and vinblastine or etoposide is the most popular regimen.[35,36,37] Complete response rates range between 25 and 36% to chemotherapy alone or to chemotherapy followed by surgical resection.

For platinum-resistant tumors, phase II drugs or high-dose chemotherapy with autologous bone marrow stem cell rescue are being investigated. In a research trial of thirty-three patients, 21% (7) died of complications related to treatment, 44% (14) had an objective response, and only 12% (4) sustained complete remission.[38]

In another study, twenty-nine patients refractory to cisplatin underwent high-dose chemotherapy with carboplatin and etoposide with or without cyclophosphamide, plus autologous bone marrow stem cell rescue. Fifty-two percent had complete response, with 34% disease-free at the time of the report. One patient died from treatment-related complications. This second group of patients was considered to have received the more favorable regimen because of fewer prior treatments.[39]

In recurrent stromal tumors, secondary debulking followed by combination chemotherapy is recommended. Radiation has been used for isolated metastases, and prolonged survival has been associated with smaller fields of intense radiation. Stromal tumors can be hormonally active, but experience using hormone therapy for recurrent disease is limited. The management of these patients with persistent or recurrent disease after primary treatment is a complicated issue, and clinical trials are ongoing.[28]

LONG-TERM FOLLOW-UP

For patients with both malignant germ cell and ovarian stromal tumors, long-term follow-up includes physical and pelvic exams and monitoring serum tumor markers, if appropriate, every three months for the first two years. The interval may then increase at the discretion of the physician.[1] In the cases that involve conservative surgery, patients are encouraged to have the remaining female organs surgically removed when childbearing has been completed.[1] For malignant germ cell tumors in younger patients, long-term follow-up is for an indefinite period of time. Because stromal tumors are so indolent and can recur many years later, these patients must also be followed for an indefinite period of time.[3]

Late Effects of Treatment

Patients with malignant germ cell tumors no longer have a dismal prognosis, because of the evolution of effective chemotherapy. Consequently, attention can now turn to the long-term effects of surgery, radiation, and chemotherapy. There is little information on this subject in the gynecologic oncology literature. Most of the available information has been extrapolated from testicular cancer research. In addition, the long-term psychological effects of living with a diagnosis of cancer, the anxiety associated with the possibility of recurrence, loss of fertility, and impact on sexuality and/or body image are even more difficult to quantify.

Late Effects of Surgery

Patients with malignant germ cell tumors all undergo at least one surgical procedure, if not more. There have been reports in the literature on the possible negative effect on fertility from pelvic surgery as a result of peritoneal and tubal adhesions, even in the case of conservative surgery to preserve fertility.[40] Another obvious cause of loss of fertility is the unnecessary removal of a normal ovary and/or uterus, which is performed by inexperienced surgeons who are unfamiliar with the natural history of these tumors.[12] As more knowledge is gained and disseminated, this practice should decrease. Surgical colleagues are becoming more educated concerning the concepts of conservative surgery, avoidance of unnecessary operative procedures (e.g., biopsy of a normal contralateral ovary), and the practice of meticulous surgical technique to decrease adhesion formation. The success of chemotherapy in these diseases makes fertility-preserving surgery a realistic option.[11]

Late Effects of Radiation Therapy

The literature regarding the long-term effects of radiation therapy has been obtained from long-term survivors of childhood cancers, Hodgkin's disease, and non-Hodgkin's lymphoma.[41] Common side effects from abdominal/pelvic irradiation include bladder irritation resulting in cystitis, bleeding, susceptibility to infection, changes in bladder tone affecting volume capacity, and vesicovaginal fistula; and bowel mucosa changes resulting in abdominal cramping, diarrhea, sensitivity to high-fiber foods, adhesions leading to bowel obstruction, radiation enteritis, and rectovaginal fistula.[42] Most early reactions are transient and easily managed with conservative measures. Delayed complications that involve the GI and GU systems generally occur six to twenty-four months after completion of irradiation. These sequelae may vary from mild symptoms with minimal mucosal changes or mucous discharge and bleeding, to necrosis and ulceration or stenosis, perforation, and fistula that require surgery. In an MD Anderson study, there was no significant difference between patients who received radiation and age-matched controls in the area of bladder function, but there was a slight increase in bowel problems and sexual dysfunction (dyspareunia) and a major increase in fertility problems.[41] No mention of lower-extremity edema or circulation problems appears in the literature, although these have been seen in clinical practice. It was concluded by Mitchell et al.[41] that radiation therapy is well tolerated in terms of minimal late effects, but it has a significant impact on fertility.

Ovarian malfunction has been well documented in the literature. Ovarian transposition (moving the ovaries out of the radiation field) done at the time of the first surgery or ovarian shielding techniques may decrease the dose of radiation patients receive.[10] However, scatter radiation may still cause ovarian failure.[1] As chemotherapy replaces radiation therapy for dysgerminomas, though, the long-term effects of radiation will become less of an issue.

Late Effects of Chemotherapy

Acute effects of chemotherapy include anemia, thrombocytopenia, and myelosuppression, which may persist months after completion of the therapy. But this delay in the return of marrow function to normal does not imply that the patient will experience any long-term hematopoietic effects. However, if the patient requires further treatment with marrow-toxic drugs, it is likely that the marrow reserve will be limited.

Many other reports are available on the long-term effects of chemotherapy. The most serious toxicity is the development of a second malignancy, especially in cases of long-term use of alkylating agents, as in Hodgkin's disease and testicular cancer.[13] Several studies have demonstrated an increased risk of developing nonlymphocytic leukemia.[43,44] A number of studies on the use of PVB in testicular cancer also demonstrate increased risk of leukemia development.[45] With chemotherapy regimens changing to fewer courses, however, the chronic side effect of developing acute leukemia should decrease.[12]

Gonadal function also has been shown to be affected by chemotherapy. But although ovarian dysfunction or failure can occur, most long-term survivors can expect a return of normal menstruation and reproductive function. Long duration of therapy, greater cumulative dose, and older age at the initiation of chemotherapy appear to have an adverse effect on future gonadal function. Successful pregnancies in patients with malignant ovarian germ cell tumors are documented in the literature,[12,46] with no major birth defects.[47]

Pulmonary toxicity, as a result of bleomycin, can manifest as subacute or chronic interstitial pneumonitis. This inflammatory process can progress to a fibrotic stage, with consequent significant impairment of pulmonary function. Studies are being conducted to evaluate the possibility of discontinuing bleomycin from the BEP regimen.

Other reports on chemotherapy's long-term effects are obtained from the testicular cancer literature. Patients treated with PVB may experience high-tone hearing loss, neurotoxicities, Raynaud's disease, ischemic heart disease, hypertension, and renal dysfunction.[42] As more patients with ovarian germ cell tumors survive, they too may encounter these toxicities.

✳ NURSING MANAGEMENT

Women with nonepithelial ovarian cancer require nursing intervention during all stages of their disease, from diagnosis and surgery, to adjuvant chemotherapy and/or radiotherapy, to long-term follow-up. Although the illness can affect postmenopausal women, most patients are young adults, whose physical and psychological needs can differ from those of older patients. Nurses must have knowledge about nonepithelial ovarian cancers, their treatment, and the management of acute and long-term effects. Nurses must also serve as patient advocate, counselor, and teacher. Patient education is crucial in this population, to relieve fears and concerns and ensure understanding of the rationale for treatment. Emotional support and counseling are imperative to address the issues of living with a diagnosis of cancer, compliance with treatment, sexuality, and fertility.

Preoperative teaching includes the basic principles of the anatomy and physiology of the female reproductive system, details regarding the extent of surgery, and assurance of quality care to relieve any symptoms after surgery. Postoperative care includes all the standard nursing care for any patient undergoing abdominopelvic surgery. In addition, the nurse must continue to be sensitive to the needs of the younger patient, recognizing that this may be the first surgery or major illness she has experienced. The potentially significant impact surgery has on the patient's body image and self-concept must be considered. Emotional support is needed to assure the patient that she is still

TABLE 7.4

Diagnostic Cluster

Diagnostic/Preoperative and Postoperative Periods

COLLABORATIVE PROBLEMS
Potential Complication: Bleeding/hemorrhage
Potential Complication: Thromboembolic event
Potential Complication: Infection/sepsis
Potential Complication: Fluid/electrolyte imbalance
Potential Complication: Atelectasis/pneumonia
Potential Complication: Bowel dysfunction
Potential Complication: Urinary dysfunction

NURSING DIAGNOSIS
1. Potential altered health maintenance related to insufficient knowledge of condition, diagnostic tests, prognosis, and treatment options
2. Decisional conflict related to insufficient knowledge of treatment options
3. Anxiety/fear related to impending surgery and insufficient knowledge of preoperative routines, intraoperative activities, and postoperative self-care activities
4. Anxiety/fear related to insufficient knowledge of potential impact of condition and treatment on reproductive organs and sexuality
5. Grieving related to potential loss of fertility and perceived effects on lifestyle
6. Potential altered respiratory function related to immobility secondary to imposed bed rest and pain
7. Potential fluid volume deficit related to losses secondary to surgical wound or gastrointestinal dysfunction
8. Altered comfort related to effects of surgery, disease process, and immobility
9. Potential for infection related to susceptibility to bacteria secondary to wound, invasive vascular access, and/or urinary catheter
10. Potential altered nutrition: less than body requirements related to disease process, wound healing, and decreased caloric intake
11. Impaired physical mobility related to surgical interruption of body structures, incisional site pain, and activity restriction
12. Potential bowel dysfunction related to decreased peristalsis secondary to surgical manipulation of bowel, effects of anesthesia and analgesia, and immobility
13. Potential urinary dysfunction related to loss of sensation of bladder distention secondary to surgical and/or pharmaceutical interventions
14. Potential impaired skin integrity related to surgical wound, decreased tissue perfusion, ostomy stomas, drain sites, and/or immobility
15a. Potential sexual dysfunction related to disease process, surgical intervention, fatigue, and/or pain

TABLE 7.4 *(continued)*

15b. Potential moderate or possible permanent alterations in sexual activity related to disease process, surgical intervention, fatigue, and/or pain

15c. Severe or permanent inability to engage in genital intercourse

16. Alteration in coping related to infertility

17. Potential altered health maintenance related to insufficient knowledge of dietary restrictions, medications, activity restrictions, self-care activities, symptoms of complications, follow-up visits, and community resources

---

Treatment Period

COLLABORATIVE PROBLEMS
Potential Complication: Preexisting medical conditions
Potential Complication: Fluid/electrolyte imbalance

NURSING DIAGNOSIS
1. Anxiety/fear related to loss of feelings of control of life, unpredictability of nature of disease, and uncertain future

2. Anxiety/fear related to insufficient knowledge of prescribed chemotherapy and/or radiotherapy, and necessary self-care measures

3. Potential for infection related to immunosuppression neutropenia secondary to chemotherapy and/or radiation therapy

4. Potential for bleeding related to immunosuppression thrombocytopenia secondary to chemotherapy and/or radiation therapy

5. Potential alteration in skin integrity related to treatment modality and/or disease process

a woman. The nurse should also allow patients time to express fears and concerns. A referral for counseling or a support group may be necessary.

After surgery, chemotherapy is usually indicated (see Table 7.3).[22] Because nonepithelial ovarian cancers are rare, many patients are asked to participate in clinical trials. Nursing care then focuses on clarification of the patient's involvement in the trial as well as education regarding the chemotherapy regimen, the rationale for treatment, and common acute and long-term side effects. Being in a clinical trial can be anxiety-provoking to a patient; she will need to be assured that her treatment is within ethical guidelines.

Patient and family teaching related to chemotherapy includes information regarding the treatment regimen, potential side effects of the chemotherapeutic agents, and the necessity of laboratory tests. Close monitoring during therapy by the nurse and medical team should include encouraging the patient and her family to ask questions and report side effects. A detailed calendar may demonstrate to the patient that the treatment is time-limited and that other important activities and plans can be arranged during the same period.

After the completion of chemotherapy, the patient needs to understand the importance of short- and long-term follow-up examinations. The purpose of follow-up is to monitor the patient's improvement from acute side effects, assess for and treat long-term side effects, and assess for early signs of recurrent disease. Follow-up includes appropriate blood marker assays and radiologic exams every three months for two years, every six months for three years, and yearly thereafter.

After completing all treatment, some patients experience increased anxiety because the regularity of contact with the health care team ends. Nurses should alert patients to this potential reaction and assure them that they are free to contact the physician or nurse with questions and concerns. Sexuality and fertility, which may not have been a priority during treatment, may now be addressed. As patients begin to return to prediagnosis lifestyles, questions may arise regarding these issues. Nurses must communicate openly by asking questions about sexual health, even if the patient does not initiate the discussion. A trusting and caring relationship between patient and nurse is paramount for providing a level of comfort and assurance that these topics may be discussed when the patient is ready. Fertility options should be discussed, and a referral to a reproductive endocrinologist may be indicated to monitor hormone replacement therapy and discuss fertility further. If a patient has become infertile, grief reactions and anger may occur. Counseling services should be made available if necessary.

Changes in self-concept and body image and issues related to being a cancer survivor may take place. Referrals for psychological support or posttreatment support groups can be made. In addition, some patients welcome the opportunity to serve as a resource to other patients who may be newly diagnosed. Nurses should encourage this; it usually is a positive experience.

✖ SUMMARY

The most important issues to most women with nonepithelial ovarian cancer are body image changes and preservation of fertility. It is important to discuss these issues with patients to help decrease anxiety and provide realistic expectations. These young women may have less familiarity with gynecologic care than older women and may thus need to be educated on the basic anatomy and physiology of the female reproductive system.

As the treatment of cancer may be a prolonged and emotionally taxing experience, the nurse must include significant family and friends in patient-teaching sessions and in the development of individualized nursing care plans. Nursing care focuses on diminishing knowledge deficits and helping patients and their families cope with the physical, psychosocial, and spiritual effects of cancer therapy.

※ REFERENCES

1. Barber, H.K. (1993). *Ovarian Carcinoma: Etiology, Diagnosis and Treatment.* New York: Masson.
2. Langman, J., & Sadlier, T.W. (1985). Urogenital system. *Langman's Medical Embryology* 5th ed. Baltimore: Williams & Wilkins.
3. Slayton, R.E. (1984). Management of germ cell and stromal tumors of the ovary. *Semin Oncol, 11*(3), 299–312.
4. Rana, M.W. (1984). *Key Facts in Embryology.* New York: Churchill Livingstone.
5. Guyton, A. (1991). *Textbook of Medical Physiology.* Philadelphia: Saunders.
6. Tortora, G., & Anagnostakos, N.P. (1987). *Principles of Anatomy and Physiology.* New York: Harper & Row.
7. Teilum, G. (1948). Tumors of germinal origin. *Ovarian Cancer: International Union Against Cancer Monograph* vol. 2. New York: Springer Verlag.
8. Barber, H.R.K. (1988). Embryology of the gonad with reference to special tumors of the ovary and testis. *J Pediatr Surg, 23*(10), 967–972.
9. Hughesdon, P.E., & Bennett, M.H. (1986). The oocytic origin of dysgerminoma. *Int J Gynecol Pathol, 5*(1), 52–62.
10. Gershenson, D. (1993). Update on malignant ovarian germ cell tumors. *Cancer, 71*(suppl. 4), 1581–1590.
11. Thomas, G., Dembo, A.J., & Hacker, N.F. (1987). Current therapies for dysgerminomas of the ovary. *Obstet Gynecol, 70*(2), 268–275.
12. Williams, S. (1991). Treatment of germ cell tumors of the ovary. *Semin Oncol, 18*(3), 292–296.
13. Price, F.V., & Schwartz, P.E. (1993). Management of ovarian stromal tumors. *Ovarian Cancer* (pp. 405–423). New York: McGraw-Hill.
14. Lappohn, R.E., Burger, H.G., Bouma, J., et al. (1989). Inhibin as a marker for granulosa cell tumors. *N Engl J Med, 321*(12), 790–793.
15. Brenner, W.J. (1989). Inhibin: From hypothesis to clinical application. *N Engl J Med, 321*(12), 826–827.
16. Williams, S.D., Gershenson, D.M., Horowitz, C.J., & Scully, R.E. (1992). Ovarian germ cell and stromal tumors. In W.J. Hoskins, C.A. Perez, & R.C. Young, eds., *Principles and Practice in Gynecologic Oncology* (pp. 715–730). Philadelphia: Lippincott.
17. Serov, S.F., Scully, R.E., & Robin, I.H. (1973). Histological typing of ovarian tumors. *International Histological Classification of Tumors* (no. 9). Geneva: World Health Organization.
18. Gershenson, D.M., Copeland, L.J., Kavanaugh, J.J., et al. (1985). Treatment of nondysgerminomatous germ cell tumors of the ovary with vincristine, actinomycin-D, and cyclophosphamide. *Cancer, 56*(12), 2756–2761.
19. Slayton, R.E., Park, R.C., Silverberg, S.G., Shingleton, H., & Creasman, W.T. (1985). Vincristine, dactinomycin, and cyclophosphamide in the treatment of malignant germ cell tumors of the ovary: A Gynecologic Oncology Group study (final report). *Cancer, 56*(2), 243–248.
20. Williams, S.D., Birch, R., Einhorn, L.H., et al. (1987). Treatment of disseminated germ cell tumors with cisplatin, bleomycin, and either vincristine or etoposide. *N Engl J Med, 316*(23), 1435–1440.
21. Williams, S.D., Blessing, J.A., Moore, D.H., Homesley, H.D., & Adcock, L. (1989). Cisplatin, vinblastine, and bleomycin in advanced recurrent ovarian germ cell tumors. *Ann Intern Med, 111*(1), 22–27.
22. Williams, S.D., Blessing, J.A., Hatch, K.D., & Homesley, H.D. (1991). Chemotherapy of advanced dysgerminoma: Trials of the Gynecologic Oncology Group. *J Clin Oncol, 9*(11), 1950–1955.
23. Kurman, R.J., & Norris, H.J. (1976). Endodermal sinus tumor of the ovary: A clinical and pathological analysis of seventy-one cases. *Cancer, 38*(6), 2404–2418.
24. DePalo, G., Zambetti, M., Pilotti, S., et al. (1992). Nondysgerminomatous tumors of the ovary treated with cisplatin, vinblastine, and bleomycin: Long term results. *Gynecol Oncol, 47*(2), 239–246.
25. Norris, H.J., Zirkin, H.J., & Benson, W.L. (1976). Immature malignant teratoma of the ovary. *Cancer, 37*(5), 2359–2372.
26. Peterson, W.F. (1956). Solid histologically benign teratomas of the ovary: A report of four cases and review of the literature. *Am J Obstet Gynecol, 72*(8), 1094–1102.
27. Scully, R.E. (1982). Special ovarian tumors and their management. *Int J Radiat Oncol Biol Phys, 8*(8), 1419–1421.
28. Schwartz, P.E., & Smith, J.P. (1976). Treatment of ovarian stromal tumors. *Am J Obstet Gynecol, 125*(3), 402–411.
29. Fox, N., Agrawal, K., & Langley, F.A. (1975). A clinicopathologic study of ninety-two cases of granulosa cell tumor of the ovary with special reference to the factors influencing prognosis. *Cancer, 35*(1), 231–241.
30. Stenwig, J.T., Hazelcamp, J.T., & Beecham, J.B (1979). Granulosa cell tumors of the ovary: A clini-

cal pathological study of 118 cases with long term follow-up. *Gynecol Oncol, 7*(2), 136.

31. Ohel, G., Kameti, H., & Shenker, J.G (1983). Granulosa cell tumors in Israel: A study of 172 cases. *Gynecol Oncol, 15*(2), 278–286.

32. Young, R.H., Dickersen, G.R., & Scully, R.E. (1984). Juvenile granulosa cell tumor of the ovary. *Am J Surg Pathol, 8*(8), 575.

33. Gershenson, D.M., Kavanaugh, J.J., Copeland, L.J., et al. (1986). Treatment of malignant nondysgerminomatous germ cell tumors of the ovary with vinblastine, bleomycin, and cisplatin. *Cancer, 57*(9), 1731–1737.

34. Gershenson, D.M., Morris, M., Cangir, A., et al. (1990). Treatment of malignant germ cell tumors of the ovary with bleomycin, etoposide, and cisplatin (BEP). *J Clin Oncol, 8*(4), 715–720.

35. Loehrer, P.J., Lauer, R., Roth, B.J., et al. (1988). Salvage therapy in recurrent germ cell cancer: Ifosfamide and cisplatin plus either vinblastine or etoposide. *Ann Intern Med, 109*(7), 540–546.

36. Loehrer, D.J., Einhorn, L.H., & Williams, S.D. (1986). VP-16 plus ifosfamide plus cisplatin as salvage therapy in refractory germ cell cancer. *J Clin Oncol, 4*(4), 528–536.

37. Motzer, R.J., Cooper, K., Geller, N.L., et al. (1990). The role of ifosfamide plus cisplatin-based chemotherapy as salvage therapy for patients with refractory germ cell tumors. *Cancer, 66*(12), 2476–2481.

38. Nichols, C.R., Tricot, G., Williams, S.D., et al. (1989). Dose-intensive chemotherapy in refractory germ cell cancer: A phase I/II trial of high dose carboplatin and etoposide with autologous bone marrow transplantation. *J Clin Oncol, 7*(7), 932–939.

39. Motzer, R.J., Gulati, S.C., Crown, J.P., et al. (1992). High dose chemotherapy and autologous bone marrow rescue for patients with refractory germ cell tumors. *Cancer, 69*(2), 550–556.

40. Bateman, B.G., & Taylor, P.T. (1991). Reproductive consideration during abdominal surgical procedures in young women. *Surg Clin North Am, 71*(5), 1053–1065.

41. Mitchell, M.F., Gershenson, D.M., Soeters, R.P., et al. (1991). The long term effects of radiation therapy on patients with ovarian dysgerminomas. *Cancer, 67*(4), 1084–1090.

42. Rubin, S.C., Markman, M., & Nori, D. (1992). Management of late effects of treatment. *Gynecology Oncology.* Philadelphia: Lippincott.

43. Reimer, R.R., Hoover, R., Fraumeni, J.F., & Young, A.C. (1977). Acute leukemia after alkylating agent therapy of ovarian cancer. *N Engl J Med, 297*(4), 177–181.

44. Greene, M.H., Harris, E.L., Gershenson, D.M., et al. (1986). Melphalan may be a more potent leukemogen than is cyclophosphamide. *Ann Intern Med, 105*(3), 360–367.

45. Van Imhoff, G.W., Sleyfer, D., Breuning, M.H., et al. (1986). Acute nonlymphocytic leukemia five years after treatment with cisplatin, vincristine, and bleomycin for disseminated testicular cancer. *Cancer, 57*(5), 984–987.

46. Wu, P., Huang, R., Lang, J., et al. (1991). Treatment of malignant germ cell tumors with preservation of fertility: A report of twenty-eight cases. *Gynecol Oncol, 40*(2), 2–6.

47. Gershenson, D. (1988). Menstrual and reproductive function after treatment with combination chemotherapy for malignant ovarian germ cell tumors. *J Clin Oncol, 6*(2), 270–276.

CHAPTER 8

Gestational Trophoblastic Neoplasia

Linda W. Carter, RN, MSN, AOCN
Suzy Lockwood-Rayermann, RN, MSN

✻ OVERVIEW

Gestational trophoblastic neoplasia (GTN) encompasses a spectrum of diseases characterized by growth disturbances of the human trophoblast. The terms *gestational trophoblastic disease* and *gestational trophoblastic tumors* are also used to refer to GTN. There are four clinicopathologic forms: complete and partial hydatidiform moles, invasive moles, choriocarcinomas, and placental site trophoblastic tumors (PSTT). At one time the prognosis of GTN was considered poor; however, with the advent of a sensitive marker, the beta subunit human chorionic gonadotrophin (hCG), for monitoring disease and efficacious chemotherapy, most patients today can be cured.

✻ ANATOMY AND PHYSIOLOGY

Conception occurs in the uterine tube about fourteen days before a menstrual period. The sperm and ovum unite and develop to form the zygote, which moves down the uterine tube to the endometrial cavity in three to five days and implants itself in the endometrium in another one to two days. The conceptus divides during this journey and, by the time of implantation, forms the blastocyst, a single layer of cells surrounding a hollow cavity. One wall thickens to a depth of three to four cells and eventually becomes the embryo. Trophoblastic cells develop from the surface of the blastocyst and enable the cell to burrow into the endometrium between the fifth and tenth days. This maneuver facilitates implantation of the fetus and assists in establishing nutrition. On day 10, the chorion, the secretory source of hCG, forms, later developing into villi, which become part of the fetal circulation. Development usually continues to produce a normal fetus, but in some instances GTN develops (Figure 8.1).

Normal trophoblastic tissues are able to invade maternal deciduae, vessels, and myometrium.[1] In addition, normal trophoblasts continuously embolize from the endometrial sinuses into the maternal venous circulation, where the trophoblastic cells are filtered by the pulmonary circulation, but further spread by way of the systemic circulation is minuscule.[2] These functions are exaggerated in GTN.

Pathophysiology

GTN is composed of both benign and malignant diseases of the chorionic portion of the placenta. Hydatidiform mole is the benign form of GTN and consists of two distinct entities: complete hydatidiform mole and partial hydatidiform mole. Hydatidiform moles have some malignant potential, as they can cause local proliferation, myometrial invasion, and systemic metastasis.[2] Invasive mole and gestational choriocarcinoma are the malignant gestational trophoblastic neoplasias. Placental site tumors can be benign or highly malignant.[3]

There are three types of trophoblast cells: cytotrophoblast, syncytiotrophoblast, and intermediate trophoblast. Proliferation of cytotrophoblast and syncytiotrophoblast,

FIGURE 8.1. Development of the fertilized ovum and the relationship to the spectrum of gestational trophoblastic neoplasias.

Source: Cook, R., & Hager, E. (1991). Gestational trophoblastic neoplasia. In *Fundamentals of Gynecologic Oncology*. Educational Pre-symposium conducted at the Society of Gynecologic Nurse Oncologists Annual Symposium, Orlando, FL.

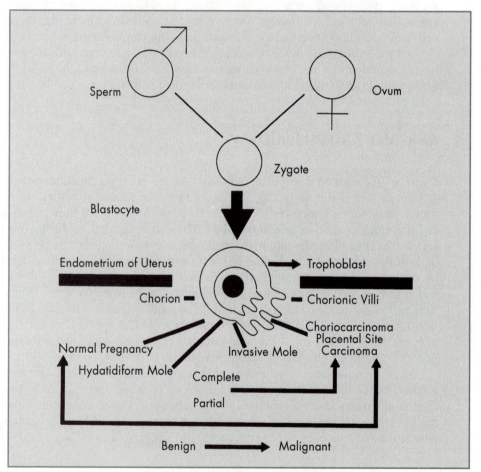

Conception occurs in the uterine tube about 14 days before a menstrual period. The sperm and ovum unite and develop to form the zygote, which moves down the uterine tube to the endometrial cavity in 3–5 days and implants itself in the endometrium in another 1–2 days. The conceptus (the products of the conception) divides during this journey and, by the time of implantation, forms the blastocyst, a single layer of cells surrounding a hollow cavity. One wall thickens to a depth of 3–4 cells and eventually becomes the embryo. Trophoblastic cells develop from the surface of the blastocyst and enable the cell to burrow into the endometrium between the 5th and 10th days. This maneuver facilitates implantation of the fetus and assists in establishing nutrition. On day 10, the chorion, the secretory source of beta human gonadotrophic hormone (beta hCG), forms and later develops into villi, which become part of the fetal circulation. Development usually continues to produce a normal fetus, but in some instances gestational trophoblastic neoplasia.

which secrete hCG, occurs in complete and partial hydatidiform mole, invasive mole, and choriocarcinoma. The placental site tumor is derived from intermediate cytotrophoblast cells, which secrete human placental lactogen (hPL) and low levels of hCG.[4]

The morphologic features of complete hydatidiform mole are generalized edema of the chorionic villi, widespread hyperplasia of cytotrophoblast and syncytiotrophoblast elements, and absence of an embryo or fetus;[5] the embryo dies within three to five weeks of development. The complete mole has been known, on very rare occasions, to occur as a partner in a twin pregnancy.[6]

The partial hydatidiform mole, in contrast, is characterized by the presence of a fetus. However, it usually has chromosomal abnormalities with growth retardation characteristic of triploidy (69 chromosomes), and usually dies during the first trimester. The fetus rarely survives into the second semester and only exceptionally reaches term.[6] The placenta is characterized by focal villous edema, trophoblastic hyperplasia usually involving the syncytium, and villous scalloping with trophoblastic inclusions.

Invasive mole is a hydatidiform mole that has extended into the myometrium. Histologically, invasive mole is characterized by edema of the villi and proliferative trophoblasts invading the myometrium or venous system. Invasive mole is seldom diagnosed histologically because most patients are treated without excising the uterus.

Choriocarcinoma, a highly malignant tumor, arises from the trophoblast of any type of gestation and shows a biphasic proliferation of cytotrophoblast and syncytiotrophoblast.[7] The most diagnostic cell of choriocarcinoma is syncytiotrophoblast. Chorionic villi are not a component of this type of GTN. PSTT can be distinguished from choriocarcinoma, as the former is composed of intermediate trophoblast and the latter, a biphasic proliferation. Again, villi are typically not present.

Cytogenetic studies have demonstrated that 90% of complete hydatidiform moles have a 46XX (diploid) karyotype and that the molar chromosomes are entirely of paternal origin.[8] The maternal haploid component is lost by an unknown mechanism; there is fertilization of an "empty egg" by a single sperm with 23 chromosomes. This sperm then duplicates its own chromosomes, resulting in the 46 karyotype. In contrast, partial hydatidiform moles usually have a triploid karyotype (69 chromosomes). A normal egg is fertilized by two sperm, with retention of the maternal haploid set, and can carry the sex chromosome XXY, XYY, or XXX genotype. The extra haploid set of chromosomes usually is of paternal origin. Since the triploid mole also has a full set of maternal chromosomes, fetal or embryonic tissues are commonly present. The central theory of the genetic makeup of molar disease appears to be an excessive number of paternal chromosomes.[9]

✕ ETIOLOGY

There are certain risk factors associated with GTN. Many studies have documented an increased risk of hydatidiform mole for women at extreme ranges of reproductive life.[4]

Bagshawe et al. reported a 411-fold increased risk for women older than age 50 and a sixfold increased risk for women younger than 15 years, compared with the expected risk in women between the ages of 25 and 29.[10] Parazzini et al.[11] reported a paternal age–associated risk of 4.9 above the age of 45 for complete mole. They did not find a maternal or paternal age–associated risk for partial hydatidiform mole. The risk for maternal advanced age (over 40 at the time of pregnancy) is greater for choriocarcinoma than for hydatidiform mole.[12]

Prior hydatidiform mole increases the risk of GTN in subsequent pregnancies, with an approximate tenfold increase in risk reported.[12] Other risk factors suggested include nutritional factors (deficiencies of dietary fat, protein, vitamin A, and carotene), low socioeconomic status, professional occupation, history of prior abortions, marital status, ABO blood groups, contraceptive history, and mean number of months from last pregnancy to index pregnancy.[8,13] The ABO blood groups of the parents have not been found to be a risk factor for hydatidiform mole but appear to be a factor in choriocarcinoma.[12] Risk factors for PSTT are not yet defined because of the small number of cases reported. In general, women of reproductive age are at risk, although several cases in women over the age of 50 have been reported.[7]

Incidence

In the United States, the incidence of hydatidiform mole is approximately 1 in 1,000 to 2,000 pregnancies and 1 in 600 therapeutic abortions.[4] The incidence of hydatidiform mole varies worldwide, with the lowest incidence in the developed countries of the Western world and the highest incidence in Asian countries.[14] In the Far East the incidence is reported to be 1 in 120 pregnancies.[8] Similarly, the incidence of choriocarcinoma varies widely throughout the world. Choriocarcinoma occurs in 1 in 20,000 to 40,000 pregnancies in the United States and Europe.[7] In Asia, Africa, and Latin America, however, the incidence is the highest reported, approximately 1 in 500 to 1,000 pregnancies. Approximately 50% of all gestational choriocarcinomas follow hydatidiform moles, 25% follow abortions, and 25% develop after term pregnancies.[8] Invasive mole develops in 15% of patients following molar evacuation and less frequently after other types of gestations.[15] The incidence of placental site tumor is unknown, as it is a rare GTN. DiSaia and Creasman[8] noted that 55 such patients have been reported in the English literature.

❋ COLLABORATIVE MANAGEMENT

History and Physical Assessment

An accurate history, including the chief complaint, past medical and surgical history with emphasis on menstrual and obstetrical history, and review of systems is critical for the diagnosis of GTN. In addition, physical examination and diagnostic testing provide valuable information for diagnosis and management. The signs and symptoms

---

TABLE 8.1

Signs and Symptoms of Hydatidiform Mole

Signs	Excessive uterine size
	Theca lutein cysts of the ovary
	Preeclampsia in the first trimester
	Hyperemesis gravidarum
	Hyperthyroidism
	Beta-hCG greater than anticipated for gestational age
	Trophoblastic embolization
Symptoms	Vaginal bleeding
	Nausea and vomiting
	Abdominal pain
	No fetal movement
	Passage of vesicular tissue

---

of hydatidiform mole are presented in Table 8.1. Most patients with complete mole have delayed menses and a postive pregnancy test, which they equate with pregnancy. But vaginal bleeding is the most common presenting symptom in patients with complete hydatidiform mole. In fact, bleeding occurs in 97% of the cases and may produce anemia (hemoglobin <10 g/100 ml).[15] The bleeding usually occurs during the first trimester and may range from dark brown to bright red. It is caused by the separation of molar tissue from the uterine wall, which exposes the maternal vascular channels. Molar vesicles, which are grapelike in appearance, may be passed along with blood clots. Nausea and vomiting can also occur; these are often confused with the symptoms of a normal pregnancy. Hyperemesis gravidarum occurs in approximately 25% of patients with complete mole and may require antiemetics or intravenous therapy.[4] Other common presenting symptoms are a lack of fetal movement and passage of vesicular tissue.

About 50% of patients with complete mole have a larger than expected uterine size relative to gestational age, although approximately one-third of patients have a uterine size smaller than gestational age.[8] The endometrial cavity may be enlarged secondary to blood and chorionic tissue. The uterus may feel doughy on palpation as a result of the vesicles. First trimester preeclampsia occurs in approximately 27% of patients with complete mole.[8] Proteinuria, hypertension, and hyperreflexia may be common, but convulsions rarely occur. Excessive uterine size, hyperemesis, and preeclampsia occur primarily in patients with markedly elevated hCG levels.

Patients may present with clinically evident hyperthyroidism with tachycardia, fever, warm skin, tremor, and thyroid enlargement. Clinical hyperthyroidism has been reported in less than 1% to as high as 7% of patients. Hyperthyroidism in complete mole is caused by a thyrotropinlike compound produced by the molar tissue.[8] Increased levels of thyroid hormones are frequently found in asymptomatic patients with hydatidiform mole but usually return to normal after evacuation.

Unilateral or bilateral ovarian enlargement caused by theca lutein cysts develops in 25 to 33% of patients with complete hydatidiform moles, which may be related to increased hCG levels.[16] Theca lutein cysts contain amber-colored or serosanguineous fluid and are usually multilocular. These cysts may be difficult to palpate on exam because of excessive uterine size but can be detected on ultrasound. Patients with theca lutein cysts may present with symptoms of acute abdominal pain due to cystic rupture or torsion. The occurrence of such cysts may signal the potential development of malignant sequelae of trophoblastic disease. Theca lutein cysts normally regress spontaneously in two to four months following evacuation.

Patients may also present with signs and symptoms of trophoblastic embolization: chest pain, dyspnea, tachycardia, tachypnea, diffuse rales, and bilateral pulmonary infiltrates. Pulmonary trophoblastic embolization occurs in approximately 2% of patients with complete mole.[15] Signs and symptoms usually resolve within 72 hours of supportive treatment. Approximately 20% of patients with complete moles have malignant sequelae after evacuation, and 10 to 20% of these have metastatic disease.[4] Most patients with malignant sequelae have invasive or persistent mole, and approximately 25 to 33% have choriocarcinoma.[17]

Patients with partial hydatidiform mole usually do not present with the same signs and symptoms as those with complete mole. For example, they usually do not present with theca lutein cysts, hyperemesis, hyperthyroidism, toxemia, excessive uterine size, or respiratory distress. Malignant sequelae are diagnosed in less than 10% of patients and are nonmetastatic.[18] Instead, patients generally present with the signs and symptoms of missed or incomplete abortion, and the diagnosis of partial mole is made only after a thorough histopathologic evaluation of the tissue. The main presenting symptom is vaginal bleeding.

Uterine bleeding after evacuation of a hydatidiform mole is the most common symptom of invasive mole. Some patients may have bleeding from a vaginal lesion, and others may present with pleuritic pain and hemoptysis from pulmonary metastasis. Theca lutein cysts and uterine enlargement may be present. The trophoblastic tumor may perforate the myometrium, causing hemorrhage or intraperitoneal bleeding.

Abnormal uterine bleeding is also one of the most frequent presentations of choriocarcinoma. Occasionally, however, symptoms related to metastasis are the first indication of the disease. These patients may present with dyspnea, hemoptysis, pleuritic pain, and cough, as the lungs are the most frequent site for hematogenous lesions. Symptoms related to hemorrhagic events may occur. Melena or gastrointestinal hemorrhage may signify gastrointestinal involvement. Focal neurologic signs similar to brain tumor or cerebrovascular accident may indicate spinal or intracranial metastasis. Patients may present with hematuria from renal involvement or with right upper quadrant abdominal pain from liver metastasis. Choriocarcinoma can also present as delayed postpartum bleeding or can occur years later following a pregnancy, hysterectomy, or tubal ligation.[7]

Patients with PSTT may present with vaginal bleeding or amenorrhea along with uterine enlargement. Since PSTT has the potential to exhibit malignant behavior, patients may present with signs and symptoms of metastasis. Vaginal bleeding after amenorrhea for a variable period of time and uterine enlargement have been reported. The antecedent pregnancy may be normal, a spontaneous abortion, or molar. Erythrocytosis, spider angiomata, and splenomegaly have been described in association with PSTT.[19]

Diagnostic Testing

Ultrasound is a reliable and sensitive test for the diagnosis of complete hydatidiform mole. The characteristic "snow storm" pattern is present, without a normal gestational sac or fetus. Ultrasound may also contribute to the diagnosis of partial mole by noting focal cystic spaces in placental tissues.[15] A transducer that is moved over the patient's skin surface produces an ultrasound beam to the tissues and involves no radiation exposure. Patients need to be instructed to have a full bladder (usually drinking three 8-ounce cups of water or coffee $1^1/_2$ hours before the exam) prior to pelvic ultrasound, and possibly a vaginal probe may need to be used for a transvaginal exam to evaluate for theca lutein cysts.

Human chorionic gonadotropin is secreted by both normal and neoplastic trophoblastic tissue, and the amount produced correlates with the amount of trophoblastic tissue in the patient. A continued rise in hCG levels after the fourteenth week of a single pregnancy is an indicator of molar pregnancy.[14] Commonly, a combination of ultrasound and beta-subunit (B-hCG) is used to determine the presence of hydatidiform mole. The B-hCG assay is currently the most specific and reliable technique for monitoring hCG production. The hCG levels are usually lower in patients with partial moles than in those with complete moles. The diagnosis of malignant GTN is established when the patient has rising or plateaued amounts of hCG relative to its mass and produces human placental lactogen (hPL).

Once a diagnosis of hydatidiform mole is made, the patient is evaluated for her medical condition and risk status. Complete blood count and platelet count determine if there is anemia or a coagulopathy present. Thyroid function tests are performed to evaluate for the possibility of hyperthyroidism. If the patient is experiencing nausea and vomiting, serum electrolytes are obtained for evaluation of fluid and electrolyte imbalances. Urinalysis and serum renal function studies are useful for patients with toxemia. In addition, liver function tests are used to help select the anesthetic agent. A chest X-ray should be taken to evaluate for preexisting lung disease and trophoblastic embolization. The patient may need to be transfused with red blood cells for anemia or possible hemorrhage; therefore, a blood type, antibody screen, and cross match are needed.

Malignant GTN requires a thorough assessment of the extent of disease prior to initiation of treatment since it can metastasize to the lung, liver, and brain. Along with history and physical examination, the laboratory studies mentioned above are performed. In addition, a metastatic work-up, which may include chest X-ray or computed tomography (CT); CT or magnetic resonance imaging (MRI) of the head, abdomen, and pelvis; and occasionally selective angiography of abdominal-pelvic organs should be performed. CT is a radiologic study that provides cross-sectional views of soft tissue; thus, the patient may be given an oral, an intravenous, or possibly a rectal contrast agent. An allergy history is obtained prior to the scan, and the patient is questioned specifically concerning reactions to iodine, shellfish, and contrast agents. Then she is placed in a large circular chamber and asked to lie still for approximately thirty minutes to an hour. A sensation of warmth and/or slight nausea may be experienced as the contrast agent is injected.

MRI uses magnetic fields and radio waves to create images of soft tissue, muscle, fat, and internal organs.[20] Before the procedure, the patient is asked if she has any type of prosthesis such as a joint, plate, clip, pacemaker, or implanted venous access device. All metallic objects must be removed. The patient is placed in a semienclosed chamber for 30 to 60 minutes, during which time she must lie still. The MRI has been capable of detecting myometrial invasion and small foci of disease in a small number of patients.

Stage of Disease

Currently there are three principal classification systems for malignant GTN: the prognostic scoring system adopted by the World Health Organization (WHO) (Table 8.2); the International Federation of Gynecology & Obstetrics (FIGO) staging system (Table 8.3); and a clinical classification system separated into two broad categories based on risk factors (Table 8.4).

The WHO prognostic index score assigns a weighted score to each factor; the sum of the scores is used to determine the patient's risk. Patients with a score of 4 or less are considered low risk, those with a score of 5 to 7 are intermediate risk, and those with scores of 8 or greater are high risk. The total prognostic score has been shown to correlate with both prognosis and response to treatment.[21]

The original FIGO staging system was based on anatomic site involvement and did not take into account other factors that may affect disease outcome.[21] However, in 1991 FIGO revised the staging system to include two prognostic factors, which are shown in the table.

The clinical classification system most frequently used in the United States is based on risk factors.[22] There are two broad categories: nonmetastatic disease and metastatic disease. Patients with metastatic disease are further subdivided into those with low-risk disease, considered to have a good prognosis, and those with high-risk disease, considered to have a poor prognosis. Once the patient has been staged, a regimen of therapy is selected.

Nonmetastatic disease is the most common form of malignant GTN. This category includes predominantly persistent hydatidiform mole and invasive mole, with rare occurrences of choriocarcinoma. Usually, the exact histology is unknown at the time of treatment, as a tissue specimen from hysterectomy is lacking. The single most effective means of diagnosis is detection of abnormal serum hCG regression after a molar pregnancy.[23] All of the classification systems use the immediate pretherapy level of hCG to determine risk.

TABLE 8.2

World Health Organization Prognostic Score for Gestational Trophoblastic Neoplasia

Prognostic Factors	Score 0	Score 1	Score 2	Score 4
Age	≤ 39 yrs.	> 39 yrs.		
Antecedent Pregnancy	Hydatidiform mole	Abortion	Term	
Months from Last Pregnancy	4 months	4–6 mo.	7–12 mo.	12 mo.
hCG (IU/L)	< 103	10^3–10^4	10^4–10^5	> 10^5
ABO (Female × male)		O × A A × O	B AB	
Largest Tumor (cm)		3–5	> 5	
Site of Metastases		Spleen Kidney	GI Liver	Brain
Number of Metastases		1–4	4–8	> 8
Prior Chemotherapy			Single drug	2 or more drugs

Low risk: less than or equal to 4; middle risk: 5–7; high risk: greater than or equal to 8

Source: Reproduced with permission from American College of Obstetricians and Gynecologists. *Management of Gestational Trophoblastic Neoplasia* (Technical Bulletin No. 178). Washington, D.C.: ACOG, © 1993.

Following staging work-up, patients with metastatic disease are further divided into low-risk/good prognosis and high-risk/poor prognosis (Table 8.4). The duration of malignant GTN, as measured by the time from the determination of the previous pregnancy event to the initiation of treatment, reflects the potential for tumor differentiation, spontaneous mutation, and growth.[24] Significantly lower remission rates have been seen in patients with metastatic GTN with a time interval exceeding four months.[24] Progression of malignant GTN proceeds initially into the myometrium, followed by pulmonary and vaginal metastases, and later into the brain, liver, and kidney. Metastatic sites are the basis for the FIGO staging. The site of metastatic involvement has the most significant impact on survival,[4] but the type of antecedent pregnancy has two effects on prognosis. First, GTN after a nonmolar pregnancy is almost always choriocarcinoma, whereas GTN arising after hydatidiform mole is usually invasive or

TABLE 8.3

FIGO Staging System for Gestational Trophoblastic Neoplasia
(1991)

Stage	Definition
I	Disease confined to the uterus
a	Disease confined to the uterus with no risk factors
b	Disease confined to the uterus with one risk factor
c	Disease confined to the uterus with two risk factors
II	GTT extends outside of the uterus but is limited to the genital structures (adnexa, vagina, broad ligament)
a	GTT involving genital structures without risk factors
b	GTT extends outside of the uterus but limited to genital structures with one risk factor
c	GTT extends outside of the uterus but limited to the genital structures with two risk factors
III	GTT extends to the lungs with or without genital tract involvement and with no risk factors
a	GTT extends to the lungs with or without genital tract involvement and with no risk factors
b	GTT extends to the lungs with or without genital tract involvement and with one risk factor
c	GTT extends to the lungs with or without genital tract involvement and has two risk factors
IV	All other metastatic sites
a	All other metastatic sites without risk factors
b	All other metastatic sites with one risk factor
c	All other metastatic sites with two risk factors

GTT: Gestational trophoblastic tissue

Risk factors affecting staging include the following: (1) hCG > 100,000 MIU/ml; (2) duration of disease > 6 months from termination of the antecedent pregnancy. The following factors should be considered and noted in reporting: (1) prior chemotherapy for known GTT; (2) placental site tumors should be reported separately; (3) histological verification of disease is not required.

Source: Reproduced with permission from DiSaia, P.J., & Creasman, W.T. (1993). *Clinical Gynecologic Oncology 4th ed.* (p. 222). St. Louis, MO: Mosby–Year Book.

TABLE 8.4

Clinical Classification of Gestational Trophoblastic Neoplasia

Classification	Definition
I	Nonmetastatic disease: no evidence of disease outside the uterus
II	Metastatic disease: any disease outside uterus
a	Good prognosis metastatic disease 1. Short duration (last pregnancy < 4 months) 2. Low pretreatment hCG titer (<100,000 IU/24 hr or <40,000 mIU/ml) 3. No metastasis to brain or liver 4. No significant prior chemotherapy
b	Poor prognosis metastatic disease 1. Long duration (last pregnancy > 4 months) 2. High pretreatment hCG titer (>100,000 IU/24 hr or >40,000 mIU/ml) 3. Brain or liver metastasis 4. Significant prior chemotherapy 5. Term pregnancy

Source: Reproduced with permission from Hammond, C.B., Borchert, L.G., Tyrey, L., et al. (1973). Treatment of metastatic trophoblastic disease: Good prognosis and poor prognosis. *American Journal of Obstetrics & Gynecology,* 115, 451–455.

persistent mole. Second, patients with GTN from a nonmolar pregnancy often experience a delay in diagnosis until symptoms initiate further investigation. Several studies reviewed by Soper[4] have confirmed that patients with malignant GTN after a term pregnancy have a worse outcome than after other types of pregnancy. In addition, the size and number of metastatic sites have an adverse effect on outcome, increasing the risk of failure of therapy.[4] Finally, patients whose primary chemotherapy has failed are high risk and have a poor prognosis.

Metastatic GTN occurs in about 4% of patients after molar evacuation.[15] Metastasis is generally associated with choriocarcinoma but can occasionally occur with invasive mole. Choriocarcinoma usually disseminates rapidly and is widespread. The most common site of metastasis is the lung; pulmonary lesions are detected on presentation in 80% of patients with metastatic GTN.[15] Trophoblastic pulmonary involvement produces four principal radiographic changes in the lung: (1) the alveolar or "snow storm" pattern; (2) discrete, rounded densities; (3) pleural effusion; and (4) an embolic pattern due to pulmonary arterial occlusion.[15] Some patients may have minimal or no gynecologic symptoms because the reproductive organs are free of trophoblastic tissue.

Vaginal metastases are present in 30% of patients with metastatic GTN and occur in the fornices or suburethral area.[15] Trophoblastic implants are often friable, vascular, and bleed easily. Hepatic metastasis occurs in 10% of patients with metastatic GTN and may be hemorrhagic and friable. Ten percent of metastatic disease involves the brain; this may also undergo spontaneous hemorrhage. Other possible but infrequent metastatic sites are the bowel, kidney, and spleen.

Treatment and Intervention

Surgical Management

The primary management of hydatidiform mole is surgical evacuation. Suction curettage is the method of choice for evacuation of a mole in patients who desire to preserve fertility. It is usually performed under general anesthesia, but local anesthesia may be used if the uterus is small. Intravenous pitocin may be given for several hours postevacuation. For women who desire no further pregnancies and in whom sterilization is desired, a primary hysterectomy may be performed. Although hysterectomy decreases the risk of malignant sequelae, the chance of malignant GTD after hysterectomy is approximately 3 to 5%.[25] Theca lutein cysts usually regress to normal as the hCG level returns to normal. Therefore, the adnexa are not removed unless the patient is perimenopausal or there is other clinical pathology.

Complications of surgery for hydatidiform mole are infrequent (Table 8.5). Uterine perforation, during primary suction D&C or due to a defect in the uterine wall from invasive mole, occurs rarely. Although some of these patients require hysterectomy, several studies[4] have suggested that some patients with invasive mole can be treated with segmental resection and repair of the affected myometrium.

Theca lutein cysts, usually bilateral, are found in about half of the patients with hydatidiform mole. Most of these are detected before molar evacuation, but they can also develop in the first week after evacuation.[4,17] Theca lutein cysts may either rupture spontaneously or cause torsion of the ovary, requiring oophorectomy. These cysts usually disappear in approximately eight weeks, although about 30% develop a secondary enlargement with post-molar GTN.[4,17]

TABLE 8.5
Complications of Hydatidiform Mole
Uterine hemorrhage Uterine perforation Respiratory disease Hyperthyroidism with thyroid storm Ovarian torsion or rupture

Pulmonary complications occurring following evacuation of hydatidiform mole include high-output congestive heart failure and trophoblastic embolization. The former can be caused by anemia, hyperthyroidism, preeclampsia, and iatrogenic fluid overload. These complications are managed by monitoring with an arterial line and ventilatory support. A postevacuation chest X-ray is usually recommended to evaluate pulmonary complications. Patients are told to report signs and symptoms of respiratory distress: shortness of breath, chest pain, difficulty in breathing, cyanosis, or confusion.

Surgical treatment of nonmetastatic GTN has a role in selected patients. Primary hysterectomy, if the patient desires sterilization, along with adjuvant single-agent chemotherapy, may be performed as the primary treatment. The reasons for this approach are to destroy microscopic metastases that are undetected at the time of surgery and to maintain a cytotoxic level of chemotherapy in the bloodstream and tissues in case viable tumor cells are disseminated at surgery.[15] Chemotherapy can be safely administered at the time of surgery without increased risk of bleeding, sepsis, or wound complications.[15] Continued chemotherapy is mandatory until hCG levels return to normal.

A hysterectomy may be performed in those patients with drug-resistant tumor in order to achieve cure. Often an intrauterine nodule of choriocarcinoma or invasive mole is found encased in dense fibrosis, which limits tissue perfusion and thus exposure to chemotherapy.[4]

Primary and secondary hysterectomy are utilized in the treatment of metastatic low-risk GTN in selected patients. Primary hysterectomy in combination with chemotherapy has been shown to reduce the time required to induce remission and limit the number of cycles of treatment in several studies.[4] Secondary hysterectomy is performed in those patients who have a drug-resistant focus of residual disease in the uterus. Hysterectomy for high-risk metastatic disease may be used in a few selected cases, although it is not as beneficial as in patients with low-risk metastatic GTN.

Other surgical procedures for metastatic disease can be performed in highly selected patients. Removal of metastatic vaginal lesions is difficult due to their friability and potential for hemorrhage. Resection of solitary pulmonary and cerebral lesions may be more successful. A pulmonary nodule may be resected in a patient who has drug-resistant disease; several studies have reported complete, sustained remissions after thoracotomy to resect a solitary resistant metastasis.[4] Thoracotomy with pulmonary wedge resection is the surgical procedure used most often. But these patients must be carefully selected, as radiographic evidence of tumor regression may lag behind hCG level response. Infrequently, craniotomy with excision of a solitary brain metastasis is performed to remove a drug-resistant focus. However, craniotomy for cerebral hemorrhage is always necessary for decompression.

Placental site tumors can be either a locally proliferative disease or a locally invasive disease that metastasizes. These tumors are not sensitive to chemotherapy; therefore, hysterectomy is the primary treatment method.

Nonsurgical Management

Nonmetastatic Disease. Nonmetastatic GTN is diagnosed most frequently following evacuation of hydatidiform mole. Serum hCG levels fall progressively after evacuation and, if the GTN is benign, return to normal in approximately eight to twelve weeks. Following term deliveries, ectopic pregnancies, miscarriages, and elective terminations, the hCG level should be undetectable in three to six weeks. A plateau in the hCG level for three or more consecutive weeks, or a rise in the hCG level following evacuation of hydatidiform mole, supports the diagnosis of persistent GTN. A persistent hCG elevation following termination of a nonmolar pregnancy beyond three to six weeks can indicate choriocarcinoma.

Use of prophylactic chemotherapy at the time of evacuation is controversial. Several studies have reported its efficacy in reducing trophoblastic sequelae,[26,27] but the risk of post-molar GTN is not eliminated altogether. In addition, only 20% of patients with hydatidiform mole develop trophoblastic sequelae, so prophylactic chemotherapy given to all patients would expose 80% to potentially toxic therapy unnecessarily. Therefore, prophylactic chemotherapy is not routinely recommended following evacuation of hydatidiform mole. Instead, weekly hCG levels can be obtained for close monitoring of these patients.

Single-agent chemotherapy is the treatment of choice for nonmetastatic GTN in those patients who want to retain fertility (Table 8.6). Methotrexate and dactinomycin have been the principal drugs used. Results of studies reviewed by Soper et al.[4] reported overall remission rates of 90 to 100% for methotrexate and dactinomycin regimens. Several different protocols have been used for both drugs.

TABLE 8.6

Chemotherapy for Nonmetastatic and Low-Risk Metastatic GTN

Agent	Recommended Dose
Methotrexate	0.4 mg/kg IV or IM daily for 5 days every 12–14 days
Methotrexate	30 mg/m² IM weekly
Methotrexate	1 mg/kg IM on days 1, 3, 5, and 7 with folinic acid, 0.1 mg/kg IM on days 2, 4, 6, and 8 every 15–18 days. (Folinic acid is given 24 hr after each methotrexate dose.)
Dactinomycin	10–12 micrograms/kg daily for 5 days. Repeat in 14-day cycles.
Dactinomycin	1.25 mg/m² IV bolus every 14 days

Source: Adapted from Lurain, J. (1990). Chemotherapy of gestational trophoblastic neoplasia. In G. Deppe, ed., *Chemotherapy of Gynecologic Cancer* 2nd ed. (p. 279). New York: Wiley & Sons.

Methotrexate 0.4 mg/kg IM or IV daily for 5 days, with cycles repeated every 12 to 14 days depending on toxicity, has been traditionally used, with excellent cure rates reported. Other methotrexate regimens have been developed to reduce toxicity. Methotrexate 1.0 mg/kg IM on days 1, 3, 5, and 7, alternating with folinic acid 0.1 mg/kg IM on days 2, 4, 6, and 8, with cycles repeated every 7 days depending on toxicity, has been found to reduce toxicity when compared with the 5-day methotrexate regimen, according to several studies reviewed by Lurain.[28] Even though some patients failed to respond to the methotrexate and methotrexate and folinic acid regimens, alternative therapy produced remission rates of 99.7 to 100% in the review of studies.[4,28]

The Gynecologic Oncology Group (GOG) evaluated methotrexate initially given at 30 mg/m^2 IM weekly, with a progressive increase in dose to 50 mg/m^2. This regimen produced decreased toxicity and was cost-effective.[29]

Dactinomycin 10 to 12 micrograms/kg IV daily for 5 days, repeated in 14-day cycles depending on toxicity, has been used for primary therapy and as sequential therapy in patients who develop resistance or excessive toxicity to methotrexate regimens. This regimen can produce alopecia and more gastrointestinal toxicity, and has the potential for extravasation. Several researchers have also studied the pulse administration of dactinomycin 1.25 mg/m^2 administered every 2 weeks. In comparison to the 5-day regimen, pulse dactinomycin is reported to have similar or lower toxicity and primary remission rates of 80 to 100%.[4] Overall, although dactinomycin has acceptable remission rates and is cost-effective, it has a higher toxicity profile, so it is frequently used for salvage therapy in those patients in whom first-line methotrexate fails. If patients have abnormal liver or renal function, methotrexate is not used, in which case dactinomycin is the drug of choice. Smith[30] has advocated the use of alternating courses of dactinomycin and methotrexate, since the two drugs have different mechanisms of action and slightly different toxicity profiles.

The most common side effects of these drugs are anorexia, nausea and vomiting, stomatitis, diarrhea, bone marrow depression, alopecia, skin rash, and hepatic dysfunction. Close monitoring of toxicity is critical, as is adherence to the treatment regimen.

Chemotherapy is continued until hCG levels have returned to normal, and one additional course is given thereafter. Patients whose hCG levels have plateaued or are rising should be switched to the alternate single-agent regimen. The failure of second-line, single-agent chemotherapy or the appearance of new metastases requires combination chemotherapy.

Low-Risk Metastatic Disease.   Patients with low-risk/good-prognosis metastatic GTN can be treated with single-agent chemotherapy with methotrexate or dactinomycin, as described above and in Table 8.6. One to two courses of chemotherapy are given after the first normal hCG level. Patients who develop resistance to the first drug are then given the second drug. If resistance to both single-agent chemotherapy regimens develops, combination chemotherapy is administered. A study conducted by

Mangili, Garavaglia, Frigerio, et al. (1996) demonstrated efficacy in the administration of etoposide (VP16) as a second-line treatment in patients who are drug resistant.[31] Patients in their study were treated with 100 mg/m^2 VP16 IV for 5 consecutive days every 10 days with an average of five courses. All participants achieved remission. Essentially all patients with low-risk GTN are cured with chemotherapy whether single agent or combination.

High-Risk Metastatic Disease.   Combination chemotherapy is the treatment of choice for high-risk metastatic disease. But many patients require a multimodal approach, utilizing radiation therapy and surgery in combination with chemotherapy. Until recently methotrexate, dactinomycin, and either chlorambucil or cyclophosphamide (MAC) was the standard regimen. Bagshawe[32] formulated the EMA-CO regimen (Table 8.7), which consists of etoposide, methotrexate, dactinomycin, cyclophosphamide, and vincristine. Studies by Bower et al.[33] and Bolis et al.[34] have reported an overall response rate of 78% and 36%, respectively, to this regimen. One of its advantages is that the EMA portion can be given during a two-day hospitalization and the CO portion can be administered outpatient. The main side effects of this regimen are bone marrow depression, alopecia, stomatitis, anorexia, nausea, vomiting, diarrhea, constipation, skin rash, hemorrhagic cystitis, peripheral neuropathies, and tissue damage from extravasation.

TABLE 8.7

EMA-CO Chemotherapy*

Schedule	Agents/Doses
Course 1 (EMA)	Etoposide 100 mg/m^2 IV infusion over 30 min
Day 1	Dactinomycin 0.5 mg IV bolus
	Methotrexate 100 mg/m^2 IV bolus
	or
	Methotrexate 200 mg/m^2 IV infusion over 12 hr
Day 2	Etoposide 100 mg/m^2 IV infusion over 30 min
	Dactinomycin 0.5 mg IV bolus
	Folinic acid 15 mg IM or orally every 12 hr for 4 doses beginning 24 hr after start of methotrexate
Course 2 (CO)	Vincristine 0.8 mg/m^2 IV stat (max 2 mg)
Day 8	Cyclophosphamide 600 mg/m^2 IV infusion over 30 min

*This regimen consists of two courses. Course 1 is given on days 1 and 2. Course 2 is given on day 8. These courses can usually be given on days 1 and 2, 8, 15 and 16, 22, etc., and the intervals should not be extended without cause.

Source: Reproduced with permission from Bagshawe, K.D. (1984). Treatment of high risk choriocarcinoma. *Journal of Reproductive Medicine, 29,* 813–817.

Combination chemotherapy should be given every three weeks until the patient has at least three consecutive normal hCG levels. The additional courses of chemotherapy are given following normal hCG levels to reduce the risk of relapse.

High-risk GTN patients in whom chemotherapy has failed have a poor prognosis. But cisplatin and etoposide are also active in the treatment of resistant GTN and are used in combination with the EMA portion of EMA-CO. Another possibility is cisplatin, etoposide, and EMA-CO alternating with EMA-CE as salvage therapy (Table 8.8). Previous chemotherapy must be reviewed in order to determine possible active agents that have not yet been tried.

Placental site tumor has the potential for metastasis and an aggressive course. In contrast to GTN, this tumor appears to be insensitive to most chemotherapy. Combination chemotherapy is generally given for the treatment of metastatic disease. Although the optimal regimen has not been determined, two complete remissions have been reported in patients with metastatic PSTT who received EMA-CO.[33,34]

Radiation Therapy

If central nervous system metastases are present, whole-brain irradiation (3000 cGy in 10 fractions) is given simultaneously with combination chemotherapy. Com-

---

TABLE 8.8

EMA-CE Chemotherapy*

Schedule	Agents/Doses
Course 1 (EMA) Day 1	Etoposide 100 mg/m^2 IV infusion over 30 min Dactinomycin 0.5 mg IV bolus Methotrexate 100 mg/m^2 IV bolus or Methotrexate 200 mg/m^2 IV infusion over 12 hr
Day 2	Etoposide 100 mg/m^2 IV infusion over 30 min Dactinomycin 0.5 mg IV bolus Folinic acid 15 mg IM or orally every 12 hr for 4 doses beginning 24 hr after start of methotrexate
Course 2 (CO) Day 8	Vincristine 1.0 mg/m^2 IV bolus Cisplatin 80 mg/m^2 IV infusion

*This regimen consists of two courses. Course 1 is given on days 1 and 2. Course 2 is given on day 8. Course 1 might require an overnight hospital stay; course 2 does not. These courses usually can be given on days 1 and 2, 8, 15 and 16, 22, etc., and the intervals should not be extended without cause.

Source: Reproduced with permission from Surwit, E.A., & Childers, J. (1991). A new dose intensive multiagent chemotherapy for high-risk gestational trophoblastic disease. *Journal of Reproductive Medicine, 46,* 45–48.

plications of cerebral lesions may be cerebral edema and acute hemorrhage, with subsequent neurologic changes. Dexamethasone is usually prescribed in an attempt to reduce the swelling and associated symptomatology. In a recent review of the literature by DiSaia and Creasman,[8] 58% of patients with brain metastasis achieved a complete remission. Some researchers recommend intrathecal methotrexate for CNS lesions, along with an increase in the intravenous dose of methotrexate in the chemotherapy regimen.

Liver metastasis carries a poor prognosis, as most patients have extensive disease when they present with liver involvement. Treatment is directed at reducing the potential for hemorrhage, which is a grave problem in these highly vascular lesions. Whole-liver irradiation with 2000 cGy in combination with multiagent chemotherapy has been recommended.[35]

Monitoring during Treatment and Follow-up

Prior to each course of chemotherapy, CBC, differential, platelet count, and blood chemistries to assess liver and renal function are obtained. Weekly serum B-hCG levels are monitored to assess the response of the tumor to chemotherapy. Periodic physical examinations and chest X-rays are obtained as indicated.

Complete remission is diagnosed if three consecutive weekly hCG levels are normal and there is no clinical or radiological evidence of disease. Following remission, hCG levels are generally obtained every two weeks for approximately six weeks to three months, then monthly for the rest of the first year of remission (Table 8.9). The risk of recurrence after one year is less than 1%, but late recurrences several years after treatment have been reported.[36] Thus repeat hCG levels every six months for an indefinite period may be recommended. Physical examinations and chest X-rays may be performed at six- to twelve-month intervals, also indefinitely. Surveillance following chemotherapy varies according to institutional preferences.

Contraception should be used for at least one year, and unless contraindicated, oral contraceptives should be given. Patients may become pregnant following a one-year remission, as there appears to be no increase in congenital anomalies or complications of pregnancy and patients can expect normal reproduction in the future. When a patient becomes pregnant following GTN, however, a pelvic ultrasound is rec-

TABLE 8.9	
Follow-up Surveillance after Remission in GTN	
Serum hCG	Every 2 weeks for 6 weeks to 3 months, then every month for the first year of remission, then every 6 months indefinitely thereafter
Clinical Exam	Depends on status of each patient; may be every 3 months for 1 year, then every 6 months, then every year
Contraception	Effective contraception for at least 1 year

ommended at eight to ten weeks' gestation to assess for normal gestational development, since these patients are at increased risk for another trophoblastic event. After delivery of the neonate, the products of conception and the placenta should be sent to pathology for a histologic exam to rule out abnormal trophoblastic tissue. An hCG level should be obtained six to eight weeks following completion of the pregnancy.

✖ NURSING MANAGEMENT

Assessment

Gestational trophoblastic neoplasia is a malignancy that affects young adult women during their reproductive years. In addition, it is the direct outcome of their reproductive desires and efforts that results in this biopsychosocial crisis. Thus GTN is not only a life-threatening malignancy but a threat to the woman's psychosocial development.[37]

The woman with GTN presents a full biopsychosocial spectrum of needs: physical, psychosocial, spiritual, and educational. Each of these needs requires careful consideration and planning, both to support the patient throughout the coming months of treatment and to facilitate her personal growth throughout the cancer experience.[37,38]

Physical Considerations

Potential physical considerations of the woman with GTN include bleeding or hemorrhage, respiratory dysfunction, and life-threatening complications, as well as the management of treatment side effects. Excessive bleeding may occur as uterine contents are expelled or may be related to the method of uterine evacuation, such as a suction curettage or routine D&C. In the evacuation process, too, uterine rupture may occur, leading to intra-abdominal bleeding. Finally, bleeding may result from torsion or rupture of ovarian cysts, leaving torn blood vessels open. Hypertension or preeclampsia may further aggravate this problem.[14,39]

Nursing assessment of the woman at risk for bleeding or hemorrhage includes color and amount of vaginal discharge, pad count, and pad weight. Tachycardia, tachypnea, and hypotension should be anticipated with excessive blood loss and decreased blood volume. In addition, skin color, temperature, and moisture, as well as cognitive changes, should be noted as the available blood volume shifts to maintain vital organ function. Abdominal pain, tenderness, or rigidity should be reported immediately as possible indicators of uterine or ovarian cyst rupture.

Respiratory dysfunction suggests pulmonary metastasis or embolization due to a thrombus or villi.[14,36] In the case of metastasis, assessment findings may include dyspnea and cough, shortness of breath with exertion, activity intolerance, or diminished breath sounds with scattered rales and rhonchi on auscultation. Tachypnea and tachycardia are also likely. In the case of pulmonary emboli, sudden chest pain, respiratory distress with diaphoresis, and anxiety would also be present, as the pulmonary artery may become partially or totally occluded.[14,40]

Other life-threatening complications that may occur with GTN are sepsis, hemorrhage, cerebrovascular accident, and cardiac failure.[14,39] Vaginal hemorrhage is defined as blood loss greater than 500 cc, or the amount of one unit of blood. Blood loss that soaks more than one perineal pad per hour for longer than twelve hours could suggest hemorrhage. This rate of blood loss accompanied by a drop in systolic blood pressure greater than 10 mm of mercury soon leads to volume depletion and possibly hypovolemic shock.

The hallmark of sepsis is fever, with or without shaking chills. A fever of 100.5°F that occurs twice within a four-hour period, or a one-time fever of 101°F, suggests sepsis. Septic fever may occur postoperatively or at the chemotherapy nadir. All septic fevers should be treated as an emergency, before the signs and symptoms of shock emerge, especially in the neutropenic patient. The signs and symptoms of septic shock include hypotension; oliguria or anuria; tachycardia with weak, thready pulse; cold, clammy extremities; and changes in cognition.[41,42]

Clients experiencing a cerebrovascular accident may report dizziness, headache, or syncope at the onset; visual deficits; numbness, tingling, or weakness; motor or sensory losses; aphasia; seizures; unequal pupil size; incontinence; weakness or paralysis; and changes in proprioception.[40,43,44]

Cardiac failure may be reported as weakness, fatigue, dyspnea with rest or activity, nausea, diaphoresis, dizziness, and changes in mentation. These changes may or may not be accompanied by a sudden onset of chest pain.[40]

The side effects of chemotherapy for malignant GTN introduce new assessment needs. Methotrexate has been the long-term mainstay of chemotherapy, and more recently dactinomycin has become a useful agent. Other agents that may be used in combination therapy include cyclophosphamide, vincristine, etoposide, and doxorubicin.[8,45,46] Side effects most commonly experienced include nausea and vomiting, stomatitis, bone marrow depression, and alopecia.

Anxiety and anticipation prior to treatment may cause some women to experience nausea even before chemotherapy has been administered. In addition, the chemotherapy agent may cause nausea and vomiting during the treatment period, and some agents may have delayed effects for as long as one week. In each of these cases, the nursing assessment must determine when the nausea and vomiting occurs for each woman so as to develop appropriate interventions.[46,47,48]

Stomatitis may be a severe effect of the antimetabolite agents. This usually occurs five to seven days after administration. Early symptoms are oral dryness and burning, which then progress to painful ulcerations of the lips and oral mucosa. Ulcerations not only may interfere with routine oral hygiene but are prone to infection by opportunistic microbes that may be swallowed, causing esophagitis, or inhaled, causing pneumonia.[44]

Both nausea and vomiting and the oral pain of stomatitis may compromise nutritional and fluid intake; therefore, assessment in these areas is important. The nurse should conduct a 24-hour dietary history, including fluid intake, to determine these needs. The patient should maintain a minimum fluid intake of two liters per day to help excrete the products of cellular destruction following chemotherapy. If not eliminated, these products may contribute to anorexia and nausea. A diet high in protein and calories should also be maintained to facilitate cellular and oral tissue repair.[42]

One of the most serious consequences of chemotherapy, and thus one of the most important areas of assessment, is bone marrow depression. Assessment of the patient at risk for neutropenia should include the most common sites of infection: the skin, oral cavity, lungs, urinary tract, and perirectal area. A central line, venous access device, or peripheral intravenous site should also be assessed for signs of inflammation. It is important to remember that the neutropenic patient may not be able to mount the full inflammatory response; therefore, any pain or tenderness should be investigated.[41,42,46]

The early signs and symptoms of thrombocytopenia include small petechiae on the extremities or abdomen. However, any report of easy bruising, epistaxis, gingival oozing, or the presence of blood in urine or stool should raise the suspicion of a low platelet count until proven otherwise.[43,46]

Anemia is most commonly manifested by fatigue and generalized weakness; however, shortness of breath, chest pain, or cognitive changes may also occur. In combination, these symptoms may lead to a reduced ability to perform the normal activities of daily living and overall compromised quality of life.[46]

Psychosocial and Spiritual Considerations

In addition to physical changes, the woman diagnosed with GTN also experiences psychosocial and spiritual changes that challenge her ability to cope. These include disruption of her life-stage development, the loss of a pregnancy, and the impact of the cancer diagnosis and treatment.

The woman with GTN has many educational needs related to her malignancy and treatment, yet she is also grieving. While grief is the normal and expected response, the associated denial may be manifested through noncompliance with treatment and/or long-term follow-up requirements.[37,41]

Three stages of the reproductive life of women can be identified that have relevance here: early, primary, and late.[39] In the early reproductive stage, between 15 and 20 years of age, the young woman is dealing with both late adolescent and early adulthood issues.[49] GTN may conflict with the formation of a positive identity and self-image in the early years of the stage. In the later years, the young woman may experience conflict and adjustment difficulties related to the issues of autonomy and independence required to enter young adulthood.[49]

In the primary reproductive stage, between 21 and 35 years of age, issues center around intimate relationships such as marriage and family and/or establishing a career.[49] At this point in a woman's life, GTN may restrict the ability to develop intimate relationships or form primary bonds with a partner. Some women compensate by focusing exclusively on careers and neglecting personal relationships.

In the late reproductive stage, after 36 years of age, women normally begin to focus their energies outward, experiencing a need to guide and care for others.[49] The experience of GTN at this point may cause conflict as her focus becomes herself, her loss, and potential losses that could evolve in the coming months and years.

At any point in a woman's development, the loss of a pregnancy is a significant psychosocial issue with at least three implications that need to be assessed. First, this loss is an interruption of a normal life-cycle event—the expectation of a normal, healthy child. Second, the loss is complicated by the lack of a tangible object to mourn. A lost pregnancy may initiate grieving over the loss of hopes and dreams, but normally there is an actual "baby" to mourn. That is, the presence of a fetus helps to reconcile the loss and bring closure to the grief process.[39] These processes are more difficult when a pregnancy results in a "tumor" instead of a baby. The third implication builds on the second one. The lack of an actual baby invalidates the pregnancy. In other words, the perceived pregnancy was never a reality. Therefore, the potential mother is deprived of warm support she may have received earlier from family and friends, who also may be disappointed and shocked.

In combination, these three implications may leave the woman feeling isolated, confused, disillusioned, and grieved about herself, her role, her relationships, and her future. During this developmental and personal crisis, both the woman and her partner need sensitive, competent care to clarify misunderstandings, facilitate the grief process, and prevent long-term depression. Additional care is needed to support the couple and their relationship until they can find ways to provide comfort and support to one another again.

This process may become further complicated by the diagnosis of cancer. All women diagnosed with GTN are closely monitored in the weeks following uterine evacuation. Blood titers are conducted weekly for hCG levels to rule out malignant GTN.[8] If these titers do not subside to normal levels in the expected length of time, the diagnosis of cancer precipitates yet another interpersonal crisis for the woman. The anxiety and uncertainty around the diagnosis and prognosis bring realization of the woman's mortality into sharp focus. Some women also begin to feel that they are being punished by God for some past activities. In addition, issues of sexuality and intimate relationships, as well as of self-concept and a sense of wholeness, may emerge again.[39] In this case, even the woman who has been able to cope with the molar pregnancy and wishes to move on with her life by trying to conceive again faces yet another obstacle—cancer, which threatens her existence.

The prescribed chemotherapy necessitates adjustment of the woman's lifestyle to accommodate the required administration schedule. In addition, if she experiences the side effect of alopecia, it represents yet another insult to her body image and serves as a constant reminder of the pregnancy loss and cancer diagnosis for months to come.

Assessment of the life-stage disruptions and loss of a desired pregnancy as well as the impact of the cancer diagnosis and treatment on the individual woman provides important data for development of the plan of care. Issues commonly identified in this population include fear, anxiety, guilt, grief, sexuality concerns, spiritual distress, and body image disturbance.[39] One of the most helpful initial nursing interventions is to communicate to the woman that her thoughts and feelings are very normal in this situation.

Fear and anxiety are similar to one another; however, it is important for the nurse to understand the differences. Fear is the psychological and physical response to something tangible and known, such as fear of harm in a dangerous situation. Anxiety is the psychological and physiological response to something that is not known, such as the cancer prognosis.[40] Anxiety is similar to fear but cannot be attached to anything specific or concrete. By knowing the difference, the nurse can intervene appropriately to empower the woman and facilitate coping.

One method to facilitate coping with fear and anxiety is to identify successful strategies used by the woman in the past. When confronted with new and overwhelming anxieties and fears, people often need to be reminded that they have demonstrated successful coping in the past. Once identified, the nurse can develop interventions to promote and reinforce these strategies.[40]

In addition to the use of known coping strategies, the nurse should use educational interventions to reduce the anxiety and uncertainty of unknowns. Information and education are powerful weapons against anxiety. The therapeutic use of the self

---

TABLE 8.10

Books and Articles on Pregnancy Loss

Berezin, N. (1982). *After a Loss in Pregnancy*. New York: Fireside/Simon & Schuster.

Berg, B.J. (1981). *Nothing to Cry About*. New York: Seaview Books.

Borg, S., & Lasker, J. (1981). *When Pregnancy Fails*. Boston: Beacon Press.

Colgrove, M., Bloomfield, H.H., & McWilliams, P. (1991). *How to Survive the Loss of a Love*. Los Angeles: Prelude Press.

Fout, C. "Stillbirth: The Silent Tragedy." *Family Circle*, February 19, 1980.

Friedman, R. (1982). *Surviving Pregnancy Loss*. New York: Little, Brown.

Grollman, E.A. (1970). *Talking About Death*. Boston: Beacon Press.

Ilse, S. (1982). *Empty Arms*. PO Box 165, Long Lake, MN 55356.

Jimemez, S. (1982). *The Other Side of Pregnancy*. Englewood Cliffs, NJ: Prentice-Hall.

Kushner, H.S. (1981). *When Bad Things Happen to Good People*. New York: Schocken Books.

Peppers, L., & Knapp, R. (1985). *How to Go on Living after the Death of a Baby*. Atlanta: Peachtree Publishers.

Pizer, H., & O'Brien Palinski, C. (1980). *Coping with a Miscarriage*. New York: New American Library.

Quindlen, A. "The Truth about Miscarriage." *Glamour*, June 1981.

Welch, M.S., & Hermann, D. "Why Miscarriage Is So Misunderstood." *MS.*, February, 1980.

Source: Adapted with permission from *Molar Pregnancy*, Magee-Womens Hospital, Pittsburgh, PA (1986).

TABLE 8.11

Diagnostic Cluster

Diagnostic/Preoperative and Postoperative Period

COLLABORATIVE PROBLEMS
Potential Complication: Bleeding/hemorrhage
Potential Complication: Thromboembolic event
Potential Complication: Infection/sepsis
Potential Complication: Fluid/electrolyte imbalance
Potential Complication: Atelectasis/pneumonia

NURSING DIAGNOSIS

1. Potential altered health maintenance related to insufficient knowledge of condition, diagnostic tests, prognosis, and treatment options

2. Decisional conflict related to insufficient knowledge of treatment options

3. Anxiety/fear related to impending surgery, and insufficient knowledge of preoperative routines, intraoperative activities, and postoperative self-care activities

4. Anxiety/fear related to insufficient knowledge of potential impact of condition and treatment on reproductive organs and sexuality

5. Grieving related to potential loss of fertility and perceived effects on lifestyle

6. Potential altered respiratory function related to immobility secondary to imposed bed rest and pain

7. Potential fluid volume deficit related to losses secondary to surgical wound or gastrointestinal dysfunction

8. Altered comfort related to effects of surgery, disease process, and immobility

9. Potential for infection related to susceptibility to bacteria secondary to wound, invasive vascular access, and/or urinary catheter

10. Potential altered nutrition: less than body requirements related to disease process, wound healing, and decreased caloric intake

11. Impaired physical mobility related to surgical interruption of body structures, incisional site pain, and activity restriction

12. Potential bowel dysfunction related to decreased peristalsis secondary to surgical manipulation of bowel, effects of anesthesia and analgesia, and immobility

13. Potential urinary dysfunction related to loss of sensation of bladder distention secondary to surgical and/or pharmaceutical interventions

14. Potential impaired skin integrity related to surgical wound, decreased tissue perfusion, ostomy stomas, drain sites, and/or immobility

15. Potential impaired tissue integrity/infection related to lymphedema secondary to surgical removal of lymph nodes

---

TABLE 8.11 *(continued)*

16c. Severe or permanent inability to engage in genital intercourse

17. Alteration in coping related to infertility

18. Potential altered health maintenance related to insufficient knowledge of dietary restrictions, medications, activity restrictions, self-care activities, symptoms of complications, follow-up visits, and community resources

---

Treatment Period

COLLABORATIVE PROBLEMS
Potential Complication: Preexisting medical conditions
Potential Complication: Fluid/electrolyte imbalance

NURSING DIAGNOSIS

1. Anxiety/fear related to loss of feelings of control of life, unpredictability of nature of disease, and uncertain future

2. Anxiety/fear related to insufficient knowledge of prescribed chemotherapy and necessary self-care measures

3. Anxiety/fear related to insufficient knowledge of prescribed radiation therapy and necessary self-care measures

4. Potential for infection related to immunosuppression neutropenia secondary to chemotherapy and/or radiation therapy

5. Potential for bleeding related to immunosuppression thrombocytopenia secondary to chemotherapy and/or radiation therapy

6. Potential alteration in skin integrity related to treatment modality and/or disease process

---

may also minimize fears of procedural events. In other words, simply by "being there," the nurse provides a source of strength and coping to the fearful patient.[42]

The nurse needs to communicate that the patient has permission to discuss both spiritual and sexual concerns, and then needs to provide adequate time and privacy for these discussions to occur. The use of cognitive reframing may be useful to restructure punitive thoughts and spiritual distress. For instance, "I don't know why God did this to me" may be reframed as, "Maybe He didn't do this; maybe He is helping you deal with this now." By reframing a thought, a negative perception can be changed to one that is positive and supportive.[42]

Sexual concerns and questions may also be addressed simply and honestly. This can be accomplished by acknowledging the woman's fears and emotional pain and by giving the woman permission to try again when she feels well and comfortable.

Sexual and spiritual issues may be influenced by feelings of guilt over the terminated pregnancy, especially if the woman has strong moral or religious convictions about abortion. These feelings may also prevent progression and resolution of the grief process. Communicating acceptance of the woman's feelings while gently reminding her of her urgent medical needs may help to refocus her thoughts and support the belief that she did nothing wrong. Spiritual issues may also be ameliorated by the hospital chaplain or her own clergy. Sexual counseling may be initiated during hospitalization to promote successful adjustment of the couple, and psychiatric consultation may also be useful to prevent long-term depression.[39]

Body image disturbances may become intensified with alopecia, a side effect of some chemotherapeutic agents. When alopecia is anticipated, the woman should be counseled in advance to purchase wigs and scarves. Several programs are available to help women through this difficult time. One program, sponsored by the American Cancer Society and entitled "Look Good, Feel Better," provides make-up, wigs, and trained personnel to teach women creative ways to cope with hair loss. Another benefit of this program is the personal, individualized attention the woman receives to her own needs in the one-to-one session.

Many nursing interventions can be implemented to assist the woman with GTN through her psychosocial and spiritual crisis. But the most important role of the nurse is to generate hope. Once considered a deadly combination of pregnancy and malignancy, today GTN is one of the most curable gynecologic cancers.[8] With accurate diagnosis and staging, surgical management, chemotherapy, and close follow-up, the patient will most likely be cured and move on to a normal life thereafter. Until that time, the role of the nurse is to communicate this hope and to guide, coach, and support the woman through the maze of unknowns until she feels safe, secure, and confident in her life again.

Educational Considerations

Numerous educational needs exist throughout the initial hospitalization and diagnostic period. First, the woman needs to be prepared for procedures such as suction curettage.[8] At this time, the nurse needs to provide technical information as well as sensory details to reduce anxiety and fear and to promote coping. As psychosocial and spiritual concerns are expressed, the nurse can teach the woman that her thoughts and feelings are very normal in this situation. The ability of the nurse to "be with" the woman and accept her need to express her feelings and grief can create a pathway for emotional healing to begin and emotional pain to be reduced.[42]

Discharge Planning

In preparation for discharge, it can be helpful to teach the woman and partner together. At this time, the nurse should reinforce the critical need for follow-up care with the physician, including blood titers for hCG, and the necessity of reliable contraception to prevent pregnancy. The nurse needs to prepare the woman for the chemotherapy experience, if planned, and teach her how to manage the expected side effects.

Finally, the woman should be provided with a list of community resources for additional support after discharge. Suggested resources include local American Cancer Society support groups, pregnancy loss support groups such as RESOLVE and SHARE, and the Lamaze parent-to-parent telephone support service. Books and articles on pregnancy loss may also be helpful, some of which are listed in Table 8.10. The telephone number of the nearest community mental health center may also be useful to both the woman and her partner. The needs of the woman with GTN have numerous implications that challenge both the woman and the nurse. The various physical, psychosocial, sexual, spiritual, and educational needs call on the nurse to creatively orchestrate the collaboration of the multidisciplinary team to ensure that the woman benefits from the expertise of each team member and obtains the best possible disease outcome.

✳ REFERENCES

1. Pijnenborg, R., Bland, J.M., Robertson, W.B., et al. (1981). The pattern of interstitial trophoblast invasion of the myometrium in early human pregnancy. *Placenta, 2,* 303.
2. Covone, A.E., Johnson, P.M., Mutton, D., et al. (1984). Trophoblast cells in peripheral blood from pregnant women. *Lancet, 2,* 841.
3. Szulman, A.E. (1988). Trophoblastic disease: Clinical pathology of hydatidiform moles. *Obstet Gynecol Clin North Am, 15,* 433.
4. Soper, J., Hammond, C., & Lewis, J. (1992). Gestational trophoblastic disease. In W.J. Hoskins, C.A. Perez, & R. Young, eds., *Principles and Practice of Gynecologic Oncology* (pp. 795–825). Philadelphia: Lippincott.
5. Szulman, A., & Surti, U. (1978). The syndromes of hydatidiform moles II: Morphologic evolution of the complete and partial mole. *Am J Obstet Gynecol, 132,* 20–27.
6. Szulman, A. (1987). Complete hydatidiform mole: Clinicopathologic features. In A. Szulman & H. Buchsbaum, eds., *Gestational Trophoblastic Disease.* New York: Springer-Verlag.
7. Mazur, T., & Kurman, R. (1987). Choriocarcinoma and placental site trophoblastic tumor. In A. Szulman & H. Buchsbaum, eds., *Gestational Trophoblastic Disease.* New York: Springer-Verlag.
8. DiSaia, P., & Creasman, W. (1993). *Clinical Gynecologic Oncology* 4th ed. St. Louis, MO: Mosby–Year Book.
9. Berkowitz, R., Goldstein, D., & Bernstein, M. (1991). Evolving concepts of molar pregnancy. *J Reprod Med, 36,* 40–43.
10. Bagshawe, K.D., Dent, J., & Webb, J. (1986). Hydatidiform mole in England and Wales, 1973–1983. *Lancet, 2,* 673.
11. Parazzini, F., LaVecchia, C., & Pampallona, S. (1986). Parental age and risk of complete and partial hydatidiform mole. *Br J Obstet Gynaecol, 93,* 582.
12. Buckley, J. (1987). Epidemiology of gestational trophoblastic disease. In A. Szulman & H. Buchsbaum, eds., *Gestational Trophoblastic Neoplasia.* New York: Springer-Verlag.
13. Morrow, C., & Townsend, D. (1987). *Synopsis of Gynecologic Oncology* 3rd ed. New York: Wiley.
14. Currie, T. (1990). Gestational trophoblastic neoplasia. *Semin Oncol Nurs, 6,* 228–236.
15. Berkowitz, R., & Goldstein, D. (1989). Gestational trophoblastic neoplasia. In J. Berek & N. Hacker, eds., *Practical Gynecologic Oncology.* Baltimore: Williams & Wilkins.
16. Berkowitz, R.S., Goldstein, D.P., DuBeshter, B., et al. (1987). Managment of complete molar pregnancy. *Obstet Gynecol, 66,* 677.
17. Morrow, C.P., Klezky, O.A., DiSaia, P.J., et al. (1977). Clinical and laboratory correlates of molar pregnancy and trophoblastic disease. *Am J Obstet Gynecol, 128,* 424.
18. Szulman, A.E., & Surti, U. (1982). The clinicopathologic profile of the partial hydatidiform mole. *Obstet Gynecol, 59,* 597.
19. Brewer, C., Adelson, M., & Elder, R. (1992). Erythrocytosis associated with a placental site trophoblastic tumor. *Obstet Gynecol, 79*(5), 846–849.
20. Chernecky, C. (1991). *Cancer: Diagnostics and Chemotherapy.* Philadelphia: Saunders.

21. American College of Obstetrics and Gynecology (1993). *Management of Gestational Trophoblastic Neoplasia* (no. 178). Washington, DC: ACOG.

22. Hammond, C.B., Borchert, L.G., & Tyrey, L., et al. (1973). Treatment of metastatic trophoblastic disease: Good prognosis and poor prognosis. *Am J Obstet Gynecol, 115,* 451–455.

23. Soper, J., & Hammond, C. (1988). Nonmetastatic gestational trophoblastic disease. *Obstet Gynecol Clin North Am, 15*(3), 505–519.

24. Miller, S., & Lurain, J. (1988). Classification and staging of gestational trophoblastic tumors. *Obstet Gynecol Clin North Am, 15*(3), 477–489.

25. Curry, S., Hammond, C., Tyrey, L., Creasman, W., & Parker, R. (1975). Hydatidiform mole: Diagnosis, management, and long term follow up of 347 patients. *Obstet Gynecol, 45,* 1–8.

26. Goldstein, D. (1974). Prevention of gestational trophoblastic disease by use of actinomycin-D in molar pregnancy. *Obstet Gynecol, 43,* 475–479.

27. Kim, D., Moon, H., & Kim, K. (1986). Effects of prophylactic chemotherapy for persistent trophoblastic disease in patients with complete hydatidiform mole. *Obstet Gynecol, 67,* 690–694.

28. Lurain, J. (1990). Chemotherapy of gestational trophoblastic neoplasia. In G. Deppe, ed., *Chemotherapy of Gynecologic Cancer* 2nd ed. New York: Wiley & Sons.

29. Holmesley, H., Blessing, J., Schlaerth, J., Rettenmaier, M., & Mayor, F. (1990). Rapid escalation of weekly IM methotrexate for nonmetastatic GTD: A GOG study. *Gynecol Oncol, 39,* 305–308.

30. Smith, J. (1975). Chemotherapy in gynecologic cancer: Malignant trophoblastic tumors. *Clin Obstet Gynecol, 18,* 113–116.

31. Mangili, G., Garavagila, E., Frigerio, L., Candotti, G., & Ferrari, A. (1996). Management of low-risk gestational trophoblastic tumors with Etoposide (VP16) in patients resistant to methotrexate. *Gynecol Oncol, 61,* 218–220.

32. Bagshawe, K. (1984). Treatment of high risk choriocarcinoma. *J Reprod Med, 29,* 813–825.

33. Bower, M., Newlands, E., Holden, L., et al. (1997). EMA/CO for High-Risk Gestational Trophoblastic Tumors: Results from a cohort of 272 Patients. *J Clin Oncol, 15*(7), 2636–2643.

34. Bolis, G., Bonazzi, C., Landoni, F., et al. (1988). EMA/CO regimen in high risk GTT. *Gynecol Oncol, 31,* 439–443.

35. Barnard, D.E., Woodward, K.T., Yancy, S.G., et al. (1986). Hepatic metastases of choriocarcinoma: A report of fifteen patients. *Gynecol Oncol, 25,* 73.

36. Jones, W., & Lewis, J. (1985). Late recurrence of GTD. *Gynecol Oncol, 20,* 83–91.

37. Sherwin, L.N., Scoloveno, M.A., & Weingarten, C.T. (1991). *Nursing Care of the Childbearing Family* (pp. 1090–1092). Norwalk, CT: Appleton & Lange.

38. Bobak, I.M., Jensen, M.B., & Lowdermilk, D.L. (1993). *Maternity and Gynecologic Care: The Nurse and the Family* 5th ed. (p. 1396). St. Louis: Mosby–Year Book.

39. Cook, R., & Hager, E. (1991). Gestational trophoblastic neoplasia. In *Fundamentals of Gynecologic Oncology,* Education presymposium, Society of Gynecologic Nurse Oncologists Annual Symposium, Orlando, FL.

40. Carpenito, L.J. (1993). *Nursing Diagnosis* 5th ed. (pp. 518–539). Philadelphia: Lippincott.

41. Brandt, B. (1990). Nursing protocol for the patient with neutropenia. *Oncol Nurs Forum, 17*(1, suppl.), 9–15.

42. Carter, L.W. (1993). Influences of nutrition and stress on people at risk for neutropenia: Nursing implications. *Oncol Nurs Forum, 20,* 1241–1250.

43. Lewis, S.M., Collier, I.C., & Heitkemper, M.M. (1996). *Medical Surgical Nursing: Assessment and Management of Clinical Problems* 4th ed. St. Louis: Mosby–Year Book.

44. Kidd, P.S., & Wagner, K.D. (1992). *High Acuity Nursing.* Norwalk, CT: Appleton & Lange.

45. Martin, L.K., & Braly, P.S. (1991). Gynecologic cancers. In S. Baird, R. McCorkle, & M. Grant, eds., *Cancer Nursing* (pp. 532–534). Philadelphia: Saunders.

46. Baird, S., McCorkle, R., & Grant, M. (1991). *Cancer Nursing.* Philadelphia: Saunders.

47. Winningham, M.L. (1988). The effect of aerobic exercise on patient reports of nausea. *Oncol Nurs Forum 15,* 447–450.

48. Page, M.A. (1992). Coke syrup for relief of nausea and vomiting. *Oncol Nurs Forum, 15.*

49. Levinson, D.J. (1996) *The Seasons of a Woman's Life.* New York: Random House.

Gynecologic Sarcomas

Susan Vogt Temple, RN, MSN, ETN

✖ INTRODUCTION

A sarcoma is defined as a tumor arising in connective or muscle tissue. Connective and muscle tissue tumors are named after their tissue of origin; for example, a cancer in a smooth muscle is a leiomyosarcoma. They are further classified according to how many cell types they contain and whether the different cell types originate from more than one germ layer.

To review, an embryo is composed of three layers of tissue, from which all body tissues are formed. The three (germ) layers are: (1) ectoderm, or outer layer, from which skin cells, hair follicle cells, skin, sweat glands, and cells of the nervous system are derived; (2) mesoderm, or middle layer, containing muscle, bone, fascia, and connective tissue cells; and (3) endoderm, or inner layer, from which the mucosa of the genital, gastrointestinal, and respiratory tracts are formed.

In classifying tumor cells, a simple neoplasm is one in which dividing cells closely resemble one another and are composed of a single cell type. Most tumors fall into this category. Mixed tumors contain more than one cell type, but the different cells originate from a single germ layer. Compound tumors contain a variety of cell types from different layers.[1]

Sarcomas of the female genital tract are very rare; the vast majority of tumors are carcinomas. The most common site for gynecologic sarcomas is the uterus, although they may also be found in the ovaries, cervix, fallopian tubes, vagina, and vulva. Because gynecologic sarcomas are so rare, data regarding effective therapy are often unclear. Studies are often limited by small sample size or data combining different tumor types.

Treatment for sarcomas may include surgery, radiation therapy, chemotherapy, and hormonal therapy. Surgery is the primary treatment and ranges from wide local excision to total abdominal hysterectomy and bilateral salpingo-oophorectomy or radical hysterectomy and vaginectomy. Radiation therapy is used for control of pelvic metastasis or prevention of recurrence. Chemotherapy is used for adjuvant treatment and metastatic disease. Chemotherapeutic agents considered active against uterine sarcomas include doxorubicin, dacarbazine, ifosfamide, and cisplatin, with many responses being partial and of short duration.[2–6]

✖ UTERINE SARCOMA

Classification

Sarcomas comprise less than 1% of gynecologic malignancies and about 3 to 5% of all uterine malignancies. These tumors arise primarily from two tissues: mesodermal (muellerian) and stromal sarcomas from the endometrial epithelium and leiomyosarcomas from the uterine muscle itself. Other sarcomas, arising in supportive tissue, such as angiosarcoma and fibrosarcoma, are rare.[7]

The most common histologic types of uterine sarcomas are carcinosarcoma, also known as malignant mixed mesodermal or mullerian sarcoma (MMMT) (50%), leiomyosarcoma (30%), and endometrial stromal sarcoma (15%).[4,7,8,34]

Clinical Manifestations

Most frequently, women present with the complaint of irregular or postmenopausal vaginal bleeding (Table 9.1). An enlarged, irregular uterus is the most common finding on physical examination. Tumors, especially carcinosarcomas, may form polypoid masses that can be seen protruding from the cervix. Other, less common symptoms include abdominal pain, abdominal mass, weight loss, and vaginal discharge.[4,9,10]

An enlarging pelvic mass may be a presenting sign, since uterine sarcomas are sometimes found in association with a benign leiomyoma.[10] Distinguishing between benign and malignant leiomyomas remains difficult. Preoperative diagnostic imaging (Table 9.2), such as ultrasound, CT scan, and MRI, and endometrial sampling and intraoperative frozen sections do not always provide definitive information.[11] For this reason, a rapidly enlarging uterine mass is a definite indication for hysterectomy with thorough intra-abdominal inspection.[7,9,12]

Women with uterine sarcoma are predominantly postmenopausal. Obesity, hypertension, and diabetes are commonly associated clinical findings.[7,9,13] The only known etiological factor, which applies to 10 to 25% of these malignancies, is previous pelvic irradiation, often administered for benign uterine bleeding approximately twenty-five years earlier.[9]

TABLE 9.1	
Potential Presenting Symptoms of Gynecologic Sarcoma	
Objective Symptoms	Subjective Symptoms
Irregular, enlarged uterus	Irregular vaginal bleeding
Rapidly growing myoma	Postmenopausal bleeding
Pelvic mass	Pelvic discomfort
Obesity	Pelvic pressure
Hypertension	Abdominal pain
Ascites	Vaginal discharge
Vaginal discharge	Weight loss
Vaginal bleeding	Bone pain
	Dysuria
	Dyspareunia
	Cough and/or dyspnea

TABLE 9.2

Diagnostic Evaluation Procedures

Endometrial biopsy/endocervical curettage
Fractional dilation and curettage
Transvaginal ultrasound
Magnetic resonance imaging
Computed tomography

Staging

There is no official staging system for uterine sarcomas. It is usual to use the Federation of Gynecology & Obstetrics (FIGO) system for uterine corpus carcinoma,[9,14] listed in Table 5.2.

Treatment

It is recommended that patients with a history of irregular or postmenopausal bleeding have an endometrial biopsy sampling or fractional D&C prior to hysterectomy for histologic evaluation.[4,8,9] In patients who are medically stable and in whom a preoperative diagnosis of sarcoma has been made, the treatment is total abdominal hysterectomy and bilateral salpingo-oophorectomy with pelvic and para-aortic selective lymphadenectomy. Cytologic washings are obtained from the pelvis and abdomen. Thorough examination of the diaphragm, omentum, and upper abdomen is performed. However, there are no good data concerning the importance of oophorectomy in the treatment of sarcoma. In premenopausal women, ovarian conservation does not appear to adversely affect survival.[15]

Data concerning the role of radiation therapy indicate that it does not typically influence ultimate survival. But adjuvant external beam pelvic irradiation may reduce the incidence of recurrence in the pelvis and increase the disease-free interval in certain patients.[11,16,17]

Active chemotherapeutic agents for carcinosarcomas include ifosfamide and cisplatin as single agents; combination chemotherapy with these drugs resulted in a higher response rate, greater toxicity, and no improvement in survival when compared to ifosfamide alone in the recent Gynecologic Oncology Group clinical trial. Agents that have been previously evaluated include: doxorubicin, etoposide, taxol, mitoxantrone, piperazinedione, aziridinylbenzoquinone, and aminothiadiazole.[2,3,8,13,17,18]

Antineoplastics under investigation as systemic therapy for leiomyosarcoma include: taxol, trimetrexate, doxorubicin, cyclophosphamide, ifosfamide, cisplatin, etoposide, mitoxantrone, piperazinedione, aziridinylbenzoquinone, and aminothiadiazole. Only doxorubicin and dacarbazine have been conclusively identified as active agents in leiomyosarcoma.[5,6]

Soft tissue sarcomas may be treated with ifosfamide, vincristine, actinomycin D, cytoxan, adriamycin, methotrexate, dacarbazine, and topotecan. Ongoing studies of aggressive dosing, regimens, and schedules with these drugs seek to increase patient response and improve the disease-free interval.[17,19]

The incorporation of new agents with novel mechanisms of action may improve disease response and long-term survival. Ongoing Phase II and Phase III clinical trials under the auspices of the Gynecologic Oncology Group continue to provide a scientific basis for selection of chemotherapeutic agents for patients with uterine sarcomas.

There is currently no standard therapy for patients with recurrent disease. Eligible patients should be offered the opportunity to participate in clinical trials when available.

The role of hormonal therapy appears to be limited to patients with low-grade stromal sarcomas, in which high-dose progesterone therapy may be of some benefit.[20]

Prognosis

The prognosis for uterine sarcoma is primarily dependent on the extent of the disease at the time of diagnosis and, in stage I and stage II, the depth of myometrial invasion.[8,21] The more advanced the disease appears at diagnosis, the shorter the interval until treatment failure.[10] For stage I disease, an approximate five-year survival rate of 50% has been reported.[10,14] The five-year survival rate when the disease has spread beyond the uterus is estimated at 10%.[14] Almost 90% of patients who do not show a response to therapy die of their disease within two years.[9,22]

Patterns of Metastasis

Metastasis commonly occurs by the tumor infiltrating the myometrium and spreading locally. Sarcomas also have a tendency for early hematogenous and lymphatic spread. Lymphatic dissemination occurs in about 35% of patients with disease clinically confined to the uterus and cervix.[23] The result is that, of the patients who have recurrence, 85% will have distant metastasis.[9]

Sites of metastasis include the peritoneal cavity, lung, brain, pelvic and para-aortic lymph nodes, skin, bone, heart, pericardium, and adrenal gland. Distant sites of metastasis are found independent of lymphatic involvement or positive cytologic findings.[23]

✳ CERVICAL SARCOMA

Among the primary neoplasms originating in the cervix, sarcoma is the most rare, with a reported incidence of 0.2 to 0.55%.[16] Currently there is no universally accepted histologic classification for cervical sarcomas. One classification system divides the tumors into two groups, leiomyosarcomas (primary or secondary) and stromal sarcomas (including homologous, heterologous, sarcoma botryoides, adenosarcoma, and mixed muellerian tumors).[24]

Leiomyosarcoma

Cervical leiomyosarcomas are smooth muscle sarcomas confined to and/or arising in the cervix. They are categorized on the basis of whether the tumors arise originally in the cervix (primary) or in a preexisting leiomyoma (secondary). The tumors have been reported in women aged 18 to 77 years, with an average age of 47 years. The major presenting symptom is abnormal vaginal bleeding.[24]

Because the number of reported cases is small, there are no definitive data regarding the most effective therapy. Reported treatments include total abdominal hysterectomy (TAH), radiation therapy, and chemotherapy. The prognosis is poor regardless of therapy.[24]

Stromal Sarcoma

Cervical stromal sarcomas arise from the basic paramesonephric stroma (mesoderm). Irregular vaginal bleeding is again the most common presenting symptom. Surgery (TAH) is the primary therapy, but radiation and chemotherapy have also been used in these patients.

Sarcoma Botryoides

Sarcoma botryoides, also called embryonal rhabdomyosarcoma, is a type of cervical cancer that occurs in the uterine corpus in older females, the cervix of women of reproductive age, and the vagina in infants and younger children. Patients range in age from 10 weeks to 75 years, with an average age of 27 years.

These malignancies arise from the growing tip of the muellerian tubercle in the patient under five years of age. The term *botryoides* is derived from the Greek *botrys*, or "grapes," which describes the tumor's typical appearance as a large, reddish, irregular, polypoid growth extending from the cervical canal.

Reported therapy is not uniform but consists of surgery with adjunct radiation. In general, survival is poor, but a few long-term survivors have been reported.[24]

Carcinosarcoma

Carcinosarcomas, also known as mixed muellerian tumors, have been reported in patients ranging from 15 to 72 years, with an average age of 54.5 years. Vaginal bleeding, vaginal discharge, and amenorrhea have all been reported as presenting symptoms. Treatment may be surgery (TAH) with or without radiation therapy or radiation therapy alone. Prognosis is poor due to frequent recurrence and distant metastasis.[24]

Adenosarcoma

Adenosarcoma is a type of malignant mixed muellerian tumor. Presenting symptoms include abnormal vaginal bleeding and asymptomatic polypoid lesions. Treatment ranges from total abdominal hysterectomy with bilateral salpingo-oophorectomy, to wide local excision and radical hysterectomy with partial vaginectomy. Recurrence appears to be rare in these tumors.[24]

✳ OVARIAN SARCOMA

Similar to other gynecologic sarcomas, sarcomas arising in the ovary are aggressive tumors associated with a poor prognosis.

These tumors are very rare, representing approximately 1% of all ovarian cancers at one center,[25] and are difficult to classify histologically. Fibrosarcoma, leiomyosarcoma, rhabdomyosarcoma, carcinosarcoma, stromal sarcoma, and teratomas with sarcomatous elements have all been reported.[25,26]

Patients may range in age from 3 to 93 years; the median age is 56. Teratoid tumors tend to occur in children and young adults, stromal tumors occur at any age, and carcinosarcomas occur in older, postmenopausal women.

Primary presenting symptoms include abdominal discomfort, increase in abdominal girth, and change in gastrointestinal or urinary habits. Abnormal vaginal bleeding is very rarely seen.

Treatment ranges from unilateral salpingo-oophorectomy in young patients with teratoid sarcomas, to total abdominal hysterectomy and bilateral salpingo-oophorectomy with omentectomy and multiple biopsies. Chemotherapy is necessary for preventing or treating recurrence outside the pelvis, and radiation therapy is helpful in controlling isolated metastasis.[26]

Survival is poor, comparable to all other ovarian cancers, and tends to be related to stage at diagnosis. There is no correlation between cell type and survival.[26] Distant metastasis is common.

✳ VULVAR SARCOMA

Sarcomas represent 1 to 2% of vulvar malignancies. Many histologic types have been described, but the most commonly seen are leiomyosarcoma and malignant fibrous histiosarcoma.[27]

Leiomyosarcoma

Leiomyosarcomas are the most common of the vulvar sarcomas. Most patients present with an enlarging, often painful mass, usually in the labia majora. The average age at diagnosis is 45 years. In general, the lesions tend to recur locally, with a rare incidence of lymphatic metastasis. Although any lesion may recur, risk increases if the lesion is larger than 5 cm, has a high mitotic count, and has infiltrating rather than pushing margins.[28] Radical local excision is the usual treatment.

Vulvovaginal Rhabdomyosarcoma

Also known as *sarcoma botryoides*, vulvovaginal rhabdomyosarcoma (RMS) is a highly malignant tumor seen in the vagina in infancy and childhood.

The patient commonly presents with enlarging polypoid lesions protruding from the vagina or vaginal bleeding. Currently, most children with vulvar or vaginal RMS can be treated by localized resection of the lesions and systemic combination chemotherapy. If complete remission is not achieved, localized brachytherapy (interstitial or intracavitary application) followed by combination chemotherapy, can be used. Brachytherapy may be used to provide local control. Combination chemotherapy regimens incorporating vincristine, dactinomycin, cyclophosphamide, doxorubicin, taxol, topotecan, and/or ifosfamide/mesna are under investigation.[19,29]

✖ VAGINAL SARCOMA

Vaginal sarcomas such as fibrosarcomas and leiomyosarcomas are rarely seen. They tend to be bulky tumors that occur most commonly in the upper vagina, with surgical excision being the primary treatment. Cure is likely in low-grade tumors with clean surgical margins. For large, unresectable, and high-grade tumors, lymphatic and hematologic disseminations are common.[2]

✖ FALLOPIAN TUBE SARCOMA

Fallopian tube sarcomas are extremely uncommon. They have been reported in adolescents as well as the elderly, but they occur mainly in the sixth decade and are typically advanced at the time of discovery. Histologic types include leiomyosarcoma and carcinosarcoma. Usual treatment is surgery (total abdominal hysterectomy and bilateral salpingo-oophorectomy) followed by chemotherapy (usually doxorubicin).[7] Survival is poor, with most patients dying of their disease within two years.[2]

✖ NURSING ISSUES RELATED TO GYNECOLOGIC SARCOMAS

Patients with gynecologic sarcomas present many nursing challenges throughout the course of the disease. Due to the high mortality associated with the disease, the goal of

TABLE 9.3
Patient and Family Education

1. Signs and symptoms of treatment complications
2. Signs and symptoms of treatment side effects
3. Management of treatment complications and side effects
4. Pain management
5. Sexuality, specifically: concerns, resources for further information, and ongoing problems
6. Community cancer support groups
7. Management of shortness of breath
8. Signs and symptoms of recurrence

nursing management is to maximize quality of life for the patient and family. This is accomplished by providing counseling and education (Table 9.3), as well as physical care to minimize side effects of treatment and disease complications (Table 9.4).

Distant Metastasis

One of the unique characteristics of gynecologic sarcomas is their propensity for distant metastasis. Although the lung is the most common site of metastasis, metastases have been reported in almost every organ. Uterine leiomyosarcomas have been found to metastasize to the abdomen, hip, face, liver, vagina, and buttocks.[30]

Since most other gynecologic tumors tend to metastasize locally, management of distant site metastases may pose a challenge to gynecologic oncology nurses. When recurrent disease is discovered, it may be the most distressing time in the course of the illness. Patients frequently describe the feeling of having developed "another" cancer separate from their primary gynecologic malignancy. The woman may experience uncertainty, grief, feelings of failure, injustice, fear, and anger. In addition, there may be spiritual concerns, concerns with coping, and problems with communication between the woman and her partner about cancer recurrence.[30] Often patients describe the recurrence as more upsetting than the initial diagnosis. The threat of death is "more real," decisions regarding treatment more difficult, side effects more severe, fear of uncontrollable pain greater, and fatigue intensified. At the time of recurrence, many patients express dissatisfaction and anger with the initial treatment choices that were made.[31]

Nurses can encourage patients to direct their energy toward living with the disease rather than focusing on cure. Various treatment options with the goals of disease control and comfort may be presented to the patient at this time. The patient and her family face difficult decisions trying to determine which possible treatments may prolong life versus those that would only postpone death while adding discomfort.[30]

TABLE 9.4		
Assessment Criteria for Gynecologic Sarcomas		
Specific System	*Subjective Criteria*	*Objective Criteria*
General Health	Past medical/surgical history Current medications Allergies	
Cognitive/Sensory	Awareness of health problems Past hospitalizations or surgical experience Ability to problem-solve Anxiety level	Vision Hearing Orientation to time, place, and person Comprehension Mood/affect
Self-Concept Relationships	Body image concerns Role responsibilities (children, employment) Sexuality Spiritual beliefs Family dynamics Stress tolerance Support systems Financial resources	

Rest/Comfort	Sleep patterns, problems, supportive aids
	Pain
	    location
	    characteristics
	    intensity
	    duration
	    exacerbated and relieved by
		Muscle tension, guarding

Skin	Lesions, problems	Skin color, temperature Skin lesions Nails, clubbing and capillary refill

Neurologic	Mental changes
	    abstract reasoning
	    poor recent memory
	    personality or intellectual changes
	Reported seizure
	    activity
		Level of consciousness
		Pupils
		    size
		    equality
		    constriction

(continued)

TABLE 9.4 *(continued)*

Specific System	Subjective Criteria	Objective Criteria
	Motor dysfunction 　vertigo 　dizziness 　loss of balance Headache, especially at night and on waking Speech disorders 　aphasia 　word finding Sensory dysfunction Visual changes Nausea/vomiting	Seizure activity Reflexes Motor functioning Sensory perception Cerebellar function Cranial nerves
Respiratory	Smoking Preexisting respiratory diseases Shortness of breath Dyspnea Cough Requirement for supplemental oxygen	Respiratory rate, quality Breath sounds Secretions Areas of dullness on per- cussion Diaphragmatic excursion Elevated temperature Tactile fremitus Apical pulse rate, character Radial pulse rate, character Peripheral pulses Blood pressure Peripheral edema Lymphadenopathy
Nutrition/ Elimination	Appetite Abdominal pain, bloating Nausea/vomiting Weight loss or gain last year Elimination patterns—change in 　flatulence 　constipation 　dysuria 　urgency 　frequency	Oral lesions Abdominal distention Bowel sounds Ascites Abdominal tenderness, guarding, mass effect Blood in stool Colostomy/urostomy Urine characteristics

	TABLE 9.4 *(continued)*	
Specific System	*Subjective Criteria*	*Objective Criteria*
Activity/Exercise	Independence in ADL Fatigue Backache	Range of motion Gait, posture Mobility Weakness Paralysis

Reproductive	Breast lumps, pain, discharge
	Breast self-examination
	Last gyn exam
	Menses
	LMP
	  menopause
	  pregnancies
	  children
	  bleeding
	  spotting or vaginal discharge
	  pelvic pain, pressure
	  lumps
	Pregnancy, family planning
	Sexual
	  activity
	  dyspareunia
	  concerns
	  informational needs
		Breast exam
		External genitalia
		Uterus
		  irregularity
		  enlargement
		Cervix, lesions
		Vagina, lesions

During this time, family members may disagree as to the aggressiveness of treatment desired. Often husbands and children encourage the woman to proceed with treatment, in the hope of a response, while the woman herself expresses the desire to stop. In trying to protect each other, family members may not openly discuss their feelings. The nurse can be an important spokesperson to make sure the patient's wishes become heard and understood and to facilitate open, honest communication. Support groups may be valuable during this time.

Pain management is a priority during this phase of the illness in order to allow the patient to maintain quality of life. Patients need to be taught that pain control is a realistic goal of care and that they are not expected to suffer. Performing a thorough assessment of pain and teaching the patient to adequately report her pain are necessary initial steps to accomplishing this goal. The nurse should explain the role of opiates in cancer pain management, since about two-thirds of patients with advanced cancer require this therapy.[32]

TABLE 9.5

Diagnostic Cluster

Diagnostic/Preoperative and Postoperative Period

COLLABORATIVE PROBLEMS

Potential Complication: Bleeding/hemorrhage
Potential Complication: Thromboembolic event
Potential Complication: Infection/sepsis
Potential Complication: Fluid/electrolyte imbalance
Potential Complication: Atelectasis/pneumonia
Potential Complication: Bowel dysfunction
Potential Complication: Urinary dysfunction

NURSING DIAGNOSIS

1. Potential altered health maintenance related to insufficient knowledge of condition, diagnostic tests, prognosis, and treatment options

2. Decisional conflict related to insufficient knowledge of treatment options

3. Anxiety/fear related to impending surgery, and insufficient knowledge of preoperative routines, intraoperative activities, and postoperative self-care activities

4. Anxiety/fear related to insufficient knowledge of potential impact of condition and treatment on reproductive organs and sexuality

5. Potential altered respiratory function related to immobility secondary to imposed bed rest and pain

6. Potential fluid volume deficit related to losses secondary to surgical wound or gastrointestinal dysfunction

7. Altered comfort related to effects of surgery, disease process, and immobility

8. Potential for infection related to susceptibility to bacteria secondary to wound, invasive vascular access, and/or urinary catheter

9. Potential altered nutrition: less than body requirements related to disease process, wound healing, and decreased caloric intake

10. Impaired physical mobility related to surgical interruption of body structures, incisional site pain, and activity restriction

11. Potential bowel dysfunction related to decreased peristalsis secondary to surgical manipulation of bowel, effects of anesthesia and analgesia, and immobility

12. Potential urinary dysfunction related to loss of sensation of bladder distention secondary to surgical and/or pharmaceutical interventions

13. Potential impaired skin integrity related to surgical wound, decreased tissue perfusion, ostomy stomas, drain sites, and/or immobility

TABLE 9.5 *(continued)*

14a. Potential sexual dysfunction related to disease process, surgical intervention, fatigue, and/or pain

14b. Potential moderate or possible permanent alterations in sexual activity related to disease process, surgical intervention, fatigue, and/or pain

14c. Severe or permanent inability to engage in genital intercourse

15. Potential altered health maintenance related to insufficient knowledge of dietary restrictions, medications, activity restrictions, self-care activities, symptoms of complications, follow-up visits, and community resources

---

Treatment Period

COLLABORATIVE PROBLEMS

Potential Complication: Preexisting medical conditions

Potential Complication: Anasarca

Potential Complication: Fluid/electrolyte imbalance

NURSING DIAGNOSIS

1. Anxiety/fear related to loss of feelings of control of life, unpredictability of nature of disease, and uncertain future

2. Anxiety/fear related to insufficient knowledge of prescribed radiation therapy and necessary self-care measures

3. Anxiety/fear related to insufficient knowledge of prescribed gynecologic radiation implant: conventional afterloading procedure

4. Anxiety/fear related to insufficient knowledge of prescribed chemotherapy and necessary self-care measures

5. Potential for infection related to immunosuppression neutropenia secondary to chemotherapy and/or radiation therapy

6. Potential for bleeding related to immunosuppression thrombocytopenia secondary to chemotherapy and/or radiation therapy

7. Potential alteration in skin integrity related to treatment modality and/or disease process

8. Potential alteration in respiratory function related to abdominal distention, decreased lung capacity, and/or lung metastasis

9. Potential for injury related to neurologic dysfunction secondary to brain metastasis

Lung Metastasis

Patients experiencing lung metastasis commonly experience dyspnea, pain, anxiety, weakness, and fatigue.[33,34] Dyspnea is defined as difficult, uncomfortable, labored breathing. Like pain, it is a multidimensional, subjective response.[33] Pulmonary obstructive and restrictive disorders are the most common cause of its development in cancer patients with lung involvement. Dyspnea may be decreased by a change in position, practicing relaxation techniques, minimizing energy expenditure, and, occasionally, oxygen therapy. Positions that help alleviate the sensation include the semi-Fowler's position or sitting with the head slightly forward and elbows resting on a chair. Progressive relaxation, meditation, and imagery are all techniques that can be taught to patients to elicit a relaxation response and lead to a sense of calm. Personalized relaxation tapes reflecting what is most important and pleasant to the individual, and addressing the particular pain and dyspnea concerns may be especially helpful.[33] Humidifiers or vaporizers may loosen secretions by increasing moisture, and low-flow oxygen may help ease breathing.

The use of opiates may provide palliation for respiratory distress. Dyspnea can often be improved with low doses of morphine sulfate, without significant respiratory depression or sedation. Glucocorticoids and sedatives may also be used.[35]

Cough is a symptom of tissue irritation resulting from infection, inflammation, or tumor. The cause of the cough needs to be determined so that appropriate treatment is prescribed. Untreated, persistent cough may lead to aggravation of existing pain, development of new pain, insomnia, anorexia, hemoptysis, and exhaustion. Treatment may include antibiotics, cough suppressants, increasing oral fluids, and the use of humidifiers to loosen secretions.

If a thoracic tumor causes venous or lymph obstruction, or if tumor seeds the pleura, reabsorption of pleural fluids may be impeded. The resulting effusion may be a cause of dyspnea. Lack of breath sounds at the lung bases and dullness on percussion are clinical cues. Diagnosis is made with a lateral decubitus chest X-ray. Treatment may include insertion of a chest tube for the drainage of fluid, followed by pleurodesis, or the sealing of the pleura with a sclerosing agent. Radiation therapy may also be used palliatively to treat the tumor.[36]

Brain Metastasis

Metastatic brain lesions frequently occur with gynecologic sarcomas. The cerebrum is the most common site, but lesions may also develop in the cerebellum or brain stem.[37] The patient may present with a wide range of symptoms, including headache, seizures, mental status or personality changes, nausea, vomiting, or lethargy.[37,38] The diagnosis is confirmed by CT scan or MRI.

Cerebral metastasis is often treated with radiation therapy, although systemic and intrathecal chemotherapy and surgery may also be used. Glucocorticosteroids are administered to decrease intracranial pressure and provide relief from symptoms such as headache and vomiting. Analgesics and antiemetics may also provide symptomatic relief. Phenytoin or phenobarbital may be administered prophylactically for seizure prevention.

Nursing management of the patient with brain metastasis is directed at minimizing symptoms of the tumor and side effects of the treatments. Performing a neurological assessment to identify actual and/or potential neurological deficits is an important first step in nursing care. Neurological assessment includes evaluation of level of consciousness, mentation, motor function, sensory function, and integrated regulatory function.[39,40]

The neurological changes associated with brain metastasis have implications for nursing care. Maintenance of patient safety is of primary concern. Careful assessment of the patient can reveal the specific safety interventions necessary, which may include full siderails, restraints, and assistance with activities of daily living. Seizure precautions may be indicated.

Weakness or immobility may also result from neurologic changes. These patients and their families require education regarding measures to maintain skin integrity and prevent further complications of immobility.

Discharge Planning

In-hospital management represents a small fraction of the care of gynecologic sarcoma patients. The majority of time during the illness is spent at home. Thus intensive planning and education are necessary during hospitalization periods to maximize the patient's and family's skills and resources and enable them to manage successfully at home.

A multidisciplinary team approach is required to meet the various demands posed by this disease. The services frequently utilized by sarcoma patients include rehabilitation services, social work, nutrition, pastoral care, medicine, and nursing (including case manager, enterostomal therapy, home care, and hospice). The nurse remains the primary communication link between all of these disciplines.

Summary

Patients with gynecologic sarcomas pose multiple nursing challenges. They require consistent support and education and aggressive nursing management to control symptoms. Although length of survival may be limited for many women, quality of life can remain minimally affected with the consistent intervention of knowledgeable, caring health care professionals.

✖ REFERENCES

1. Bristol-Myers Oncology Division (1985). *Oncology: Programmed Modules for Nurses*. Syracuse, NY: Bristol-Myers Oncology Division.
2. Hacker, N.F. (1989). Uterine cancer. In J.S. Berek & N.F. Hacker, eds., *Practical Gynecologic Oncology* (p. 317). Baltimore: Williams & Wilkins.
3. Sutton, G.P., Blessing, J.A., Manetta, A., et al. (1992). Gynecologic Oncology Group studies with ifosfamide. *Semin Oncol, 19*(6, suppl. 12), 31–35.
4. Curtin, J.P., Silverberg, J., Thigpen, T., & Spanos, W. Corpus: Mesenchymal tumors. In W.J. Hoskins, C.A. Perez, & R.C. Young, eds., (1997). *Principles*

and Practice of Gynecologic Oncology 2nd ed. (pp. 897–917). Philadelphia: Lippincott-Raven.

5. Resnick, E., Chambers, S.K., Carcangiu, M.L., et al. (1995). A phase II study of etoposide, cisplatin, and doxorubicin chemotherapy in mixed mullerian tumors of the uterus. *Gynecol Oncol, 56,* 370–375.

6. Keohan, M.L., Taub, R.N. (1997). Chemotherapy for advanced sarcoma: Therapeutic decisions and modalities. *Semin Oncol, 24,* 572–579.

7. DiSaia, P.J., & Creasman, W.T. (1992). *Clinical Gynecologic Oncology* 5th ed. (pp. 169–179). St. Louis, MO: Mosby–Year Book.

8. Arrastia, C.O., Fruchter, R.G., Clark, M., Maiman, M., et al. (1997). Uterine carcinosarcomas: Incidence and trends in management and survival. *Gynecol Oncol, 65,* 158–163.

9. Jones, H.W. (1988). Sarcoma of the uterus. In H.W. Jones, A.C. Wentz, & L.S. Burnett, eds., *Novak's Textbook of Gynecology* (pp. 761–772). Baltimore: Williams & Wilkins.

10. Salazar, O.M., Bonfiglio, T.A., Patten, S.F., et al. (1978). Uterine sarcomas: Natural history, treatment, and prognosis. *Cancer, 42,* 1152–1160.

11. Schwartz, L.B., Diamond, M.P., & Schwartz, P.E. (1993). Leiomyosarcomas: Clinical presentation. *Am J Obstet Gynecol, 168*(1), 180–183.

12. Oláh, K.S., Gee, H., Blunt, S., et al. (1991). Retrospective analysis of 318 cases of uterine sarcoma. *Eur J Cancer, 27*(9), 1095–1099.

13. Zelmanowicz, A., Hildesheim, A., Sherman, M., Sturgeon, S., et al. (1998). Evidence for a common etiology for endometrial carcinomas and malignant mixed mullerian tumors. *Gynecol Oncol 69,* 1253–1258.

14. Shepard, J.H. (1989). Revised FIGO staging for gynaecological cancer. *Br J Obstet Gynaecol, 96*(8), 889–892.

15. Gallup, D.G., & Cordray, D.R. (1979). Leiomyosarcoma of the uterus: Case reports and a review. *Obstet Gynecol Surv, 34*(4), 300–311.

16. Larson, B., Silfversward, L., Nilsson, B., & Pettersson, F. (1990). Mixed muellerian tumors of the uterus—prognostic factors: A clinical and histopathologic study of 147 cases. *Radiother Oncol, 17*(2), 123–132.

17. Gerszten, K., Faul, C., Kornelis, S., Huamg, Q., et al. (1998). The impact of adjuvant radiation therapy on carcinosarcomas of the uterus. *Gynecol Oncol, 68,* 8–13.

18. Antman, K.H. (1993). Uterine sarcomas. In R.C. Knapp & K.S. Berkowitz, eds., *Gynecological Oncology* 2nd ed. (p. 247). New York: McGraw-Hill.

19. Antman, K.H. (1997). Adjuvant therapy of sarcomas of soft tissue. *Semin Oncol, 24,* 556–560.

20. Katz, L., Merino, M.J., Sakamoto, H., & Schwartz, P. (1987). Endometrial stromal sarcoma: A clinicopathologic study of eleven cases with determination of estrogen and progestin receptor levels in three tumors. *Gynecol Oncol, 26*(1), 87–97.

21. Peters, W.A., Kumar, N.B., Fleming, W.P., & Morley, G.W. (1984). Prognostic features of sarcomas and mixed tumors of the endometrium. *Obstet Gynecol, 63*(4), 550–556.

22. Major, F.J., Blessing, J. A., Silverber, S.G., et al. (1993). Prognostic factors in early stage uterine sarcomas. A Gynecology Oncology Group Study. *Cancer, 71,* 1702–1709.

23. Rose, P.G., Piver, M.S., Tsukada, Y., & Lau, T. (1989). Patterns of metastasis in uterine sarcoma. *Cancer, 63* (5), 935–938.

24. Rotmensch, J., Rosenshein, N.B., & Woodruff, J.D. (1983). Cervical sarcoma: A review. *Obstet Gynecol Surv, 38*(8), 456–460.

25. Azoury, R.S., & Woodruff, J.D. (1971). Primary ovarian sarcoma. *Obstet Gynecol, 37*(6), 920–940.

26. Anderson, B., Turner, D.A., & Benda, J. (1987). Ovarian sarcoma. *Gynecol Oncol, 26*(2), 183–192.

27. Hacker, N.F. (1989). Vulvar cancer. In J.S. Berek & N.F. Hacker, eds., *Practical Gynecologic Oncology* (pp. 416–417). Baltimore: Williams & Wilkins.

28. Morrow, C.P., & Townsend, D.E. (1987). *Synopsis of Gynecologic Oncology* 3rd ed. (pp. 82–84). New York: Wiley.

29. Hicks, M.L., & Piver, M.S. (1992). Conservative surgery plus adjuvant therapy for vulvovaginal rhabdomyosarcoma, diethylstilbestrol clear cell adenocarcinoma of the vagina, and unilateral germ cell tumors of the ovary. *Obstet Gynecol Clin North Am, 19*(1), 219–233.

30. Chekyrn, J. (1984). Cancer recurrence: Personal meaning, communication, and marital adjustment. *Cancer Nurs, 7*(6), 491–498.

31. Mahon, S.M., Cella, D.F., & Donovan, M.I. (1990). Psychosocial adjustment to recurrent cancer. *Oncol Nurs Forum, 17*(3, Suppl.), 47–52.

32. Bonica, J.J. (1986). Treatment of cancer pain: Current status and future needs. *Adv Pain Res Ther, 9,* 589–616.

33. White, E.J. (1986). Home care of the patient with advanced cancer. *Semin Oncol Nurs, 3*(3), 216–221.

34. Benedict, S. (1989). The suffering associated with lung cancer. *Cancer Nurs, 12*(1), 34–40.

35. Billings, J.A. (1985). *Outpatient Management of Advanced Cancer* (pp. 80–87). Philadelphia: Lippincott.

36. Holmes Grobel, B., & Lawler, P.E. (1985). Malignant pleural effusions. *Oncol Nurs Forum, 12*(4), 34–40.

37. Billings, J.A. (1985). *Outpatient Management of Advanced Cancer* (pp. 121–125). Philadelphia: Lippincott.

38. Dollinger, M., Rosenbaum, E.H., & Cable, G. (1992). *Everyone's Guide to Cancer Therapy* (pp. 560–566). Kansas City, KS: Somerville House.

39. Saba, M.T., & Magolan, J.M. (1991). Understanding cerebral edema: Implications for oncology nurses. *Oncol Nurs Forum, 18*(3), 449–505.

40. Ryan, L.S. (1981). Nursing assessment of the ambulatory patient with brain metastases. *Cancer Nurs, 4*(8), 281–291.

Cancer of the Breast

Jacqueline Balon, RN, MSN, CS, NP, OCN
Teresa C. Wehrwein, RN, PHD, CNAA

INTRODUCTION

Breast cancer is a frequently occurring disease for which many women perceive personal vulnerability. The approximate lifetime risk for receiving a diagnosis of breast cancer is 12.3% in American women.[1] The frequency with which this disease occurs, the variety of medical treatment options available, and the psychosexual implications of the loss of a breast combine to make caring for a woman with breast cancer a challenging nursing experience.

Anatomy

The breast is a mammary gland that lies on the anterior chest wall from the second to sixth ribs and laterally between the axilla and sternum (Figure 10.1). Posterior to the breast lie the pectoralis major and minor muscles. The gland consists of fifteen to twenty lobes, which are radially arranged and connected to the nipple by way of ducts. The ducts form minute openings in the nipple. The skin of the nipple is pigmented

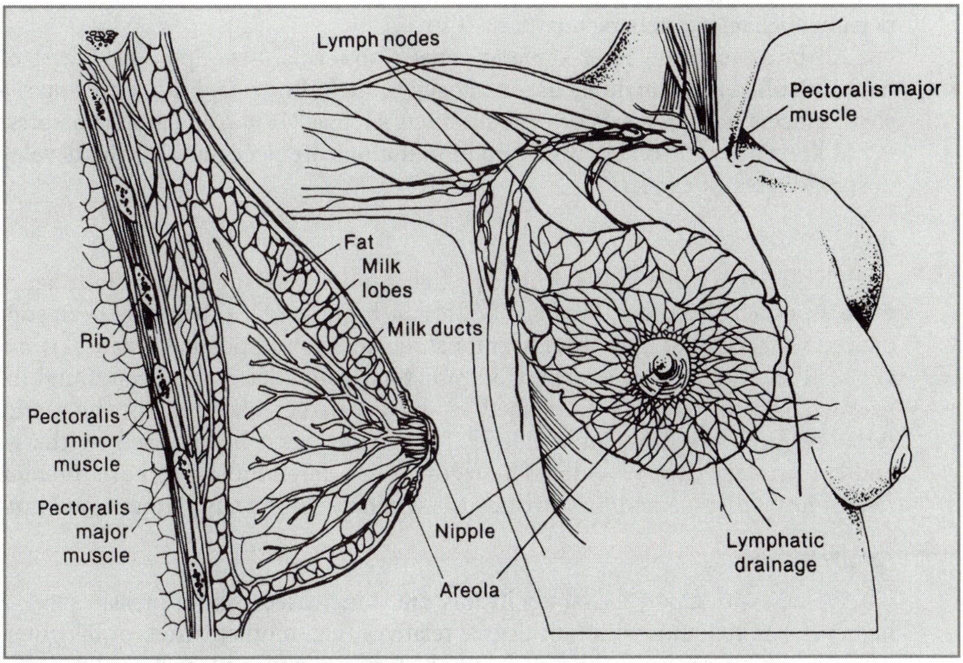

FIGURE 10.1. Anatomy of the breast.

Source: Reproduced with permission from DiSaia, P.J., & Creasman, W.T. (1993). *Clinical Gynecologic Oncology* 4th ed. (p. 469). St. Louis, MO: Mosby–Year Book, Inc.

and roughened by papillae, which extend 1 to 2 cm to form the areola. The primary lymphatic drainage sites for the breast are the axillary, infraclavicular, and supraclavicular lymph nodes. The breasts are drained medially by the internal mammary lymph nodes.

Estrogen and progesterone influence the configuration of the breast. These hormones cause an increase in the proportion of periductal connective tissue, fat deposition, ducts, lobes, and breast tissue. Familial tendency and body size influence the size and shape of the adult female breast. At menopause, the fatty tissue disappears slowly, and the breast atrophies to a pendulous fold of skin.[2]

The primary physiologic function of the breast is lactation. However, it is often associated with femininity and sexuality, especially in Western cultures.

Etiology and Incidence

The incidence of breast cancer in American women has increased from 1 in 11 to almost 1 in 8 in the past decade.[1] Increasingly young women are being diagnosed with this disease, with the greatest increase seen in young black women.[3] Although correlational data are available regarding risk factors, few definitive links have been established. Factors that appear to be most significant include family history and reproductive history. The data are less consistent in assessing risks associated with other personal behavior or characteristics.

All breast cancers have somatic genetic abnormalities. Sporadic breast cancers have identified abnormalities in several genes, including *p53*, *bcl-2*, and *c-myc*, and in some cancers normal genes or gene products such as HER-2/neu are overexpressed. It is not known what number and type of mutations are necessary for the development of sporadic breast cancer.[4]

Age

The woman's age is a significant factor, with risk increasing with age. Older women, especially those over age 55, are at highest risk. There has been some evidence to suggest that long-term hormonal replacement in postmenopausal women increases the risk of breast cancer. Contradictory results have also been found in other research. DiSaia's review of published results revealed no clear relationships, and additional research is still recommended.[5] These risks must be assessed by the woman and her primary care provider. The factors considered most often are the increased risk of heart disease and/or osteoporosis when hormone supplements are not used.

Family History

Women with a positive family history are at increased risk for breast cancer. Risk is highest for individuals with first-degree relatives (i.e., mother, sister, or daughter) who have had breast cancer. While all family history is significant, maternal relatives with breast cancer are more closely associated with a woman's risk than is disease in paternal relatives. Recent research has identified BRCA1 and BRCA2 as contributing factors for some familial breast cancers. An 85% lifetime risk of breast cancer is associated with both of these mutations. One group in which the BRCA1 mutation has been identified is Ashkenazi Jewish women. Risk of other cancers including ovarian and colon is also increased. This research is aiding in the differentiation of high-risk individuals who develop breast cancer due to hereditary disposition and not other risk factors.[6]

The psychosocial, ethical, and legal implications of genetic testing have not been fully explored. A woman's decision regarding testing may have both personal and family impact. Assessment should include both the behavioral and mood manifestations and its implications, whether the woman has tested positive or negative or has declined to be tested. Nurses are encouraged to review and consider recommendations of professional organizations in planning care for women receiving genetic testing.[7]

Other factors that contribute include country of birth. There is a higher risk for women born in North America and northern Europe. Japanese women have a lower breast cancer risk than North American women. This decreased risk is also seen in first-generation Japanese-American women, but Japanese-American women born in subsequent generations in the United States have an incidence of breast cancer more similar to the general North American rate.[8]

Reproductive History

Incidence of breast cancer is higher in both nulliparous women and those who are over 30 at the time of their first pregnancy.[9,10] Some evidence has been presented that breastfeeding decreases the risk of breast cancer,[11] but these findings have not been consistently replicated in other studies.[3] Early menarche and late menopause have also been associated with increased risk of breast cancer.[3] And a slight but significant increase in breast cancer risk is also reported for women who took diethylstilbestrol (DES) during pregnancy.[12] Use of oral contraceptives does not appear to increase risk of breast cancer, but research continues regarding the impact of prolonged use of oral contraception.

Other Personal Factors

Excess weight, a high-fat diet, and alcohol intake have been suggested as factors contributing to breast cancer risk. Consistent evidence to support the specific cause of these relationships has not been determined. Women who engage in regular, vigorous exercise have been found to have decreased risk of breast cancer compared to sedentary women.

In summary, the most significant risk factors for breast cancer include family history of the disease, especially in a mother or sister; increased age; and nation of birth. These factors are not modifiable risks but identify individuals who should receive increased screening for early detection. Research continues to attempt to identify modifiable risks that significantly impact breast cancer rates. At this point, health promotional intervention that supports maintaining normal body weight and a low-fat diet appears to be most promising.

Breast Cancer Cell Types

The cellular types of breast cancer can be characterized by both the histologic grade and nuclear grade of the tumor cells (Table 10.1). The histologic grade incorporates observed cellular growth patterns, and nuclear grade evaluates the nuclei. Histologic grade 1/nuclear grade 3 is descriptive of a well-differentiated tumor, which is associated with a better prognosis. Histologic grade 3/nuclear grade 1 is a poorly differentiated tumor, with a poorer prognosis. Women who have histologically high grade, poorly differentiated invasive breast cancer have more occurrences of axillary node involvement, develop more recurrences, and are more likely to die of metastatic disease than women with low-grade tumors.[13] This grading system is similar to that employed for other cancers. However, in breast cancer, the stage of the disease is more significant than the histologic grade.

Breast cancers that arise in epithelial tissue are classified as adenocarcinomas. There are several histologic types, and they are classified as either ductal or lobular. The most common type is infiltrating ductal, which comprises approximately 80% of breast cancers. The grade can range from well differentiated to poorly differentiated, the latter having the least favorable prognosis. On appearance, this tumor is a strong, hard mass and has a gritty texture. Infiltrating ductal carcinoma most commonly affects women in their 50s. Invasive lobular is the second most common type of breast cancer. It occurs most frequently in women 55 years and older. The invasive lobular subtype accounts for 5 to 10% of breast cancers. The two types are similar in prognosis and nodal involvement, with the exception that lobular carcinoma more frequently develops in both breasts, and there are some differences in common metastatic sites between the two forms. Lobular carcinomas tend to spread to meningeal and serosal surfaces, and ductal carcinomas spread to bone or sites in the lung, liver, and/or brain.[14]

TABLE 10.1

Comparision of Histologic and Nuclear Grading

Histologic Grade	Nuclear Grade	
Grade 1	Grade 3	Well differentiated
Grade 2	Grade 2	Intermediate
Grade 3	Grade 1	Poorly differentiated

Source: Adapted with permission from Fisher, B., Osborne, C.K., Margolese, R., & Bloomer, W. (1993). Neoplasms of the breast. In J.F. Holland, E. Frei, R.C. Bast, et al., eds., *Cancer Medicine* 3rd ed. (pp. 1752–1775). Philadelphia: Lea & Febiger.

The less common types of adenocarcinomas are the medullary and mucinous/colloid types. Medullary carcinomas constitute 5 to 7% of all breast cancers. They are soft in texture, may be large, have a rapid growth rate, and are common in younger women. Mucinous carcinomas, which constitute about 2% of breast cancers, are slow growing, tend to metastasize late, and occur in women 60 to 70 years of age. Another type of breast cancer is tubular carcinoma, which makes up around 2%. They are usually well-differentiated adenocarcinomas. A characteristic of tubular carcinomas is microcalcifications, which can be detected early on mammography. Both axillary lymph node involvement and distant metastasis are uncommon.[15]

Inflammatory carcinoma is characterized by a red-purplish color, warmth, edema, and induration of the skin (the so-called peau d'orange appearance, which resembles an orange skin; Figure 10.2). A palpable tumor is not generally present. The prognosis for these patients is poor even though there may be no sign of metastatic disease at the time of diagnosis.[14]

Paget's disease is found in 1 to 4% of all breast cancer patients. In this disorder, the nipple area is scaly and eczematous. It may be accompanied by the following additional signs and symptoms: burning, discharge, itching, and bleeding. The underlying carcinoma is palpable in about two-thirds of the patients.[14] The specific histologic type of tumor tissue determines the prognosis.

Disease Pattern

The breast is divided into four quadrants. Most tumors occur in the upper-outer quadrant (there is more tissue in this area), followed by the upper-inner quadrant, lower-

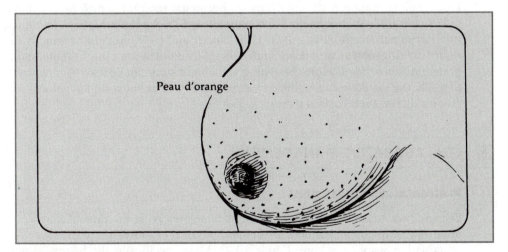

FIGURE 10.2. Peau d'orange appearance.

Source: Dr. Susan Love's Breast Book. (Figure 17–3, p. 233), © 1991 by Susan M. Love, M.D. Reprinted by permission of Addison-Wesley Publishing Company, Inc.

outer quadrant, and then the lower-inner quadrant. Approximately 17% of tumors are found around the areola. The exact tumor location does not convey useful prognostic information.[16]

Breast cancer spreads regionally via the lymphatic system and systemically via the blood system. The original concept of tumor spread, described by Haagensen, stated that breast cancer begins as a local disease, then spreads chronologically from the original site to the regional lymph nodes before distant sites.[14] However, later research, supported by the National Surgical Adjuvant Breast and Bowel Project (NSABP), has found that this may not be true. There may be involvement of the supraclavicular and infraclavicular nodes without disease present in the axillary nodes.[15] There is a strong correlation between distant metastatic disease and involvement of the supraclavicular nodes. If the primary lesion is located in the medial aspect of the breast, the internal mammary lymph nodes, which receive about 25% of the lymph fluid leaving the breast, may also be affected. If these nodes are involved, chances of recurrence are greater compared to individuals with only axillary node involvement.[15] In other words, breast cancer may metastasize to a distant location before, during, or after it spreads to local lymph nodes.

Breast cancer is a highly unpredictable, complex disease. Subclinical metastasis may be present at the time of diagnosis. In individuals who were treated with apparently curative surgery (with or without radiation therapy) there may be delayed onset of metastasis. Metastasis may also be found at the time of diagnosis, early in the disease, or after a long disease-free interval. The most common sites of metastasis are bone, lung, liver, and brain. One of the risk factors associated with the spread of disease is tumor size at diagnosis. There is about a 25% risk of metastasis for a 1 cm tumor and a 50% risk for a 3 to 4 cm tumor. Along with tumor size, histology, histologic grading, lymph node involvement, hormonal receptor status, and menopausal status play a role in prognosis. Flow cytometry of DNA ploidy–S-phase fraction, peptide hormonal receptors (c-erB-2 (HER-2/neu) and p 53) and cathepsin D are still under investigation as prognostic indicators. Standardization of techniques and interpretation is necessary before these prognostic indicators can be used as measurements to guide the management of breast cancer patients. The most important indicator of risk for distant metastasis is lymph node status.[4]

❈ COLLABORATIVE MANAGEMENT

Pretreatment Assessment

Because breast cancer is often systemic or disseminated at the time of diagnosis, it is important to obtain a complete history and physical examination when a woman presents with a suspicious lump (Table 10.2). More specifically, the history should include breast and axillary symptoms, medical history of breast disease, reproductive history, and family history. The physical examination should include careful assessment of the musculoskeletal and respiratory systems as well as of the breast and ax-

TABLE 10.2		
Nursing Assessment Criteria		
Medical/Surgical History	History of breast disease or biopsies	
Family History	History of breast cancer in mother, daughter, sister, aunt(s), or grandmother	
Reproductive History	Age at onset of menses and/or menopause Age at first pregnancy Number of pregnancies History of breast feeding	
Breast/Axillary Symptoms (Date)	Breast mass Nipple or skin discharge Nipple or skin retraction Axillary swelling or pain	
Additional Symptoms (Metastatic Spread)	Bone pain Respiratory problems	
Psychosocial Assessment	Support system Sexuality Spirituality	
Physical Examination	Breast mass Skin changes Nipple changes/discharge Axillary nodal status	
Mammogram	Diagnostic Digital mammography CAD (computer-assisted diagnosis)	
Biopsy	Type of breast cancer Cell growth rate Hormone receptor tests	
Radiologic	Sonogram Chest X-ray Bone scan CT (if abnormal laboratory studies)	
Other Lab	Chemistries	

illa.[14] A malignancy is most frequently located in the upper-outer quadrant or beneath the nipple, and more often in the left breast than in the right. A palpable mass that is fixed and has less discrete boundaries is more likely to be malignant than a movable, distinct mass. Other characteristics of a malignancy include nipple retraction or elevation, skin dimpling or retraction, skin edema, and ulceration of the skin.

After the physical exam, a bilateral mammogram is performed. This should take place before a biopsy is obtained. The mammogram can often give a more definitive look at the breasts before surgery and disclose the presence of unsuspected lesions. However, if a mass is palpated, a biopsy should still be performed even in the case of a negative mammogram.[14] Computer tomography (CT scans), magnetic resonance imaging (MRI), and ultrasound may facilitate lesion identification but cannot detect small lesions. The use of a positron emission tomography (PET) scan may be useful in identifying smaller tumors and may differentiate between a viable tumor and scar tissue, and even between benign and malignant axillary nodes.[15]

Mammography is most effective in postmenopausal women, who have less dense breast tissue. Routine mammography in this age group is most likely to identify tumors too small to be found by palpation. Ultrasound is frequently used in conjunction with mammography to determine the nature (cystic vs. solid) of a suspicious area.

Ninety percent of all palpable breast lumps are discovered by the woman herself. These are usually accidental findings with no symptoms. The mass may be tender, but it is often painless. A painful mass, however, is not always benign.[17]

Mammography is least accurate in premenopausal women, and controversy continues as to the timing of initial screening. Women with suspicious masses or a history of fibrocystic disease that is not visualized on mammography would still be biopsied.[14]

Before any treatment can be initiated, a confirmation of the diagnosis must be obtained. Aspiration and open biopsy are two mechanisms for determining a breast malignancy (Figure 10.3). The two types of cytologic studies are fine-needle aspiration and core-needle tissue-sampling. Incisional and excisional biopsies are the two forms of open biopsies that are also performed. These studies are all used for diagnostic purposes. Core biopsies provide tissue for evaluation of hormonal receptor levels. Estrogen and progesterone receptor levels assist in the determination of a treatment plan and prognosis.

Two new strategies for obtaining biopsies for nonpalpable and/or small tumors are stereotactic needle-guided biopsy and wire localization biopsy. The stereotactic needle-guided biopsy is done to target and identify mammographically detected nonpalpable lesions in the breast. Very small tumors, areas of calcifications, superficial lesions, and lesions that are extremely lateral or medial do not benefit from this type of procedure. Wire localization is similar, but its goal is to locate nonpalpable lesions for the purpose of minimizing the deformity during surgical excision of the lesion. After the biopsy a specimen mammogram is performed to ensure that all of the area of abnormality has been removed.[15]

There are no definitive biologic markers for breast cancer. However, if levels are elevated before treatment is initiated, several serum tumor markers have been used for follow-up. The most common of these are carcinoembryonic antigen (CEA) and CA 15–3. Both CEA and CA 15–3 levels have frequently been shown to be elevated with metastasis and/or recurrence. CA 15–3 has also been shown to be elevated in benign breast and gastrointestinal diseases.[14] An abdominal CT scan is performed when an elevated CEA or elevated liver enzymes are detected, to investigate potential metastatic

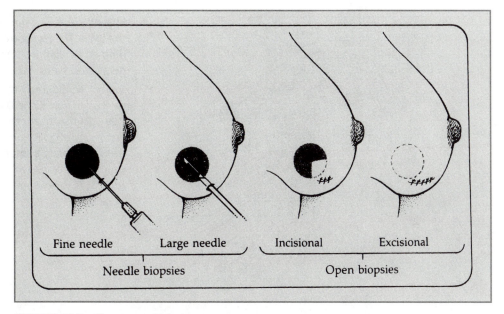

FIGURE 10.3. Biopsy procedures.

Source: Dr. Susan Love's Breast Book (Figure 10–1, p. 124), © 1991 by Susan M. Love, M.D. Reprinted by permission of Addison-Wesley Publishing Company, Inc.

disease in the liver. A bone scan is performed as a baseline and/or if there is some evidence of bony disease, bone pain, or an unexplained increase in alkaline phosphatase.

Another indicator of disease spread is axillary lymph node and/or supraclavicular lymph node involvement. Palpable nodes do not always mean spread of disease.[14] Histologic involvement is more significant than enlargement. The more proximal the lymph node involvement, the better the prognosis. The axilla is divided into three levels (Figure 10.4). Level I (proximal) is the tissue located inferior to the lower edge of the pectoralis minor muscle. Level II (middle) includes tissue beneath the pectoralis minor. Level III (distal) is the tissue that is superior to the pectoralis minor.[14] Prognosis is dependent on both the level and number of lymph nodes involved. However, studies have concluded that prognosis is more closely related to the number of involved lymph nodes than their location.[13]

Late signs and symptoms (Figure 10.5) can be exhibited as gross local spread of primary tumor and/or distant metastasis. Skin retraction, or dimpling of the skin, is often associated with cancer, although fat necrosis and plasma cell mastitis can produce the same signs. Other late signs are asymmetry of the breasts, scaling or edema of the skin, nipple erythema, peau d'orange skin, bloody discharge from the nipple, and ulceration of the breast.

Distant metastases may sometimes be found at the time of diagnosis. After biopsy, the staging work-up should include a chest X-ray, a baseline bone scan, and liver

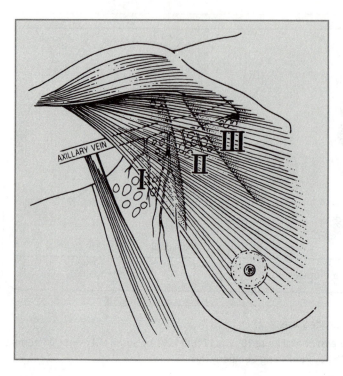

FIGURE 10.4. Anatomy of the axilla. The levels are defined in relation to the pectoralis minor muscle.

Source: Reproduced with permission from Kinne, D.W. (1991). Primary treatment of breast cancer. In J.R. Harrris, S. Hellman, I.C. Henderson, & D.W. Kinne, eds., *Breast Disease* 2nd ed. (p. 357). Philadelphia: J.B. Lippincott.

chemistries. An abdominal CT scan is not done unless the liver enzymes are elevated or the liver is enlarged. Studies of the brain (CT or MRI scans) are done only in the presence of central nervous system symptoms.

Another important parameter to include in the assessment is the psychosocial status of the patient. In exploring quality of life issues in women with breast cancer, Ferrell discovered four primary domains that need to be investigated: physical well-being, psychological well-being, social concerns, and spiritual well-being.[18] It is important to explore the patient's and family's concerns regarding the impact of the disease on their lives. The woman with breast cancer and her significant others are confronting both a potentially fatal and disfiguring disease. Assessment should include the patient's general knowledge of breast cancer and its treatment, and personal experience with friends or relatives with any cancer, but with breast cancer in particular.[19] Preconceptions related to cancer and its treatment should be assessed. There may be not only loss of a body part, but also a change in self-esteem. Individuals who place a priority on appearance may have a higher anxiety level than those who do not.[20] It is also very important to investigate the individual's coping strategies and how she has dealt with stress in the past, and the woman's support systems. Finally, it has been found that anxiety can interfere with the ability to think clearly and make decisions.[21] Gathering this information and being aware of these factors enable the nurse to understand the individual's response to her disease.

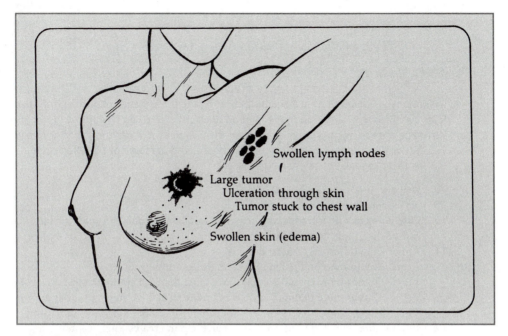

FIGURE 10.5. Advanced breast cancer.

Source: Dr. Susan Love's Breast Book (Figure 17–2, p. 233), © 1991 by Susan M. Love, M.D. Reprinted by permission of Addison-Wesley Publishing Company, Inc.

The factors in the baseline assessment need to be taken into account not only at the time of diagnosis but in continual assessments while caring for such patients. Northouse and colleagues' longitudinal study of breast cancer patients showed that, eighteen months after diagnosis, patients reported an improvement in both mood disruption and role function, regardless of the stage of the disease, but their concerns and worry did not decrease with time.[22]

Staging

Breast cancers are grouped according to the extent of disease, which includes size of tumor, nodal involvement, and distal spread. Staging of disease requires an accurate clinical and pathologic exam. Clinical staging is useful in determining the therapeutic approach and serves as a baseline. It includes not only a physical exam but laboratory and radiologic findings. The pathologic staging is based on the results of biopsy and study of resected tissue, including the size of the mass and the number of lymph nodes involved.

Staging helps define the natural progression of the disease. The most widely used staging system is the tumor-node-metastasis (TNM) system (Table 10.3), which is ad-

TABLE 10.3

TNM Classification System for Breast Cancer

Primary Tumor (T)

Definitions for classifying the primary tumor (T) are the same for clinical and for pathologic classification. The telescoping method of classification can be applied. If the measurement is made by physical examination, the examiner will use the major headings (T1, T2, or T3). If other measurements, such as mammographic or pathologic, are used, the examiner can use the telescoped subsets of T1.

TX Primary tumor cannot be assessed
T0 No evidence of primary tumor
Tis Carcinoma *in situ:* Intraductal carcinoma, lobular carcinoma *in situ,* or Paget's disease of the nipple with no tumor
T1 Tumor 2 cm or less in greatest dimension
   T1mic Microinvasion 0.1 cm or less in greatest dimension
   T1a   Tumor more than 0.1 cm but not more than 0.5 cm in greatest dimension
   T1b   Tumor more than 0.5 cm but not more than 1 cm in greatest dimension
   T1c   Tumor more than 1 cm but not more than 2 cm in greatest dimension
T2 Tumor more than 2 cm but not more than 5 cm in greatest dimension
T3 Tumor more than 5 cm in greatest dimension
T4 Tumor of any size with direct extension to (a) chest wall or (b) skin, only as described below
   T4a   Extension to chest wall
   T4b   Edema (including peau d'orange) or ulceration of the skin of the breast or satellite skin nodules confined to the same breast
   T4c   Both (T4a and T4b)
   T4d   Inflammatory carcinoma (See the definition of inflammatory carcinoma in the introduction.)
Note: Paget's disease associated with a tumor is classified according to the size of the tumor.

Regional Lymph Nodes (N)

NX Regional lymph nodes cannot be assessed (e.g., previously removed)
N0 No regional lymph node metastasis
N1 Metastasis to movable ipsilateral axillary lymph node(s)
N2 Metastasis to ipsilateral axillary lymph node(s) fixed to one another or to other structures
N3 Metastasis to ipsilateral internal mammary lymph node(s)

Pathologic Classification (pN)

pNX Regional lymph nodes cannot be assessed (e.g., previously removed, or not removed for pathologic study)

TABLE 10.3 *(continued)*

pN0 No regional lymph node metastasis
pN1 Metastasis to movable ipsilateral axillary lymph node(s)
  pN1a   Only micrometastasis (none larger than 0.2 cm)
  pN1b   Metastasis to lymph node(s), any larger than 0.2 cm
      pN1bi   Metastasis in 1 to 3 lymph nodes, any more than 0.2 cm
            and all less than 2 cm in greatest dimension
      pN1bii   Metastasis to 4 or more lymph nodes, any more than 0.2
            cm and all less than 2 cm in greatest dimension
      pN1biii Extension of tumor beyond the capsule of a lymph node
            metastasis less than 2 cm in greatest dimension
      pN1biv   Metastasis to a lymph node 2 cm or more in greatest
            dimension
pN2 Metastasis to ipsilateral axillary lymph nodes that are fixed to one another or to
    other structures
pN3 Metastasis to ipsilateral internal mammary lymph node(s)

Distant Metastasis (M)

MX   Presence of distant metastasis cannot be assessed
M0   No distant metastasis
M1   Distant metastasis (includes metastasis to ipsilateral supraclavicular lymph node(s))

Stage Grouping

Stage	T	N	M
Stage 0	Tis	N0	M0
Stage I	T1*	N0	M0
Stage IIA	T0	N1	M0
	T1*	N1**	M0
	T2	N0	M0
Stage IIB	T2	N1	M0
	T3	N0	M0
Stage IIIA	T0	N2	M0
	T1*	N2	M0
	T2	N2	M0
	T3	N1	M0
	T3	N2	M0
Stage IIIB	T4	Any N	M0
	Any T	N3	M0
Stage IV	Any T	Any N	M1

Note: T1 includes T1mic.

**Note:* The prognosis of patients with N1a is similar to that of patients with pN0.

Source: American Joint Committee on Cancer. (1998). *Breast* (pp. 159–170). Philadelphia: Lippincott Raven.

vocated by the American Joint Committee on Cancer (AJCC). This system distinguishes between two staging groupings: postoperative-pathologic and clinical-diagnostic. Both of these are used to assist with the treatment and prognosis of this disease.

Prognosis

In addition to the AJCC staging classification, which is based on anatomical findings, other tumor characteristics are influential in determining prognosis and survival (Tables 10.4 and 10.5). These factors include growth rate (proliferative activity), differentiation of the tumor, metastatic potential of the tumor, hormonal receptors, and patient characteristics.[13]

The proliferation of tumor cells is measured by the thymidine labeling index and flow cytometry. The thymidine labeling index is an important prognostic factor. Various studies have shown that the index correlates with the histologic features of the tumor but not the size or presence of nodal involvement. Thus the index has been shown to be a significant prognostic factor for node-negative patients,[14] helping to explain that stage I patients do not have 100% survival rate with treatment. The disadvantage of this test is that viable tumor tissue is needed, and it usually takes about ten days to obtain the results.

Flow cytometry studies the percentage of tumor cells in the DNA synthesis (S-phase) fraction. Specimens for this test can be taken from fresh or frozen tissue,

TABLE 10.4		
Survival Status by Stage of Breast Cancer		
Stage	*5 Years*	*10 Years*
Stage I	90%	76%
Stage II	68	58
Stage III	52	37
Stage IV	10	5

Source: Adapted with permission from Harris, J., Morrow, M., & Bonadonna, G. (1993). Cancer of the breast. In V.T. DeVita, S. Hellman, & S. A. Rosenberg, eds., *Cancer: Principles and Practice of Oncology* 4th ed. (pp. 1264–1332). Philadelphia: J.B. Lippincott.

TABLE 10.5

Survivor Status
by Lymph Node
Involvement

Axillary Status	5 Years	10 Years
None (0)	78%	65%
Node (+)	47	25
1–3 Nodes	62	38
4+ Nodes	32	13

Source: Adapted with permission from Fisher, B., Osborne, C.K., Margolese, R., & Bloomer, W. (1993). Neoplasms of the breast. In J.F. Holland, E. Frei, R.C. Bast, et al., eds., *Cancer Medicine* 3rd ed. (pp. 1752–1775). Philadelphia: Lea & Febiger.

paraffin blocks, or cells from fine-needle aspirations (which are more easily obtainable). Flow cytometry shows the degree of abnormality (aneuploidy) of the DNA content in the tumor cells.[14] A correlation has also been shown between a high S-phase and poorly differentiated, receptor-negative, and aneuploid tumors, all of which are associated with poor long-term outcome.[23]

Hormonal receptor status is important to prognosis. Estrogen receptor (ER+)– and progesterone receptor (PR+)– positive levels are associated with better prognosis. Postmenopausal women with a positive estrogen receptor status have a better prognosis than premenopausal women with negative estrogen (ER–) receptor status. A controversy still exists regarding the need for treatment with tamoxifen in estrogen/progesterone receptor–positive women with very small tumors (<1.0 cm) who do not have node involvement but have a high S-phase fraction tumor.[14] The high S-phase fraction would tip the scales in favor of treatment despite the otherwise favorable prognostic factors. But positive hormonal receptors are a good prognostic indicator whether or not lymph node involvement has been found.[14] Estrogen receptor–positive tumors more frequently have recurrence in the bone, whereas estrogen receptor–negative tumors recur frequently in soft tissue or the viscera.[15]

Age, weight, and race have also been correlated with survival rates. Although studies on age have been controversial, one done in the 1980s by Hibberd found that women aged 20 to 34 years had survival rates of 37, 35, and 35% at 10, 20, and 30 years, respectively, whereas the 55 to 64 year age group had lower survival rates: 35,

22, and 19% at the same intervals.[24] However, causes of death other than breast cancer may be implicated in the decrease in survival in the latter age group.[14]

Weight and cholesterol have been shown to play a role in survival. A reduced five-year survival was found for obese patients, patients weighing more than 150 pounds, and women with an elevated cholesterol level.[25] Overweight patients have also been shown to have a higher incidence of positive lymph nodes and disease recurrence compared to age-matched normal weight patients.[26]

Race may be a factor in breast cancer survival. Black women have been shown to present at more advanced stages than white women. Caucasian women are more frequently diagnosed with smaller tumors and with node-negative disease. These phenomena may be related to health care access issues rather than any physiologic tendency. However, research in this area is in progress.

Treatment Strategies

Noninvasive Cancer

There are two main types of noninvasive carcinoma: lobular carcinoma in situ (LCIS) and ductal carcinoma in situ (DCIS). These two diseases are different in presentation and treatment options. LCIS has no distinct clinical characteristics, is not found on a mammogram, and does not present as a palpable mass. It is usually an incidental finding by a pathologist investigating a specimen for a benign condition.[27] It is shown to be bilateral in about 20 to 30% of the cases. If untreated, it may lead to cancer in one or both breasts. The abnormal cells occur within the lobules of the breast. There are three options for treatment: observation, ipsilateral mastectomy, or bilateral mastectomy if both breasts are involved. Radiation and systemic therapy are not indicated.[14] In the case of mastectomy, breast reconstruction is a viable option. If observation is the choice, close follow-up through a yearly mammogram is indicated.

Unlike LCIS, DCIS often presents with a positive mammogram finding or bloody nipple discharge. It rarely involves the lymph nodes, but lymph node dissection is recommended when the lesion is >5 cm.[28] There are three treatment options: wide excision (lumpectomy), wide excision with radiation therapy (preferred method), and total mastectomy.[14] In this type of disease, the nipple-areola should also be removed because of the risk of microscopic Paget's disease. Breast reconstruction is an option for the women who elect a mastectomy. It has been shown that DCIS may be a precursor lesion, since invasive cancer can develop in the same area as the noninfiltrating lesion.[14]

Invasive Cancer

The overall treatment regimen for early stage I or II disease has changed over the past five years as knowledge has improved regarding the mechanism of breast cancer spread. Traditionally, surgery was the method of choice and was done quickly. This is because it was once believed that the natural history of the cancer was that it started in the breast, slowly enlarged, invaded the lymph node chain into the axilla, and finally spread throughout the body. However, data currently exist showing that cancers can be present for eight to ten years before diagnosis and may micrometastasize prior to diagnosis.[29] Thus systemic therapy for potential micrometastases is now the primary therapy for early stage invasive breast cancer. It has been shown to increase survival by 30% in Stage I node-negative women, especially in women with larger tumors. Women who have the lowest risk of recurrence are individuals whose tumor is less than 2 cm, are ER and PR positive, have a histologic grade of I, and have a low proliferation rate.[30]

The two components of therapy for early stage disease are local therapy and systemic therapy. The purpose of local therapy for early stage breast cancer is to eliminate cancer within the breast and prevent local recurrence. Local therapy involves a mastectomy or lumpectomy followed by radiation therapy.[27]

In this regard, the National Institutes of Health has stated, "Breast conservation treatment (excision of the primary tumor plus radiation therapy) is an appropriate method of primary therapy for the majority of women with stage I or II breast cancer, and is preferable because it provides survival equivalent to total mastectomy and axillary dissection while preserving the breast. However, there may be times when this option will not be the best form of treatment and mastectomy may be the preferred option.[31] The criteria used to recommend mastectomy are found in Table 10.6.

The choice of systemic therapy is dependent on menopausal status, hormonal receptor status, and stage of disease. If there is direct evidence or a high probability of metastatic disease, then systemic therapy may be done before local treatment is initiated. Systemic treatment can be either chemotherapy or hormonal therapy. It is a fact that women do not die of cancer in the breast but rather of cancer that spreads to vital organs.

Locoregionally advanced disease is classified as stage III. These patients have large tumors and/or positive axillary nodes that have become attached to each other or the surrounding tissue (IIIa). More advanced disease entails infraclavicular, internal mammary, and/or supraclavicular node extension, skin involvement, ulceration, and edema in the breast (IIIb). Stage IIIa is managed, for the most part, like Stage II, that is, with surgery and radiation, surgery and chemotherapy, or a combination of all three treatment modalities. Stage IIIb had been considered inoperable in most cases. Recent studies have shown that more than 65% of women receiving preoperative chemother-

---

TABLE 10.6

Criteria for Recommending Mastectomy

High tumor/breast size ratio

Inability to obtain clear margins of resection in the lumpectomy specimen

Multifocal involvement

Previous breast irradiation

Inability of lung to tolerate radiation

apy or hormonal therapy decreased their tumors more than 50%. Most previously inoperable tumors become operable. Locoregional treatment in nonoperable cases can be made more effective by surgical removal of the primary tumor. However treatment is, for the most part, palliative and the goal is to obtain a response.[30]

By definition, Stage III does not include patients with distant metastases. But the poor results of local and regional treatment may indicate that the majority of these patients have occult distant micrometastases at the time of diagnosis.[29] Locoregional treatment in nonoperable cases can be made more effective by surgical removal of the primary tumor.

Inflammatory adenocarcinoma is generally found in Stage IIIb, and inflammatory disease is considered inoperable. The usual treatment is multiagent systemic chemotherapy along with local-regional irradiation. Mastectomy for these women does not improve survival. However, local control of disease may be recommended for palliation if there is ulceration at the primary tumor site.

Stage IV is classified as clinical evidence of distant metastases. Radical surgery is not the therapy of choice for this disease. A simple mastectomy may be performed to reduce tumor burden prior to radiation therapy. Systemic chemotherapy and hormonal therapy are used to provide palliation and keep the disease under control.[14]

Surgical Options

Various types of surgical procedures can be performed to provide locoregional control of breast cancer (Figure 10.6). Table 10.7 categorizes and defines the terminology used for the various surgical procedures. Neither the quadrantectomy nor simple mastectomy is commonly performed.

Frequently, mastectomy specimens demonstrate multifocal involvement. This potential must be considered at the time of planning the surgical procedure and follow-up treatment. The modified radical mastectomy (total mastectomy) has been the treatment of choice in the past; however, current lumpectomy procedures with external irradiation have produced equivalent survival rates.[13]

Lymph Node Dissection. Axillary lymph node dissection is the removal of lymph nodes on the affected side of the breast lesion. It has been used for both staging purposes and providing prognostic information. Recent studies, however, have indicated that either irradiation of the nodes or observation of the lymph nodes until there is evidence of lymph node involvement produces results equivalent to initial lymph node dissection.[14]

Axillary lymph node dissection provides prognostic information but has little therapeutic benefit especially in women who are lymph node negative. It is also responsible for an increase in morbidity (lymphedema) associated with breast surgery. A new procedure, sentinel node mapping, has been found to be highly effective in the hands of a surgeon experienced with this technique. This procedure has spared patients with clinically negative axillary lymph nodes of an axillary dissection if the sentinel node was found to be negative.[32] An alternative technique is to do axillary lymph node sampling as opposed to axillary lymph node dissection, which reduces the chance of lymphedema.[30]

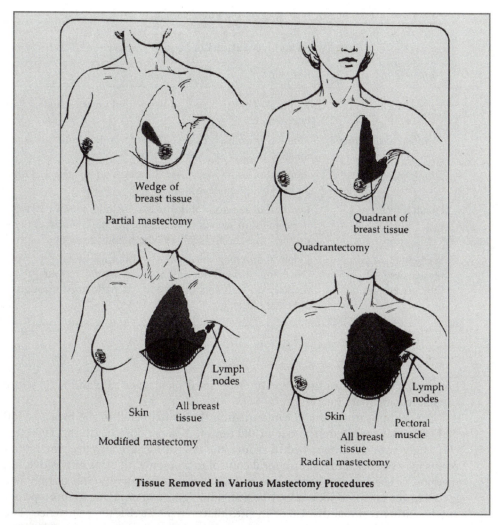

Wedge of
breast tissue

Partial mastectomy

Quadrant of
breast tissue

Quadrantectomy

Lymph
nodes

Skin   All breast
tissue

Modified mastectomy

Lymph
nodes

Skin

Pectoral
muscle

All breast
tissue

Radical mastectomy

Tissue Removed in Various Mastectomy Procedures

FIGURE 10.6. Surgical procedures for breast cancer.

Source: Dr. Susan Love's Breast Book (Figure 21–2, p. 285), © 1991 by Susan M. Love, M.D. Reprinted by permission of Addison-Wesley Publishing Company, Inc.

Radiation Therapy

Radiation therapy is similar to surgery in that they both act as local therapy for the breast cancer patient. Radiation with lumpectomy is an alternative to mastectomy. It is also used in conjunction with surgery for locoregional control of breast cancer. With lumpectomy, it is the primary mode of therapy for women whose disease is limited to the breast and local lymph nodes.[13] Radiation therapy and lumpectomy have been shown to be as effective as mastectomy for stage I and II disease. Lumpectomy alone,

TABLE 10.7

Terms and Definitions in Breast Surgery

Surgery Term	Definition
Radical mastectomy	Removal of entire breast, skin, pectoral muscles, and axillary lymph nodes
Modified radical/total mastectomy	Removal of entire breast, skin, and pectoralis minor muscle, and axillary lymph nodes
Simple mastectomy	Removal of entire breast and pectoralis minor muscle without axillary lymph node dissection
Quadrantectomy	Removal of a quarter of the breast. Includes removal of the overlying skin, sheath covering the pectoral muscle, entire pectoral muscle, and axillary lymph node dissection
Segmental/partial mastectomy, lumpectomy, tylectomy	Removal of tumor and small rim of normal tissue. Overlying skin and underlying fascia are not excised. Axillary node dissection, if done, is performed through a separate incision.

however, has shown an unacceptably high local recurrence rate and is therefore not considered adequate treatment.[13]

The amount of external beam radiation that is delivered to the breast is 4500 to 5000 cGy, depending on the size of the tumor. A boost dose of around 1000 to 1500 cGy is given to the tumor bed to reduce the risk of local recurrence. Interstitial implants may be added to increase local control in women with close or positive surgical margins.[14] The therapy begins two to four weeks after surgery and usually is completed in about five to six weeks. Interstitial implants can be added to this type of therapy for either residual disease or in sites that may be at risk for recurrence. The implants are in place for about two to three days. Also, electron boosts to the scar area may be added to decrease the risk of recurrence at that site.

Radiation in conjunction with chemotherapy has been used preoperatively for large, bulky tumors to reduce tumor burden prior to surgery. It is also used after mastectomy for stage III and stage IV disease for control of disease on the chest wall. Studies have shown continuing debate on the sequencing of chemotherapy and radiation therapy after surgery. The recent randomized trials revealed that administering chemotherapy prior to radiation has reduced the incidence of distant metastasis, while others support the opposite order to reduce local recurrence.[30]

There are both early and late reactions to radiation therapy. One early reaction involves the skin. Skin changes depend on the dose and may vary from hyperpigmentation and dry skin to moist desquamation. In addition, skin turgor changes to a rubbery consistency and sometimes becomes very firm and/or fibrotic. This reaction can make it difficult to palpate for recurrence. Fatigue is another reaction that generally occurs with radiation therapy.

Late reactions include radiation pneumonitis, rib fractures, and lymphedema. These reactions may occur anywhere from three months to years after therapy.

Adjuvent Chemotherapy

Women with involved lymph nodes, hormone receptor–negative tumors, and/or aggressive metastatic disease in the liver or respiratory system often receive single or multiagent chemotherapy. Combination chemotherapy is the preferred regimen. Cyclophosphamide, methotrexate, and 5-fluorouracil (CMF), with or without prednisone, and cyclophosphamide, doxorubicin (Adriamycin), and 5-fluorouracil (CAF) were commonly used regimens. Both have been shown to have a 50 to 70% response rate, and responses typically last for about nine to twelve months. The complete response rate is 10 to 20%. The most effective single agent in the treatment of breast cancer is doxorubicin (Adriamycin).[13] New studies have shown that adjuvant therapy with four cycles of Adriamycin and cyclophosphamide followed by four cycles of taxol have had an increase in survival in women who are node positive than with the previous regimens. It has also been shown that women who are node negative and ER and PR negative have benefited from four cycles of Adriamycin and cyclophosphamide.[30]

The use of adjuvant chemotherapy has been shown to increase survival in premenopausal and perimenopausal women when a four- to six-month course of chemotherapy is given after definitive primary treatment. This is true in both node-negative and node-positive women, but the magnitude of the effect is greater in the node-positive group.[13]

New treatment modalities that are being studied include chemoimmunotherapy, chemohormonal therapy, and hypothalamic hormone analogs. Combination of chemotherapy and tamoxifen in premenopausal women has been recommended especially for women with a high risk of recurrent disease. The use of HER-2 overexpression has shown some promise to predict a breast cancer patient's responsiveness to chemotherapy or hormonal agents in the adjuvant or metastatic settings but remains controversial. Methods of standardization and techniques for testing are not fully established. A new drug, an anti-HER-2 antibody (Herceptin) has been shown to be promising in women who have failed standard chemotherapy and have the overexpression of this gene.[30] Other therapeutic investigations include alternating drug combinations, preoperative adjuvant chemotherapy, and cell-cycle synchronization.[34] High-dose chemotherapy and peripheral stem cell transplant are presently being used to treat advanced cases of breast cancer in both the adjuvant and metastatic setting. Clinical trials are used to continue to evaluate the effectiveness of this treatment.

High-dose chemotherapy and autologous bone marrow or peripheral stem cell transplantation have been used in patients who have a good performance status but have shown poor response to traditional treatments, and in patients unlikely to benefit from conventional treatment. The latter have been identified as either stage II with at least ten positive axillary lymph nodes or stage III by the Eastern Cooperative Oncology Group in trial EST2190.[17] But transplantation has been shown to have high morbidity and mortality rates. Side effects include not only hemorrhage, infection, and organ failure, but also quality of life and psychological issues.[35]

The clinical course in the treatment of metastatic breast cancer is dependent on a number of factors such as variations in the tumor growth rate and responsiveness to systemic therapy. Chemotherapy, hormonal therapy, radiation therapy, and limited surgery are all used in the treatment of metastatic breast cancer. Today the taxanes (second generation) and vinorelbine (third generation) drugs have shown some promise and the response rate ranges from 30 to 40%. New drugs, anti-HER-2 antibody (Herceptin) and capecitabine (Xeloda), have also shown promise in women with advanced disease. The main goals are palliation and prolonging life with treatment that will obtain maximum control of symptoms, prevent serious complications, and promote quality of life (Table 10.8).[30,36]

Chemoprevention. In 1992 the National Surgical Adjuvant Breast and Bowel Project (NSABP) initiated a five-year tamoxifen trial to determine if this antiestrogen agent could lower the primary occurrence of breast cancer in high-risk individuals. Another goal of this study was to determine whether tamoxifen lowers the incidence of myocardial infarction or bone fractures. The double-blind study's aim was to accrue 16,000 high-risk women 35 years or older, who were then randomized between the tamoxifen group and the placebo group. Women between the ages of 35 and 59 years were evaluated for eligibility to determine if, based on a combination of risk factors (number of first-degree relatives with breast cancer; history of lobular carcinoma in situ; history of atypical hyperplasia; history of previous breast biopsies; nulliparity; age at first live birth; age at menarche), their risk of developing breast cancer is at least that of a 60-year-old woman. For each woman, the annual and lifetime probability of developing breast cancer was estimated utilizing the Gail model of risk assessment. In this study, placebo or tamoxifen was administered for at least five years. Toxicity and compliance monitoring, quality of life assessment, lipid and lipoprotein evaluation, and other studies were major components of this trial.[37,38]

In 1994 the accrual of new subjects for this study was temporarily suspended due to internal problems in the NSABP. Although the risk associated with developing uterine cancer secondary to tamoxifen use is uncertain, women in the study were exposed to this potential risk factor. Thus the study was revised to include a prestudy endometrial sampling with yearly follow-up for five years.[38]

The primary objective of NSABP was to determine if tamoxifen could reduce the incidence of invasive breast cancer in women with a prior history of lobular carcinoma in situ and atypical hyperplasia. The results showed tamoxifen to be beneficial. There was an approximate 50% reduction in the incidence of both invasive and noninvasive breast cancer in the premenopausal women studied. Research is continuing to determine optimum length and timing of preventative tamoxifen therapy.

Prophylactic use of tamoxifen therapy is not without risks. An increased incidence of endometrial cancer was found. However, for very high risk individuals, the benefit seems to outweigh the risk.[39]

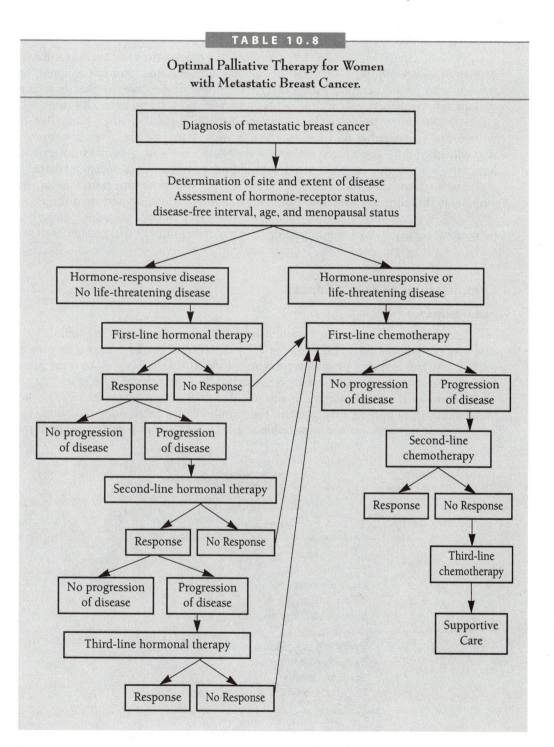

TABLE 10.8

Optimal Palliative Therapy for Women
with Metastatic Breast Cancer.

Hormonal Therapy

Adjuvant tamoxifen therapy has significantly reduced the risk of recurrence in women of all age groups. Hormonal therapy has been a major form of treatment for women who have systemic breast cancer with hormone-positive disease. First-line therapy for postmenopausal women with metastatic disease who have ER+ tumors is tamoxifen (an antiestrogen). The maximum benefit is greatest when tamoxifen is given for five years rather than for one to three years. It may also be given in conjunction with chemotherapy. Recent analysis of the NSABP trials suggest that women who have estrogen receptor–negative tumors should not be treated with hormonal therapy. If tamoxifen becomes ineffective, other hormonal agents, such as megestrol acetate or aminoglutethimide, and arimidex (aromatase inhibitors) can be added to the therapy.[15] Other agents such as trioxifene (an antiestrogen that does not appear to be hepatocarcinogenic in rats) and anastrozole (an aromatase inhibitor that has not been associated with weight gain) are also being used.[15,30]

Complications of Breast Cancer

Bone Metastasis

Bone metastasis is the most common complication of breast cancer (Table 10.9). The first symptom is pain in the area of bony destruction by the tumor. The pain is usually constant and gets progressively worse. Laboratory studies may be done prior to X-ray and bone scans to evaluate pain, specifically serum chemistries including an alkaline phosphatase and calcium levels. Alkaline phosphatase levels are usually elevated in the event of bone involvement. Calcium level may be elevated if there is significant bone destruction. A complete blood count (CBC) is also performed, and re-

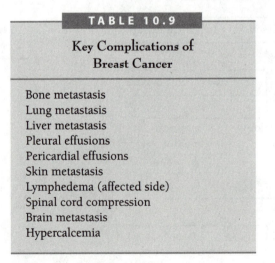

TABLE 10.9

Key Complications of
Breast Cancer

Bone metastasis
Lung metastasis
Liver metastasis
Pleural effusions
Pericardial effusions
Skin metastasis
Lymphedema (affected side)
Spinal cord compression
Brain metastasis
Hypercalcemia

sults showing anemia, leukocytosis, thrombocytopenia, and immature forms of circulating nucleated red blood cells may be indicative of bone marrow involvement.[17]

The metastatic infiltrate in the bone may not be seen on plain X-ray until the lesion is at least 1.0 to 1.5 cm in diameter with a 30 to 50% loss of bone mineral content. A bone scan is often performed to determine the full extent of the osseous metastases throughout the body.[14] A bone biopsy may also be necessary to document metastatic breast disease in the bone. This is especially important if there is a long disease-free interval or no evidence of metastatic disease.

Painful fractures may result from destruction of the bone by the metastatic lesion. These fractures may cause immobility and vascular and neurologic damage. Radiation therapy is usually given to the involved bony lesion for pain relief and recalcification of bone. If the bony involvement is widespread, only the symptomatic areas may be irradiated; other lesions are treated with hormones and/or chemotherapy. Anti-inflammatory agents such as prednisone and nonsteroidal pain medications such as ibuprofen can be given for pain relief.[17] The use of biphosphonates (pamidronate and clodronate) added to the present regimen has been shown to reduce pain and the incidence of complications and to prolong survival free of bone-related complications.[40]

Palliative surgery may be indicated for impending fractures. Stabilization of the fracture is done to keep the individual mobile. Immobility secondary to lytic lesions in the bone contributes to the development of pneumonia, deep-vein thrombosis, and hypercalcemia. Range-of-motion activities, turning/positioning, and leg exercises can aid in preventing these complications.

Hypercalcemia

Hypercalcemia is a complication caused by immobility and metastatic disease in the bone. This problem is due to excess bone resorption and impaired renal calcium excretion. The symptoms are nonspecific, numerous, and vague. Hypercalcemia develops slowly. Common symptoms include vomiting, polyuria, polydipsia, nausea, anorexia, weakness, bone pain, confusion, and fatigue. Early identification of symptoms is important to reduce the risk of irreversible renal failure, coma, or cardiac arrest.[17]

Treatment initially consists of correcting renal function, generally by aggressive hydration with normal saline, with or without furosemide, and an antihypercalcemic agent such as pamidronate disodium.[14] The underlying cause of the bone resorption and osteoclast activity should be treated, if possible, with an antineoplastic drug. Urgent treatment is required when corrected serum calcium levels are greater than 13.0 mg/dl or when the patient is symptomatic. Asymptomatic patients with a lower calcium level also require treatment, but not with the same urgency. If the disease cannot be controlled, then the goal of treatment is palliative.

Spinal Cord Compression

Another oncologic emergency associated with breast cancer is spinal cord compression. This situation needs an immediate response because of the potential for paralysis. Spinal cord compression can be due to an epidural tumor or a lytic lesion in the vertebrae. The symptoms initially are subtle. Pain may be present for a period of time before the patient develops any neurologic deficits, which might include bowel or bladder dysfunction, increase in back pain, gait disturbances, and weakness, as well as paralysis.[17]

An MRI scan of the spine is performed to determine the exact location of the compression. Once determined, radiation to the affected area and corticosteroids are used for treatment. Depending on the neurologic damage, the patient may be able to regain body functions and ambulate. A decompression laminectomy can also be performed in a selective population whose neurologic deficits worsen while on radiation therapy. However, only about 50% of patients are expected to regain lost motor functions.[14]

✖ DISCHARGE TEACHING

Teaching patients about their postoperative care should begin at the preoperative assessment visit. While providing support and information to assist the woman in her treatment decision process, the nurse can begin to provide information and hands-on demonstration of postoperative care. Preparation and practice prior to surgery can increase patients' confidence in their ability to provide self-care in the home.

Physical Care

The woman who has had either a mastectomy or lumpectomy with axillary lymph node dissection is at risk for the development of lymphedema in the affected arm. A drain for the collection of fluid is usually inserted during the surgical procedure that includes lymph node dissection. During hospitalization, the nurse may need to empty the drainage device and record both the amount and characteristics of the drainage. If the drain ceases to function during the hospitalization, it may indicate that the device is obstructed, in which case the patient should be observed for development of pain and edema in the affected arm.

Prior to discharge, the patient requires instruction on a number of topics (Table 10.10). One is the correct method to empty the device. Identifying ways to secure the drain to clothing can facilitate mobility without increasing pressure on the drain or incision line. Additional teaching includes observation to detect increasing lymphedema or infection. The drain is usually removed by the surgeon at the first office visit after discharge. The patient should notify the physician if the drainage stops and fluid begins to accumulate in her arm and axilla, or if she detects signs of infection.

The patient also needs to be instructed on exercises to decrease swelling and improve mobility. The extreme form of edema that used to be associated with radical mastectomy procedures is rarely seen today, but mild forms persist for many women. Formal exercise regimens are generally not started until the drainage device is removed and the wound is healed. However, a mild form of exercise can be practiced in the immediate postoperative period by instructing the woman to use her affected arm

TABLE 10.10

Patient Education

Potential for Recurrence

1. Reinforce follow-up with physician for additional treatment as needed.
2. Encourage maintenance follow-up examination and scheduled mammography.
3. Reinforce BSE techniques and encourage monthly checks.
4. Encourage patient to notify physician of any lump or thickening found during BSE, or if bone pain, unexplained weight loss, cough or hoarseness, changes in menses, or gastrointestinal or neurologic symptoms develop.

Potential for Infection

1. Teach signs and symptoms of infection, and encourage inspection of arm and axilla on affected side.
2. Avoid injury, including burns from cooking or skin irritation from cleaning.
3. Avoid sunburn through use of sunscreen and loose, long-sleeved clothing.
4. Use electric razor to shave under arms. Use extreme caution initially, as sensitivity may be increased.
5. Use gloves when gardening or using strong cleaners.
6. Never cut cuticles. Push back gently with lotion to soften.
7. Use a thimble when sewing.

Potential for Injury

1. Carry heavy bags and shoulder bags on unaffected side.
2. Have all injections, blood draws, and blood pressure readings done on unaffected side.
3. Wear loose-fitting watches and jewelry on affected side.
4. Avoid elastic-banded sleeves on clothing.
5. Use insect repellent to avoid bites and stings.
6. Do exercises to retain range of motion and strength when approved by physician.

when brushing her hair or teeth and while showering. Formal exercises to increase strength and range of motion include arm swings, pulley motion, wall climbing, and rope turning (Figure 10.7). In addition to exercises, many women find it more comfortable to elevate the arm when sitting or reclining. Making a pumping motion with the affected hand by squeezing a ball or other soft object can also assist in decreasing edema.

With the removal of the axillary lymph nodes, a woman is at increased risk for infection in the arm on the affected side. The National Cancer Institute's publication *After Breast Cancer: A Guide to Follow-up Care*[41] provides a list of recommendations on how patients should protect the affected arm. Precautions are avoiding burns,

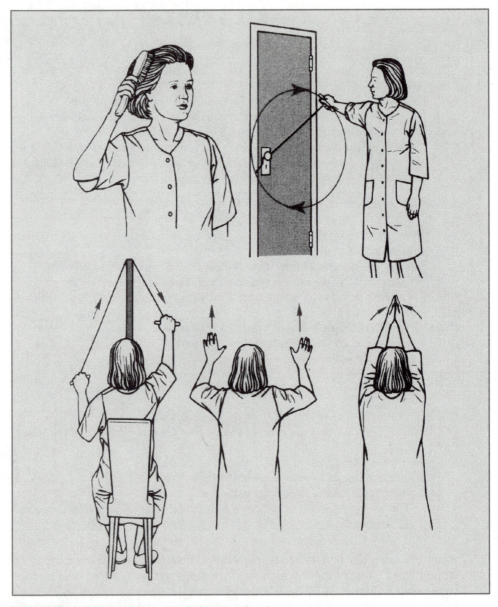

FIGURE 10.7. Postoperative mastectomy exercises.

Source: Reproduced with permission from Lewis, S.M., & Collier, I.C. (1992). *Medical Surgical Nursing* 3rd ed. (p. 1392). St. Louis, MO: Mosby–Year Book.

sunburn, and insect bites; cleaning and treating all cuts promptly; avoiding cutting cuticles and using caution with nail care; carrying heavy objects on the unaffected side; and notifying the health care provider promptly at any signs of inflammation.

Most women do not require home nursing care after surgery. But predischarge instructions should include recommendations to ensure adequate rest to allow for recovery. Care related to the chemotherapy or radiation that may be used for these patients is discussed in Chapters 11 and 13.

In addition to routine postsurgical follow-up, most women also have some postsurgical treatment. Following completion of treatment, examinations may initially be scheduled every three months. The interval between visits is gradually increased as the disease-free interval increases. Recurrences, however, may be seen many years after initial diagnosis, so lifetime follow-up is a must. Annual mammography, chest X-ray, blood studies, and professional breast examinations are routinely included in long-term follow-up care.

Monthly breast self-examination (BSE) should continue to be stressed in patient teaching (Figure 1.2). Observe the woman's technique during teaching and watch for signs of hesitancy to examine the affected side or the unaffected breast. Review the patient's technique with her and encourage her to perform regular BSE. Women who have had a mastectomy should be instructed to examine the chest wall skin on the affected side, as well as the unaffected breast.

Many breast cancer patients choose to add complementary therapies including mental imaging, meditation, diet, and nutritional supplements to their treatment regimen. While practice varies widely concerning the addition of complementary therapies within traditional care settings, nurses should obtain information on these modalities, including dosage and frequency of nutritional supplements.

Psychosocial Planning

The woman diagnosed with breast cancer may experience a grief reaction related to both the loss of a body part and the potential for death from the disease. Breast cancer may increase feelings of vulnerability in individuals who value their ability to control their lives, and for some women this can be more threatening than the physical changes. After surgery, assessing the woman for her perceptions of losses associated with the disease needs to be ongoing. Discharge planning may include instruction that some women experience delayed anger or depression in response to the disease and treatment, delays that can vary in length from days to months. Counseling or support groups should be offered to the woman who needs long-term emotional support. Caution the patient that at times family or friends may not be the most supportive people to whom to verbalize fears or concerns. These individuals may also be traumatized by her disease and thus unable to respond in a manner the woman would need or like.

Community groups are available to assist patients following breast cancer. Reach for Recovery, sponsored by the American Cancer Society, and Y-ME, sponsored by the YWCA, are two such groups. These agencies have volunteers who have

TABLE 10.11

Diagnostic Cluster

Diagnostic/Preoperative and Postoperative Period

COLLABORATIVE PROBLEMS
Potential Complication: Bleeding/hemorrhage
Potential Complication: Thromboembolic event
Potential Complication: Infection/sepsis
Potential Complication: Atelectasis/pneumonia

NURSING DIAGNOSIS
1. Potential altered health maintenance related to insufficient knowledge of condition, diagnostic tests, prognosis, and treatment options
2. Decisional conflict related to insufficient knowledge of treatment options
3. Anxiety/fear related to impending surgery, and insufficient knowledge of preoperative routines, intraoperative activities, and postoperative self-care activities
4. Potential for anticipatory grieving related to change in body image following proposed surgical interventions
5. Altered comfort related to effects of surgery, disease process, and immobility
6. Potential for infection related to susceptibility to bacteria secondary to surgical wound and lymphadenectomy
7. Potential for grieving related to loss of all or portion of breast
8. Potential for impaired physical mobility related to decrease in strength and discomfort of affected arm
9. Potential for self-care deficit: dressing and grooming related to loss of breast and limitation in movement of affected arm
10. Potential for alteration in tissue perfusion, tissue integrity/infection related to lymphedema secondary to surgical removal of lymph nodes
11a. Potential sexual dysfunction related to disease process, surgical intervention, fatigue, and/or pain
11b. Potential altered sexual pattern related to physical changes and emotional connection of breast with female sexuality
11c. Disturbance in self-concept: body image related to loss of all or portion of breast
12. Potential altered health maintenance related to insufficient knowledge of dietary restrictions, medications, activity restrictions, self-care activities, symptoms of complications, follow-up visits, and community resources

Treatment Period

COLLABORATIVE PROBLEMS
Potential Complication: Lymphedema
Potential Complication: Hypercalcemia

TABLE 10.11 *(continued)*

Potential Complication: Pathologic fracture
Potential Complication: Pleural effusions

NURSING DIAGNOSIS

1. Anxiety/fear related to loss of feelings of control of life, unpredictability of nature of disease, and uncertain future
2. Anxiety/fear related to insufficient knowledge of prescribed radiation therapy and necessary self-care measures
3. Anxiety/fear related to insufficient knowledge of prescribed chemotherapy and necessary self-care measures
4. Potential for infection related to immunosuppression neutropenia secondary to chemotherapy and/or radiation therapy
5. Potential for bleeding related to immunosuppression thrombocytopenia secondary to chemotherapy and/or radiation therapy
6. Potential alteration in skin integrity related to treatment modality and/or disease process
7. Potential for alteration in comfort related to side effects of therapy and/or disease process

personally experienced breast cancer meet with newly diagnosed individuals. Volunteers are frequently matched with patients on the basis of both disease-related and social variables. Issues such as how others respond to the patient, sexuality, clothing, and the use of prostheses are discussed. Volunteers receive formal training before visits and are provided with current written materials to share with the woman.

The use of a prosthesis is an individual decision for each woman. In addition to total mastectomy prosthetics, partial prostheses are available for patients who have elected conservative surgery. Purchase of a permanent prosthesis is usually deferred for six to eight weeks after surgery to allow for healing and decrease of postoperative edema. But the woman can be temporarily assisted with a soft, fiberfill prosthesis and advised to wear loose-fitting clothing, which may be more comfortable. Clothing advice may be especially important for women for whom physical appearance is a major issue.

Breast Reconstruction

Most women have the option of either wearing an external prosthesis or having reconstructive surgery following mastectomy. The choice of procedure varies from implantation of a silicone or saline prosthesis under the musculofascial layer to translo-

cation of a flap of skin and muscle tissue to the chest wall. Reconstruction is contraindicated in progressively metastatic, locally advanced, and inflammatory breast
cancer. Women who are obese, smoke, had previous abdominal surgery, or have conditions that impair circulation may not be candidates for autologous reconstruction
techniques.

Reconstruction may be done immediately or delayed until the completion of radiation and/or chemotherapy. Immediate reconstruction does not normally delay adjuvant treatment. It may decrease body image disturbance and eliminate the need for
an additional anesthetic induction. Comparable cosmetic results, however, can be
achieved with delayed reconstruction. Preoperative counseling should include discussion of reconstructive options and consultation with a plastic surgeon for specific procedural recommendations. Supporting the woman's decision regarding reconstruction
or her decision to delay her choice regarding reconstruction is an important part of the
nursing role during the preoperative period. Postprocedural photographs can assist

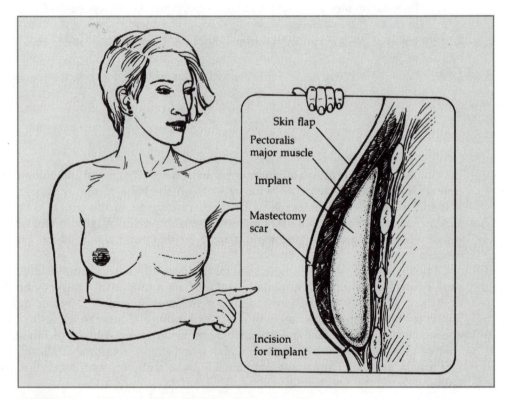

FIGURE 10.8. Silicone implant for breast reconstruction.

Source: Dr. Susan Love's Breast Book (Figure 25–2, p. 351), © 1991 by Susan M. Love, M.D. Reprinted by
permission of Addison-Wesley Publishing Company, Inc.

the patient to make an informed decision about the type of reconstructive surgery she wishes to have.[15]

Much controversy has recently centered around the use of silicone implants. After investigating the side effects of such implants, the FDA rescinded approval of their use in April 1992 except by breast cancer patients.[14]

Either implant is positioned behind the pectoralis muscle. A silicone prosthesis (Figure 10.8) cannot expand, so small-breasted women generally have more cosmetically acceptable results with one. The saline implant (Figure 10.9) can be expanded over time to stretch the muscle and skin, and can later be replaced by an appropriately sized permanent silicone sack. The latter process is often uncomfortable and takes several months to complete.

There are several different reconstructive procedures using the woman's own tissue. Three procedures that were generally used were the latissimus dorsi muscle flap, rectus (abdominal) muscle flap, and the gluteus maximus musculocutaneous flap and microsurgical transfer (Figures 10.10 and 10.11). The TRAM (transverse rectus abdominal muscle) flap and free tram flap are more commonly used today. The free tram flap is the newest technique in reconstruction and has been shown to reduce complications, require a shorter hospital stay, and provide a better cosmetic outcome.[15] Postprocedural photographs can assist the patient to make an informed decision about the type of reconstructive surgery she wishes to have.

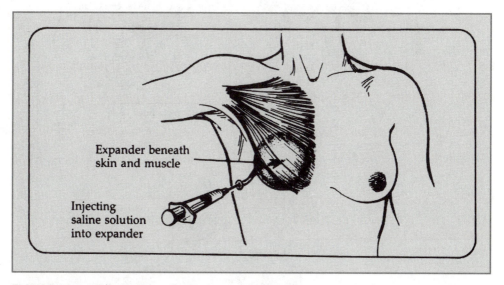

FIGURE 10.9. Saline implant for breast reconstruction.

Source: Dr. Susan Love's Breast Book (Figure 25–3, p. 352), © 1991 by Susan M. Love, M.D. Reprinted by permission of Addison-Wesley Publishing Company, Inc.

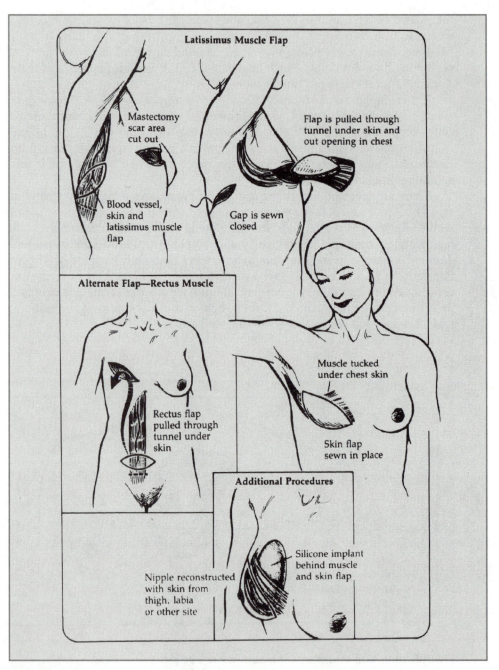

FIGURE 10.10. Latissimus muscle flap and rectus muscle flap reconstructive techniques.

Source: Dr. Susan Love's Breast Book (Figure 25–4, p. 354), © 1991 by Susan M. Love, M.D. Reprinted by permission of Addison-Wesley Publishing Company, Inc.

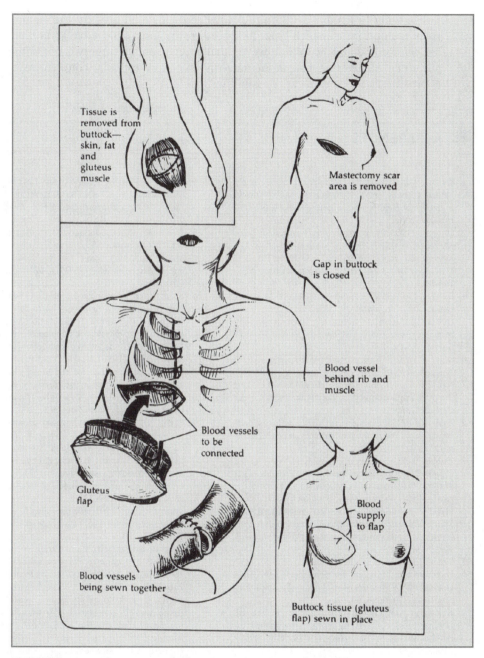

FIGURE 10.11. Gluteus muscle flap reconstructive technique.

Source: Dr. Susan Love's Breast Book (Figure 25–5, p. 356), © 1991 by Susan M. Love, M.D. Reprinted by permission of Addison-Wesley Publishing Company, Inc.

In order to make a decision regarding reconstructive surgery, the woman may be given the options of which types of procedure are most acceptable and/or available to her. She should also be told, however, that reconstructive surgery is not without complications. Hematoma, soft-tissue necrosis, infection, capsular contracture, extrusion of prosthesis, and seroma are possibilities.

❈ REFERENCES

1. Ries, L., Miller, B., et al. (1973–1991). *SEER Cancer Statistics Review* (p. 124). Bethesda, MD: National Institutes of Health, US Department of Health and Human Services.
2. Gray, H. (1985). *Anatomy of the Human Body* 13th ed. (pp.1581–1587). Boston: Jones and Bartlett.
3. Kelsey, J.L., & Gammon, M.D. (1991). The epidemiology of breast cancer. *Cancer J Clin, 41*(3), 146–165.
4. Ravdin, P.M. (1997). Prognostic factors in breast cancer. *Am J Clin Oncol, 39,* 217–227.
5. DiSaia, P.J. (1996). Hormone replacement therapy in gynecologic and breast cancer patients. *Cancer Control, 3,* 101–106.
6. Daly, M. (1994). New perspectives in breast cancer: The genetic revolution. *Oncol Nurs, 1*(6), 1–10.
7. Nguyen, A.D. (1997). The genetics of breast cancer: Provider implications. *Innovations in Breast Cancer Care, 2*(4), 70–77.
8. Buell, P. (1973). Changing incidence of breast cancer in Japanese-American women. *J Natl Cancer Inst, 51*(5), 1479–1483.
9. Pathak, D.R., Speizer, F.E., Willett, W.C., et al. (1986). Parity and breast cancer risk: Possible effect of age at diagnosis. *Int J Cancer, 37*(1), 21–25.
10. Layde, P.M., Webster, L.A., Baughman, A.L., et al. (1989). The independent associations of parity, age at first full term pregnancy, and direction of breast-feeding with risk of breast cancer. *J Clin Epidemiol, 42*(10), 963–973.
11. Byers, T., Graham, S., Rzepkait, A., et al. (1985). Lactation and breast cancer: Evidence for negative association in premenopausal women. *Am J Epidemiol, 121*(5), 664–674.
12. Colton, T., Greenburg, E.R., Noller, K., et. al. (1993). Breast cancers in mothers prescribed diethylstilbestrol in pregnancy. *JAMA, 269,* 2069–2100.
13. Fisher, B., Osborne, C.K., Margolese, R., & Bloomer, W. (1993). Neoplasms of the breast. In J.F. Holland, E. Frei, R.C. Bast, et al., eds., *Cancer Medicine* 3rd ed. (pp. 1752–1775). Philadelphia: Lea & Febiger.
14. Harris, J., Morrow, M. & Norton, L. (1997) Cancer of the Breast. In V.T. DeVita, S. Hellman, S. Rosemburg, eds. *Cancer: Principles and Practice of Oncology* 5th ed. (pp. 1557–1616).
15. Chapman, D., & Goodman, M. (1997). Breast cancer. In Groenwald, S.L., Frogge, M.H., Goodman, M., & Yarbo, C.H., eds., *Cancer Nursing Principles and Practice* 4th ed. (pp. 931–932). Boston: Jones & Bartlett.
16. Black, J., & Matassaarin-Jacobs, E. (1993). Nursing care of a client with breast disorders. In J. Luckmann & K.C. Sorensen, eds., *Medical Surgical Nursing: A Psychophysiologic Approach* 4th ed. (pp. 2173–2196). Philadelphia: Saunders.
17. Donegan, W. (1988). Diagnosis. In W.L. Donegan & J. Spatt, eds., *Cancer of the Breast* 3rd ed. (pp. 125–163). Philadelphia: Saunders.
18. Ferrell, B. (1993). Overview of breast cancer: Quality of life. *Oncol Patient Care, 3*(3), 7–9.
19. Turns, D. (1988). Psychosocial factors. In W.L. Donegan & J. Spatt, eds., *Cancer of the Breast* 3rd ed. (pp. 728–736). Philadelphia: Saunders.
20. Leinster, S., Ashcroft, J., Slade, P., et al. (1989). Mastectomy versus conservative surgery: Psychosocial effects of the patient's choice of treatment. *J Psychosoc Oncol, 7,* 179–192.
21. Wainstock, J. (1991). Breast cancer: Psychosocial consequences for the patient. *Semin Oncol Nurs, 7*(3), 207–215.
22. Northouse, L., Cracchiiolo-Caraway, A., & Appel, C. (1991). Psychologic consequences of breast cancer on partner and family. *Semin Oncol Nurs, 7*(3), 216–233.
23. Meyer, J. (1988). Cell kinetics of breast and breast tissue. In W.L. Donegan & J. Spatt, eds., *Cancer of the Breast* 3rd ed. (pp. 250–266). Philadelphia: Saunders.
24. Hibberd, A.D., Harwood, L.J., & Wells, J.E. (1983). Long-term prognosis of women with breast cancer in New Zealand: Study of survival to thirty years. *Br Med J, 286,* 1777–1779.
25. Jones, D., Schatzkin, A., Green, S., et al. (1987). Dietary fat and breast cancer in the National Health

and Nutrition Examination Survey: I Epidemiologic follow-up study. *J Natl Cancer Inst, 79*(3), 465–471.

26. Ballard-Barbash, R., Schatzkin, A., Carter, L., et al. (1990). Body fat distribution and breast cancer in the Framingham study. *J Natl Cancer Inst, 82*(24), 286–290.

27. Kalinoski, B. (1991). Local therapy for breast cancer: Treatment choices and decision making. *Semin Oncol Nurs, 7*(3), 187–193.

28. Recht, A., Sadowsky, N., & Cady, B. (1990). Clinical problems in follow-up of patients after conservative surgery and radiotherapy. *Surg Clin North Am, 70*(5), 1179–1187.

29. Baum, M. (1990). Trends in primary breast cancer management. *Surg Clin North Am, 70*(5), 1187–1192.

30. Hortobagy, G. (1998). Treatment of breast cancer. *N Engl J Med, 339*(14), 974–984.

31. National Institutes of Health (1990). *Consensus Development: Conference Consensus Statement, 8*(6). Washington, DC: National Institutes of Health.

32. Sounding Board (1998). Sentinel-lymph node biopsy for breast cancer—not yet the standard of care. *N Engl J Med, 339*(14), 990–995.

33. De Valeriola, D., Awada, A., Roy, J., et al. (1997). Breast cancer therapies in development. *Drugs, 54*(3), 385–413.

34. Whedon, M. (1993). Emerging treatments. *Oncol Patient Care, 3*(3), 8–9.

35. Pryor, T., & Maher, K. (1998). Stem cell transplantation in advanced breast cancer. *Am J Nurs,* Supplement (April), 30–33.

36. Slamon, D., Leyland-Jones, B., Ahak, S., et al. (1998). Addition of Herceptin (Humanized Anti-HER2 Antibody) to First Line Chemotherapy for HER2 Expressing Metastatic Breast Cancer Markedly Increases Anticancer Activity: A Randomized, Multinational, Controlled Phase III Trial. *ASCO Annual Meeting Highlights* (pp. 6, 7).

37. Gould, K., Gates, M., & Miaskowski, C. (1994). Breast cancer prevention: A summary of the chemoprevention trial with tamoxifen. *Oncol Nurs Forum, 21*(5), 835–847.

38. National Surgical Adjuvant Breast and Bowel Project (1992, 1994). *A Clinical Trial to Determine the Worth of Tamoxifen for Preventing Breast Cancer.* Pittsburgh, PA: NSABP.

39. Wickerham, J.C., Costantino, J.C., Fisher, B., et al. (1998). The Initial Results from the NSABP Protocol P-1: Tamoxifen for Preventing Breast Cancer in Women at Increased Risk. *ASCO Annual Meeting Highlights* (pp. 1–3).

40. Diel, I.J., Solomayer, E.F., Costa, S.D., et al. (1998). Reduction in new metastases in breast cancer with adjuvant clodronate treatment. *N Engl J Med, 339*(6), 357–363.

41. US Department of Health and Human Services (1990). *After Breast Cancer: A Guide to Follow-up Care.* Washington, DC: National Cancer Institute.

Chemotherapy

Lois Almadrones, RN, MS, FNP, MPA

✻ INTRODUCTION

Most gynecologic malignancies are treated with a multimodality approach using surgery followed by chemotherapy, radiation, or both. The specialty of gynecologic oncology is unique because patients may be treated with surgery and chemotherapy by the same physician. Therefore, the nurse caring for gynecologic oncology patients must be equally familiar with the clinical management of the operative patient and the patient receiving chemotherapy. It is imperative for the nurse who practices within this discipline to understand the basic rationale for chemotherapy in the treatment of each type of gynecologic malignancy in order to adequately care for this patient population.

History of Chemotherapy in Gynecologic Oncology

The first chemotherapeutic agent to be used in the treatment of gynecologic malignancies was methotrexate, in the late 1950s, for choriocarcinoma.[1,2,3] Many of the drugs developed and produced from 1945 to 1965 are still in use for the treatment of gynecologic malignancies. These include dactinomycin, melphalan, chlorambucil, cyclophosphamide, 5-fluorouracil, methotrexate, the vinca alkaloids, and progestins.[4] Single agents, such as chlorambucil or melphalan, were standard therapy for ovarian cancer until 1978.[5] In the 1970s, cisplatin entered clinical trials for ovarian cancer. Today, cisplatin and its analogues are still considered the most active agents in the treatment of gynecologic malignancies. Doxorubicin, bleomycin, etoposide, and tamoxifen are other active agents developed during the 1970s.[4] A newer class of antineoplastic agents are the taxanes, of which paclitaxel is the prototype. This natural product was originally isolated from the bark of the Pacific yew, *Taxus brevifolia*.[6] The experimental studies with paclitaxel were completed in the late 1980s.[7] Paclitaxel, which was approved by the FDA for the treatment of refractory ovarian cancer in 1993, has been heralded as the most active agent against this disease since cisplatin. The superiority of combination paclitaxel/cisplatin over cyclophosphamide/cisplatin for initial treatment of epithelial ovarian cancer was demonstrated in the Gynecologic Oncology Group (GOG 111) trial.[8,9] Since that trial, the substitution of carboplatin for cisplatin in combination with paclitaxel in a GOG trial has demonstrated equal efficacy with decreased toxicity and increased ease of administration in the outpatinet setting.[10] Other trials have identified the paclitaxel analogue docetaxel as another active drug that may play a role in chemotherapy for women with gynecologic malignancies.[11,12,13,14]

The use of growth factors has demonstrated efficacy in accelerating hematopoietic recovery and reducing the morbidity associated with the myelosuppressive effects of cytotoxic chemotherapy.[15] Clinical trials have demonstrated the benefit of cytoprotectants in the prevention of toxicity to normal tissues induced by chemotherapy.[16–22] Approved cytoprotectants currently in use prevent or decrease hemorrhagic cystitis caused by ifosfamide, cardiotoxicty associated with doxorubicin, and renal and neurologic toxicities associated with cisplatin. These supportive therapies have led to investigational approaches to the treatment of gynecologic malignancies: dose intensity and dose intensification. These regimens include higher doses of cytotoxic agents given within shorter time intervals in an attempt to kill more cancer cells before drug resistance develops. In addition to allowing investigational trials that it is hoped will improve the survival of women with gynecologic malignancies, growth factors and cytoprotectants have increased the short- and long-term quality of life of women undergoing chemotherapy.

Goals of Treatment

The three major goals of cancer treatment for patients with gynecologic malignancies, as with all cancers, are cure, control, and palliation. The most appropriate goal is recommended by the physician to the patient after thorough diagnostic and metastatic tests and physical examinations have been completed. Considerations included in this decision are the tumor histology, stage and grade of the disease, performance status, age, other medical problems, general health, and the patient's desire to pursue and comply with the recommended treatment. The nurse's role involves understanding the goal of treatment and assessing the patient's role in the family, economic situation, beliefs, values, and cultural norms in order to determine a holistic plan of care that is suited to the patient.[23] If the goal of therapy includes chemotherapy, the nurse must have basic knowledge of the classes of chemotherapeutic agents, their mechanisms of action and efficacy in each gynecologic malignancy, the safest methods of administration, the expected side effects, and their medical and nursing management.

Cure

Most sources[24] consider cure a possibility for a particular disease when a 5- to 10-year survival rate can be achieved and the surviving patient has the same life expectancy as anyone her age and general health. Surgery, radiation, and chemotherapy may be used singly or in combination to achieve cure. Types of gynecologic cancers amenable to cure are choriocarcinoma and early-stage cervical, endometrial, and ovarian cancers. Choriocarcinoma is generally curable with single-agent chemotherapy.[4] Early-stage cervical cancer can frequently be cured by surgery or radiation. Early-stage endometrial cancer can usually be cured with surgery but may be combined with postoperative radiation. Patients with low-grade, early-stage ovarian cancer are often cured by a combination of chemotherapy and surgery. *Adjuvant therapy* is the term used to describe the treatment for a patient who receives chemotherapy after completion of a curative surgical procedure or radiation therapy but for which the risk of tumor recurrence is high.

Control

Control is the goal of treatment when disease is metastatic at the time of diagnosis. Control implies that cure is not possible but benefit may be obtained by retarding tumor growth. Ovarian cancer patients can frequently achieve the goal of control after debulking surgery and adjuvant chemotherapy. These patients frequently enjoy remission from their disease, with subsequent recurrence requiring treatment with additional chemotherapy. Control of disease may allow a patient with ovarian cancer several more optimum quality years of life which otherwise would not be possible.

Palliation

Palliation is considered when the patient has widespread disease normally not amenable to cure or control. The goal of palliation is to relieve intolerable symptoms and allow the patient the optimum quality of life for whatever time remains. The Food and Drug Administration (FDA) enhanced the definition of *palliation* by allowing approval of a drug to be used when it demonstrates beneficial effect on disease-related symptoms or a patient's quality of life. Gemcitabine was the first drug to obtain FDA approval on the basis of using clinical benefit response as the primary efficacy end point in patients with pancreatic cancer.[25,26]

✻ CLASSES OF CHEMOTHERAPEUTIC AGENTS

All cells, both normal and malignant, follow a sequence of five steps or phases as they divide and replicate. Each phase is designated by a letter and a subscript, G_O, G_1, S, G_2, and M. Figure 11.1 illustrates the cell generation cycle and the major cell function that occurs in each phase.[24] The amount of time required to complete the cell generation cycle varies depending on the type of cell. The time from beginning of the S phase to the end of M is fairly constant, but the time spent in G_1 varies from ten to thirty-one hours.[27] In general, cells that are actively dividing, that is, that have short G_1 phases, are more sensitive to the toxic effects of chemotherapy. This is true of both normal and malignant cells. This is the explanation for the untoward effects caused by chemotherapy on normal rapidly dividing cells such as bone marrow and cells in the gastrointestinal tract.

Chemotherapeutic agents are divided into two major categories defined by their mechanism of action: cell-cycle–specific agents and cell-cycle–nonspecific agents. Just as their name implies, cell-cycle–specific agents act during a specific phase of the cell's life, and the cell-cycle–nonspecific agents interfere with cell function and reproduction at any point in the cycle.

When the action of drugs on the cell cycle is considered, it is easy to see why combination therapy using drugs that act in different phases of the cell cycle is more effective than single-agent therapy. Combination therapy allows cells in different phases of the cell cycle to be affected simultaneously by agents that have different spectrums of toxicity. An example of this is the standard treatment of epithelial ovarian cancer, which uses a combination of agents, cisplatin or carboplatin (cell-cycle–nonspecific) and paclitaxel (cell-cycle–specific in M phase).

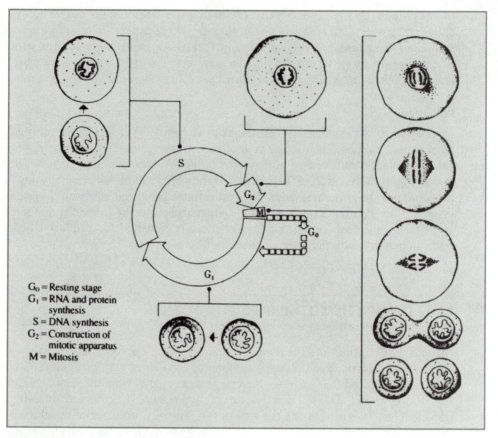

FIGURE 11.1. Cell Generation Cycle

Reproduced with permission: Goodman, M., (1992). *Cancer: Chemotherapy and Care* (3rd ed.). Princeton, NJ: Bristol-Myers Squibb.

Cell-Cycle–Specific Agents

Cell-cycle–specific agents act on cells that are in the process of proliferation during cycles G through M. Cell-cycle–specific agents commonly used in the treatment of gynecologic cancers include etoposide and bleomycin, both of which act on the G_2 phase. This is a short phase, and consequently it is often necessary to infuse these drugs over twenty-four hours or over several days in divided doses to be sure to treat the cell in the appropriate phase.

The S phase is important because it is in this phase that cellular DNA is duplicated in preparation for cell division. It is a relatively long phase, lasting almost twenty hours. Two drugs used in the treatment of gynecologic cancers that are active in the S phase are 5-fluorouracil and methotrexate.

Mitosis is that part of the cell cycle in which cell division occurs. This phase usually lasts only one hour. The vinca alkaloids (vincristine, vinblastine) are examples of cytotoxic agents that bind to microtubular proteins, thus arresting cell mitosis in the M phase.

Cell-Cycle–Nonspecific Agents

Cell-cycle–nonspecific agents used in gynecologic cancers include agents such as cisplatin, carboplatin, cyclophosfamide, ifosfamide, and chlorambucil. The antitumor antibiotics doxorubicin, mitomycin, and dactinomycin are also included in this classification. As the category implies, these agents act on the cell regardless of its cycle. Cisplatin and carboplatin are not always considered alkylating agents and may also be classified as miscellaneous alkylatorlike agents.

An example of combination agents using both cell-cycle–nonspecific and cell-cycle–specific agents is for the treatment of nonepithelial ovarian cancers. It incorporates bleomycin and etoposide (G_2 phase), and cisplatin (nonspecific phase), followed by vincristine (M phase), and actinomycin and cyclophosphamide (nonspecific phase).

Hormones

In addition to agents that act on cells during the cell cycle, some hormones are used that affect tumor cell growth. Hormone therapy generally works by changing the cellular environment, making it unfavorable for the cell to grow. Progestins such as medroxyprogesterone acetate and the antiestrogen tamoxifen citrate are hormonal agents used in the treatment of endometrial, ovarian, and breast cancer.[24,28,29] Although the response rate to hormonal agents is low (10–15%) in the gynecologic population, they are a viable option when the use of active cytotoxic agents has failed. Patients with metastatic endometrial cancer may be treated palliatively with a single agent or multiple chemotoxic agents that act in different phases of the cell cycle with limited response and survival, followed by one of the the antiestrogens, megestrol acetate or tamoxifen.

Tamoxifen therapy is associated with a significant reduction in the risk of recurrence and death in all women regardless of age or menopausal status with early-stage steroid-receptor positive breast cancer. Tamoxifen is believed to act primarily through binding to estrogen receptors in breast cancer cells, acting as an inhibitor of estrogen. Tamoxifen is recommended as adjuvant therapy for five years in this population.[30,31,32] Results of the National Surgical Adjuvant Breast and Bowel Project (NSABP) suggest a benefit of tamoxifen as preventive therapy in women at high risk for breast cancer.[33] However, the use of tamoxifen in the NSABP trial also increased the rate of endometrial cancer (risk ratio = 2.53) predominantly in women of 50 years or older. Tamoxifen use has been implicated in the development of endometrial polyps and hyperplasia in postmenopausal women.[34] Results of a prospective trial by Barakat et al. to characterize the frequency and type of abnormal pathology suggest that significant pathology requiring hysterectomy was noted in only 3 of 111 (2.7%) women while on tamoxifen who were followed with surveillance serial endometrial biopsies for five years.[35]

✳ TUMOR RESPONSE

Standardized criteria have been established to assess the efficacy of chemotherapy. These criteria include degree of response, duration of response, survival rates, and grade of toxicity by categories. The following categories are accepted as criteria for therapeutic response:[36,37]

- *Complete response (CR)*—Disappearance of all measurable or evaluable disease, signs, symptoms, and biochemical changes related to the tumor for four weeks or more following chemotherapy, during which no new lesions appear.
- *Partial response (PR)*—When compared to pretreatment measurements, a reduction of greater than 50% in the sum of the products of the perpendicular diameters of all measurable lesions lasting four weeks or more following chemotherapy, during which no new lesions appear and no existing lesions enlarge.
- *Stable disease (SD)*—A less than 50% reduction and less than 25% increase in the sum of the products of two perpendicular diameters of all measured lesions lasting greater than eight weeks or more following chemotherapy, during which no new lesions appear.
- *Progression of disease (POD)*—An increase in the product of the two largest perpendicular disease diameters of any measured lesion by greater than 25% over the size present at start of therapy.

✳ FACTORS CONTRIBUTING TO EFFICACY

Drug Resistance

Most gynecologic tumors are sensitive to the cytotoxic effects of chemotherapy, but permanent cures remain elusive. One mechanism that prevents total tumor eradication by cytotoxic drugs is referred to as *drug resistance*.[38] Drug resistance occurs most often by a process known as *acquired resistance*, in which biochemical changes occur within the cancer cell after exposure to a cytotoxic drug.[39,40] Multidrug resistance (MDR) may occur after exposure to only one natural cytotoxic agent. In addition to acquired resistance, another type of drug resistance is known as *intrinsic resistance*. This type of resistance is so called because it is intrinsic to the cell even before administration of cytotoxic agents. Intrinsic resistance is thought to have evolved as the body's own protective mechanism to prevent the exit of toxic compounds from the intestine or to remove toxic compounds through the bile and urine if they are absorbed.[41]

Tumors vary in the particular drugs to which they are resistant. The intrinsic resistance between or within drug families may be specific and related to known enzymatic or metabolic differences or may have no known explanation.[42]

Laboratory studies and clinical trials are under way to understand and overcome both intrinsic and acquired multidrug resistance. Bourhis[43] reported that MDR occurs in ovarian cancer patients after they receive doxorubicin. This research suggests that this MDR is caused by an expression of a membrane glycoprotein (P-170) that acts as an efflux pump. The P-glycoprotein is coded for the MDR-1 gene. In a study by Sikic, only 14% of ovarian cancer patients had elevations of the MDR-1 gene before treatment, but after doxorubicin treatment, 33% demonstrated high MDR-1 expression.[44] Increased MDR-1 expression also occurred in three of ten patients treated with natural products.[40,43] These results are of particular consequence because resistance to paclitaxel, another natural product that is highly active in ovarian cancer, may also be caused by increased expression of MDR-1.

Another possible explanation for acquired drug resistance has been observed in human ovarian cell lines resistant to alkylating agents, cisplatin, and irradiation. These resistant cells had increased levels of cellular glutathione (GSH), which is known to increase the cancer cell's DNA repair capacity. Restoration of drug sensitivity was observed by exposure to the synthetic amino acid buthionine sulfoximine (BSO) which inhibits gamma-glutamylcysteine synthetase, causing GSH depletion.[44,45] A phase I trial using BSO with melphalan showed that GSH was reduced by 20% of baseline.[46] Phase II clinical studies are under way to assess BSO's clinical significance in patients with ovarian cancer and melanoma.

It appears that both acquired and intrinsic resistance to platinum compounds, which are the most active drugs in the treatment of gynecologic cancers, is multifactorial. A research priority is to develop molecular probes that can diagnose a particular patient's cause of drug resistance so that treatment can be individualized to overcome it. It is clear that the development of novel chemotherapeutic agents such as the topoisomerase-1 inhibitors, which are not cross-resistant to current effective agents like cisplatin compounds and paclitaxel, will affect response to treatment and have an overall positive effect on the survival of ovarian cancer patients, which at this time remains dismal.

Dose Intensity and Dose Intensification

Dose intensity is likely to be an effective method of increasing responses to therapy while minimizing drug resistance. Dose intensity is the amount of drug administered over time.[47] The dose intensity of a regimen is computed by converting each drug in a regimen to a standard measure (e.g., $mg/m^2/week$) and comparing it to the dose intensity of the standard regimen for that tumor type. The relative intensity is expressed as a percentage of intensity greater than the standard regimen. Levin and associates, in 1987, compared response rates and overall survival in regimens used for treating ovarian cancer and reported a better outcome from the dose-intense regimens.[28]

Dose intensification is different from dose intensity. The rationale for intensification is born in the Gompertzian growth curve, which suggests that the rate of tumor regrowth increases as tumor size shrinks. Dose intensification combats the slowing rate of tumor regression during therapy by increasing the intensity of the treatments as the tumor gets smaller. This theory capitalized on the fact that tumors that have been cytoreduced are in a state of relative kinetic resistance and thus require a late intensification of therapy for their eradication.[48] Intensification applies not only to the increase in total dose but also to the shortened time interval between chemotherapy cycles and overall regimen delivery time. Use of growth factors for bone marrow support to lessen the length and severity of hematologic nadirs has increased the feasibility of dose intensification.[15,49]

Despite the hopeful results of the retrospective comparisons by Levin and Hryniuk, the Gynecologic Oncology Group (GOG) prospective dose-intense trials for suboptimally debulked ovarian cancer patients showed no improvement in disease-free survival or overall survival in the group that received the dose-intense regimen.[50]

Tumor Size and Cytoreductive Surgery

Griffiths, in 1986, described the theoretical advantages of cytoreductive surgery in the treatment of ovarian cancer.[51] Two of the advantages are directly related to the potential enhanced effect of chemotherapy after surgery. First, surgical cytoreduction removes large tumor masses, which are known to be less sensitive to the cytotoxic effects of chemotherapy. Second, the small residual tumors left after surgical debulking divide more rapidly, and their heightened kinetic state renders them more sensitive to the cytotoxic effects of chemotherapy.

The volume of residual disease after surgery has been correlated with an overall improvement in median survival of twenty-two months in patients with optimal cytoreduction compared to those whose tumors are suboptimally resected.[52]

Stage of Disease

As gynecologic cancers move out of the organ of tumor origin into adjacent pelvic organs, lymph nodes, and metastatic sites, the need for systemic management with chemotherapy increases. Not all advanced gynecologic cancers benefit from chemo-

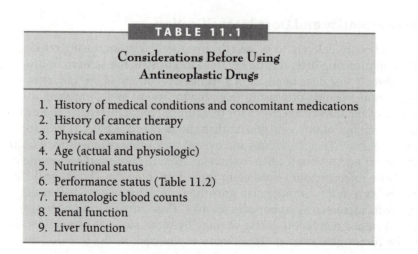

TABLE 11.1

Considerations Before Using
Antineoplastic Drugs

1. History of medical conditions and concomitant medications
2. History of cancer therapy
3. Physical examination
4. Age (actual and physiologic)
5. Nutritional status
6. Performance status (Table 11.2)
7. Hematologic blood counts
8. Renal function
9. Liver function

TABLE 11.2

Performance Status Scale

Description: Karnofsky Scale	Karnofsky Scale (%)	Zubrod Scale (ECOG)	TNM Scale (AJC)	Description: ECOG and AJC Scales
No complaints; no evidence of disease	100	0	H0	Normal activity
Able to carry on normal activity; minor signs or symptoms of disease	90			
Some signs or symptoms of disease with effort	80	1	H1	Symptoms of disease but ambulatory and able to carry out activities of daily living
Cares for self; unable to carry on normal activity or to do active work	70			
Requires occasional assistance, but is able to care for most personal needs	60	2	H2	Out of bed more than 50% of time; occasionally needs assistance
Requires considerable assistance and frequent medical care	50			
Disabled; requires special care and assistance	40	3	H3	In bed more than 50% of time; needs nursing care
Severely disabled; hospitalization indicated, although death not imminent	30			
Very sick; hospitalization necessary; requires active supportive treatment	20	4	H4	Bedridden; may need hospitalization
Moribund; fatal processes progressing rapidly	10			
Dead	0			

ECOG = Eastern Cooperative Oncology Group; AJC = American Joint Commission for Cancer Staging and End Results Reporting

Source: Reprinted with permission from *Manual of Bedside Oncology,* D.A. Casciato & B.B. Lowitz, eds. © 1983. Published by Little, Brown and Company.

therapy. The decision to use chemotherapy is based on multiple factors. Critical factors that must be considered before initiating chemotherapy are listed in Table 11.1

Based on this evaluation, the patient's overall dose will be determined. The better performance status the patient has (Table 11.2), the better chance she has to complete the regimen that favors a better response. Table 11.3 is a list of chemotherapeutic agents commonly used in gynecologic oncology and some of their characteristics.

TABLE 11.3

Chemotherapeutic Agents Commonly Used in the Treatment
of Gynecologic Cancers

Drug	Class	Mechanism of Action	Metabolism
Bleomycin Sulfate	Antitumor antibiotic	Inhibits DNA synthesis Cell-cycle–specific for G_2 phase	Renal
Carboplatin	Alkylating agent	Produces predominantly intrastrand RNA cross-links but at a slower rate than cisplatin Cell-cycle–nonspecific	Renal
Cisplatin	Alkylating agent heavy metal	Binds to DNA, producing cross-links and DNA adducts, thus preventing cell replication Cell-cycle–nonspecific	Renal Biliary

Dose Range	Administration	Gyn Tumor	Rx Goal	Principal Adverse Effects
10–20 u/m^2/day $\times$ 4 consecutive days	CVI, IV	Squamous cell carcinoma (SCC), cervix Stage IB, IIA	Adjuvant Palliation	Anaphylactoid reactions Fever Hypotension Nausea and Vomiting Delayed pulmonary toxicity
		rec/mets		
20 u/m^2 q week up to 30 u maximum per cycle lifetime maximum 400 u	CVI, IV	SCC, vulva rec/mets Germ cell tumors, ovary any stage rec/mets	Cure / control Control / palliation	
360 mg/m^2 q 4 weeks or based on AUC 6–7. Calvert formula: Dose (mg) = AUC $\times$ GFR +25	IV	Epithelial ovarian Recurrent epithelial ovarian	Cure/ control	Thrombocytopenia Pancytopenia Nausea and vomiting
		Endometrial rec/mets	Control	
		Cervical rec/mets	Control	
50–120 mg/m^2 q 3–4 weeks *or*	IV	Epithelial ovarian Cervical	Cure	Nausea and vomiting Leukopenia Thrombocytopenia
100 mg/m^2 day 1 and day 8 q 20 days	IV	Stage IB, IIA Stage IIB and above rec/mets	Adjuvant Control/ palliation Control	Anemia Electrolyte disturbance Cumulative dose-related nephrotoxicity
		Endometrial rec/mets		Cumulative dose-related neurotoxicity
100 mg/m^2 q 3–4 weeks	IP	Epithelial ovarian Persistent tumor <0.5cm	Control	Ototoxicity

(continued)

TABLE 11.3 *(continued)*

Chemotherapeutic Agents Commonly Used in the Treatment of Gynecologic Cancers

Drug	Class	Mechanism of Action	Metabolism
Cyclophosphamide	Alkylating agent	Causes cross-linkage in DNA strands thus preventing DNA synthesis and cell division Cell-cycle–nonspecific	Renal Activated by micro-somal enzymes in liver Excreted by kidneys
Dactinomycin	Antitumor antibiotic	Binds to guanine portion of DNA and blocks ability of DNA to act as a template for both DNA and RNA Cell-cycle–nonspecific, but maximal cell kill in G_1 phase	Renal Biliary
Doxorubicin	Anthracycline antibiotic	Binds to DNA and inhibits nucleic acid synthesis Cell-cycle–nonspecific, but maximal cell kill in S phase	Biliary
Doxorubicin-Liposomal (Doxil)	Liposomal anthracycline	Binds to DNA and inhibits nucleic acid synthesis. Polyethylene glycol (PEG) coating increases therapeutic half-life and its cell concentration	Liver

Dose Range	Administration	Gyn Tumor	Rx Goal	Principal Adverse Effects
600–1000 mg/m^2 q 3–4 weeks	IV	Epithelial ovarian	Cure	Hemorrhagic cystitis Neutropenia
		Endometrial rec/mets	Control	Thrombocytopenia Inappropriate anti-diuretic hormone secretion Alopecia Nausea and vomiting
400 mcg/m^2/day × 5 days q 3–4 weeks *or* 1.25 mg/m^2 q 14 days	IV	Germ cell tumors:		Leukopenia Thrombocytopenia
		ovary	Cure	Nausea and vomiting
		endo-metrium	Cure	Diarrhea Mucositis Alopecia
		GTD:		Immunosuppression
		nonme-tastatic	Cure	Maculopapular rash
		metastatic	Cure/ control	Radiation recall phenomenon Extravasation-induced tissue necrosis
60–75 mg/m^2 q 3 weeks Not to exceed 450–550 mg/m^2 lifetime maximum	IV	Endometrial rec/mets	Control	Leukopenia Thrombocytopenia Cumulative dose-related cardiomy-opathy, arrhythmias
		Epithelial ovarian	Cure	Nausea and vomiting
		Persistent ovarian	Control	Extravasation-induced tissue necrosis
40–50 mg/m^2 q 3 weeks	IV	Persistent epithelial ovarian	Control	Hypersensitivity reactions Myelosuppression Skin reactions (palmar-plantar erythro-dysesthesia) Stomatitis Cardiac events

(continued)

TABLE 11.3 *(continued)*

Chemotherapeutic Agents Commonly Used in the Treatment of Gynecologic Cancers

Drug	Class	Mechanism of Action	Metabolism
Etoposide	Plant alkaloid (Semisynthetic podophyllo-toxin derived from root of the mayapple)	Inhibits DNA synthesis Cell-cycle–specific for S and G_2 phases	Renal
5-Fluorouracil	Antimetabolite	Inhibits formation of thymidine synthetase, which is necessary for DNA synthesis. Incorporates into RNA, causing abnormal synthesis Cell-cycle–specific for S phase	Liver Renal
Hexamethylmela-mine	Alkylating agent or antimetabo-lite in S phase	Not clearly known. May inhibit incorporation of thymidine and uridine into DNA and RNA, respectively	Liver
Ifosfamide	Alkylating agent	Activated by microsomal liver enzymes Destroys DNA by binding to protein and DNA cross-linking with DNA	Liver Renal

Dose Range	Administration	Gyn Tumor	Rx Goal	Principal Adverse Effects
50–100 mg/m²/day × 5 q 3–4 weeks	IV	Germ cell tumors of the ovary	Cure	Leukopenia Thrombocytopenia Alopecia Nausea and vomiting
50 mg/day × 21 days	PO	Persistent epithelial ovarian	Control	Bronchospasms Severe hypotension with rapid infusion
200 mg/m² q 3–4 weeks	IP			
12 mg/kg/day × 4–5 days (400–600 mg/m²/day × 4 days) *or*	CVI	Persistent/mets epithelial ovarian	Control	Stomatitis Nausea and vomiting Diarrhea Leukopenia Thrombocytopenia
6 mg/kg (200–250 mg/m² every other day q 4 weeks *or* 15 mg/kg (500–600 mg/m² weekly	IV	Rec/mets cervix	Control	Rashes Alopecia Hyperpigmentation
150–260 mg/m²/ day in 3–4 divided doses × 14–21 days. Rest 7–14 days and begin next cycle	PO	Persistent epithelial ovarian	Control/ palliation	Anorexia Nausea and vomiting Diarrhea Abdominal cramps Peripheral neuropathy Central nervous system toxicity, somnolence, confusion Mild leukopenia Mild thrombocytopenia
1.2–2.0 g/m²/day × 3–5 days	IV	Persistent/mets epithelial ovarian	Control	Hemorrhagic cystitis Neutropenia Thrombocytopenia

(continued)

TABLE 11.3 *(continued)*

Chemotherapeutic Agents Commonly Used in the Treatment of Gynecologic Cancers

Drug	Class	Mechanism of Action	Metabolism
Ifosfamide (continued)			
Melphalan	Alkylating agent	Interstrand cross-links with DNA, causing miscoding and breakages Cell-cycle–nonspecific	Renal Bowel
Methotrexate	Antimetabolite, folic acid antagonist	Binds to dihydrofolate reductase, blocking reduction of this enzyme to tetrahydrofolic acid, the active form of folic acid. This in turn arrests DNA, RNA, and protein synthesis Cell-cycle–specific for activity in S phase	Renal
Mitomycin	Antitumor antibiotic	Inhibits DNA synthesis by cross-linking of DNA Cell-cycle–nonspecific, but maximum cell kill in late G_1 and early S phase	Liver

Dose Range	Administration	Gyn Tumor	Rx Goal	Principal Adverse Effects
Must be given with uroprotector mesna: 240 mg/m^2 15 min prior to and 4 and 8 hrs after ifosfamide		Advanced or rec/met cervix	Control	Central nervous system toxicity, confusion, hallucinations, depression, fatigue Alopecia Nausea and vomiting
1 mg/kg q 4–6 weeks *or* 0.2 mg/kg × 5 days q 4–5 weeks	PO or IV PO or IV	Persistent or rec/mets Epithelial ovarian	Control/ palliation	Delayed myelosuppression Addisonian-like syndrome Hyperpigmentation
15–30 mg/day × 5 days q 1–2 weeks	PO, IM	GTD	Cure	Leukopenia Thrombocytopenia Anemia
High dose: 100 mg/m^2 q 1–3 weeks with leucovorin rescue	CVI	Met squamous cell cancer, cervix	Palliation	Mucositis Nausea and vomiting Diarrhea Hepatotoxicity Nephrotoxicity Rash
Numerous dose schedules adjusted by clinical response and hematologic monitoring	IM, IT, IV			Encephalopathy Dizziness, blurred vision
Single agent: 20 mg/m^2 q 6–8 weeks	IV	Persistent epithelial ovarian	Control/ palliation	Delayed and cumulative anemia, leukopenia, thrombocytopenia
Combination: 10 mg/m^2 q 6–8 weeks		Advanced cervix	Control	Nausea and vomiting Stomatitis Extravasation-induced tissue necrosis Alopecia

(continued)

TABLE 11.3 *(continued)*

Chemotherapeutic Agents Commonly Used in the Treatment
of Gynecologic Cancers

Drug	Class	Mechanism of Action	Metabolism
Mitoxantrone	Antitumor antimetabolite	Inhibits both DNA and RNA synthesis Cell-cycle–nonspecific	Biliary
Paclitaxel	Diterpene plant product	Promotes assembly of microtubules and stabilizes them, preventing depolymerization, and thus cellular replication	Liver
Topotecan HCl	Semisynthetic derivative of plant alkaloid camptothecin	Binds to topoisomerase-1 DNA complex and prevents religation of these single-strand breaks	Liver Renal excretion
Vinblastine sulfate	Plant alkaloid	Binds microtubular proteins, thus arresting mitosis during metaphase Cell-cycle–specific in S phase and expressed in M phase	Liver

Key for abbreviations: u = units; m^2 = meters squared; mg = milligrams; cm = centimeters; CVI = continuous venous infusion; IV = intravenous; IP = intraperitoneal

Dose Range	Administration	Gyn Tumor	Rx Goal	Principal Adverse Effects
12–14 mg/m^2 q 3 weeks	IV	Persistent epithelial ovarian	Control	Leukopenia Pancytopenia Nausea and vomiting Stomatitis
10 mg/m^2 q 2 weeks	IP	Persistent epithelial ovarian tumor <0.5 cm	Control	Alopecia Cardiotoxicity
135–250 mg/m^2 q ·3 weeks	CVI	Epithelial ovarian	Cure	Leukopenia Thrombocytopenia Hypersensitivity reaction
(see premedication schedule in Table 11.4)	all treatment through non-PVC tubing	Persistent epithelial ovarian	Control	Cardiotoxicity Peripheral neuropathy Nausea and vomiting Alopecia
60 mg/m^2 weekly	IP	Persistent ovarian tumor <0.5 cm	Control	
1.5 mg/m^2 × 5 days q 3 weeks	IV	Persistent ovarian cancer	Control	Neutropenia Thrombocytopenia Anemia Nausea and vomiting Alopecia Headache Dyspnea
0.1–0.5 mg/m^2 q week	IV	Germ cell tumor, ovary	Cure	Leukopenia Thrombocytopenia Nausea and vomiting
1.5–1.7 mg/m^2/day × 5 days	IV	Rec/mets germ cell tumor, ovary	Control	Neurotoxicity Extravasation-induced tissue injury Alopecia Stomatitis Rashes

Each chemotherapeutic agent has a variety of side effects that can manifest differently in each patient. A standard nursing care plan provides information about the needs of patients who experience toxicities. Nurses must be knowledgeable in their discipline but must also understand the patient's beliefs, values, and cultural norms and use a holistic approach to each patient's care. Nursing care plans that may be used for patients receiving chemotherapy are found in the Pocket Guide to this textbook.[53]

✻ COMMONLY USED AND INVESTIGATIONAL AGENTS

Taxanes

Paclitaxel is the prototype of a novel class of agents known as taxanes. In 1967, paclitaxel, a unique compound, was isolated from the bark of the Western yew by Wani and Wall.[6] This organic compound demonstrated antineoplastic activity in murine tumors through a unique mechanism. Phase I studies began in 1983,[7] and in 1993, paclitaxel was approved for use after failure of first-line therapy or subsequent chemotherapy for the treatment of ovarian cancer.

The taxanes, paclitaxel and its semisynthetic analogue docetaxel, promote the assembly of microtubules, which are structures within cells that are vital to cell division and a variety of other critical cell functions. Taxanes also inhibit disassembly of these structures, resulting in the accumulation of abnormal bundles of nonfunctional microtubules.[54,55]

Phase II studies indicate that paclitaxel shows significant antitumor activity in patients with ovarian cancer that is refractory to platinum-containing first-line therapy or that has recurred despite an initial response. A Phase III randomized GOG trial demonstrated that a combination of cisplatin and paclitaxel led to significant improvement in clinical response over the standard therapy of cisplatin and cyclophosfamide for the initial treatment of advanced ovarian cancer (79% versus 63%, respectively; P = <0.01).[8] These results changed the clinical management of advanced ovarian cancer and led to an improvement in overall survival for patients with this disease.[56] In an effort to maintain or improve efficacy while decreasing the known neurotoxicity of the cisplatin/paclitaxel regimen, the GOG completed a trial of carboplatin for cisplatin. Results indicate that the carboplatin regimen is equally efficacious, less toxic, and able to be administered with ease in the outpatient setting.[10] Therefore, current regimens contain carboplatin.

The dose-limiting toxicity related to paclitaxel is bone marrow suppression, particularly neutropenia.[7,8,57,58] The nadir usually occurs about seven to eleven days after intravenous administration and is of short duration (less than two days). Patients who have received prior radiation therapy seem to have more severe myelosuppression. Hypersensitivity reactions have been reported to occur in 19% of all courses of paclitaxel. Symptoms usually occur during the first hour of infusion and include dyspnea, hypotension, chest pain, facial flushing, and rash. All patients should be

TABLE 11.4	
Paclitaxel Administration Guidelines	
Infusion Set-up	Glass or polyolefin containers to hold paclitaxel solution
	Deliver through polyethylene-lined IV administration set (non-PVC tubing or nitroglycerin tubing)
	In-line 20–22 µm filter at patient end of infusion set-up
Length of Infusion	3- or 24-hour continuous infusion at a steady rate using a controlled infusion device
	Paclitaxel solutions are stable for up to 27 hours after dilution
Drug Compatibilities	Known to be compatible with either 0.9% sodium chloride solution or 5% dextrose in water
	No other compatibility studies have been done
Premedication Guidelines to Prevent Hypersensitivity Reactions	Dexamethasone 20 mg PO or IV 12 and 6 hours before and 20 mg IV 30 minutes before infusion
	Diphenhydramine HCl 50 mg IV 30 minutes before infusion
	Cimetidine 300 mg or Ranitidine 50 mg IV 30 to 60 minutes before infusion

Adapted with permission: Lubejko, B., & Sartorius, S. (1993). Nursing considerations in paclitaxel administration. *Seminars in Oncology Nursing, 20*(4, suppl. 3), 26–30.

premedicated (Table 11.4) with dexamethasone, diphenhydramine, and cimetidine or ranitidine.[59]

Alopecia occurs in almost all patients. Loss of body hair, including axilla, pubic, eyebrows, and eyelashes, may occur. Nausea and vomiting, diarrhea, and mucositis have been reported to occur in 59%, 43%, and 39% of cases, respectively. Other, less severe toxicity includes peripheral neuropathy, arthralgia and myalgia, hypotension, asymptomatic bradycardia, and liver damage.[60]

Another unique nursing issue relates to the method of administering paclitaxel. The surfactant Cremophor EL is needed in the preparation of paclitaxel for intravenous use, but this combination has been known to cause leaching of the plasticizer di(2-ethylhexyl)phthalate (DEHP) from polyvinyl chloride infusion bags and administration sets. To minimize patient exposure to DEHP, diluted paclitaxel should be prepared and stored in glass or polyolefin containers and infused through polyethylene-lined intravenous administration sets.[61]

Prepared paclitaxel solution may appear hazy and may contain minute particles. It is recommended that the agent be administered through an in-line filter with a microporous membrane not greater than 0.22 microns.[59] See Table 11.4 for paclitaxel administration guidelines.

The toxicity profiles of docetaxel are similar to those of paclitaxel, with moderately severe neutropenia occurring between days five and seven and lasting five to six days. Acute hypersensitivity reactions may occur, and a premedication schedule similar to that for paclitaxel is recommended. Other adverse effects reported in these trials are mild peripheral edema, skin reactions (erythema, thickening, and desquamation), and neurotoxicity.[62,63]

Platinum Compounds

Platinum-based therapy has been the mainstay of cytotoxic treatment for epithelial and most non-eptithelial ovarian cancers for more than a decade. Cisplatin in combination with 5-fluorouracil and radiation therapy or cisplatin alone with radiation therapy is now the recommended standard for locally advanced (stages IIB, III, or IVA) carcinoma of the cervix.[64,65] Cisplatin and its analogue carboplatin also have broad activity when used in combination with other cytotoxic or hormonal agents or when used concomitantly with other modalities in the treatment of other common gynecologic malignancies, such as adenocarcinoma of the endometrium, endometrial mixed mesodermal tumors, early-stage squamous carcinoma of the cervix, and fallopian tube carcinoma.

Cisplatin is an inorganic heavy-metal complex that is usually considered to be an alkylating agent. It binds to DNA, producing cross links and DNA adducts and thus preventing cell replication. It is administered intravenously but can also be administered safely intraperitoneally. Cisplatin is the chemotherapy drug of choice intraperitoneally in women with small-volume intraperitoneal disease following second-look surgery.[66,67] Results of a cooperative group trial that assessed the efficacy of intraperitoneal cisplatin and intravenous cyclophosphamide versus conventional intravenous cisplatin and cyclophosphamide as initial combination chemotherapy for optimally debulked ovarian cancer showed a survival benefit for the intraperitoneal group.[68] In the adjunct setting, intraperitoneal cisplatin/etoposide given to patients after a negative second-look laparotomy showed a benefit in time to progression compared to matched historical controls who underwent observation only.[69]

The dose-limiting toxicity of cisplatin is peripheral neurotoxicity, evidenced by sensory loss in the distal extremities in a classic stocking-glove distribution. Peripheral neuropathy is first noted after the third cycle or at cumulative dose of 350 mg/m^2. It may increase in severity after treatment is completed. Patients with severe neurotoxicity have difficulty performing fine-motor activities such as buttoning and may also need visual cues to walk in dimly lit areas. Patients may benefit by information provided in *A Patient Guide to Peripheral Neuropathy*.[70] Other toxicities include ototoxicity with loss of high-pitch frequency, cumulative nephrotoxicity, bone marrow suppression, nausea, and vomiting. Because of cisplatin's renal toxicity the patient must receive intravenous hydration before its administration and her renal status must be carefully monitored throughout treatment.

Carboplatin is used interchangably with cisplatin in the treatment of epithelial ovarian cancer.[10] It is the drug of choice to be used in the outpatient setting because of its ease of intravenous administration. Cumulative myelosuppression, particularly thrombocytopenia, is the major dose-limiting toxicity. At high doses carboplatin may cause ototoxicity similar to that of cisplatin. Because it is a larger molecule than cisplatin, it is not as efficacious as cisplatin when given intraperitoneally.

Topoisomerase I Inhibitors

Topotecan hydrochloride and irinotecan hydrochloride are semisynthetic derivatives of camptothecin. In the 1980s camptothecin was discovered to inhibit the DNA enzyme topoisomerase I. This enzyme relieves torsional strain in DNA by inducing reversible single-strand breaks.[71] Topoisomerase-I inhibitor compounds stabilize the DNA breakage and interfere with the resealing process, allowing for the uncoiling but not the subsequent reannealing of the DNA. This interference results in permanent breakage of the replicating DNA and eventual cell death.[72]

Currently topotecan is approved for use in the salvage setting for epithelail ovarian cancer. In phase II trials it showed activity in paclitaxel/cisplatin-resistant tumors.[73] Subsequent trials confirmed response rates of 12 to 14% in previous platinum failures.[74]

Recent trials combined either sequential couplets of topotecan/cisplatin and cisplatin/paclitaxel for chemotherapy-naive patients with epithelial ovarian cancer and reported an 85% clinical response rate in the topotecan-treated patients, which is similar to that of the paclitaxel/cisplatin combination.[75] Although feasible, myelotoxicity was higher and treatment delays were more frequent in the topotecan-treated group. The disease-free and overall survival for each group has not been determined. Other phase I trials suggest that topotecan can be safely administered intraperitoneally.[76]

Irinotecan (CPT-111) is indicated for use in 5-FU refractory colorectal cancer. Recent trials suggest that, combined with mitomycin-C, the regimen showed a survival benefit in platinum refractory mucinous and clear cell carcinoma of the ovary.[77]

Dose-limiting toxicities of topoisomerase-I inhibitors vary. Myelosuppression, particularly neutropenia, is associated more often with topotecan, while early and late diarrhea occur more frequently with irinotecan. Severe myelosuppression has also been reported with iriniotecan.

Liposomal Anthracyclines

The anthracyclines, particularly doxorubicin, have been used in gynecologic regimens in the treatment of ovarian and advanced endometrial cancers. The dose-limiting toxicity has been the cardiotoxicity when the cumulative dose of doxorubicin exceeds 350 mg/m^2. Liposomal technology encapsulates the agent in a *fat body,* thus minimizing side effects while delivering higher concentrations of drug into the tumor.[78] Encapsulated doxorubicin (Doxil) is approved treatment for advanced ovarian cancer patients who have known platinum, paclitaxel, and topotecan refractory tumors ("triple refractory").[79] Phase I trials are under way to examine the use of intraperitoneal liposomal cisplatin analogue L-NDDP.[80]

The liposomal preparations are classified as irritants and have not demonstrated significant extravasation necrosis at the intravenous site of injection.[81] These agents may be administered through peripheral intravenous access in the outpatient setting. The use of in-line filters is contraindicated, because the filter may rupture the liposomal encapsulation and allow the drug to flow freely.[78]

The dose-limiting toxicity seen with liposomal anthracyclines is palmar-plantar erythrodysesthesia, or hand-foot syndrome. The syndrome may occur after the second or third course of treatment, and patients may report a rash or skin irritation in the area of skin pressure. Patients should be educated about the avoidance for seventy-two hours after administration of tape on skin, tight clothing, sun exposure, pressure on bony prominances, and vigorous activity that may cause excessive pressure on skin. Skin reactions may delay the subsequent course or require a decreased dose. If severe, grade 3 or 4, skin reactions occur, the treatment may need to be discontinued.[78]

Gemcitabine

Gemcitabine is an investigational drug that has activity in many solid tumors, including breast and ovarian cancer. It was the first drug to receive FDA approval on the basis of its clinical benefit response as first-line treatment for pancreatic cancer.[82] It may be a desirable agent in the salvage setting for ovarian cancer because it has activity when used in combination with cisplatin or paclitaxel in refractory ovarian cancer.[83] It has also demonstrated synergy with cisplatin when given intraperitoneally and may be another agent to use in ovarian cancer patients with small-volume disease after initial response to chemotherapy.[84]

Gemcitabine is a novel nucleoside analogue with a unique mode of action: it inhibits DNA synthesis through a process called *masked chain determination*. After the drug is incorporated into the DNA strand, one or more nucleotide base pairs are allowed to be inserted before the DNA chain elongation is terminated. This prevents proofreading enzymes from being able to detect, excise, and repair the DNA lesion, thereby leading to a permanent halt in DNA production within the cell.[85]

The toxicity profile is mild; patients report mild nausea and vomiting, grade 1 or 2 maculopapular rash on trunk, and flulike symptoms. The drug may be administered as a short intravenous infusion (30 minutes) in the outpatient setting, and no premedications are required.[86]

Plant Alkaloids

Etoposide is a plant alkaloid that has been used for many years in multidrug regimens for epithelial cancer, non-epithelial ovarian cancer, and gestational trophoblastic disease. It is cell-cycle–specific and inhibits DNA synthesis in the S and G_2 phases so cells do not enter mitosis.[87]

In today's cost-conscious health care market, oral etoposide is an attractive agent as second-line treatment in ovarian cancer. Studies have shown that it has a 26% overall response rate and a 12% response rate in platinum-resistant patients.[88]

Monoclonal Antibodies

The use of monoclonal antibodies in gynecologic malignancies is limited to date because known antibodies such as OC-125 against CA-125 and B72.3 against TAG-72 localize on intraperitoneal ovarian tumors, but clinical utility remains to be established.[89]

Trastuzumab (Herceptin)

In breast cancer, a recombinant DNA-derived humanized monoclonal antibody, trastuzumab (Herceptin) was approved for use. It is specific for use in patients with metastatic breast cancer whose tumors overexpress the HER2 protein (approximately 25–30% of primary breast cancers) and who have received one or more chemotherapy regimens for metastatic disease. Its recommended use is in combination with paclitaxel. In a large multicenter trial patients who were randomized to receive trastuzumab with paclitaxel had significantly longer time to disease progression, a higher overall reponse rate, a longer median duration of response, and a higher one-year survival rate. The degree of overexpression (2+ to 3+ levels of overexpression based on a 0 to 3+ scale) was a predictor of treatment effect.[90] HER2 protein overexpression can be determined using an immunohistochemistry-based assessment of fixed tumor blocks.[91]

Trastuzumab can be safely administered by intravenous infusion over 90 minutes in the outpatient setting. During the first infusion a symptom complex consisting of chills and/or fever may be observed in about 40% of patients. Usually these symptoms can be successfully treated with acetaminophen, diphenhydramine, and meperidine with or without reduction in the intravenous rate of drug infusion.[92]

Cardiotoxicity (ventricular dysfunction and congestive heart failure) is the major toxicity of trastuzumab. Candidates for this agent should undergo baseline cardiac assessment including history and physical examination and one or more of the following: EKG, echocardiogram, and MUGA scan. Patients should undergo frequent monitoring for deteriorating cardiac function. Patients with preexisting cardiac disease or prior cardiotoxic therapy (e.g., anthracyclines or radiation therapy to the chest) may have decreased tolerance to this therapy. Other adverse reactions noted in clinical trials were mild to moderate anemia and leukopenia, diarrhea, and increased mild upper respiratory infections. This therapy should be used with caution in patients with known hypersensitivity to trastuzumab, Chinese Hamster Ovary cell proteins, or any component of the compound.[92]

✖ CYTOPROTECTANTS

Cytoprotecants are agents used in conjunction with certain chemotherapeutic agents or radiation therapy to lessen or prevent the known dose-limiting toxicities. Cytoprotectants differ from growth factors and rescue agents in that they are administered be-

TABLE 11.5

Standard Cytoprotectants Used in Gynecologic Cancer Treatment

Drug and Use	Mechanism of Action	Standard Dose	Administration Route	Side Effects
Mesna Prevent hemorrhagic cystitis induced by ifosfamide or cyclophosphamide	Binds to acrolein in bladder. Produces inactive compound that is excreted in urine	20% of ifosfamide or cyclophosphamide dose given at time of administration and 4 and 8 hours after. Total, 3 doses	IV	Diarrhea Headache Fatigue Nausea Allergy Hypotension
		40% of ifosphamide or cyclophosphamide dose 4 and 8 hours after. May be mixed in flavored syrup. *Give first dose IV. Total, 3 doses.	PO	
Dexrazoxane Prevent or decrease doxorubicin-associated cardiotoxicity	Potent intracellular chelating agent. *Should not be used with first cycle of doxorubicin. It may diminish antitumor effects	10:1 ratio of dexrazoxane to doxorubicin	IV, 30 minutes prior to doxorubicin	Enhanced myelosuppression Pain on injection Nausea/vomiting Fatigue Anorexia Stomatitis
Amofostine Prevent or decrease multiple cisplatin-associated toxicities. Prevent or decrease radiation-induced xerostomia	Potent scavenger of oxygen-free radicals	910 mg/m^2 or 740 mg/m^2 in 50 ml NSS. *Prehydrate with 500–1,000 ml NSS	IV, 7 to 10 minutes prior to cisplatin IV, within 30 minutes prior to radiation	Hypotension *Contraindicated if hypertensive medication cannot be stopped within 24 hours of amofostine or if patient is dehydrated.

	Mechanism		Administration	
Drug and Use	of Action	Standard Dose	Route	Side Effects
		Radiation:		Nausea/Vomiting
		200 mg/m² daily		*Antiemetic pre-
		*Prehydrate with		medication re-
		1 liter NSS		quired
				Flushed feeling
				Sneezing
				Hypocalcemia—
				rare

TABLE 11.5 *(continued)*

fore or during chemotherapy to prevent normal tissue damage, but they do not inter-fere with the efficacy of the therapy. Their use is increasing because they improve com-pliance with the treatment plan, maximize therapeutic intent, and enhance quality of life for the patient during and after treatment.

Three cytoprotectants are approved for use: dexrazoxane (Zinecard), mesna (Mes-nex), and amofostine (Ethyol) (Table 11.5). Dexrazoxane is administered before dox-orubicin in patients who have received a cumulative dose of doxorubicin of 300 mg/m². Studies in breast cancer patients suggested that dexazoxane can interfere with antitumor activity when given with combination regimens of fluorouracil, doxoru-bicin, and cyclophosfamide.[93] For the same reason, intravenous administration of dexrezoxane should occur a full 30 minutes before initiation of chemotherapy.[22] The most common side effects are myelosuppression and pain at the injection site.

Mesna is the most widely used cytoprotectant and is indicated to prevent hemor-rhagic cystitis due to the administration of ifosfamide or cyclophosphamide. Mesna neutralizes the toxic by-product acrolein by binding to it and making it an inactive compound that is eliminated in the urine. No studies have shown that mesna inter-feres with the antitumor effects of either ifosfamide or cyclophosphamide. Mesna may be given intravenously at a dose calculated at 20% of the ifosfamide or cyclophos-phamide or orally at a dose that is 40% of the ifosfamide or cyclophosphamide dose. It is usually given 15–30 minutes before and 4 and 8 hours after administration but may also be administered as a continuous infusion with high-dose therapy at a dose of 100 to 200% of the total dose of ifosfamide or cyclophosphamide.[20,21,94] Side effects are mild and include diarrhea, headache, nausea, and fatigue. Undiluted mesna has a sul-fur odor and can be mixed with grape- or orange-flavored syrups to lessen nausea and vomiting caused by the odor.

Amofostine has emerged as the first pancytoprotectant. It was approved by the FDA in 1996[17,18] for use in reducing renal toxicity associated with the long-term use of cisplatin in patients with ovarian and non–small cell lung cancer. It may soon have a second indication for reducing xerostomia in patients receiving radiation therapy for head and neck cancer.[19] It has also shown a spectrum of protective effectiveness against neurologic and hematologic function in patients receiving chemotherapy.

Clinical trials are under way in cooperative groups to examine the efficacy of amofostine to reverse neurologic toxicity after cisplatin-based therapy.

Amofostine is a phosphorylated aminothiol pro-drug that is dephosphorylated at the tissue site by membrane-bound alkaline phosphastase to form its active metabolite, WR-1065.[95] Upon administration WR-1065 is rapidly taken up by normal cells and provides cytoprotection through the scavenging of oxygen-free radicals and other reactive species as well as through hydrogen donation to repair damaged DNA.[16,96]

When used as a cytoprotectant with cisplatin the recommended dose is either 910 mg/m^2 or 740 mg/m^2 and should be administered over five to seven minutes with the administration of the agents fifteen minutes after completion of amofostine. The most common side effects may be temporary hypotension, nausea and vomiting, somnolence, hypocalcemia, sneezing, and a warm, flushed feeling during administration.[97] By using standard antiemetic regimens and allowing the patient to receive treatment in a reclining chair, the side effects are minimal and well tolerated. If studies continue to suggest that amofostine is indeed an effective pancytoprotectant its usefulness will make it part of many standard chemotherapy and radiation therapy regimens.[16]

CHEMOTHERAPY ADMINISTRATION

Site Selection and Venipuncture

Extreme care should be exercised when preparing to infuse chemotherapeutic agents intravenously. The nurse who accesses the vein for the intravenous infusion should be experienced in intravenous access and familiar with the drug being infused.

To minimize trauma, the smallest gauge catheter or butterfly needle should be used to access the vein. Usually a no. 22 angio catheter or 21- or 23-gauge butterfly needle is adequate for infusion of any solution volume.

Vein selection is an important aspect of chemotherapy administration. Veins near joints, (e.g., wrist or elbow) should be avoided, since damage to nerves or tendons may occur if the drug extravasates. The cephalic, accessory cephalic, and basilica veins are good choices for chemotherapy infusion. The dorsum of the hand can be used if the drug is a nonvesicant, but hand veins are to be avoided in administration of vesicants, since extravasations may cause damage to nerves and tendons with resultant loss of hand function.

Extravasation

Extravasation is tissue damage caused by an infiltrated irritant or vesicant agent. The severity of the resulting injury depends on several factors, including the specific vesicant potential, drug concentration and amount extravasated, duration of exposure, the venipuncture site and device, needle insertion technique, and the patient's tissue response. Injuries range from mild to severe and include hyperpigmentation, burning, erythema, inflammation, ulceration, prolonged pain, sloughing of tissue, infection, and loss of mobility.[87,98,99]

The site of chemotherapy infusion must be constantly monitored by the nurse. The patient should be instructed to report burning or pain at the site. If the patient complains of discomfort at the site, if a blood return is absent, or if there is swelling, crepitus, or discoloration of the skin, the nurse should assume extravasation has occurred and treat the site according to the policy of the institution. It is often important to maintain the infusion catheter and attempt to aspirate any extravasated drug, and then use the catheter to infuse appropriate antidote. A cold compress is usually recommended, except for extravasation of a vinca alkaloid, in which case hyaluronidase and warm compresses are usually recommended. The Oncology Nursing Society provides guidelines for care of extravasation.[100]

Venous Access and Devices

The patient's veins should be thoroughly assessed to select the best available vein that will ensure comfort, ease, and safety of drug delivery. The vein should feel smooth and pliable, not hard or sclerotic. The most distal vein should be used first, moving proximally with each venipuncture.[87,99] Other criteria to be considered when selecting venous access are frequency of venous access, length of the planned treatment regimen, and patient preference.[101]

Venous access devices are a valuable asset in the care of many oncology patients. The most common venous access devices in use today are the tunneled atrial catheter; the nontunneled, small-gauge central venous catheter; and the implanted port.[102] Implanted ports are often preferred by patients because they are not visible, require minimal maintenance, and do not interfere with bathing, showering, or swimming. If a vesicant drug is to be used, however, a tunneled catheter may be preferable to lower the risk of extravasation.[103,104]

Safe Handling of Chemotherapeutic Agents

Chemotherapy drugs should always be prepared under a class II biological safety cabinet. The person who prepares drugs and administers chemotherapy should wear nonpowdered latex gloves and a protective gown with closed front and cuffs. After chemotherapy is administered, the empty bags, tubing, needles, and unused drug should be discarded in a leak-proof, puncture-proof container and disposed of as toxic waste. The Occupational Safety and Health Administration (OSHA) mandates national standards for safe handling,[105] which can be supplemented with the Oncology Nursing Society specific guidelines.[100]

Personnel who handle bodily fluids or excreta from patients who have received chemotherapy within the previous forty-eight hours should be instructed to wear disposable surgical latex gloves and gowns and to discard them appropriately after use. Linen that is contaminated with bodily fluids within forty-eight hours after chemotherapy administration should be placed in a specially labeled, impervious laundry bag and managed according to procedures for drug spills.[106]

Intraperitoneal Therapy

Intraperitoneal (IP) therapy is the delivery of therapeutic agents—both cytotoxic and biological response modifiers—directly into the peritoneal cavity. In the late 1970s investigators at the National Cancer Institute published pharmacokinetic calculations demonstrating that peritoneal clearance of certain antineoplastic drugs was much lower than the plasma clearance.[107] This concentration difference offered a potentially exploitable biochemical advantage, especially to tumors that are principally confined to the peritoneal cavity, such as ovarian cancer. A peritoneal tumor is exposed to high concentrations of the drug, but because the drug is metabolized in the liver before it enters the systemic circulation, there is less systemic toxicity.[66,108] See Table 11.6 for a list of agents examined for safety, pharmacokinetic advantage, and efficacy in IP treatment of ovarian cancer.

Large fluid volumes (1–2 liters) are needed to ensure adequate drug distribution within the peritoneal cavity, which in turn ensures maximal tumor exposure to the drug. The anticancer agents penetrate the tumor by means of free surface diffusion. Therefore, as expected, studies have shown that only free-floating cells or tumor nodules less than 0.5 cm benefit from this type of therapy.[66,108,109]

The side effects of intraperitoneal therapy are primarily determined by the me-

TABLE 11.6

Pharmacokinetic Advantage for Intraperitoneal Chemotherapy

Drug	Ratio of drug level in peritoneal cavity to plasma concentration	
	Peak	AUC
Cisplatin	20	12
Carboplatin	—	18
Melphalan	93	65
Mitomycin-C	71	—
Doxorubicin	474	—
Mitoxantrone	—	1400
5-Fluorouracil	298	367
Methotrexate	298	100
Paclitaxel	92	1000

AUC = area under the curve

Reprinted with permission: Markman, M. *Principles and Practices of Gynecology Oncology* (2nd ed) (1997). p. 971. W.J. Hoskins, C.A. Perez, R.C. Young, eds. Philadelphia: Lippincott-Raven.

chanical effects of distending the abdomen with large volumes of fluid and by the toxicity of the particular anticancer agent. Common side effects are bloating, abdominal pressure, urinary frequency, and shortness of breath. These effects usually subside within forty-eight hours, at which time most of the fluid volume has been absorbed.[66,110]

An ideal candidate for IP therapy is the patient who has the following characteristics:

- A tumor that demonstrates response to the agent[67,111]
- Normal or adequate liver and kidney function[112]
- Surgically documented small volume disease (<0.5 cm) that is confined to the peritoneal cavity[113]
- Good peritoneal distribution, with minimal adhesion formation[67,113,114]
- Ability to tolerate a large treatment volume (two) or more liters[67,115]

Access to the peritoneal cavity is gained through the use of one of several types of devices. One type is a temporary catheter that is placed before each IP treatment, such as a Groshong intraperitoneal catheter (Bard Access Systems, Salt Lake City, Utah). Another is a semipermanent peritoneal dialysis catheter. The device most often used is a totally implanted subcutaneous port with an attached peritoneal catheter. This port device and catheter are associated with lower complication rates and better patient acceptance than other methods.[116–121] The nursing care of the patient receiving intraperitoneal therapy is in the Pocket Guide for this textbook.[53]

✖ GYNECOLOGIC ONCOLOGY RESEARCH AND NURSING ORGANIZATIONS

The Gynecologic Oncology Group (GOG)

National cooperative groups have been established to conduct clinical research in many oncologic diseases. The GOG is the only national cooperative group whose sole purpose is to conduct clinical research in the field of gynecologic oncology. The GOG was founded in 1970 under the auspices of the National Cancer Institute.

The GOG functions as an interdisciplinary group consisting of oncologic specialists in the fields of gynecology, medicine, radiation therapy, immunology, pathology, nursing, and psychosocial psychology. These specialists are located in more than fifty "parent" medical institutions and more than 120 affiliated hospitals in the United States and Canada. Support staff consists of data managers (many of whom are nurses), statisticians, nurses, and administrative staff.

In addition to its ability to complete surgical-pathological studies on the major gynecologic neoplasms and conduct phase III studies on the most common gynecologic neoplasms (e.g., ovary, endometrium, and cervix), the GOG is the only mecha-

TABLE 11.7

Diagnostic Cluster

Diagnostic/Pretreatment Period

NURSING DIAGNOSIS

1. Anxiety-fear related to insufficient knowledge of prescribed chemotherapy (including clinical trials) and necessary self-care measures

Treatment Period

COLLABORATIVE PROBLEMS
Potential Complication: Preexisting medical conditions
Potential Complication: Fluid/electrolyte imbalance

NURSING DIAGNOSIS

1. Potential for infection related to immunosuppression neutropenia secondary to chemotherapy and/or radiation therapy
2. Potential for bleeding related to immunosuppression thrombocytopenia secondary to chemotherapy and/or radiation therapy
3. Potential alteration in skin integrity related to treatment modality and/or disease process
4. Potential alteration in sensory perception related to neurotoxicity, neurological pain and paresthesia, ototoxicity, and retinal toxicity
5. Potential injury related to acute water intoxication (SIADH)
6. Potential alteration in urinary elimination related to hemorrhagic cystitis and nephro-toxicity
7. Potential altered nutrition: less than body requirements related to nausea, vomiting, anorexia, and/or stomatitis

Treatment Period: Paclitaxel Therapy

NURSING DIAGNOSIS
(In addition to those listed above)

1. Potential for injury related to hypersensitivity and anaphylaxis during paclitaxel therapy
2. Potential alteration in comfort related to flulike syndrome, arthralgia/myalgia
3. Potential for alteration in cardiac output during paclitaxel therapy

TABLE 11.7 *(continued)*

Treatment Period: Intraperitoneal Therapy

NURSING DIAGNOSIS
(in addition to those listed above)

1. Anxiety/fear related to insufficient knowledge of prescribed intraperitoneal chemotherapy and necessary self-care measures
2. Potential for infection related to indwelling peritoneal access port (PAC) and manipulation of the system during administration
3. Potential alteration in respiratory function related to abdominal distention, decreased lung capacity, and/or lung metastasis
4. Potential alteration in comfort related to intraperitoneal instillation of fluid

nism through which less common neoplasms (e.g., germ cell tumors) of the female genital tract can be studied in a meaningful way.

The GOG has two annual meetings for its member institutions and their affiliates. One of seven scientific committees is the Nursing Committee. The three major roles of this committee are:

- to standardize nursing procedures used in the implementation of GOG studies,
- to educate gynecologic nurses with regard to GOG studies and the discipline of gynecologic oncology, and
- to develop and conduct relevant nursing research and supportive care studies that increase the scientific base for nursing practice in gynecologic oncology.

The Society of Gynecologic Nurse Oncologists

Nurses in the GOG first identified the need for a separate nursing organization for gynecologic oncology nursing. In 1980, with the assistance of Dr. Richard Boronow, the Society of Gynecologic Nurse Oncologists (SGNO) was formed with ten charter members. Today, membership includes more than 500 nurses who specialize in and practice gynecologic oncology nursing in the United States, Canada, Australia, and New Zealand.

Benefits of membership in this subspecialty organization are many. They include many opportunities to network with other nurses who specialize in the care of women with gynecologic cancers and access to the most current information regarding medical and nursing advances in the SGNO's quarterly journal, *The Journal of Gynecologic Oncology Nursing*. Professional growth opportunities include speaking at the annual symposium or writing an article for the SGNO's journal.

✖ REFERENCES

1. Knopf, M.K., Tischer, D.S., & Welch-McCaffrey, D. (1984). *Cancer chemotherapy: Treatment and care* (pp. 6–7). Boston: G.K. Hall.
2. Burchenal, J.H. (1977). The historical development of cancer chemotherapy. *Semin Oncol, 4*(2), 135.
3. DeVita, V.T. (1989). Principles of chemotherapy. In V.T. DeVita, S. Hellman & S. Rosenberg, eds., *Principles and Practice of Oncology* (pp. 276–300). Philadelphia: J.B. Lippincott.
4. Young, R. (1989). Chemotherapy. In J. Berek & N. Hacker, eds., *Practical Gynecologic Oncology* (pp. 25–26). Baltimore: Williams and Wilkins.
5. Young, R.C., Chabner, B.A., Hubbard, S.P., et al. (1978). Advanced ovarian adenocarcinoma: A prospective clinical trial with melphalan (L-PAM) versus combination chemotherapy. *N Engl J Med, 299*(23), 1261–1266.
6. Wani, M.C., Taylor, H.L., & Wall, M.E. (1971). Plant antitumor agents. The isolation and structure of taxol, a novel antileukemic and antitumor agent from *Taxus brevifolia. J Am Chem Soc, 93*, 2325–2327.
7. McGuire, W.P., Rowinsky, E.K., Rosenshein, N.B., et al. (1989). Taxol: A unique antineoplastic agent with significant activity in advanced ovarian cancer. *Ann Intern Med, 111*(4), 273–279.
8. McGuire, W., Hoskins, W.J., Brady, M.F., et al. (1993). A phase III trial comparing cisplatin/cytoxan and cisplatin/taxol in advanced ovarian cancer. *Proc Am Soc Clin Oncol, 12*, 255.
9. McGuire,W.P., Hoskins, W.J., Brady, M.F. (1996). Cyclophosphamide and cisplatin compared with paclitaxel and cisplatin in patients with stage III and stage IV ovarian cancer. *N Engl J Med, 334*(1), 1–6.
10. Ozols, R.F., Bundy, B.N., Fowler, D., et al. (1999). Randomized phase III study of cisplatin (CIS/paclitaxel PAC) versus carboplatin (CARBO/PAC) in optimal stage III epithelial ovarian cancer (OC): A Gynecologic Group Trial (GOG 158), *Proc Am Soc Clin Oncol, 1373*, 356a, (abs.).
11. Aapro, M., Pujade-Laurine, E., Lhomme, C. (1993). Phase II study of taxotere in ovarian cancer. *Proc Am Soc Clin Oncol, 12*, 256 (abs.).
12. Piccart, M.J., Gore, M., et al. (1993). Taxotere (RP56976,NSC628508): An active new drug for treatment of advanced ovarian cancer. *Proc Am Soc Clin Oncol, 12*, 258 (abs).
13. Kavanaugh, J., Kudelkai, A., Freedman, R., et al. (1993). A phase II trial of taxotere (RP56976) in ovarian cancer refractory to cisplatin/carboplatin therapy. *Proc Am Soc Clin Oncol, 12*, 259 (abs.).
14. Francis, P., Schneider, J., Hann, L., et al. (1994). Phase II trial of docetaxel in patients with advanced platinum refractory advanced ovarian cancer. *J Clin Oncol, 12*(11), 2301–2308.
15. Gabrilove, J.L.(1991). Colony-stimulating factors: Clinical status. In V.T. DeVita, S. Hellman, S. Rosenberg, eds., *Biology Therapy of Cancer* (pp. 445–463). Philadelphia: J.B. Lippincott.
16. Viele, C., Holmes, B.C. (1998). Amifostine: Drug profile and nursing implications of the first pancytoprotectant. *Oncol Nurs Forum, 25*(3), 515–523.
17. Alberts, D.S. (1996). Introduction: Applications of amifostine in cancer treatment. *Semin Oncol, 23*(suppl. 8), 1.
18. Alberts, D.S., Bleyer, W.A. (1996). Future development of amifostine in cancer treatment. *Semin Oncol, 23* (suppl, 8), 90–99.
19. Buntzel J., Schuth J., Kuttner, K., Glatzel M. (1998). Radiochemotherapy with amofostine cytoprotection for head and neck cancer. *Support Care Cancer, 6*(2),155–160.
20. Goren, M.P, McKenna, L.M., Goodman, T.L. (1997). Combined intravenous and oral mesna in outpatients treated with ifosfamide. *Cancer Chemother Pharmacol, 40*(5), 371–375.
21. Goren, M.P., Anthony, L.B., Hande, K.R., et al. (1998). Pharmacokinetics of an intravenous–oral versus intravenous mesna regimen in lung cancer patients receiving ifosfamide. *J Clin Oncol, 16*(2), 616–621.
22. Zinecard (dexrazoxane for injection) product information. (1998). Kalamazoo, MI: Pharmacia and Upjohn Company. *Physician's Desk Reference (52*, pp. 2299–2302). Montvale, NJ: Medical Economics.
23. Dorsett, D.S. (1990). Quality of care. In S.L. Groenwald, M.H. Frogee, M. Goodman, & C.H. Yarbro, eds., *Cancer Nursing: Principles and Practices* (p. 1153). Boston: Jones and Bartlett.
24. Goodman, M. (1992). *Cancer: Chemotherapy and Care* 3rd ed. (p. 33). Princeton, NJ: Bristol-Myers Squibb.
25. Carmichael, J., Fink, U., Russell, R.C., et al. (1996). Phase II study of gemcitabine in patients with advanced pancreas cancer. *Br J Cancer, 73*, 101–105.
26. Casper, E., Green, M., Kelson, D., et al. (1994). Phase II trial of gemcitabine (2',2'-difluorodeoxycytidine) in patients with adenocarcinoma of the pancreas. *Invest New Drugs, 12*(1), 29–34.

27. Tannock, I. (1978). Cell kinetics and chemotherapy: A critical review. *Cancer Treat Rep, 62*(8), 1117–1133.

28. McGuire, W.P., Rowinsky, E.K. (1991). Old drugs revisited, new drugs and experimental approaches in ovarian cancer therapy. *Semin Oncol, 18,* 255.

29. Thigpen, J.T., Vance, R.B., Balducci, L., et al. (1984). New drugs and experimental approaches in ovarian cancer treatment. *Semin Oncol, 11,* 314.

30. Robinson, E., Kimmick, G., & Muss, H. (1996). Tamoxifen in postmenopausal women: A safety perspective. *Drugs Aging, 8*(5), 329–337.

31. Davidson, N. (1999). Adjuvant endocrine therapy for early-stage breast cancer. *Proc Am Soc Clin Oncol,* 201–204.

32. Early Breast Cancer Trialists' Collaborative Group (1998). Tamoxifen for early breast cancer: An overview of the randomised trials. *Lancet 351,* 1451–1467.

33. Fisher, B., Costantino, J.P., Wickerham, D.L., et al. (1998). Tamoxifen as prevention of breast cancer: Report of the National Surgical Adjuvant Breast and Bowel Project P-1 study. *J Natl Cancer Inst, 90*(18),1371–1388.

34. Barakat, R.R. (1997). Benign and hyperplastic endometrial changes associated with tamoxifen use. *Oncology, 11,* 35–37.

35. Barakat, R.R., Gilewski, T.A., Almadrones, L., et al. (1999). The effect of adjuvant tamoxifen on the endometrium in women with breast cancer: A prospective study. *Proc Am Soc Clin Oncol, 1381,* 358a (abs.)

36. Miller, A.B., Hoogstraton, B., Statquet, M., & Winkler, A. (1981). Reporting results from cancer treatment. *Cancer, 47*(1), 207–214.

37. Schag, C.C., Heinruch, R.L., Ganz, P.A. (1984). Karnofsky performance status revisited: Reliability, validity and guidelines. *J Clin Oncol, 2*(3), 187–193.

38. Norton, L., & Simon, R. (1986). The Norton-Simon hypothesis revisited. *Cancer Treat Rep, 70*(1), 163–169.

39. Dolnick, B.J., Berenson, R.J., & Bertino, J.R. (1979). Correlation of dihydrofolate reductase elevation with gene amplification in a homogeneously staining chromosomal region in L5178Y cell. *J Clin Biol, 83,* 399–402.

40. Goldstein, L.J., Galski, H., Fojo, A., et al. (1989). Expression of multidrug resistance gene in human tumors. *J Natl Cancer Inst, 81*(2), 116–124.

41. Paston, I., & Gottesman, M. (1991). Multidrug resistance. *Ann Rev Med, 42,* 277–286.

42. Young, R. (1991). Principles of chemotherapy in gynecologic cancer. In W. Hoskins, C. Perez, & R. Young, eds., *Principles and Practices of Gynecology oncology* (pp. 333–347). Philadelphia: J.B. Lippincott.

43. Bourhis, J., Goldstien, L., Riou, G., et al. (1989). Expression of a human multidrug resistance gene in ovarian carcinomas. *Cancer Res, 49*(18), 5062–5065.

44. Ozols, R. (1991). Summary of symposium: Biology and therapy of ovarian cancer. *Semin Oncol, 18*(3), 297–306.

45. Ozols, R., Hamilton, T.C., & Masuda, H. (1988). Manipulation of cellular thiols to influence drug resistance. In P.V. Wooley & K.D. Kew, eds., *Mechanisms of Drug Resistance in Neoplastic Cells* (p. 289). San Diego: Academic Press.

46. O'Dwyer, P.J., Hamilton, T.C., LaCreta, F.P., et al. (1996). Phase I trial of buthiomine sulfoximine in combination with melphalan. *J Clin Oncol, 14*(1), 249–256.

47. Hryniuk, W.M. (1988). The importance of dose intensity in the outcome of chemotherapy. In S. Hellman, V. DeVita & S. Rosenbery, eds., *Advances in Oncology* (pp. 121–141). Philadelphia: J.B. Lippincott.

48. Levin, L. & Hryniuk, W. (1987). Dose intensity analysis of chemotherapy regimens in ovarian cancer. *J Clin Oncol, 5*(5), 756–767.

49. Aghajanian, C., Fennelly, D., Shapiro, F., et al. (1998). Phase II study of *dose-dense* high-dose chemotherapy treatment with peripheral–blood progenitor-cell support as primary treatment for patients with advanced ovarian cancer. *J Clin Oncol, 13*(5), 1852–1860.

50. McGuire, W.P., Hoskins, W.J., Brady, M.F., et al. (1995). Assessment of dose-intensive therapy in suboptimally debulked ovarian cancer: A Gynecologic Oncology Group study. *J Clin Oncol, 13*(7), 1589–1599.

51. Griffiths, C.T. (1986). Surgery at the time of diagnosis in ovarian cancer. In G. Blackledge, & K.K. Chan, eds., *Management of Ovarian Cancer.* London: Butterworths.

52. Ozols, R., Rubin, S., Dembo, A., & Robboy, S. (1991). Epithelial ovarian cancer. In W. Hoskins, C. Perez & R. Young, eds., *Principles and Practice of Gynecologic Oncology.* Philadelphia: J.B. Lippincott.

53. Moore, G., Almadrones, L. Huff, B.C., et al., eds. (1998). *Pocket Guide for Women and Cancer.* Boston: Jones and Bartlett.

54. Rowinsky, E.K., Cazenave, L.A., Donehower, R.C. (1990). Taxol: A novel investigational antimicrotubule agent. *J Natl Cancer Inst, 82*(15), 1247–1259.

55. Rowinsky, E.K., Onetto, N., Canetta, R.M., & Ar-

buck, S.G. (1992). Taxol: The first of the taxanes, an important new class of antitumor agents. *Semin Oncol, 19*(6), 646–662.

56. McGuire, W., Hoskins, W.J., Brady, M., et al. (1995). Taxol and cisplatin (TP) as compared to cytoxan and cisplatin (CP). *Proc Am Soc Clin Oncol, 14,* 771 (abs).

57. Einzig, A.I., Wiernik, P.H., Sasloff, J., & Runowicz, C.D. (1992). Phase II study and long-term follow-up of patients treated with taxol in advanced ovarian adenocarcinoma. *J Clin Oncol, 10*(11), 1748–1753.

58. Thigpen, T., Vance, R.B., McGuire W.P., et al. (1995). The role of paclitaxel in the management of coelomic epithelial carcinoma of the ovary: A review with emphasis on the Gynecologic Oncology Group experience. *Semin Oncol, 22*(6 suppl. 14), 23–31.

59. Lubejko, B., & Sartorius, S. (1993). Nursing considerations in paclitaxel administration. *Semin Oncol Nurs, 20*(4, suppl. 3), 26–30.

60. Bristol-Myers Sqibb Co. (1992). Data on file. Princeton, NJ.

61. Waugh, W.N., Trissel, L.A., & Stella, V.J. (1991). Stability, compatibility, and plasticizer extraction of taxol (NSC-125973) injection diluted in infusion solutions and stored in various containers. *Am J Hosp Pharm, 48*(7), 1520–1524.

62. National Cancer Institute. (1992, May). Taxol and related anticancer drugs. Washington, DC: National Cancer Institute Office of Communications.

63. National Cancer Institute. (1992, July). National Cancer Institute and Rhone-Poulenc Rorer agree to develop taxotere. National Cancer Institute Office of Communications.

64. Whitney, C.W., Sause, W., Bundy, B., et al. (1999). Randomized comparison of fluorouracil plus cisplatin versus hydroxyurea as an adjunct to radiation therapy in stage IIB–IVA carcinoma of the cervix with negative para-aortic lymph nodes: A Gynecologic Oncology Group and Southwest Oncology Group study. *J Clin Oncol, 17*(5), 1339–1348.

65. Rose, P.G., Bundy, B., Watkins, E.B., et al. (1999). Concurrent cisplatin-based radiotherapy and chemotherapy for locally advanced cervical cancer. *N Engl J Med, 340*(15), 1144–1153.

66. Markman, M., & Howell, S.B. (1985). Intraperitoneal cancer for ovarian carcinoma. In P.S. Alberts & E.A. Surwait, eds., *Ovarian Cancer.* Boston: Marinus Nijhoff.

67. Markman, M. (1986). Intraperitoneal antineoplastic agents for tumors principally confined to the peritoneal cavity. *Cancer Treat Rep, 13,* 219–242.

68. Alberts, D.S., Liu, P.Y., Hannigan, E.V., et al. (1996). Intraperitoneal cisplatin plus intravenous cyclophosphamide vs. intravenous cisplatin plus cyclophosphamide in stage III ovarian cancer. *N Engl J Med, 335*(26),1950–1955.

69. Barakat, R., Almadrones, L., Venkatraman, E., Spriggs, D. (1997). A phase II trial of intraperitoneal cisplatin and etoposide as consolidation therapy in patients with stage II–IV epithelial ovarian cancer following negative surgical assessment. *Proc Am Soc Clin Oncol, 16,* A1264 (abs).

70. Almadrones, L., Arcot, R. (1999). Patient guide to peripheral neuropathy. *Oncol Nurs Forum* (in press).

71. Rothenberg, M.L. (1997). Topoisomerase-I inhibitors: Review and update. *Ann Oncol, 8*(9), 837–855.

72. Sinha, B.K. (1995). Topoisomerase-I inhibitors: A review of their therapeutic potential in cancer. *Drugs, 49*(1), 11–19.

73. Kudelka, A.P., Tresukosal, D., Edwards, C.L., et al. (1996). Phase II study of intravenous topotecan as a five day infusion for refractory ovarian carcinoma. *J Clin Oncol, 14*(5), 1552–1557.

74. Gordon, A., Doherty, M., Hancock, K., et al. (1999). Phase I study of topotecan with carboplatin alternating with paclitaxel via a three hour infusion in combination with carboplatin in treatment of newly diagnosed ovarian cancer patients. *Proc Am Soc Clin Oncol, 1408,* 364a (abs).

75. Hoskins, P., Eisenhauer, B., Fisher, I. (1999). Sequential couplets of cisplatin/toptecan and cisplatin/paclitaxel as first-line therapy for advanced epithelial ovarian cancer: An NCIC clincial trials group phase II study. *Proc Am Soc Clin Oncol, 1378,* 357a (abs.).

76. Bos, A.M.E., De Vries, E.G.E., Van der Zee, A.G.J. (1999). Phase I and pharmakokinetic study of intraperitoneal topotecan. *Proc Am Soc Clin Oncol, 1404,* 363a (abs.).

77. Shimizu, Y., Umezawa, K., Ustugi, K. (1999). Combination of CPT-11 with mitomycin-C (MMC) for platinum-refractory clear cell (CCA) and mucinous (MCA) adenocarcinoma of the ovary. *Proc Am Soc Clin Oncol, 1393,* 361a (abs.).

78. Steingass, S. (1998). Liposomal anthracyclines: Doxil® and Daunoxome® administration guidelines and nursing management. Highlights from newer therapeutic agents. *Nursing Management, 3–6,* Meniscus Educational Institute.

79. Rose, P., Gordon, A., Granai, C.O., et al. (1999). Interim analysis of a non-comparitive, multicenter study of Doxil/Caelyx in the treatment of patients with refractory ovarian cancer. *Proc Am Soc Clin Oncol,1392,* 360a (abs.).

80. Verschraegan, C.F., Mansfield, P.F., Feig, B.W., et al. (1999). Phase I study of an intraperitoneal liposomal cisplatin analog L-NDDP for treatment of peritoneal carcinomatosis. *Proc Am Soc Clin Oncol, 1405,* 364a (abs.).

81. Cabriales, S., Bresnahan, J., Testa, D., et al. (1998). Extravasation of liposomal daunorubicin in patients with AIDS-associated Kaposi's sarcoma: A report of four cases. *Oncol Nurs Forum, 25*(1), 67–70.

82. O'Shaughnessy, J.A., Wittes, R.B., Burke, G., et al. (1991). Commentary concerning demonstration of safety and efficacy on investigational anti-cancer agents in clinical trials. *J Clin Oncol, 9,* 2225–2232.

83. Geersten, P., Hansen, M., Stroyer, I., et al. (1999). Combination chemotherapy with platinum, paclitaxel, and gemcitabine in patients with relapsed ovarian carcinoma. *Proc Am Soc Clin Oncol, 1395,* 391a (abs.).

84. Aghajanian, C., Sabbatini, P., Hensley, M., et al. (1999). A phase I trial of intraperitoneal cisplatin with IP gemcitabine in patients with epithelial ovarian cancer. *Proc Am Soc Clin Oncol, 1428,* 370a (abs.).

85. Plunkett, W., Huang, P., & Gandhi, V. (1995). Preclinical characteristics of gemcitabine. *Anticancer Drugs, 6*(suppl.), 7.

86. Stephens, C.D. (1998). Gemcitabine: A new approach to treating pancreatic cancer. *Oncol Nurs Forum, 25*(1), 87–93.

87. Barton Burke, M., Wilkes, G., Ingwerson, K., et al. (1996). Etoposide. In *Cancer Chemotherapy: A Nursing Process Approach* (p. 284). Boston: Jones and Bartlett.

88. Hoskins, P.J., Swenerton, K.D. (1994). Oral etoposide is active against platinum-resistant epithelial ovarian cancer. *J Clin Oncol, 12,* 60.

89. Hird, V., Marveyas, A., Snook, D., et al. (1993). Adjuvant therapy of ovarian cancer with radioactive monoclonal antibody. *Br J Cancer, 68,* 403.

90. Baselga, J., Norton, L., Albanell, J. (1998). Recombinant humanized anti-HER2 antibody (Herceptin™) enhances the antitumor activity of paclitaxel and doxorubicin against HER2/neu overexpression human breast cancer xenografts. *Cancer Res, 58*(13), 2825–2831.

91. Press, M.F., Pike, M.C., Chazin, V.R., et al. (1993). Her2/neu expression in node-negative breast cancer: Direct tissue quantification by computerized image analysis and association of overexpression with increased risk of recurrent disease. *Cancer Res, 53,* 4960–4970.

92. Genentech, Inc. (1998). Herceptin® (Trastuzumab). Manufacturers instructions for Administration.

93. Swain, S.M., Whaley, F.S., Gerber, M.C., et al. (1997). Cardioprotection with dexrezoxane for dosorubicin-containing therapy in advanced breast cancer. *J Clin Oncol, 15*(4), 1318–1332.

94. Michelotti, A., Salvadori, B., Donati, S., et al. (1997). A dose-finding study of ifosfamide by three-day continuous infusion in pretreated, advanced breast cancer patients. *Tumori, 83*(5), 826–828.

95. Capizzi, R.L. (1996). Amifostine: The preclinical basis for broad-spectrum selective cytoprotection of normal tissues from cytotoxic therapies. *Semin Oncol, 23* (suppl. 8), 2–17.

96. Peters, G.J., & van der Vijgh, W.J. (1995). Protection of normal tissues from the cytotoxic effects of chemotherapy and radiation by amofostine (WR-2721): Preclinical aspects. *Eur J Cancer, 31a* (suppl. 1), S1–S7.

97. Schuster, L.M. (1996). Guidelines for the administration of amofostine. *Semin Oncol, 223*(suppl. 8), 40–43.

98. McCaffrey, D., & Engelking, C. (1990). Ten fallacies associated with the nature and managment of chemotherapy extravasation. *Progressions, 2*(4), 3.

99. Otto, S. (1995). Chemotherapy. In S. Otto, ed., *Oncology Nursing* 2nd ed. St. Louis: Mosby–Year Book.

100. Oncology Nursing Society. (1996). *Cancer Chemotherapy Guidelines and Recommendations for Practice.* Pittsburgh: Oncology Nursing Society Press.

101. Goodman, M., & Wickman, R. (1984). Guide to vascular access devices. *Oncol Nurs Forum, 11*(5), 16–23.

102. Esparza, D. (1994). Ambulatory care. In S.L. Groenwald, M.H. Frogge, M. Goodman & C.H. Yarbro, eds., *Cancer Nursing: Principles and Practices.* Boston: Jones and Bartlett.

103. Groeger, J., Lucas, A.B., & Coit, D. (1991). Venous access in the cancer patient. In V.T. DeVita, S. Hellman & S. Rosenberg, eds., *Cancer Principles and Practices of Oncology* 3rd ed. Philadelphia: J.B. Lippincott.

104. Wickham, R., Purl, S., Welker, D. (1992). Long term central venous catheter issues for care. *Semin Oncol Nurs, 8*(2), 133–147.

105. Enviromental Protection Agency. (1991, October 9). Solid waste disposal facility criteria. EPA rules and regulations. *Fed Reg, 56*(196).

106. U.S. Department of Labor, Office of Occupational Medicine, Occupational Safety and Health Administration. (1993). *Work Practice Guidelines for Personnel Dealing with Cytotoxic (Antineoplastic) Drugs* (No. 8-1.1). Washington, DC: U.S. Government Printing Office.

107. Dedrick, R.L., Myers, C.E., Bungay, P.M., & DeVita, V.T. (1978). Pharmacokinetic rationale for peritoneal drug administration in the treatment of ovarian cancer. *Cancer Treat Rep, 62*(1), 1–9.

108. Swenson, K.K., & Eriksson, J. (1986). Nursing management of intraperitoneal therapy. *Oncol Nurs Forum, 13*(5), 33–39.

109. Hoff, S.T. (1987). Concepts in intraperitoneal chemotherapy. *Semin Oncol Nurs, 3*(2), 112–117.

110. Reichman, B., Markman, M., Hakes, T., et al. (1988). Phase I trial of concurrent intraperitoneal and continuous intravenous infusion of fluorouracil in patients with refractory ovarian cancer. *J Clin Oncol, 6*(1), 158–162.

111. Lucas, W. E., Markman, M., & Howell, S.B. (1985). Intraperitoneal chemotherapy for advanced ovarian cancer. *Am J Obstet Gynecol, 152*(4), 474–478.

112. Kraft, A.R., Tompkins, R.K., & Jesseh, J.E. (1971). Peritoneal electrolyte absorption of intraperitoneally administered compounds. *J Pharmacol Exp Ther, 178*, 562–566.

113. West, G.W., Weichselbaum, R., & Little, J.B. (1980). Limited penetration of methotrexate into human osteosarcoma spheroids as a proposed model for solid tumor resistance in adjuvant chemotherapy. *Cancer Res, 40*(10), 3665–3668.

114. Markman, M., Hakes, T., Reichman, B., et al. (1989). Intraperitoneal therapy in the management of ovarian carcinoma. *Yale J Biol Med, 62*(4), 393–403.

115. Rosenshein, N.B., Blake, D., McIntyre, P.A. (1978). The effect of volume on the distribution of substrates instilled into the peritoneal cavity. *Gynecol Oncol, 6*, 106–110.

116. Piccart, M.J., Speyer, J.L., Markman, M., et al. (1985). Intraperitoneal chemotherapy: Technical experience at five institutions. *Semin Oncol, 12*(3, suppl. 4), 90–96.

117. Rubin, S.C., Hoskins, W.H., Markman, M., et al. (1989). Long-term access to the peritoneal cavity in ovarian cancer patients, *Gynecol Oncol, 33*(1), 46–48.

118. Almadrones, L., & Yerys, C. (1990). Problems associated with the administration of intraperitoneal therapy using the Port-A-Cath system. *Oncol Nurs Forum, 17*(1), 75–80.

119. Davidson, S., Rubin, S., Markman, M., et al. (1991). Intraperitoneal chemotherapy: Analysis of complications with an implanted subcutaneous port and catheter system. *Gynecol Oncol, 41*, 101–106.

120. Makija, S., Leitao, M., Bander, N., et al. (1999). Complications associated with intraperitoneal chemotherapy catheters. *Proc Am Soc Clin Oncol, 1462*, 378a (abs.).

121. Eriksson, J., & Swenson, K. (1986). Your guide to intraperitoneal therapy. *Oncol Nurs Forum, 13*(5), 77–81.

C H A P T E R   1 2

Biologic Response Modifiers

Jane Duffy-Weisser, RN, ANP, CS
Kimberly A. Schmit-Pokorny, RN, MSN, OCN

✕ INTRODUCTION

Biological response modifiers (BRMs) are "agents or approaches that modify the host's biological response to tumor cells with resulting therapeutic benefit."[1] "BRMs are natural substances produced in small amounts in the body. They are important regulators and messengers of normal function. The action of BRMs is to boost body response to foreign substances, most notably tumor cells. They act indirectly to stimulate or enhance activity of the immune system."[2] During the 1980s, the use of BRMs to treat cancer patients rapidly increased. BRMs are now given to patients with gynecologic cancers, both as treatment and to decrease recovery time following chemotherapy and/or irradiation. Gynecologic oncology nurses must have a thorough understanding of the roles BRMs may have for their patients. This is a unique challenge as the number of BRMs continues to grow and the applications for specific BRMs continue to expand.

✕ HISTORICAL DEVELOPMENT

The work of Dr. William B. Coley, in the late 1800s, contributed to the knowledge and understanding of BRMs in the cancer patient. Coley, a surgeon, noted that patients who had a postoperative infection remained free of cancer for a longer period of time than others. He began to induce infections in patients with cancer by using live bacteria and, later, filtered toxins. Coley's toxins, used until 1975, laid the foundation for the identification of tumor necrosis factor, which is still being investigated today.[3]

In the 1960s, trials using *Bacillus Calmette-Guerin*, methanol-extracted residue, and *Corynebacterium parvum* were conducted. These substances were thought to initiate an immune response, thereby increasing the body's defenses against foreign substances.[1] The majority of these trials produced beneficial results but were difficult to replicate.

Because of this inability to replicate results, a negative attitude toward biotherapy developed in the 1970s. By the late 1970s and early 1980s, however, major advances in science, primarily the development of recombinant deoxyribonucleic acid (rDNA) technology, improved the understanding of BRMs. Better comprehension of the immune system and progress in genetic engineering also allowed for the major biotechnological advances seen in the last decade.[4]

✕ OVERVIEW OF THE IMMUNE SYSTEM

To appreciate the concept and function of BRMs, one must first have a basic understanding of the immune system and the human immune response. This means having knowledge of the components of the immune system as they relate to various organs, tissue, and blood, as well as the role lymphocytes and cytokines play in facilitating the immune response. The function of the immune system as a whole depends on the orchestrated actions of its cellular parts.

Components

Many different areas of the body can be considered components of the immune system. The largest organ is the skin. When intact, skin functions as an excellent barrier to the myriad different invading organisms with which it is constantly bombarded. Once the shield is broken, however, infection is a possibility. This point has been illustrated in surgical patient populations and those who have sustained trauma.[5]

Although skin provides an excellent barrier to invading organisms, or antigens, natural openings such as the respiratory, gastrointestinal, and urogenital tracts allow for the entry of bacteria, viruses, fungi, and parasites. However, the immune system does not leave these areas unguarded. Mucosa-associated lymphoid tissue (MALT), a general term describing tissue that is enriched with lymphocytes, lines these areas so that pathogens can be intercepted at their points of entry.[6] The unique physiologic functions of the systems themselves also assist in removal of invading pathogens. Examples of these functions are the sweeping action of the ciliated epithelium in the respiratory tract, the flushing action of the urinary tract, and the washing action of tears.

The most critical work of the immune system takes place at the cellular level, by the actions of lymphocytes (T and B cells), phagocytes (monocytes, macrophages, and neutrophils), and accessory cells (eosinophils, basophils, mast cells, platelets, and antigen-presenting cells).[7]

Lymphocytes

B Cells

These cells are a part of the humoral immune response. They develop in the bone marrow and are distributed in lymph nodes. They produce immunoglobulins, or antibodies. There are five classes of immunoglobulins, all of which are composed of proteins:

IgA is found mostly in salivary secretions and the respiratory and gastrointestinal tracts. It protects mucous membranes.

IgD is coexpressed with IgM and is found on differentiating B cells.[6] Little is known about this antibody.

IgE mediates type I hypersensitivity reactions, which are usually seen in hayfever and asthma.

IgG is the major immunoglobulin. It is responsible for long-term immunity against infectious diseases.

IgM is produced shortly after exposure to an antigen.

T Cells

These cells are also part of the humoral immune response. They develop in the bone marrow and mature in the thymus gland. They are distributed throughout the lymph system. There are four categories of T cells:

Helper cells recognize antigens and release cytokines. They facilitate the production of B cells and antibody production.
Killer cells directly destroy antigens that have been sensitized with antibody.
Suppressor cells slow down the cytotoxic action of T and B cells when the antigen is under control.
Memory cells facilitate an immediate cell-mediated, or T cell, response on exposure to a previously encountered antigen.

Phagocytes

Neutrophils

Neutrophils are the most abundant type of white blood cell, accounting for approximately 70% of the total white blood cell count. They are considered the second-line phagocyte in defense against infection. Neutrophils are used by the body primarily for extravascular phagocytosis. Neutrophils develop in the bone marrow and are distributed systemically.

Monocytes

These cells are the precursors to macrophages. They develop in bone marrow and are distributed systemically.

Macrophages

Macrophages are morphologically the largest of all the phagocytes and are considered the first-line phagocytes in defense against infection. They develop in the bone marrow and are distributed in the lungs, spleen, and secondary lymphoid tissue.

Accessory Cells

Eosinophils

These cells regulate the inflammatory response. Eosinophils develop in the bone marrow and are distributed systemically.

Basophils

Basophils are precursors to mast cells. They produce histamines and assist during inflammatory response. They develop in bone marrow, are distributed systemically, and account for less than 0.5% of the total white blood cell count.

Mast Cells

These cells assist in inflammatory response by releasing histamine. They develop in the bone marrow and are distributed in the gut, lung, and vascular circulation.

Antigen-Presenting Cells

These cells present antigens to lymphocytes in a form they can recognize. They are distributed in spleen, skin, circulation, and lymphoid tissue. Some examples of antigen-presenting cells are macrophages, Langerhans' cells, follicular dendritic cells, and dendritic cells.

Types of Immunity

Innate Immunity

The human immune system comprises two types of immunity, one of which is considered more generalized than the other and is known as *innate* or *natural immunity*. Innate immunity does not defend against specific organisms, and the immunologic ability to resist a specific organism is not improved each time this system is used.[6] The cells that are involved in innate immunity are the macrophages, neutrophils, and T cells. In addition, the complement complex, which is a system of twenty or more proteins that can further destroy invading organisms, can also be initiated during this type of response. Other, less obvious components of innate immunity include the pH of certain areas of the body, such as the high acid content of gastric secretions, which assists in the destruction of bacteria.[8,9]

Acquired Immunity

Acquired immunity is specific, and it is characterized by its ability to improve resistance to infection when the specific organism tries to invade again. There are two types of acquired immunity: cell-mediated and humoral.

Cell-Mediated.   Cell-mediated immunity is known as *T cell immunity* because it does not involve the antigen/antibody complexes that are made from B cells. In this system, helper T cells (CD4) begin to proliferate when a piece of antigen has been displayed on the surface of a nearby macrophage.[10] The T cell response results in the production of a variety of different types of cytokines, such as Interleukin-1 and Interleukin-2. These cytokines cause a proliferation of yet more T cells, including another subset known as cytotoxic (killer) T cells, which work by puncturing holes in the host cells that have become infected by the antigen. Helper cells are extremely instrumental in regulating immunity because they stimulate not only cytotoxic T cells but also the production of more macrophages, and they somehow enhance their phagocytosis.

Suppressor T cells are another subset. They help to keep the cytotoxic effects of killer T cells under control so that a large number of normal cells are not destroyed. Memory T cells also play an important role, in that they remember an antigen to which they were exposed and are able to create a stronger and faster immune response on subsequent exposure to the same antigen.

The distinguishing feature of cell-mediated response is that it recognizes antigens that are presented by a cell. That is, antigens recognized in this response are not free-floating. Instead, T cell recognition is dependent on the presentation of a macrophage. A graft-versus-host reaction is an example of a cell-mediated response.[6,11]

Humoral. Humoral response is characterized by the antigen/antibody complex, which means that the B cells are involved. However, it is helper T cells that stimulate the proliferation of B cells during a humoral response. The most mature type of B cell, known as the *plasma cell*, produces the antibodies, and each daughter cell of a single B cell produces the same type of antibodies against a particular antigen. Once the antigen/antibody complex has been formed, free-floating antigens can be directly attacked without having to first be presented by a macrophage or other antigen-presenting cell. This makes the humoral response particularly effective in eliminating foreign organisms.

Monoclonal Antibodies

The theoretical concept of monoclonal antibody production is to clone unlimited quantities of a pure antibody with a single specificity. The technique for this procedure was first accomplished in 1975 by George Kohler and Cesar Milstein. Their work revealed that malignant myeloma cells could continuously reproduce themselves in vitro; thus, they were considered immortal.[12] Antibody-presenting B lymphocytes were not considered immortal, however, as they could survive for only several days in culture medium. The monoclonal antibody (MoAb) technique involved the fusion of the immortal myeloma cells and B lymphocytes, which were taken from a mouse that had been immunized with the myeloma cells. The hybrid mix, known as a *hybridoma*, produced some antibodies that possessed qualities of the immortal cells and the specificity of the antibodies. The hybridoma thus produced unlimited growth of specific antibodies.

MoABs may be used to diagnose and treat certain malignancies. However, they still work better in theory than in clinical practice. This is due to the lack of true specificity of tumor antigens. That is, many cancer antigens share a certain amount of heterogeneity with normal tissue and other conditions that are not specific to the tumor in question.[13] An example of this is the CA-125 antigen, which is the most widely used tumor marker, or tumor-associated antigen, in gynecologic oncology. The CA-125 antigen is detected by MoAb OC 125, which was developed from an epithelial ovarian cancer line. But an elevated CA-125 value can be seen in conditions other than epithelial ovarian cancer, such as endometriosis, fibroids, pelvic inflammatory disease, pregnancy, congestive heart failure, intestinal obstruction, cirrhosis, and other cancers, such as breast cancer.[14] Although the CA-125 marker is the single most important use of MoAb OC 125, its use as a screening tool for ovarian cancer remains controversial. In 98% of postmenopausal women, an elevated CA-125 value is a positive predictor of ovarian cancer, but in premenopausal women, the positive predictor value is only 49%.[14]

Another use of MoAb OC 125 has been to immunopathologically distinguish occult mesothelial cells from ovarian cancer cells in pleural effusion fluid.[14] In the future, its use may allow for antigenic phenotyping of individual tumors obtained at the time of surgery. This may improve the specificity of tumor markers, which may in turn improve treatment and predictive prognosis.[14]

Another clinical application of MoAbs is in computerized axial tomography (CAT or CT scan imaging). This is accomplished by attaching a radioisotope to a MoAb. The advantage of this type of diagnostic, or prognostic, imaging is to determine the geometric distribution of tumor growth.[15] CAT imaging remains investigational; to date, radiolabeled isotopes remain too unreliable to replace second-look laparotomy.

Interferons

Interferons (IFNs) are a category of BRMs that have antitumor and antiviral properties. There are three subtypes, alpha, beta, and gamma,[16] all of which stimulate different types of biological responses. Antiviral effects are produced by stimulating cells infected with a virus to produce proteins that slow down viral replication. Other responses result in the inhibition of DNA and protein synthesis of cancer cells. Interferons can also stimulate the host's immune system by enhancing the production of natural killer cells.

Alpha and beta INFs are classified as type I. They are produced by macrophages and are used to treat viruses such as rhinovirus, papilloma virus, condyloma acuminata, and retrovirus. They have also been approved to treat hairy cell leukemia, Kaposi's sarcoma, and hepatitis C. Gamma INF, which is produced by T cells and natural killer cells, is classified as type II. It has recently been approved to treat chronic granulomatous disease.[2]

Other uses for IFNs are being tested in clinical trials.

Colony-Stimulating Factors

Colony-stimulating factors (CSFs), sometimes called *lymphokines*, *cytokines*, or *hematopoietic growth factors*, are glycoproteins that regulate hematopoiesis at all levels in the hematopoietic tree (Figure 12.1). CSFs may be considered for supportive treatment of patients with cancer, because they are given to treat side effects from the primary treatment. CSFs regulate and stimulate the production and maturation of red blood cells (RBCs), white blood cells (WBCs), and platelets by binding to specific receptor sites located on the cell surface. Recombinant DNA technology has allowed the production of CSFs. In the oncology setting, CSFs may be used to decrease the neutropenia, anemia, or thrombocytopenia caused by cancer therapy agents.

Lineage-Restricted versus Multilineage CSFs

CSFs can be divided into lineage-restricted (affecting one specific cell maturational or proliferational line) and multilineage (affecting more than one specific cell maturational or proliferational line) CSFs (Table 12.1). The most common CSFs are granulocyte colony–stimulating factor (G-CSF), granulocyte-macrophage colony–stimulating factor (GM-CSF), and erythropoietin (EPO).

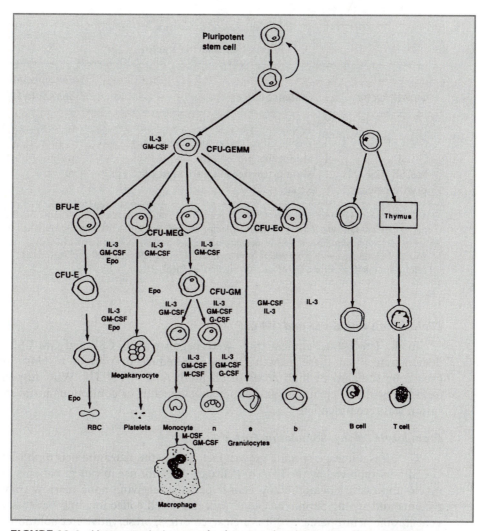

FIGURE 12.1. Hematopoietic cascade showing development of blood cells from a common progenitor to mature cells of the various lineages. Also shown are stages of development at which colony-stimulating factors (growth factors) have been found to stimulate cell proliferation, differentiation, or maturation. Abbreviations for cell types: BFU-E, burst-forming unit-erythroid; CRU-Bas, colony-forming unit-basophil; CRU-E, colony-forming unit-erythroid; CFU-Eo, colony-forming unit-eosinophil; CFU-GM, colony-forming unit-granulocyte-macrophage; CFU-Meg, colony-forming unit-megakaryocyte.

Source: Clark, S.C., & Karmen, R. (1987). The human hematopoietic colony-stimulating factors. *Science, 236*(4806), 1229–1237. Copyright © 1987 American Association for the Advancement of Science. Reprinted with permission.

TABLE 12.1

Colony-Stimulating Factors

Growth Factor	Cellular Sources	Cell Lineages Stimulated
Il–3	T cells	n, m, e, E, M
GM-CSF	T cells, fibroblasts, endothelial cells	n, m, e, E, M
G-CSF	Monocytes, fibroblasts	n
M-CSF (CSF–1)	Monocytes, fibroblasts, endothelial cells	m
Erythropoietin	Renal	E

Abbreviations: Il–3, Interleukin-3; GM-CSF, granulocyte-macrophage colony–stimulating factor; G-CSF, granulocyte colony–stimulating factor; M-CSF, macrophage colony–stimulating factor; n, neutrophils; m, monocytes; e, eosinophils; E, erythroids; M, megakaryocytes.
Source: Reproduced with permission from Vadhan-Raj, S. (1989). Clinical applications of colony-stimulating factors. *Oncology Nursing Forum, 16*(6), 21.

Clinical Trials with G-CSF and GM-CSF

In the late 1980s, clinical trials were begun with G-CSF and GM-CSF. Studies demonstrated that these growth factors can reduce or prevent myelosuppression caused by standard or high doses of chemotherapy.[17,18,19] The WBC response was found to be dose-dependent, and either subcutaneous or continuous intravenous infusion was recommended.[20]

Granulocyte Colony–Stimulating Factor

G-CSF is a lineage-specific growth factor that stimulates the neutrophil lineage.[21] G-CSF was approved by the FDA in February 1991 for use in cancer patients receiving myelosuppressive chemotherapy, cancer patients receiving bone marrow transplants, patients undergoing peripheral blood progenitor cell collection, and patients with severe chronic neutropenia.[22,23] It is a clear, colorless, preservative-free solution that can be diluted with dextrose solutions, but not saline solutions. G-CSF can be given intravenously (IV) or subcutaneously (SQ). Unused portions should be discarded, and vials should be refrigerated. The recommended dose of G-CSF is between 5 and 10 mcg/kg, and this may be increased by 5 mcg/kg with each chemotherapy cycle.[24] If the absolute neutrophil count (ANC) reaches 10,000 cells/mm^3, the G-CSF should be decreased or discontinued. Once G-CSF is stopped, the WBC may fall by 50%. The administration of G-CSF should be started twenty-four hours after the completion of chemotherapy; otherwise, the initial burst of cells could be destroyed by the chemotherapy.[24]

Within five minutes of IV administration of G-CSF, the neutrophil count decreases. In four hours, a rise in the circulating neutrophils occurs. No constant changes in hemoglobin, hematocrit, or platelet counts have been noted. Some morphological changes in granulocytes, including Dohle bodies and toxic granulations, have been reported.[25]

Granulocyte-Macrophage Colony–Stimulating Factor

GM-CSF is a multilineage colony-stimulating factor.[25] It is active at much earlier stages in the hematopoietic stem cell lineage than other factors. Currently, GM-CSF is indicated and approved to stimulate myeloid engraftment following induction chemotherapy in acute myelogenous leukemia, for use in mobilization and following transplantation of autologous peripheral blood progenitor cells, for myeloid reconstitution after autologous and allogeneic bone marrow transplantation, and for use in bone marrow transplantation failure or engraftment delay.[23,24]

GM-CSF is supplied as a sterile, preserved, liquid, injectable solution (500 mcg/ml), and as a preservative-free white powder to which 1.0 cc of sterile water is added. GM-CSF should be diluted with normal saline according to the package insert. Vials should be stored in a refrigerator. Unused portions of open vials should be discarded. To prevent foaming, the sterile water should be injected and directed toward the side of the vial.

After administration of GM-CSF, neutrophil counts immediately increase. In three to seven days, the WBC plateaus. After this plateau, there is another increase in WBC and another plateau. Cellular changes include toxic granulations in the neutrophils and an increase in eosinophils and monocytes.[25]

The recommended dosage is 250 mcg/m^2/day for 21 days. If the ANC reaches 20,000 or greater, the drug should be decreased or discontinued.

Erythropoietin

Erythropoietin (EPO) is produced mainly by the kidney to stimulate red blood cell production. It was first purified from human urine by Dr. Eugene Goldwasser at the University of Chicago in 1976. In 1985, clinical trials were begun, and in 1989, EPO was approved by the FDA for use in decreasing anemia produced by chronic renal failure. In April 1993, EPO was approved by the FDA for the treatment of anemia caused by chemotherapy.

The commercially available product is colorless and preservative-free and may be administered IV or SQ. For patients receiving chemotherapy, the recommended dosage is 150 units/kg three times weekly. After two months, if the response is not satisfactory, the dose may be increased to 300 units/kg three times weekly. The hematocrit should be monitored, with a reduction in dose for a hematocrit of greater than 40%.

Before starting EPO, the patient's serum ferritin levels should be evaluated. If the serum ferritin is less than 100 ng/ml, the patient should be given iron supplements to maximize the effect of the EPO. Blood pressure should be monitored, as EPO may cause an elevation.

Other Cytokines

Many cytokines are in clinical trials. Interleukin-3 (IL-3), a multilineage growth factor; PIXY321, a fusion of GM-CSF and IL-3; Interleukin-6, stem cell factor; and FLT3 Ligand are several.

CSFs hold great potential for oncology patients. Many of the risks of chemotherapy or radiation can be decreased or avoided through their use, allowing higher doses of therapy to be given. Nurses must understand the rationale for using CSFs and possess a thorough knowledge of their potential functions.

✻ NURSING MANAGEMENT

Assessment

It is important for nurses to perform a thorough assessment of the patient who is to undergo BRM therapy. The assessment should include pretreatment considerations (Table 12.2),

---

TABLE 12.2

Pretreatment Considerations in the Nursing Assessment of Patients Receiving Biological Response Modifiers

Prior experience with chemotherapy and/or BRMs
Medical/surgical history
Informed consent
Treatment protocol details
Physical
   Weight and height
   Vital signs
      Blood pressure
      Heart rate
      Respiratory rate
      Temperature
   Skin
      Turgor
      Color
      Integrity (scars, rashes, varicosities)
   Neurologic
      Peripheral sensation
      Mental status
      Memory
      Reflexes
      Sensory perception
   Cardiovascular
      Heart sounds
      Edema
      Angina
   Respiratory
      Breath sounds

TABLE 12.2 *(continued)*

Cough
    Sputum production
    History (e.g., pleural effusion)
Genitourinary
    Patterns of elimination
    Characteristics of urine (color, amount)
    Frequency patterns
    Symptoms of infection (dysuria, urgency, frequency)
Nutritional status
    Weight
    Diet
    Food intolerances
    Nausea (frequency, precipitating patterns)
    Vomiting (frequency, color, amount)
    History of recent weight loss/gain
Gastrointestinal
    Evaluation of abdomen
    Character of bowel sounds
    History of pain
    History of abdominal distention (e.g., ascites)
    Evaluate stool for blood
Laboratory values
    Electrolytes
    BUN
    Creatinine
    Uric acid
    Magnesium
    Calcium
    Complete blood count with differential
Psychosocial anxiety related to:
    Diagnosis
    Disease status
    New treatment modality
    Side effects
    Efficacy of treatment
Knowledge deficit related to:
    Rationale for new treatment modality
    Self-injection technique
Financial and health insurance resources

Sources: Adapted with permission from Yasko, J., & Dudjak, L. (1990). *Biological Response Modifier Therapy Symptom Management* (pp. 190–191). New York: Park Row Publishers, Cetus Corporation. Mayer, D. (1990). Biotherapy: Recent advances and nursing implications. *Nursing Clinics of North America,* 25(2), 296–301.

TABLE 12.3		
Management of BRM Side Effects		
System	Side Effect	Assessment/Management
Neurological/ Psychological	Confusion Disorientation Combativeness Psychosis Anxiety Irritability	Assess before starting Reassurance Patient/family education Provide for patient safety Support/encouragement Relaxation techniques Avoid alcohol
Renal	Oliguria Increased creatinine Increased BUN Proteinuria	Monitor I/O Monitor BUN/Cr Adequate hydration
Hematologic	Anemia Thrombocytopenia Leukopenia	Monitor CBC and platelet count Assess petechiae, bruising, bleeding gums, other bleeding Test stool, urine, emesis for blood No rectal thermometers, suppositories Assess for infection Possible transfusions
Hepatic	Increased bilirubin LDH, SGOT, SGPT	Monitor bilirubin LDH, SGOT, SGPT
Skin	Rash Pruritus Dryness Dermatitis Erythema Alopecia	Prophylactic diphenhydramine hydrochloride Avoid scrubbing, pat dry Apply water-based lotion
Gastrointestinal	Nausea Vomiting Diarrhea Mucositis Reduced appetite Taste alterations	Nutritional assessment Monitor I/O Prophylactic antiemetic Antidiarrheal Good oral hygiene Assess oral mucosa Small, frequent meals Monitor weight

System	Side Effect	Assessment/Management
Cardiovascular/ Pulmonary	Hypo/hypertension Weight gain Peripheral edema Ascites Arrhythmia Pulmonary edema Dyspnea Tachycardia Cough Pallor Cyanosis Tachypnea	Monitor vital signs Monitor I/O Elevate extremities Oxygen Monitor weight
Flulike Syndrome	Fever Chills Headache Malaise Nasal congestion Fatigue Bone pain Weight loss	Prophylactic acetaminophen and prn Monitor temperature Meperidine hydrochloride Warm clothing, blankets Keep well hydrated Schedule rest periods Prioritize activities Decrease infusion rate Cold or warm compresses

TABLE 12.3 *(continued)*

Sources: Adapted with permission from Yasko, J., & Dudjak, L. (1990). *Biological Response Modifier Therapy Symptom Management* (pp. 190–191). New York: Park Row Publishers, Cetus Corporation. Mayer, D. (1990). Biotherapy: Recent advances and nursing implications. *Nursing Clinics of North America, 25*(2), 296–301.

which necessitates knowledge of the patient's history, current treatment plan, and any chemotherapy protocol details.[27] In addition, a thorough physical examination should be done prior to therapy and intermittently throughout the regimen.

The side effects of the different BRMs are similar to one another. Nurses need to be able to assess the patient for side effects and initiate management strategies to lessen them (Table 12.3).

Discharge Planning

Home Care Preparations

Because more gynecologic cancer patients are being treated with dose-intensive schedules of chemotherapy, it is imperative that they comply with adjuvant treat-

TABLE 12.4

Patient Education: How to Take Growth Factors at Home

Supplies	Vials of medication Syringes Needles Alcohol preps Storage container for used syringes and needles
Medical Direction	Dosage in milligrams Volume of medication to be drawn up into the syringe Frequency Preferred time of day Know sites of injection (provide patient with charts of subcutaneous sites) Hygiene (hand-washing)
Storage	Store medicine vials in a safe place Keep medicine vials refrigerated Allow medicine to come to room temperature before injecting Discard entire vial and any unused portions after self-injection
Self-Injection Technique	Choose a clean and well-lighted area to set up supplies and self-inject Make sure all equipment is in front of you before you attempt to self-inject Wash and dry hands thoroughly before starting Choose a subcutaneous site that is free of rash, bruise, varicosity, or other skin breakdown Properly dispose of needles and syringes after use
Common Side Effects	Fatigue Flulike syndrome
Contacts	Know the telephone number of your attending physician. Know the telephone number of your local emergency room. Call your nurse or doctor with any questions regarding your medication.

ments, such as self-administering colony-stimulating factors following chemotherapy (Table 12.4). Nurses play a crucial role in ensuring that patients and their families understand the various rationales for their treatments and that protocol details are followed conscientiously. Thorough and professional educational techniques, along with follow-up evaluation, may also decrease the morbidity associated with chemotherapy and related BRMs.

TABLE 12.5
Diagnostic Cluster

Treatment Period

COLLABORATIVE PROBLEMS
Potential Complication: Preexisting medical conditions
Potential Complication: Fluid/electrolyte imbalance

NURSING DIAGNOSIS
1. Anxiety/fear related to loss of feelings of control of life, unpredictability of nature of disease, and uncertain future
2. Anxiety/fear related to insufficient knowledge of prescribed biotherapy and necessary self-care measures
3. Potential for infection related to immunosuppression neutropenia secondary to chemotherapy and/or radiation therapy
4. Potential for bleeding related to immunosuppression thrombocytopenia secondary to chemotherapy and/or radiation therapy
5. Potential altered nutrition: less than body requirements related to nausea, vomiting, anorexia, and/or stomatitis
6. Potential alteration in comfort related to flulike syndrome and/or arthralgia/myalgia
7. Potential for alteration in comfort related to side effects of therapy and/or disease process
8. Potential for alteration in quality of life related to fatigue

Psychosocial Preparations and Resources

Nurses must keep in mind the burden and anxiety that are placed on patients when we ask them to physically participate in their own cancer therapy, using skills that have traditionally belonged only to their nurses and doctors. Self-injecting with colony-stimulating factors is such a case. This requires us to refine our psychosocial skills. We must find out who our patients really are and what resources are available to them, including health care resources covered by their insurance companies, resources in their communities, and their connections with family and friends.

✳ REFERENCES

1. Abernathy, E. (1987). Biotherapy: An introductory overview. *Oncol Nurs Forum, 14*(suppl. 6), 13–15.
2. Wujak, D. (1993). An odyssey into biologic therapy. *Oncol Nurs Forum, 20*(6), 879–887.
3. Goodfield, J. (1984). Dr. Coley's toxins. *Science, 84,* 68–73.
4. Jassak, P. (1987). Future trends in biotherapy. *Oncol Nurs Forum, 14*(suppl. 6), 38–40.

5. Schnefider, R., Christou, N.V., Meakins, J.L., & Norh, C. (1991). Humoral immunity in patients with and without trauma. *Arch Surg, 126,* 143–148.

6. Male, D. (1991.) *Immunology: An Illustrated Outline* 2nd ed. (pp. 14–37). London: Gower.

7. Abernathy, E. (1987). How the immune system works. *Am J Nurs,* (April), 455–459.

8. Gallucci, B. (1987). The immune system and cancer. *Oncol Nurs Forum, 14*(6), 2–12.

9. Morstyn, G., & Dexter, M.T. (1994). *Filgrastim in Clinical Practice.* New York: Marcel Dekker.

10. Guyton, A. (1991). *Textbook of Medical Physiology* 8th ed. (pp. 374–384). Philadelphia: Saunders.

11. Galluci, B., & McCarthy, D. (1995). The immune system. In P. Trahan, ed., *Biotherapy: A Comprehensive Overview* (pp. 32–34). Boston: Jones and Bartlett.

12. Kohler, G., & Milstein, C. (1975). Continuous culture of fused cells secreting antibodies of predefined specificity. *Nature, 256,* 495–497.

13. Smith, L., Nelson, N., & Teng, H. (1987). Clinical applications of monoclonal antibodies in gynecologic oncology. *Cancer, 60*(8), 2068–2074.

14. Rubin, S. (1993). Monoclonal antibodies in the management of ovarian cancer: A clinical perspective. *Cancer, 71*(4), 1602–1612.

15. Smith, L., & Yin, A. (1992). Human monoclonal antibody recognizing an antigen associated with ovarian and other adenocarcinomas. *Am J Obstet Gynecol, 166*(2), 634–645.

16. Yasko, J., & Dudjak, L. (1990). *Biological Response Modifier Therapy Symptom Management* (pp. 49–163). New York: Park Row Publishers, Cetus Corporation.

17. Gutterman, J. (1988). Clinical studies of granulocyte-macrophage colony–stimulating factor. *Semin Oncol, 5*(suppl. 5), 52–53.

18. Vadhan-Raj, S., Keatting, J., & LeMaistre, A. (1987). Effects of recombinant human granulocyte-macrophage colony–stimulating factor on myelodysplastic syndromes. *N Engl J Med, 317*(25), 1547–1552.

19. Antman, K., Griffin, J., & Elias, A. (1988). Effect of recombinant human granulocyte macrophage colony–stimulating factor on chemotherapy-induced myelosuppression. *N Engl J Med, 319*(14), 593–598.

20. Herrmann, F., Schulz, G., & Lindemann, A. (1989). Hematopoietic responses in patients with advanced malignancy treated with recombinant human granulocyte-macrophage colony–stimulating factor. *J Clin Oncol, 7*(2), 159–167.

21. Morstyn, G., & Burgess, A. (1988). Hemopoietic growth factors: A review. *Cancer Res, 48*(20), 5624–5637.

22. Shoemaker, D. (1992). Recombinant granulocyte colony–stimulating factor in patients receiving chemotherapy for small-cell lung cancer: Clinical findings and case management. In R. Carroll-Johnson, *A Case Management Approach to Patients Receiving G-CSF* (p. 14019). Pittsburgh, PA: Oncology Nursing Press.

23. Ortho Biotech, Inc. (1998). Package insert for Procrit® (epoetin alfa). Raritan, NJ: Ortho Biotech, Inc.

24. Wujcik, D. (1992). *Practical Questions and Answers for Oncology Nurses.* New York: Triclinica Communications.

25. Gabrilove, J. (1991). Colony-stimulating factors: Clinical status. In V. DeVita, S. Hellman, & S. Rosenberg, eds., *Biologic Therapy of Cancer* (pp. 445–463). Philadelphia: Lippincott.

26. Stewart, S. (1992). Colony-stimulating factors—Helping blood cells grow. *BMT Newsletter.* Highland Park, NJ: BMT Newsletter.

27. Irwin, M. (1987). Patients receiving biological response modifiers: Overview of nursing care. *Oncol Nurs Forum, 14*(6), 32–37.

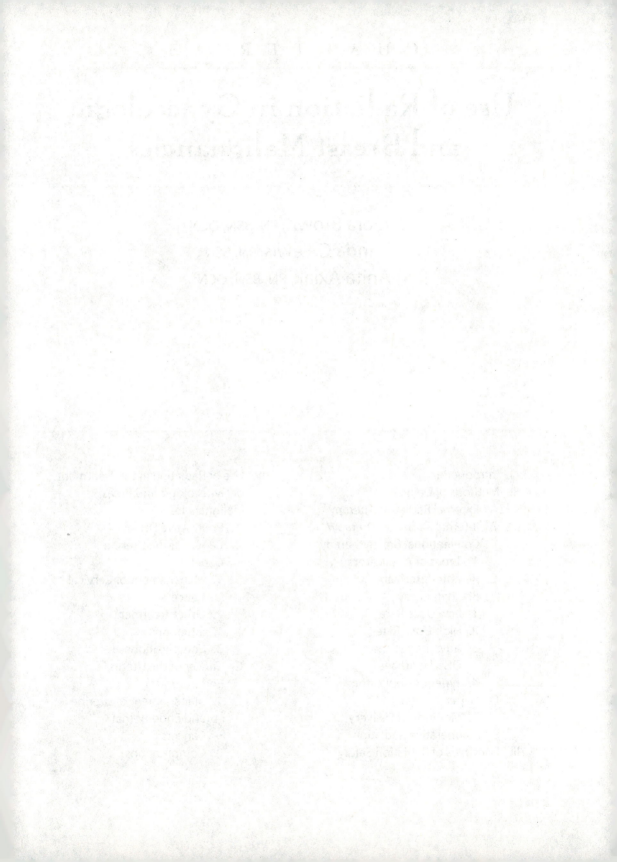

Use of Radiation in Gynecologic and Breast Malignancies

Debra Brown, RN, BSN, OCN

Linda C. Lewis, RN, BSN

Anita Axiak, RN, BSN, OCN

✳ INTRODUCTION

Radiation oncology is a discipline that uses radiation therapy (radiotherapy) as a mode of treatment in the clinical and scientific management of patients with cancer and some benign diseases.[1] Treatment may be carried out either alone or in collaboration with other disciplines and treatment modalities. The goal of radiation therapy is to deliver a prescribed dose of high-energy radiation, defined as ionizing radiation, to the tumor or affected areas with minimal injury to surrounding normal tissue.[2]

The biological effects of ionizing radiation were not recognized until the late 1890s, after Roentgen described X-rays (1895), Becquerel discovered radioactivity (1898), and the Curies reported the discovery of radium (1898). Following extensive experimentation and the first report of patient cure in 1899, radiation therapy became very popular.[3] It was used clinically to treat numerous benign and malignant diseases between 1900 and 1920, marking the beginning of a method of treatment that has since become of prime importance in the management of gynecologic and other cancers. In 1910, Wickham reported the treatment of 1,000 women with cervical cancer, as well as the development of an umbrella-type applicator for treatment delivery.[2] Greater interest was generated by Bumm and Doderlein, who published reports in 1913 about the use of radium to treat cancer of the uterus.[3]

Kilovoltage or deep therapy X-ray machines were developed between 1920 and 1940, after the invention of the vacuum X-ray tube. During the early 1930s, a frac-

---

TABLE 13.1

Units of Measure

- *Rad.* An acronym for *radiation absorbed dose,* indicating the amount of ionizing energy absorbed by matter per kilogram. This term indicates the amount or dose of radiation given.
- *Gray (Gy).* Replaces the rad. 1 Gray = 100 rads; 1 centiGray (cGy) = 1 rad.
- *Rem.* An acronym for *radiation equivalent man;* expresses the amount of absorbed dose and the variable biological effects on tissues and organs occurring from exposure to different levels of radiation. *Rem* is the term used to express numerically how much radiation an individual has been exposed to and how the tissues are affected.

---

tionated daily dose schema was devised, which continues to be the basis of radiotherapy today. Table 13.1 refers to some commonly used units of measure for radiation therapy. A treatment method using brachytherapy applicators, known as the Manchester System, was developed, and rules for dose distribution were also formulated at this time.[2] Radiation is delivered in specific amounts (doses), similar to medications. The terminology, however, is different.

The megavoltage era began following 1940.[4] More sophisticated machinery was developed, such as the betatron and the linear accelerator, leading to greater treatment capabilities. The availability of radioisotopes, made possible by the advent of the nuclear reactor in the 1950s and 1960s, enhanced the scope of radiation therapy practice. Heyman, another pioneer, began using afterloading techniques with brachytherapy in the 1950s, resulting in decreased exposure to radiation by hospital personnel.

During the 1960s and 1970s, as teletherapy (external radiation therapy) became more popular, brachytherapy (internal radiation therapy) was used less frequently. Since the 1980s, however, interest in brachytherapy has been renewed and is now used either alone or as a combined modality to treat disease. Both types of radiation therapy play an important part in the treatment of gynecologic cancers. Radiation oncology continues to grow and progress through increasing knowledge of radiobiology, new treatment methods, improved machinery for delivery, and refinement of current treatment techniques.

Sixty percent or more of cancer patients receive some form of radiation therapy during the course of their disease. Treatment may be given with the intent of cure, adjuvant therapy/prophylaxis, control, or palliation. Table 13.2 provides a profile of each role. As radiation therapy is an integral part of the treatment plan for many gynecologic cancers, it is essential for the nurse caring for this patient population to have an understanding of the basic principles of radiation therapy, as well as the biologic effects on patients and treatment goals. Patients are frequently fearful when told that ra-

TABLE 13.2

Role of Radiation Therapy in Gynecologic Cancer Management

Role	Purpose	Expected Outcome	Example
Cure	Primary treatment to cure disease	Normal/extended life span expected	Early cervical cancer (stages Ia–IIa)
Adjuvant Therapy/ Prophylaxis	Therapy: Before, during or after surgery. Enhance alone, in combination with chemotherapy to assist local control	Normal/extended life span or disease-free interval expected	Early stage breast cancer following lumpectomy Early stage cervical (stages Ib–IIa) following surgery Early stage uterine cancer having greater than one-third myometrial invasion
Control	Limit growth and spread of disease	May result in remission of disease for variable periods of time	Breast, late stage Late stage uterine, cervical cancers
Palliation	Relieve symptoms/ complications	No expected effects on extending life span. May improve quality of life. May receive numerous courses to different cancer sites	Pain caused by Organ compression Bone metastasis Tissue/organ invasion Nerve damage Obstruction Bowel Ureters Malignant effusions Pleural Abdominal ascites Pericardial Bleeding Neurological symptoms Brain metastasis Spinal cord compression

diotherapy will be included in their treatment plan and often look to the nurse for information, clarification of information obtained from physicians, and support. The nurse who is knowledgeable about this treatment modality can be more effective in reducing anxiety and providing for improved quality of care for the total patient. In some instances, personal concerns about working around radioactive devices may also be decreased.

✳ METHODS OF DELIVERY

External Radiation Therapy

External radiation therapy, or teletherapy, literally means "therapy given from a distance." The source of energy is located outside of the body and delivers electromagnetic radiation in the form of waves (electron beams) from specialized machines having various capabilities, or from rays emitted by a radioactive source (for example, cobalt-60). Higher energy machines (betatrons, linear accelerators; Figure 13.1) have

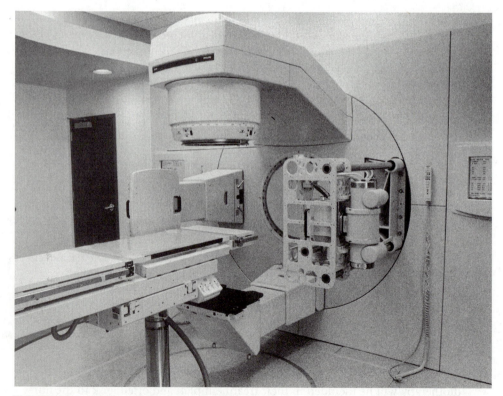

FIGURE 13.1. Phillips-SI linear accelerator.

Source: Courtesy of Dr. Alvaro Martinez, Chairman, Department of Radiation Oncology, William Beaumont Hospital, Royal Oak, MI.

the advantage of deeper penetration, greater skin sparing, and sharper beam definition. As a result, fewer side effects are experienced.

Radiation therapy is a complex treatment modality based on a number of factors:[3,5] tumor stage and prognosis, tumor size and location, histology and other tumor characteristics, routes of spread, goal of treatment, potential side effects, physical status of the patient, types of equipment available and their capability, use of additional treatment modalities in the treatment plan, and age. The initial evaluation of the patient is extensive. A history is obtained and a thorough general physical examination is performed. Once the work-up has been completed and the extent of disease defined, treatment planning begins. The radiation treatment plan includes decisions about the total amount of radiation (cGy) needed to control the tumor (target dose prescription), how much radiation is to be given each day (daily dose), the schedule, and the arrangement of the rays (beams) to include the affected tissue area (field) but spare normal tissue.[6] In order to establish an effective treatment plan, radiographic studies and simulation are necessary to identify the target volume as well as the surrounding anatomical structures.

Simulation or treatment planning usually begins after the consultation visit. Data from the work-up are fed into a computer, and several treatment plans are generated. Variations in the number and directions of beams as well as dose intensities influence the shape of the fields and are customized to fit the patient. The plan that provides the best dose distribution within the target field while simultaneously having minimal effect on surrounding tissue is selected. Protective devices called *blocks*, composed of various metal alloys, are developed to shield sensitive tissues and organs during treatment. Additional devices, such as molds and wedges, may be used to assist the radiologist in positioning the patient in order to accurately reproduce the treatment each day. Simulation films are taken several times prior to treatment. They are also taken periodically throughout the schedule for verification of the treatment field, and may be repeated if the area to be treated changes in size or location. The skin is marked with ink to define the fields during treatment, and is later tattooed to permanently identify the fields. The tiny tattoo dots serve to delineate the radiation fields for future reference and are readily identified by other professionals who become involved in the care of the patient.

During radiation treatment, the patient lies on a hard X-ray table. This may be uncomfortable for elderly patients or those who are thin, have back problems, or are experiencing pain. Occasionally, mild analgesics may be prescribed to alleviate this problem. Once the patient is positioned, she is left alone in the room; voice contact is maintained via intercom and TV screen. There are no sensations associated with the treatment. When instructing patients about the procedure, the nurse can compare the experience to that of a conventional X-ray with the exception that the time period is longer (several minutes). Some patients may feel claustrophobic because they must remain immobile during the treatment. An antianxiolytic taken one hour prior to treatment is helpful in this case. Most centers schedule treatment at the same time each day. This allows patients to arrange schedules and minimizes interruptions in lifestyle.

Internal Radiation Therapy/Conventional Brachytherapy

Internal radiation therapy is defined as radiation placed near or into the tumor tissue. Internal radiation therapy or brachytherapy has a long history. It first came into use at the turn of the century shortly after the discovery of radium by the Curies in 1898. Margaret Cleeves used radium to treat cervical cancer as early as 1902. This method allows a high dose of radiation to be delivered directly to the tumor. The radiation dose falls off sharply outside the implanted area, decreasing irradiation of normal tissue or organs surrounding the implant. Brachytherapy can be used in several ways. Radioactive liquids (^{131}I) or colloidal suspensions (^{32}P), for example, are unsealed sources of radioactivity; that is, they are absorbed or metabolized by the body. Sealed sources, such as iridium and cesium, are solid substances sealed inside small platinum capsules or, in some instances, seeds. The sealed sources are either permanently or temporarily placed within body tissues or cavities.

In the 1950s, Henshke and Hilaris, at Memorial Hospital in New York, developed the afterloading technique.[7] Afterloading technique allows hollow needles, tubes, and intracavitary applicators to be inserted in the operating room without the radioactive source in place. Once the position of the applicator is verified by X-ray, the patient is returned to her room and the applicator loaded with radioactive sources, thus the name *afterloading*. Afterloading technique reduces the exposure of personnel to radiation. The technique is done in one of two ways: either conventional afterloading, where the applicator is manually afterloaded, or remote afterloading, where special equipment afterloads the applicator. Remote afterloading is recognized as an effective treatment modality for many gynecological cancers. The nurse's responsibilities include ensuring that the best quality of patient care and education is provided to the brachytherapy patient and family or significant others, before, during, and after treatment.

Brachytherapy is used alone for local control or combined with external radiation to attain control in adjacent tissues and organs as well as regional lymph nodes. It is also used in combination with surgery and chemotherapy. In gynecology, the type of implant chosen depends on the cancer site and anatomical characteristics.

The initial consultation and treatment planning are similar to that for external radiation. A history, thorough physical examination, and extensive diagnostic work-up are conducted to determine the extent of disease, type of treatment, and applicator to be used. Once the type of applicator is determined, the radioactive source and strength are selected to produce a field shaped to meet treatment requirements. The radioactive sources most frequently used are cesium, iodine, and iridium. Each source is calibrated into a specific number of milligrams (e.g., 10 mg). The dose is expressed either in milligram-hours (the total number of milligrams times the number of hours of the implant) or in rads. Great care must be exercised in the dose prescription because of the proximity of the applicator to the bowel and bladder and its contact with the vaginal mucosa. There is strong potential for tissue damage to all three organs.

Once the applicator or needles are inserted in the operating room, verification films are taken before the patient is returned to her room. Final dose calculations are

FIGURE 13.2. The Delclos applicator consists of a hollow metal rod, plastic dome, and discs. Radioactive sources are interspaced with "dummy" sources within the metal rod. The plastic discs are sized to fit snugly within the vagina.

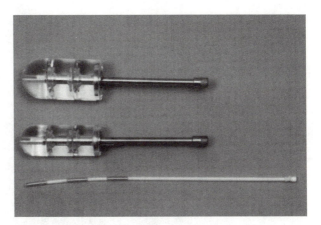

obtained from the computer using the verification films. The patient is transported back to her room and the applicator is then afterloaded.

Types of Applicators

The *Delclos* applicator consists of a hollow metal rod and clear plastic discs (Figure 13.2). Since vaginas vary in size, the diameter of the discs used is chosen to fit snugly inside. The procedure is simple and relatively noninvasive, and may be done in an operating room or radiation oncology suite. It is used in patients with vaginal cancers and postoperatively in patients who have had hysterectomy for cervical or endometrial cancers.

Fletcher-Suit applicators consist of a tandem (long hollow rod with a curved end) for insertion into the uterus; two ovoids, or colpostats (cylindrical chambers located at the ends of hollow rods) that fit into the vagina on either side of the cervix, into the fornices; and plastic caps that fit over the colpostats to attain a better fit and desired dose (Figure 13.3). The colpostats contain tungsten shields on the medial, lateral, and posterior sides to protect the bladder and rectum without affecting irradiation of essential tissue. Fletcher-Suit applicators are inserted in the operating room under spinal or general anesthesia. The Fletcher-Suit applicator is used for the treatment of cervical and uterine cancers. The *Minicolpostat* and the *Henschke* applicators are two similar instruments used to treat uterine and cervical cancers when the vagina is small, narrow, or anatomically distorted by tumor.[1]

Heyman capsules, small plastic containers attached to long plastic tubes, are another type of applicator used in the treatment of uterine cancers. When this method is used, the uterus is packed with the capsules to expose the entire wall to radiation. Capsules are also placed in the endocervical canal and ovoids in the vaginal fornices to ensure complete exposure of the whole uterus and surrounding tissue.

The *Syed-Neblett* template consists of two plastic plates held together by screws and containing openings in the plates to hold numerous hollow stainless steel needles.

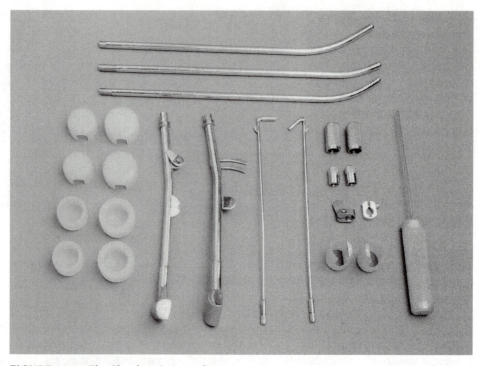

FIGURE 13.3. The Fletcher-Suit applicator.

Source: Courtesy of Dr. Alvaro Martinez, Chairman, Department of Radiation Oncology, William Beaumont Hospital, Royal Oak, MI.

A plastic vaginal cylinder containing grooves for additional needles is placed into a circular opening in the center of the template (Figure 13.4). The template is useful in the interstitial treatment of vaginal cancers, advanced or recurrent cervical cancers, and in some gynecologic cancers for which intracavitary treatment is suboptimal.[8]

Patients manage well with internal implants despite the extreme invasiveness of the procedures. Patient-controlled analgesia and epidural analgesics are effective in maintaining comfort initially; later, oral forms of pain medications are used. Once the applicators are removed, recovery is usually uneventful.

Chromic phosphate (^{32}P) is an unsealed colloidal suspension of radioactive phosphorus. It is sometimes used as adjuvant therapy for ovarian cancer. The beta energy radioactivity emitted by ^{32}P has little penetrating power; it does not extend beyond the level of the abdominal wall. The patient is often medicated prior to the procedure. A peritoneal dialysis catheter is inserted into the abdomen, usually in the nuclear medicine department, or left in after second-look surgery.[9] Approximately 500 ml of normal saline is instilled, followed by technetium and additional fluid totaling 1 liter. The abdomen is radiographically examined to determine the free flow of fluid throughout the abdomen. If loculation or any impairment of fluid distribution occurs,

FIGURE 13.4. The Syed-Neblett template.

Source: Courtesy of Dr. A. Chen, Radiation Oncology Department, Allegheny General Hospital, Pittsburgh, PA.

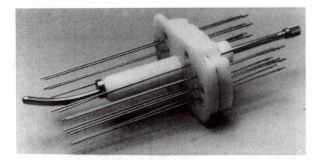

the procedure is discontinued, but otherwise 15 to 20 millicuries of ^{32}P are instilled into the abdomen. The patient is then rotated back to side to abdomen to side to back every 15 minutes for approximately 2 hours, using the same procedure as that used for sclerosing the abdomen, to disperse the ^{32}P as evenly as possible. Other than some abdominal distention from the volume of fluid instilled and occasional reports of shoulder pain, little discomfort is experienced.[9]

The effectiveness of treatment with ^{32}P is still under investigation. It is currently used in the treatment of stage I or II cancers of the ovary when minimal residual tumor remains or after negative second-look surgery for consolidation treatment. The risk of significant complications is low; however, severe late complications, particularly small bowel obstruction, are higher than with adjuvant chemotherapy.[10] Low-dose intraperitoneal ^{32}P treatment in conjunction with platinum analogue chemotherapy is a promising approach for the treatment of disseminated intraperitoneal ovarian cancer.[11]

Remote Afterloading Brachytherapy

Low Dose Rate

Remote afterloading systems are available for both interstitial and intracavitary placements. Low dose rate (LDR) remote afterloading utilizes radioactive isotopes, ^{192}Ir ribbons or wires, or ^{137}Cs ribbons (see Figure 3.5). These sources are widely used for gynecologic tumors. They provide internal radiation treatment with no radiation exposure to staff members. These systems can be connected to either rigid or flexible applicators, and the applicators are placed during surgery with the patient under anesthesia. The patient remains hospitalized for the entire treatment time. The necessary treatment planning and source preparation can be extremely time-consuming for the physics staff because each patient's treatment is planned individually and the activity of the sources has to be taken into consideration.

Once the planning is complete, however, the programming of the radiation delivery machine is a relatively simple process for the physics staff, and the treatment is started with the push of a button. A cable-driven mechanism transfers the source into the applicator. A specific dose of radiation is prescribed by the physician and delivered

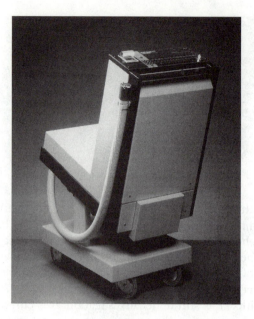

FIGURE 13.5. LDR remote afterloader.

Source: Courtesy of Nucletron Corporation, Columbia, MD.

over a specific time frame. The dose prescribed is generally less than 100 cGy/hour delivered over 24 to 96 hours. The treatment can be interrupted at any time for patient care or visitors.

The patient remains on bed rest for the entire duration of treatment and is encouraged to do isometric exercises while on bed rest. Alternating-pressure stockings are put on the patient's legs to promote adequate venous flow from the lower extremities. Patients are encouraged to bring in materials from home, such as books or magazines, to help pass the time. A telephone and television are also made available to them.

Once the treatment is completed, the patient is disconnected from the treatment machine. She is then premedicated and the applicator is removed in the patient's room. Any packing is removed from the vaginal canal, and pressure is applied to the area, as in the case of an interstitial implant, to minimize the amount of bleeding and decrease the chances of a hematoma developing. A dressing is applied to the area and the patient is assisted in gradually increasing her activity level. She is usually discharged within the next 24 hours.

High Dose Rate

High dose rate (HDR) techniques are widely used in the treatment of many gynecologic tumors. HDR remote afterloading systems (Figure 13.6) are capable of intraluminal, interstitial, intracavitary, and intraoperative treatments. A high-energy radioactive source, ^{192}Ir (a 10 Ci source), is utilized with rigid or flexible plastic applicators. These systems are designed primarily for treatments to be done on an outpatient basis. However, depending on the applicator used, the patient may or may not be hospitalized for initial placement of the applicator.

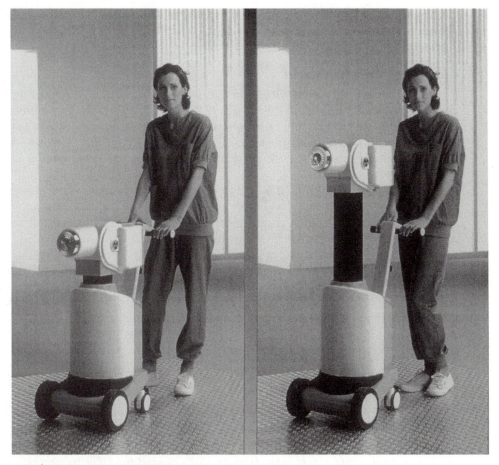

FIGURE 13.6. HDR remote afterloader.
Source: Courtesy of Nucletron Corporation, Columbia, MD.

Source preparation is not necessary prior to each treatment. But the high-energy source decays over time and is replaced by the physics staff approximately every three months. Programming the treatment machine is a relatively simple process, but the treatment planning for each patient is individual, requiring additional time for the physics staff. As with the LDR machine, the HDR system utilizes a cable-driven mechanism to transfer the source into the applicator that has been placed into the patient. A specific dose of radiation is prescribed by the physician and delivered over a short period of time. The dose prescribed is generally greater than 10 cGy per minute, giving a treatment time of less than ten minutes per treatment. The treatment can be interrupted at any time for patient care. Once the treatment dose is delivered, the applicator is removed and the patient goes home. No extended bed rest is necessary, and no medications are needed prior to the removal.

Advantages and Disadvantages

The advantages of remote afterloading are many. LDR remote afterloading techniques provide less exposure to the physics staff in preparing and loading sources, and no exposure to the medical and nursing staffs taking care of the patient. There is also less risk to visitors and ancillary staffs (e.g., housekeeping, dietary). Patients are no more uncomfortable with remote afterloading than with conventional afterloading brachytherapy.

The greatest advantage of HDR remote afterloading techniques is to the patients. This newest technology provides shorter treatment times and allows treatments to be done on an outpatient basis. It eliminates the need for extended hospitalized bed rest and is available for patients who are poor surgical risks.

But remote afterloading is not without disadvantages. There are radiation exposure risks should a machine malfunction or a source become lodged in the tubing/machine with the system on (see Table 13.3). The treatments can be more time-consuming for departmental staff, since they involve a nurse, a physicist, a physician, a dosimetrist, and a radiation therapist. Another disadvantage specific to HDR treatments is that the patient may need to make multiple visits to the hospital for treatment. Cost effectiveness may also be an issue; it is currently being debated among the groups that utilize remote afterloading.

Types of Applicators

As with conventional brachytherapy, remote afterloading techniques can be used alone or in combination with external beam therapy. In gynecologic cancers, the type of applicator used depends on the site to be treated and anatomical parameters.

The *vaginal cylinder applicator* (Figure 13.7) is used for HDR treatments to the vaginal cuff or apex postoperatively for endometrial cancers and vaginal lesions. The applicator consists of a single hollow metal tandem, a perineal bar, and several different sized clear plastic cylinders. The treatment is divided into several fractions. The first treatment involves taking the patient to the simulation room, where she is placed in the lithotomy position, a Foley catheter is placed into the bladder, and a marker is placed in the rectum. An applicator sized to fit the patient's vaginal canal is then inserted. Once placement is verified with X-ray films, the patient is taken to the treatment room and connected to the HDR treatment machine, and the prescribed dose of radiation is delivered. For subsequent treatments, the patient is supine on the treatment table, but the applicator is placed by the physician, and its placement is verified under fluoroscopy.

The *ring applicator* (Figure 13.8) is an applicator set that consists of a hollow tandem curved at the end for insertion through the cervix into the uterus, a tandem with a ring curvature at the end for insertion up to the cervix, a plastic cap that snaps onto the ring, a rectal retractor, and a perineal bar that helps to keep the applicator in place.

TABLE 13.3

Emergency Procedures for microSelection-HDR [192]Ir
If the Source Fails to Return to the Safe

1. Depress **RED EMERGENCY STOP BUTTON** on emergency stop switch in control room. If the source retracts, go to step 5, otherwise, step 2.

2. Enter the treatment room with a hand-held survey meter.
   - **Push** down on the access panel on top of the treatment unit to access the **GOLD** hand crank. Turn it in the direction of the arrows until it stops.
   - If the source retracts, go to 5, otherwise step 3.

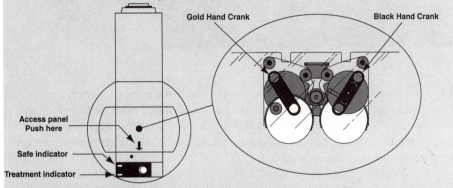

Access Panel Location   **Gold Hand Crank Location**

3. Remove the applicator from the patient. **DO NOT** disconnect any transfer tubes from the machine or applicators. Place the applicator, still attached to the machine, into the shielded emergency container. (See Specific Instructions)

4. If a survey still shows radiation in the room, move the patient to the anteroom, and survey the patient. If there is no radiation in the patient, remove the patient from the room. Otherwise, activate Surgical Emergency Procedures.

5. Retain the treatment data printout, and record the time the source was removed from the patient, and estimated exposure time of employees. Contact the following:

Physicist: _____ Phone#: _____ B#: _____

Physician: _____ Phone#: _____ B#: _____

RSO: _____ Phone#: _____ B#: _____

Nucletron Representative:

_____ B#: _____

Nucletron Phone #: _____

The unintended radiation dose to which those present have been subjected should be estimated and recorded by the RSO and/or a suitable qualified person.

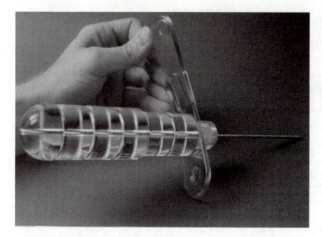

FIGURE 13.7. Nucleton vaginal cylinder applicator.

Source: Courtesy of Dr. Alvaro Martinez, Chairman, Department of Radiation Oncology, William Beaumont Hospital, Royal Oak, MI.

Prior to placement of the applicator, the patient has a cervical sleeve, or stint, sutured into the cervix, which allows for easier and reproducible placement of the tandem into the uterus. The tandems and retractors are made in several different angles, and the applicator is custom fit to the patient's anatomy. After verification films are taken, the patient is treated. The sleeve is removed after the course of treatment is completed.

The *Martinez endometrial applicator* consists of two hollow tandems, which are inserted into the uterus, and a plastic cylinder that fits closely along the vaginal mucosa (Figure 13.9). The patient needs to have the cervix dilated surgically, manually, or with medication prior to each placement. Once the applicator is in place, films are taken to verify placement and the treatment is given. The applicator is removed once the course of treatment is completed.

The *Martinez universal perineal interstitial template (MUPIT)* consists of a two-part plastic template with a cover plate secured with screws, a rectal cylinder, a vaginal cylinder, a cylinder adapter for needles, and cover plate fillers to accommodate additional needles and catheters (Figure 13.10). The template is designed for use in locally

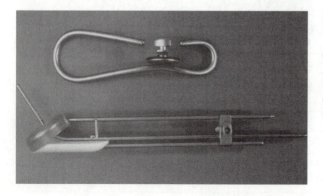

FIGURE 13.8. Nucleton ring applicator set.

Source: Courtesy of Dr. Alvaro Martinez, Chairman, Department of Radiation Oncology, William Beaumont Hospital, Royal Oak, MI.

FIGURE 13.9. The Martinez endometrial applicator.

Source: Courtesy of Dr. Alvaro Martinez, Chairman, Department of Radiation Oncology, William Beaumont Hospital, Royal Oak, MI.

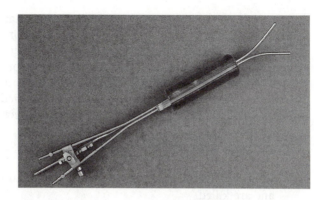

advanced or recurrent disease. This procedure is done in the operating room using a perineal approach. The needles are placed through the template into the perineum, and their placement is verified by fluoroscopy in the operating room. A CT scan is done postoperatively for treatment planning. The patient is then transferred to a private room where she is connected to the LDR remote afterloader (Figure 13.5). The patient remains on strict bed rest for the duration of the treatment. The template and needles are removed in the patient's room and the patient is generally discharged within 24 hours.

Hyperthermia

Hyperthermia is a method of using heat to treat cancer in which tumor-bearing areas are elevated to temperatures ranging from 41 to 45 degrees Celsius (106 to 112 degrees Fahrenheit). The objective of hyperthermia is to produce sufficient heat to kill

FIGURE 13.10. The Martinez universal perineal interstitial template (MUPIT).

Source: Courtesy of Dr. Alvaro Martinez, Chairman, Department of Radiation Oncology, William Beaumont Hospital, Royal Oak, MI.

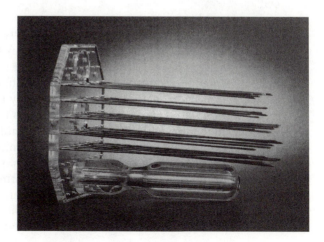

cancer cells without damaging normal cells. Generally scheduled every 72 hours, heat treatments are not cumulative in effect and therefore are not toxic.

Hyperthermia treatments are given as an adjunct to radiation therapy, chemotherapy, and surgery, or used for palliation in tumors where local and regional control rates with conventional therapy have been poor. Heat and the synergistic effects of hyperthermia and radiation therapy have been studied for many years.[12,13,14] Hall and Roizin-Towle describe the following biological effects of heat on tumor cells:[15]

1. Heat is cytoxic to tumor cells, yet well tolerated within the therapeutic range by normal cells.
2. Cells in S phase, which are usually radioresistant, become radiosensitized by heat and are killed.
3. Cells characterized by lower pH and nutritional deficiency, namely hypoxic cells, are more sensitive to heat.
4. When heat and radiation are used in combined therapy, the amount of radiation required is reduced.
5. Repair from radiation damage is impaired by heat.

In addition, the increased blood flow in normal tissue and subsequent tissue cooling is not found in growing tumors after hyperthermia.[16] Instead, tumor blood flow remains relatively stable, resulting in heat retention and thus higher tumor tissue temperature. This in turn leads to cellular and tissue hypoxia, decreased acidity, and nutritional deprivation, which potentially lead to cellular death.

Methods of Delivery

Three methods of administering hyperthermia are local treatment, used for superficial or well defined tumors; regional treatment, where there is involvement of surrounding tissue; and whole-body treatment for widespread disease.[17] Several electromagnetic methods as well as ultrasound are used to provide local heating to the tumor bed.

External Treatment. Ultrasound transmits sound (pressure) waves through a water bolus to the treatment area (see Figure 13.11). A conducting jelly is placed on the skin to act as a seal between the transducer and the skin. The pressure waves via the transmitted transducer cause tissue vibration, resulting in heat. Temperature monitoring and measurement, however, are done by temperature probes, which are invasive devices. Treatments are usually given over a period of 65 minutes, followed by external beam therapy within approximately 30 minutes, while the tumor is still warm.

The patient's vital signs and status are monitored continuously by the nurse for complications that may necessitate interruption or discontinuation of treatment. Mild to moderate discomfort and the sensation of warmth felt by the patient can sometimes be managed by relaxation techniques rather than discontinuing treatment.

The most frequent side effects and complications of external hyperthermia are skin irritations, blisters, and pain. The long-term side effects associated with hyper-

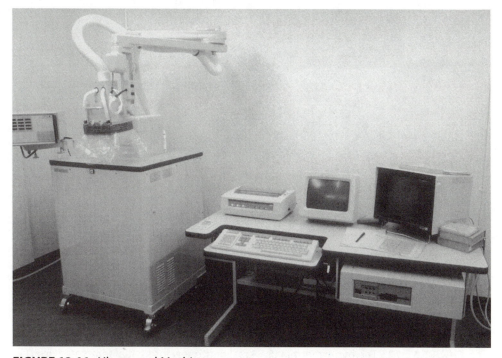

FIGURE 13.11. Ultrasound Machine.

Source: Courtesy of Dr. Alvaro Martinez, Chairman, Department of Radiation Oncology, William Beaumont Hospital, Royal Oak, MI.

thermia include tissue necrosis, severe enough in some cases to require skin grafting. But the discomfort associated with the treatment disappears as soon as the hyperthermia is discontinued. Mild analgesics are used to maintain comfort. Heavy sedation is not used or recommended because the patient must be alert in order to inform the nurse should the treatment become too warm and uncomfortable. Patients taking pain medication at home are instructed to take it prior to coming in for treatment.

Interstitial Hyperthermia. Many aspects of interstitial hyperthermia are similar to those of external hyperthermia. A major difference between the two treatments is the type of applicator used to deliver the heat. The interstitial applicator (Figure 13.12) consists of a flat template that is used to guide needles or antennae into the tumor area. A cover plate that resembles an electronic circuit board is placed over the template and secured to it once needle placement is completed. The cover plate is connected to a computer system via two cables on the top and bottom of the plate. Thermosensors are also placed into the tumor to record internal temperatures. Once the computer is programmed for the specific patient, the treatment is started. The heat is conducted through metal needles or antennae to the tumor area. Interstitial hyper-

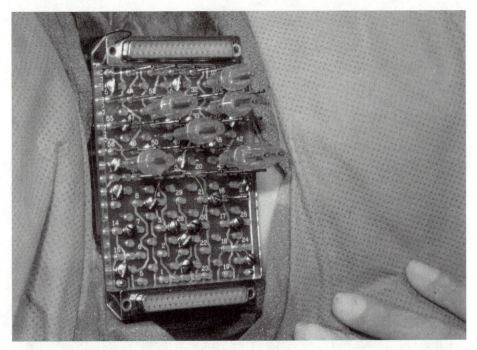

FIGURE 13.12. The hyperthermia universal peritoneal interstitial template (HUPIT).

Source: Courtesy of Dr. Alvaro Martinez, Chairman, Department of Radiation Oncology, William Beaumont Hospital, Royal Oak, MI.

thermia is generally done in combination with brachytherapy, and the applicator remains in place during the entire treatment time of the brachytherapy, usually 24 to 72 hours.

Hyperthermia does not have the same unpleasant side effects that may accompany radiation therapy or chemotherapy. Because hyperthermia involves the use of heat, minor skin irritations or blisters occasionally occur, but they do not usually delay the course of treatment.

The nurse's role in hyperthermia includes side effect/symptom management, patient teaching, and pain control as the primary concerns. Research is under way at many institutions to further define the role and potential of hyperthermia in cancer treatment.

Intraoperative Radiation

Intraoperative radiation therapy (IORT) is the delivery of a single high dose of radiation to the tumor during an operative procedure or as a boost with surgery and external radiation.[18,19] The goal is to attain better control of a localized tumor. This technique enables the surgeon to manually move surrounding organs away from the tumor site and expose the tumor to direct radiation. It is also possible to protect tissue underlying the tumor. Normal tissues are thus spared while a very high dose of radiation is delivered to the tumor.

IORT is performed in either the operating room or the radiation department (RD), depending on institutional facilities.

Common complications of IORT are enteritis, bowel obstruction, and hemorrhage. Nursing care and patient education are tailored to the operative procedure and individual needs.

❋ PRINCIPLES OF RADIATION SAFETY

Rules, regulations, and standards of radiation safety are set by the National Council on Radiation Protection (NCRP) and enforced by the Nuclear Regulatory Commission (NRC) to protect radiation workers and others from excessive exposure to ionizing radiation. Recommendations stress that exposure dose should remain "as low as reasonably achievable" (ALARA).

Radiation is present throughout our entire environment, and this type is referred to as background radiation.

In order to function safely and securely around patients receiving conventional brachytherapy, the nurse must incorporate three essential principles into her practice:

1. *Time.* Limit the time spent in direct contact with the patient. This is the one controllable factor in patient care. Less time means less exposure and less absorption of radiation. It is also important to note that as radiation dose increases, exposure time should decrease. The physicist/dosimetrist designates the time allowed for direct patient contact.
2. *Distance.* Maximize the distance between the nurse and the source.
3. *Shielding.* Use the appropriate types of shielding depending on the source.

Additional effective guidelines for protection that can be utilized by the nurse are found in Table 13.4.

❋ USE OF RADIATION IN THE TREATMENT OF GYNECOLOGIC AND BREAST MALIGNANCIES

Preinvasive Disease

Ideally, intraepithelial tissue abnormalities (dysplasia) of the cervix, uterus, vagina, and vulva can be detected early, during regular periodic physical examinations, before

TABLE 13.4

Guidelines for Radiation Implant Safety

- Adhere to general precautions. Assign the patient to a private room. Keep a lead container and long-handled forceps in the room at all times. *DO NOT* handle any dislodged radioactive sources by hand.
- Organize patient care to limit time and direct contact with the patient. Save all linen and trash in the room until the radioactive source is removed and inventoried. Then dispose of everything according to institutional policy.
- Work behind the lead shield as much as possible. Place a "Radiation in Place" sign on the door. Do not provide care for brachytherapy patients if you are, or think you may be, pregnant. Know the emergency procedure should cardiac arrest or another emergency occur. (Precautions are normally ignored and CPR initiated.) If the patient dies, do not remove the body until the radioactive source has been removed and permission is given by the Radiation Department. Limit visitors per agency policy. Do not allow pregnant women or others 18 years or younger to visit. Do not allow ancillary staff to clean or enter the room. Rotate staff assigned to brachytherapy patients.

symptoms occur. Treatment is some type of local excision and does not include radiotherapy. (A thorough discussion of preinvasive disease can be found in Chapter 2.)

Cancer of the Uterine Cervix

Management of Cervical Cancers

The management of cervical cancers is dependent on numerous factors, including physical status, stage of disease, type of lesion, and histology of the tumor. Many gynecologic oncologists prefer using a team approach, collaborating with the radiation oncologist. The goal of treatment, particularly in early disease (carcinoma in situ, stage I through stage IIa) is cure. In late stage disease (stage IIb through stage IV), the goal remains cure, although five-year survival rates decrease considerably. When cure is not possible, the goal is to control disease, provide optimal quality of life, and prolong survival. Chemotherapy can also be given prior to or concurrently with radiation. Severe toxicities have resulted from combination therapy, including intestinal obstruction, perforation, and fistula formation. External radiation is given to the pelvis in a boxlike shape to include the essential organs and tissues. If lymph nodes are positive, then extended field irradiation is used to include the affected nodes. Internal radiation can be delivered by several different applicators, depending on the anatomic and tumor characteristics.

Other Treatment Situations

Recurrent Cancer of the Cervix.   Approximately 35% of all patients previously treated can be retreated in several ways.[20] Because of the limitation of normal tissue tolerance to radiation, patients must be very carefully evaluated for further treatment if the recurrence is within the original treatment field. In some instances, small doses of external or internal treatment may be given. When the original treatment has been surgery alone, or recurrence is outside the original field, then treatment may be effectively accomplished with irradiation. Frequently, however, recurrence is in a previously irradiated area. Additional surgery, if possible, or chemotherapy then becomes the treatment of choice. In any case, recurrent disease has a discouraging outlook.

Suboptimal Surgery.   This situation occurs infrequently and results from the incidental discovery of cervical cancer during hysterectomy or in an emergency situation. In either case, additional surgery is the treatment of choice; in most cases, it offers a better prognosis. When bulky tumor is present, preoperative irradiation has been found to decrease pelvic recurrence.[20]

Cancer of the Cervical Stump.   This is rarely seen today. It responds better to surgical intervention.

Cancer of the Cervix in Pregnancy.   This circumstance has been shown to have no negative effects on pregnancy. Short delays in treatment, particularly if the patient is in the late stages of pregnancy, are acceptable.[21] Several factors influence treatment decisions, including stage of disease, duration of pregnancy, religious beliefs, and desires of the patient concerning the pregnancy. In early pregnancy, that is, the first or second trimester up to 24 weeks' gestation, it is recommended that the pregnancy be terminated and treatment begun. If the cancer is discovered in late pregnancy, 24 weeks' gestation or longer, treatment is frequently delayed until the fetus is able to survive outside the uterus. A cesarean section is then performed and treatment initiated.

Palliation.   The need for palliation of pain or bleeding is another frequent goal of radiation therapy in cervical cancers. Either external beam or brachytherapy may be used with satisfactory outcome. Schedule and dose are dependent on previous irradiation, site, and objective of treatment.

Complications

Table 13.5 provides a profile of complications resulting from radiation treatment of cervical cancers. Acute complications often resulting from therapy are proctosigmoiditis manifested by diarrhea, cramps, and tenderness. Enteritis, resulting from whole-abdomen and extended field irradiation, is often severe enough to result in dehydration and electrolyte imbalance requiring hospitalization and extended treatment. Bone marrow suppression from pelvic irradiation may also occur. Postradiation vaginitis, an almost inevitable side effect of vaginal radiation, requires meticulous teaching and follow-up care to prevent vaginal stenosis.

Delayed complications include chronic proctitis, sigmoiditis, bowel obstruction, fistula formation, and injuries to the urinary tract and intestine.

TABLE 13.5		
Complications of Cervical Cancer from Radiotherapy		
Site	Acute	Chronic
General	Radiation skin reaction Fatigue Pain	Pain
Vaginal	Vaginitis	Vaginal dryness Vaginal stenosis Vaginal necrosis Sexual dysfunction
Intestinal	Proctitis Enteritis Rectal ulcers	Chronic proctitis Chronic enteritis Diverticulitis Malabsorption Small bowel obstruction Small bowel perforation Rectovaginal and other fistulas Rectal/sigmoid stricture or perforation
Urinary	Cystitis Bladder ulcer	Chronic cystitis Bladder dysfunction Ureteral/bladder fistulas Urethral stricture Incontinence Cystocele
Other	Pelvic abscess/infection Leg edema Thrombophlebitis Thrombosis of pelvic blood vessels Pulmonary embolism Hemorrhage Lymphocyst	Leg edema Neuropathy Arteriosclerosis Subcutaneous fibrosis

Cancer of the Uterus/Endometrium

Management of Uterine and Endometrial Cancers

When planning treatment for uterine cancers, prognostic factors and the physical status of the patient are strong determinants. A small number of patients may be treated initially or primarily with radiation because of institutional policy, oncologist preference, or physical status of the patient. These patients are usually clinically staged using FIGO criteria. When using clinical criteria for staging, documentation must state the method used.

Stage I disease can be treated with surgical intervention alone for low-grade disease limited to the uterus. In high-grade disease, with or without positive peritoneal cytology, adjuvant radiation is added to the treatment plan. Uterine packing with Heyman capsules or Fletcher-Suit applicators, either before or after surgery, are additional options. If preoperative irradiation is performed, surgery takes place within a week of the final treatment. The disadvantage of the preoperative method is that the lymph nodes frequently receive less than therapeutic levels of irradiation. External radiation may then be required again after surgery.

Stage II disease is treated similarly to stage I disease, except more extensive surgery is performed. In late stage disease (III and IV), treatment becomes individualized. When tumors are large but well described and nonadherent to the pelvic walls, both external irradiation and brachytherapy may be given to decrease tumor volume, followed by surgical intervention. Large tumors fixed to the pelvic wall and other critical structures are usually treated by both internal and external radiation alone. The goal of treatment then becomes tumor control or palliation.

Radiation therapy alone is sometimes used to treat uterine cancers. Most frequently, the medical status of the patient influences this treatment decision. Patients with stage I disease who are treated in this manner appear to have survival outcomes dependent on the same prognostic factors as patients treated surgically.[22] Park et al., in a survey of the literature, found that stage II patients had an approximately 50% five-year survival rate of those given combined therapy.[23] Survival of stage III patients ranged from 8 to 40%, independent of the method of treatment. Five-year survival of stage IV patients was also highly variable. Treatment focused on palliation of symptoms.

Regardless of stage, radiation therapy can consist of external radiation to the whole pelvis plus two initial intracavitary or interstitial treatments or intracavitary treatment alone. In addition, chemotherapy and progestin treatment are usually added to the treatment plan.

Recurrent disease found in the vagina is usually treated with surgery alone or combined with radiation. When recurrence is limited to a single site within the vagina, the five-year survival rate is 25 to 50% whether proximal or distal portions of the vagina are involved.[24] The majority of recurrences, however, are in either the pelvis and/or the lung and periaortic lymph nodes. Patients with single site recurrences are more responsive to treatment than those with multiple metastases. Treatment is managed surgically, if possible, followed by radiation if the site has not been irradiated previously or if limited radiation has been used. Recently, Randall et al. explored the use of interstitial implants in patients who had previously received external beam radiation therapy.[25] His results indicate that interstitial radiation may be an effective alternative in providing tumor control in a select population who cannot tolerate radical surgery.

Chemotherapy is also used in addition to radiation therapy and surgery. Hormonal therapy may also be added, if hormonal receptor status is positive for progesterone and estrogen.

Sarcomas of the uterus are uncommon (3–5% of all uterine tumors) but aggressive tumors. Primary treatment of sarcoma is surgical intervention. Radiation may be used

preoperatively or postoperatively to assist with control, for recurrence, and for palliation. If no operative procedure is done, an increased radiation dose of both external
radiation and intracavitary treatment is given.[3,20] Approximately 50% of stage I sarcomas and 90% of stage III through IV sarcomas recur.

Complications

Acute and chronic cystitis and proctitis occur, as well as symptoms similar to
those experienced by patients receiving radiation for cervical cancers. The concomitant physical problems in this more elderly population may cause increased risk of infection and fistula formation.

Cancer of the Vulva

Management of Vulvar Cancer

Vulvar cancer is managed primarily by surgical treatment. Prognostic factors (size
of tumor, depth of invasion, cell type, vascular and lymph node involvement) are essential considerations in the treatment plan. Radiation is given as adjunctive treatment, and until recently, has been used primarily in advanced disease in the following
situations:

- Preoperative treatment to decrease tumor volume and consequently the extent of
  surgery necessary as radical vulvar surgery can be exceptionally disfiguring
- Postoperative treatment to prevent recurrence when there is nodal involvement
- Alternative treatment due to patient inability to tolerate surgery

Radiation alone in the treatment of vulvar cancer is controversial. The controversy
centers around the belief that vulvar tissue cannot tolerate high doses of radiation
(>6000 cGy) without development of wet desquamation and late complications, for
example, fistula, bone necrosis, and stenosis of the vagina and urethra. An overview of
numerous studies indicates that radiation alone may be more useful in advanced or recurrent cancers.[26]

The goal of treatment today is cure in both primary and recurrent cancers. Tumor
control or palliative treatment becomes the goal when disease disseminates outside
the pelvis. Lymph node involvement is a major factor in disease outcome. Patients
with three or more positive lymph nodes have a high incidence of local, regional, and
systemic recurrence.[20] Overall survival is reported as follows: 90% in node negative
women, 75% with one or two positive unilateral nodes, 25% with bilateral or more
than three positive unilateral nodes, and 10% with pelvic node metastasis.[27]

Complications

Patients receiving radiation therapy to the vulva develop severe wet desquamation of the skin and mucosa. Management of skin reactions is challenging to both
the physician and nurse. Other effects commonly seen are infection, bone or tissue
necrosis, leg edema, and edema of the vulva. Late effects include persistent edema

of the labia, ulceration of the vulva, fistula formation, and stenosis of the vagina or urethra.

Cancers of the Vagina

Management of Vaginal Cancers

Radiation provides good tumor control and is the treatment of choice for invasive vaginal cancer. It is used alone or in combination with surgery and/or chemotherapy. The goal of treatment is cure. Although good tumor response is obtained with radiation, prognosis is poor for all but stage I.

Treatment is individualized according to stage, location, and size of the tumor and age of the patient.

Localized carcinoma in situ (CIS) is preferably treated by surgical excision. If brachytherapy is selected for CIS, treatment of the entire vagina via intracavitary cylinder is recommended because of the multicentric nature of the tumor.

Stage I vaginal cancers located in the upper third of the vagina may be treated similarly to cancer of the cervix using a tandem and ovoids. Intracavitary cylinder treatments, interstitial therapy, and external radiation for aggressive tumors are some other treatment options.

Stage II vaginal cancers may be treated with a combination of interstitial and intracavitary implants. External radiation is given with bulky tumors. Stage III and IV disease may be treated with a combination of interstitial and intracavitary implants and external radiation. Larger tumors and tumors located in the upper vagina have been associated with a worse prognosis because of the proximity to adjacent organs. Interstitial implants may be placed by means of laparotomy into specific cancer sites to maximize radiation to tumor-invaded tissue. When the tumor is located close to the vaginal opening, metastasis to the inguinal lymph nodes is suspected. Then a lymph node dissection may be done, followed by radiation therapy. Careful planning must be done to avoid damage to the bladder and rectum.

Complications

Numerous treatment effects result from vaginal radiation. Vaginal dryness, fibrosis, and stenosis are common. Acute proctitis frequently occurs as a transient problem. Late effects include rectovaginal and other fistula formations, vaginal necrosis, chronic proctitis, and strictures of the vagina, rectum, and urethra.

Cancer of the Ovary

Management of Ovarian Cancers

The role of radiation therapy in ovarian cancer is controversial. Surgery and chemotherapy are the current standard of treatment, but little improvement in five-year survival has resulted from use of the combined modalities. Numerous studies have been reported in the literature about the effectiveness of external and internal radiation as an alternative method of treatment.[28,29] Several factors have emerged that impact on the selection of patients to be treated with radiotherapy and the success or failure of the treatment. They are as follows.

External Radiation Treatment. Potish points out that whole-abdomen radiation does not necessarily provide irradiation of the entire abdomen.[30] Sensitive organs (liver, kidneys) are shielded, protecting portions of the abdomen and tumor cells hidden within these areas from lethal levels of radiation. In addition, larger tumor volumes require higher levels of radiation to provide adequate tumor control.[31] Normal cells within the abdomen tolerate maximum doses specific to the organ of origin. Higher doses of radiation to normal tissues cause severe, potentially life-threatening complications. It has also been noted that low-grade, well to moderately well-differentiated tumors respond better to treatment and that tumors recur when radiation is limited to the pelvis.[32] Other factors influencing the effectiveness of treatment were the presence of dense adhesions and ascites.[29] Based on the above information, the following criteria have been found to be important in the selection of patients for primary adjunctive treatment of ovarian cancer with abdominal pelvic irradiation:

1. Residual disease or tumor size ≤2 cm
2. Tumor site contained within the radiation field
3. Cell type and grade (important prognostic indicators)
4. Early stage (indicates better prognostic outlook)
5. Physical status able to tolerate abdominal-pelvic radiation

Abdominal-pelvic radiation is delivered by one of several open field techniques. Open field technique delivers radiation to the entire abdomen and pelvis and then provides a boost (extra dose of radiation) to the lower abdomen and appropriate areas (see Table 13.6). The liver and kidneys are shielded. Other open field techniques include manipulation of shields/blocks and fields to achieve the acceptable distribution of radiation. Recurrence is usually in the pelvis, abdomen, or distant areas, particularly the chest and lungs.

Brachytherapy. Internal radiation has also been used for the management of ovarian cancer. A colloidal suspension of radioactive phosphorus (^{32}P), a pure beta emitter, is used. Beta radiation is fairly weak and does not penetrate beyond the skin level of the abdominal wall, yet has better tumor-penetrating ability than radioactive gold (^{198}Au) as well as a longer half-life (14 days vs. 2 days, respectively). Radioactive gold is no longer used in the United States because of the danger to staff caretakers from exposure to the dangerous levels of gamma radiation emitted during treatment. The use of ^{32}P is limited to patients with minimal or no residual gross disease and where there are no adhesions or other situations that could prevent free distribution of

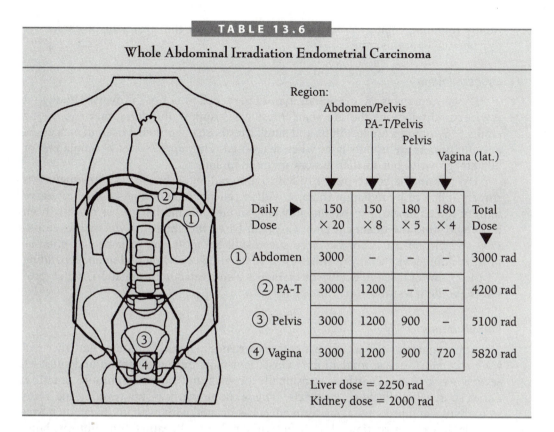

TABLE 13.6

Whole Abdominal Irradiation Endometrial Carcinoma

Region:
Abdomen/Pelvis
PA-T/Pelvis
Pelvis
Vagina (lat.)

Daily Dose ▶	150 × 20	150 × 8	180 × 5	180 × 4	Total Dose ▼
① Abdomen	3000	–	–	–	3000 rad
② PA-T	3000	1200	–	–	4200 rad
③ Pelvis	3000	1200	900	–	5100 rad
④ Vagina	3000	1200	900	720	5820 rad

Liver dose = 2250 rad
Kidney dose = 2000 rad

the fluid throughout the abdomen. Reports on treatment with intra-abdominal ^{32}P therapy are similar to those on external treatment. Patients with minimal or no residual disease and early stage disease have higher survival rates than patients with advanced and/or high-grade disease.

Combined Chemotherapy and Radiation. Most patients with ovarian cancer receive surgical treatment followed by chemotherapy, with or without second-look laparotomy with whole abdomen-pelvic radiation used as salvage treatment. Radiation is poorly tolerated at this point, which is attributed to either bone marrow toxicity intensified by numerous courses of earlier chemotherapy or chronic radiation enteritis.[31] Although hope was renewed with the advent of cisplatin treatment, no further improvement has been noted in treatment outcome. The current opinion of some researchers following laboratory experiments is that when resistance to drugs develops, a cross resistance to radiation also develops and is responsible for poor tumor response.[31] Surgery and chemotherapy remain the treatment of choice for ovarian cancer at this time.

Dysgerminoma

Dysgerminoma is an uncommon type of germ cell tumor of the ovary. Although it can occur throughout the life span, most cases appear in adolescents and young adults.[20] Symptoms are insidious and similar to those of epithelial ovarian cancer. As a result, tumors are usually large when diagnosed. They appear as either unilateral or bilateral growths, but smaller tumors are often unilateral.

Dysgerminoma is exceptionally sensitive to radiation. In the past, treatment was surgery followed by radiation therapy, with excellent results. In an effort to preserve fertility and childbearing capability in young women, chemotherapy has recently been introduced into the treatment plan. Cisplatin-based therapy using vincristine, etoposide, and bleomycin (VEB) has been successful. Radiotherapy remains an option as primary adjunctive therapy to either the ipsilateral side or whole abdomen, depending on the extent of disease. Recurrent disease is also treated with radiation, which produces excellent results.

Complications

Approximately 75% of all patients experience nausea, vomiting, and diarrhea from abdominal-pelvic irradiation.[33] Onset is usually during treatment and subsides several weeks later. Diarrhea occasionally persists and becomes chronic enteritis. Other short-term effects are anorexia, fatigue, bone marrow suppression, and transient cystitis and proctitis. Long-term effects associated with ovarian cancer are bowel damage, bowel obstruction, chronic enteritis, radiation hepatitis, lung fibrosis, bone necrosis, and secondary malignancies such as leukemia, breast cancer, and melanoma.

Gestational Trophoblastic Disease

Radiation plays no significant part in the treatment plan for gestational trophoblastic disease, with the exception of two circumstances. When metastasis to the liver occurs, external beam radiotherapy is used, with the goal of eradicating disease. And in the event of brain metastasis, the patient is treated with external beam radiotherapy or, in some cases, intrathecal chemotherapy, also with the goal of cure. Otherwise chemotherapy and/or surgical interventions are the treatment of choice for this spectrum of diseases.

Cancer of the Breast

Women have an estimated 1:8 lifetime risk of developing breast cancer, depending on multiple risk factors.[34] The reader is referred to Chapter 10 for a complete discussion of breast cancer.

Management of Breast Cancer

Radiation was first used as a treatment for breast cancer in the early part of this century, shortly after the discovery of X-rays by Roentgen.[35,36] A single treatment was given to produce erythema to the skin in the belief that the breast cancer would be cured. This belief was rooted in a physician's observations of a student who developed severe dermatitis and resulting skin damage following exposure to X-rays. In the 1920s, technological developments resulted in treatment using tangential fields. Of particular significance were the results obtained by Dr. Jeffrey Fields from the use of radium needles to treat recurrent and, later, primary cancers, which were comparable to radical mastectomy. In the 1930s Baclesse began to treat patients with preoperative radiation over 8 to 13 weeks, with positive results. The use of preoperative radiation lasted until the 1950s. The work done by Baclesse was important because he established the relationship among dose, control, and tumor size.[35] McWhirter first used simple mastectomy followed by radiation in 1941. His results were comparable to those of radical mastectomy. McWhirter's work was a turning point in the management of breast cancer because it "justified the use of less radical surgery."[35]

Radiation therapy is an essential component of the management of breast cancers. The goal for treatment of breast cancer is cure in stages I to III, and disease control or palliation for stage IV. Recurrence, if localized and discovered early, can also be treated with the goal of cure. A second goal is to preserve the cosmetic appearance of the breast (cosmesis) as much as possible. Other goals of radiotherapy in the intact breast are to prevent recurrence, expose the minimum amount of lung, spare the mediastinum, and deliver homogeneous doses to the target tissue.[37]

Preoperative Irradiation.   Historically, radiation as a treatment modality for breast cancers indicated that local control was attainable either by implant or external beam. Breast cancer was once considered to be a local disease, and as radiation therapy is a local treatment, it was the treatment of choice. Large or inoperable tumors were treated to decrease the size and enable resection.[38] But as more information about breast cancer emerged, revealing the systemic nature of the disease, radiation therapy was replaced by chemotherapy. The same or better results have been obtained at the tumor site, and chemotherapy is also able to treat systemic micrometastasis. Although radiation is effective as preoperative treatment, it reduces positive lymph nodes by 50%, thus eradicating one of the most effective prognostic indicators available.[37] The above two factors have resulted in infrequent use of radiotherapy preoperatively.

Postoperative Irradiation of Modified Radical or Radical Mastectomy.   Postoperative radiation therapy following surgical removal of the breast has not been routinely practiced in many institutions in recent years, except for patients who fit the following specific criteria:[39] tumors that are centrally or medially located (irradiation of internal mammary nodes only); positive internal mammary, supraclavicular, and axillary apex nodes (all areas with positive nodes); greater than 20% positive lymph nodes (receive chest wall radiation in addition to nodes plus peripheral nodes); or primary tumors greater than 5 cm (poor prognostic sign) and the presence of tumor margins and/or perineural or vascular space invasion (receive radiation to the chest wall).

Because only a small number (5–10%) of node-negative patients have recurrences following surgery and most node-positive patients receive chemotherapy, it has been generally believed that radiation therapy is unnecessary. Recently, however, this practice has been under scrutiny. Several studies cited by Mendenhall et al. report that significant local control of recurrence is attained with postoperative radiation, while chemotherapy has had little or no effect on local recurrence.[39] Bonadona et al. and Stefanich et al. have found no differences in local recurrence between patients receiving chemotherapy and patients receiving only mastectomy.[40,41] Recurrence has been associated, however, with size of the primary tumors (>5 cm) and the number of positive axillary nodes (>4).[42] It has also been reported that Duke University Medical Center routinely irradiates the chest wall of patients receiving bone marrow transplants because it is the site of frequent local failure even when high-dose chemotherapy is given.[42]

Postoperative Radiation Following Breast-Conserving Surgical Procedures. The dread of breast removal as a result of breast cancer has historically had considerable psychological impact on women.[43] As more knowledge about the behavior of breast cancer has accumulated from clinical trials, women have become more conscious of health care practices. Considerable change has taken place in order to provide effective treatment, yet respect the need to preserve a positive self-image.

The results of many clinical trials comparing mastectomy to wide local tumor excision and radiation in women with early breast cancer have shown no difference in 15-year survival using any technique.[44] However, breast irradiation has been shown to improve local control of disease. In a five-year study conducted by the National Surgical Adjuvant Breast Protocol (NSABP) of women randomized to receive mastectomy, segmental resection alone, or segmental resection followed by radiation therapy, Fisher et al. found a recurrence rate of 35% in women who received no radiation compared to 5% in irradiated breasts.[45] Although other studies in the literature support these findings, not all women are advised to receive treatment with radiation following conservation therapy. Patient selection includes a number of criteria:[44] adequate physical status, mammography, sufficient normal tissue surrounding the tumor to provide adequate margins, and therapeutic doses of radiation to sterilize remaining breast tissue of potential residual microscopic disease, yet preserve normal tissue. The criteria that may exclude patients are[44] large tumors (≥5 cm), nipple discharge or subareolar mass, extent of intraductal invasion, lupus erythematosus–incurred sensitivity to irradiation, and pregnancy.

In general, the tumor is excised and the lymph nodes are either sampled or removed via axillary lymph node dissection Then two to four weeks later radiation therapy is initiated. Figure 13.13 illustrates the techniques used for irradiation of the breast. Treatment is usually given by external beam therapy, with a boost (added dose) to the tumor bed. Boost therapy is done by external beam electron therapy or intersti-

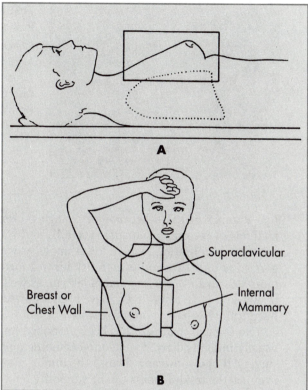

FIGURE 13.13. Treatment fields for intact breast radiotherapy. Note the small crescent of underlying lung that is included (in **A**). Pneumonitis is a frequent side effect of lung irradiation.

Source: Reproduced with permission from McCall, A. (1993). Radiation therapy in the treatment of breast cancers. In J. Isaacs, ed., *Textbook of Breast Disease* (pp. 271–272). St. Louis, MO: Mosby–Year Book, Inc.

tial brachtherapy implant (see Figure 13.14). In some cancer centers, breast brachytherapy alone, HDR, or LDR afterloading technique is used as primary treatment for breast cancer.[46]

In a study in France, Spitalier et al. reported a 20-year survival rate of 61% in patients who received conservative treatment.[47] Forty-five percent of the patients were treated with radiation alone, and 55% with wide local excision followed by radiation. In the United States, current estimates indicate that approximately 30% of newly diagnosed patients with breast cancer are treated with conservative treatment.[43] The use of concomitant chemotherapy as neoadjuvant or adjunctive treatment has been successful in obtaining local control, enhancing surgical removal, and controlling distant metastasis.

Local recurrences in the tumor bed, incision, or adjacent tissue have been reported in approximately 5 to 10% of patients.[43] Most recurrences take place within two to five years; these are considered to be true recurrences. Tumors found after five years are elsewhere in the breast and suggest new primary tumors.[39]

Locally Advanced Breast Cancers. The frequency of locally advanced breast disease (LABD) is approximately 10 to 20%.[47] It has been difficult to estimate the ac-

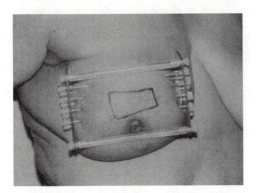

FIGURE 13.14. HDR breast implant.

Source: Courtesy of Dr. Alvaro Martinez, Chairman, Department of Radiation Oncology, William Beaumont Hospital, Royal Oak, MI.

tual number of cases because of changing classification systems and inconsistent methods of recording statistics. Stage III and stage IV epithelial tumors, infiltrating ductal and infiltrating lobular, for example, as well as inflammatory cancers, are categorized as LABD and are at high risk for treatment failure. Failure rates of 44% for tumors ≤8 cm and 76% for tumors >8 cm, as well as decreased five-year survival rates of 30% and 40%, respectively, have been reported.[47] Inflammatory-type breast disease historically has had a poor prognosis.

No optimal treatment has been described for any advanced cancers. Treatment is usually individualized to include chemotherapy and radiotherapy, with or without surgery. If chemotherapy shrinks the tumor enough to provide clearance for surgical margins, the residual mass can be surgically removed and, optimally, eradicated. Initiation of radiation is dependent on the type of surgery performed. In the intact breast, radiation therapy is started two to three weeks after the tumor is excised. When mastectomy is performed, radiation therapy is begun three to four weeks later. The techniques used are the same as those for conservative treatment. If risk of recurrence in the axilla is high, a boost to the midaxilla is considered. Special attention is paid to providing adequate radiation to the skin, since many relapses occur within the scar tissue.

Metastatic Disease.   Radiation is effective in controlling or palliating most metastatic breast disease. Sites commonly affected are bone, brain, spinal cord, and lung. Large doses of radiation are administered over a short period of time to palliate symptoms. Pain from bone metastasis is relieved within three to four weeks of beginning radiation therapy in the majority of patients. Spinal cord compression, an oncologic emergency, is effectively treated with a short course of radiation to the site. Functional impairment is spared if the complication is recognized and treated early. Brain metastasis and neurologic symptoms respond well to treatment with radiation and steroids, used to decrease resulting cerebral edema, irritation, and inflammation. When the skin is invaded by tumor, nodules or open lesions may develop and bleeding from friable tissue occurs. In some instances, it is possible to control nodular development and the bleeding with radiation. Lung metastasis is also frequently treated with radiation therapy in an attempt to obtain control. As patients are able to live with recurrent diseases for extended periods of time, it is essential that the individual be carefully assessed for customization of treatment, not only to meet physical needs but to provide optimal quality of life.

Breast Reconstruction Following Irradiation

Breast reconstruction is possible after radiation to the breast. Several reconstructive methods, such as tissue expanders alone or later replaced by implants, implants alone, and autogenous transplants (transabdominus rectus, latissimus, or gluteal flaps), are currently employed.[48] The method used depends on the posttreatment defect.[49]

Complications

A number of acute effects result from radiation treatment to the breast (see Table 13.7). The most obvious and inevitable effects are those on the skin. This is because the rapidly dividing epithelial cells experience cumulative damage from daily exposure to radiation. Approximately two to three weeks after treatment is started, the skin becomes dry, scaly, and itchy. A slight redness may appear, and the breast may become swollen and tender. The nipple and areola may also become tender. In heavy women or women with pendulous breasts, the skin folds beneath the breast are at great risk for wet desquamation and skin breakdown. If the higher doses of radiation are given, more intense skin reactions are seen. The skin often becomes blistered, and wet desquamation and peeling of the entire breast area may occur. Transient hyperpigmentation, or a brown-tanned appearance, lasting several months, occurs.

Moisturizing, water-based creams or cornstarch is used to relieve minor reactions. Because cornstarch is a plant substance, careful assessment of the area must be ongoing since fungal infections may occur in the presence of moist skin or wet desquamation. Silver sulfadiazine cream, gel dressings, and analgesics are some measures frequently employed to manage the painful effects of more intense reactions.

Transient pneumonitis, characterized by a dry, hacking cough, shortness of breath, and possibly fever lasting for two to three weeks, may develop. It results from the unavoidable irradiation of a small portion of the lung included in the radiation field. Occasionally, the pneumonitis persists and must be treated with steroids.[39] Other transient effects are hoarseness, sore throat, and dysphagia from radiation to the supraclavicular nodes[50] and adjacent tissue, as well as bone marrow suppression.

Long-term effects may occur months to years following treatment. Arm edema is a common occurrence. Patients must be closely followed to maintain as much control of the edema as possible. The incidence of arm edema is directly related to the amount of lymph node dissection and radiation therapy given to the affected area.[44] Entrapment of the brachial plexus is another occasional late effect, which causes considerable distress to the patient.[50] The brachial plexus is included in the field when the supraclavicular nodes are irradiated. Later, tissue fibrosis can occur, causing pressure on or entrapment of the nerves, with resulting pain, paraesthesias, and decreased motor function. Other late complications might include cardiac damage, rib fractures, and myositis.

TABLE 13.7

Radiation Oncology Acute Toxicity Flowsheet
Breast/Chest Wall Malignancies

PATIENT NAME							I.D.#			
TIME	PRE TX	WK 1	WK 2	WK 3	WK 4	WK 5	WK 6	WK 7	WK 8	FINI
DATE										
WBC (x1000)										
HGB (GM%)										
PLT (x1000)										
NEUT. (x1000)										
WEIGHT (kg)										
PERF. SCALE										
BREAST EDEMA										
PAIN										
SKIN										
OTHER										
INITIALS										

(Left side label: PARAMETERS)

SIGNATURE		INITIALS	SIGNATURE		INITIALS

TREATMENT RELATED MEDICATIONS	DOSE	DATE BEGAN	TREATMENT RELATED MEDICATIONS	DOSE	DATE BEGAN

TREATMENT RELATED NURSING INTERVENTIONS	

TABLE 13.7 *(continued)*

HEMATOLOGIC

WBC	HGB	PLT	NEUTROPHILS
0 - > 4.0	0 - > 11	0 - > 100	0 - > 1.9
1 - 3.0 - < 4.0	1 - 11 - 9.5	1 - 75 - < 100	1 - 15 - < 1.9
2 - 2.0 - < 3.0	2 - < 9.5 - 7.5	2 - 50 - < 75	2 - 1.0 - < 1.5
3 - 1.0 - < 2.0	3 - < 7.5 - 5.0	3 - 25 - < 50	3 - 0.5 - < 1.0
4 - < 1.0	4 - _____	4 - < 25 or spontaneous bleeding	4 - < 0.5 or sepsis

PERFORMANCE SCALE

100 - normal; no complaints; NED
 80 - normal activity with effort; some s/s of disease
 60 - requires occasional assistance, but is able to care for most personal needs
 40 - disabled; requires special care and assistance
 20 - very sick; hospitalization necessary; active support treatment is necessary
 10 - moribund; fatal processes progressing rapidly

BREAST EDEMA

0 - no change
1 - mild; asymptomatic and causes only minor increase in breast size
2 - moderate; readily apparent disparity between breasts and accompanied by features of peau
   d'orange
3 - severe; causes significant symptoms such as pain **or** increase in breast size ✕ one cup

PAIN

0 - no change
1 - aware of discomfort; **no** medication required
2 - non-narcotics required
3 - oral narcotics required
4 - parenteral narcotics required
5 - uncontrollable; requires hospital admission for pain control

SKIN

0 - no change over baseline
1 - follicular, faint or dull erythema, epilation, dry desquamation, decreased sweating
2 - tender or bright erythema, patchy moist desquamation, moderate edema
3 - confluent, moist desquamation other than skin folds, pitting edema
4 - ulceration, hemorrhage, necrosis

TABLE 13.8

Assessment Criteria for the Patient Receiving Radiation Therapy

Body System	Examination Requirements
Neurological	Mental alertness (agitated, dull, lethargic) Pain (restless, tense) Coordination

Integumentary	Turgor
	Integrity
	    Perianus
	    Eyes (sunken or soft to touch)
	    Periocular area (dark)

Cardiovascular	Vital signs Hematology (decreased hemoglobin and hematocrit, abnormal WBC, differential, platelets) Blood chemistry profile (electrolyte imbalance) Monitor for shock (hypovolemic or septic)
Respiratory	Chest and lung sounds (character, rate, rhythm of respirations) SOB or dyspnea
Gastrointestinal	Observe abdomen (distention, cramping) Auscultate bowel sounds (hyper or hypo) Palpate (pain, tenderness, guarding, rigidity) Assess stool (number, frequency, character, odor) Assess for nausea and vomiting (amount, frequency, character) Assess nutritional status (fluid intake, anorexia, cachexia) Assess for rectal bleeding (duration, amount, character) Assess weight status (loss or gain)
Genitourinary	Assess output (amount, frequency, pain, color) Monitor specific gravity Assess vaginal integrity (dryness, irritation, pruritis, dyspareunia) Perform sexual assessment
Musculoskeletal	Skeletal assessment (pain, edema) Muscle tone, strength, presence of cramps
General	Sleep patterns Weakness, malaise, fatigue Activity patterns Social habits (alcohol, tobacco)
Psychosocial	Assess knowledge related to disease, treatment, diagnostic studies Functional status and self-care capabilities

TABLE 13.8 *(continued)*	
Assessment Criteria for the Patient Receiving Radiation Therapy	
Body System	*Examination Requirements*
	Perceived threats on mortality, lifestyle, and family
	Anxiety concerning family, job, friends, treatment outcome
	Coping skills; decision-making styles
	Self-image
	Potential and perceived impact of treatment on self-image, self-esteem, parenting
	Concerns regarding finances and health insurance resources
	Impact of disease on life stage
	Support network
Spiritual	Source and strength of religous beliefs
	Impact on and relationship of illness to belief and practices
	Feelings of hope/hopelessness, trust, and feelings of power/control/powerlessness

✻ NURSING MANAGEMENT

Psychological Effects

The nursing management of the patient receiving radiation therapy is concerned with the total patient, thus requiring equal focus on education, emotional, psychosocial/psychosexual concerns, and the physical effects of treatment (Table 13.8). Welsh-McCaffrey states that the educational needs of patients change throughout the course of disease, which in turn requires continual assessment of the care plan and nursing care to keep pace with the patient's changing status.[51] Individual factors, personal stressors, timing, readiness, coping mechanisms, and extent of desired information, for example, play an important part in the patient's informational needs. To answer the question of what kind of information is most desired by patients with cancer, Derderian studied perceived threats and disruptions to life and lifestyle, the importance of information, and the scope of information deemed necessary to a group of cancer patients.[52,53] Results indicated that patient perception of the amount, degree, and imminence of anticipated threats/harm had a direct bearing on informational needs, particularly when physical/physiological survival was in question. As radiation therapy is frequently perceived by the public (and many health care professionals) as a threat to survival (associated with incurability and death) and a cause of "burning," mutilation, disfigurement, pain, or transformation into a radioactive entity, it is essential that patients and families are evaluated for their misconceptions, understanding, and expectations of this treatment modality.[54] Furthermore, a specific plan of patient education must be developed and implemented to foster a fundamental understanding by the patient of the treatment goal, procedure, expected effects, and available support services.

Extensive support services are essential for the patient receiving radiation therapy. Fear of sterility; loss of sexuality; rejection by a spouse, family, and friends; feelings of shame, guilt, and punishment; and loss of self-esteem as well as body image cause severe psychological and psychosexual concerns.[54] Establishing a close rapport through maintaining open lines of communication with the multidisciplinary team is an important aspect of the nurse's supportive patient care. Patients frequently disguise true feelings in behavior such as anger, excessive humor, apathy, or denial. Others appear to be coping well but in reality are experiencing severe psychological pain. Whether newly diagnosed or experiencing recurrence of disease, many patients express a feeling of lack of control, hopelessness, and powerlessness. It is therefore necessary to provide a strong support staff to strengthen coping styles and behaviors. By establishing good communication and trust and imparting a sense of caring to patients, the nurse in radiation therapy is in a key position to assist in managing patient concerns and complex problems, either alone or in collaboration with the multidisciplinary team.

Anxiety

In this chapter, anxiety is addressed as a prime consideration in the nursing management of patients receiving radiation therapy. Adult learners must be willing and ready to learn in order to "hear" and assimilate helpful information. Anxiety and fear can immobilize patients and prevent learning from taking place, thus setting up a cycle that can only increase depression and despair. By addressing the anxiety associated with radiation treatment first, a sequence of events can be initiated that may disarm the distress associated with the problem, thus increasing the patient's ability to learn. Once the patient is able to hear, learning is more possible. And once learning begins and the patient becomes more knowledgeable, anxiety and fear can frequently be decreased and the patient's energy can be focused on recovery and rehabilitation.

Biological Effects

The biological effects from radiation therapy result from damage to normal cells and tissue. The severity of side effects is directly related to dose, size of the field irradiated, length of time exposed, source of radiation, and individual factors such as concomitant treatment or medical conditions. The effects of radiation are classified as general side effects, acute/local effects, or late/chronic effects. General and acute effects usually occur within ten days to two weeks of treatment onset and resolve within weeks to several months once treatment is completed. Chronic effects develop months to years after treatment and are usually permanent. Table 13.9 cites some common key

TABLE 13.9		
Side Effects of Radiation Therapy in Gyncologic and Breast Cancers		
General and Side Effects	Radiation skin reactions	G & B
	Fatigue	G & B
	Anorexia	G & B
Acute/Local Side Effects	Diarrhea	G
	Cystitis	G
	Proctitis	G
	Enteritis	G
	Pneumonitis	B
	Nausea and vomiting	G
	Esophagitis	B
	Dysphagia	B
	Vaginitis	G
Chronic/Late Side Effects and Complications	Vaginal dryness	G
	Vaginal stenosis	G
	Vaginal vault necrosis	G
	Sexual dysfunction	G
	Fistula	G
	Chronic cystitis	G
	Arm and leg edema	G & B
	Bowel obstruction	G
	Chronic proctitis	G
	Pulmonary fibrosis	B

B: breast; G: gynecologic

side effects of gynecologic and breast cancers. (See also Table 13.14, which provides a diagnostic cluster dividing common side effects into collaborative and nursing diagnoses to assist in establishing foci of care.)

General Side Effects

Although radiation therapy is a local treatment and side effects are limited to the field of radiation, several general/systemic effects may occur.

Fatigue is one side effect frequently experienced to some degree. The pathophysiology of fatigue is unclear but has been associated with the by-products of cellular destruction resulting from therapy and the increased metabolism from the tumor burden. One study indicates that weight loss, depression, pain, and length of treatment contribute to the problem.[55] Other factors cited as potential causes are recent surgery, chemotherapy, tumor burden, nutritional status, medications, treatment visits, attempt to maintain lifestyle, pain, anemia, and respiratory compromise.[56] Management of the problem focuses on increasing the frequency of rest periods, prioritizing and pacing activities, and initiating a mild exercise program.[57]

Anorexia and *nausea* are two additional general symptoms often experienced by patients receiving radiation treatment. Nausea, frequently occurring one to two hours following treatment, is often transient and managed by omitting oral intake for several hours. Anorexia may be persistent and may escalate during the course of treatment, resulting in physical debilitation, fatigue, cachexia, and depletion of visceral proteins. Nutritional counseling regarding maintenance of protein intake is essential. Measures such as frequent small feedings and intake of high-protein foods and protein supplements are useful in assisting with this problem. Another helpful strategy is to serve foods cool or at room temperature to decrease food odors, which are frequently noxious to the patient. Although the mechanism of anorexia is not understood, it is believed to be associated with the presence of the by-products of cellular destruction in the blood stream, as well as other extraneous factors, for example, transportation for treatment and concomitant medical problems.[58]

Acute/Local Side Effects

Diarrhea develops in many women who receive radiation therapy to the pelvis. The rapid reproduction of the cells comprising the villi and microvilli lining the intestine cause them to be particularly sensitive to radiation. The effects can be detected as soon as twelve hours after the first treatment.[59] Consistent daily exposure to radiation prevents cellular replacement and results in damage or destruction of the villi and consequent inability of the small intestine to ingest nutrients and absorb fluids. The large intestine also loses its ability to absorb fluids and electrolytes, although to a lesser extent than the small intestine. The majority of women receiving radiation to the pelvis for gynecologic cancers have been reported to develop diarrhea, the cardinal symptom of enteritis, within the first few weeks of treatment.

Acute radiation enteritis is transient, usually beginning during treatment and resolving several weeks after treatment ends. Factors directly affecting the severity of the injury are dose, fractionation, volume of treatment area, tissue characteristics, and treatment techniques.[60] Predisposing factors, such as earlier surgery, pelvic inflammatory disease, and peritonitis, may cause adhesions and increase the risk of severe disease. Medical problems such as hypertension, diabetes, and poor nutrition impair blood supply to the bowel and may also potentiate risk for severe disease.

Diagnosis is based on clinical presentation of symptoms varying from increased numbers of stools to loose, watery diarrhea, cramping, colicky pain, and possibly nausea and vomiting. When symptoms are more severe, dehydration, electrolyte imbalance, and weight loss occur from malabsorption of fluid and essential nutrients. Excoriation of the skin surrounding the rectum and tenesmus, the constant urge to defecate, may also be present. Treatment includes dietary modification and use of antidiarrheal agents and anticholinergics.

Nursing management focuses on patient education, symptom management, and support. Teaching emphasizes the likelihood of enteritis, expected symptoms, and self-care strategies. Implementation of a low-residue diet decreases irritation to the bowel.[61] Patients are instructed to omit whole grain cereals and bread, milk and milk products, and raw fruits and vegetables, with the exception of peeled apples and bananas, from the diet. Pectin, a natural substance found in apples, is an effective antidiarrheal agent. Fats, caffeinated coffee, spicy foods, and alcohols are among other foods excluded from the diet. A lactose-free diet may also be implemented and nutritional supplements added to the diet. Antidiarrheal medications may be ordered to control diarrhea. Codeine or tincture of opium are helpful in managing severe diarrhea unresponsive to other medication as well as the cramping associated with the problem. Assessment by the nurse is important to determine the functional status of the patient and the effectiveness of the regimen, and to assist in tailoring the treatment to provide better control and teach the patient how to maintain adequate hydration and nutrition.

Maintaining skin integrity of the perianal area is another concern for the nurse. Many patients are embarrassed and reluctant to address the issue unless it is tactfully approached by the nurse. The use of protective ointments can assist in relieving the burning, itching, and pain from excoriated tissue. (See Table 13.10.)

Support is an important part of the nursing care of the patient with radiation enteritis. Support is needed by all patients, who frequently become frustrated and require patience and understanding. Reassurance, allowing the patient time to talk, and taking the time to listen are helpful supportive interventions. Sharing supportive efforts with other members of the multidisciplinary team is also important.

Tenesmus, a constant urge to defecate or urinate, occasionally develops during treatment due to sphincter irritation. The problem may persist for several weeks after radiation is completed. Tenesmus may result in interference with the patient's rest and lifestyle as well as an increase in stress and tension. Gastrointestinal and urinary antispasmodics may be of help in resolving the problem. Steroid suppositories are also useful if other medications are ineffective. Extensive psychological support is needed to minimize feelings of powerlessness and depression during this period.

Cystitis is an infrequent side effect resulting from irradiation of the bladder and may be either infectious or noninfectious.[58] The presence or absence of bacterial infection is established through urine culture and sensitivities tests. Medical management is usually initiated using urinary antiseptics, antibiotics, and, in some cases, antispasmodics. In cases where bladder spasm is unrelieved by antispasmodics, one or two small bladder instillations via Foley catheter of xylocaine diluted in sterile normal saline may be helpful in providing relief. Increased fluid intake is urged. Additional acute/local side effects are listed in Table 13.9.

Chronic/Late Side Effects and Complications

Chronic/late side effects and complications occur months to years after radiation treatment has ended. Damage occurs from the direct release of toxic waste products into the tissue resulting from cellular destruction. Inflammation then develops in

TABLE 13.10

Caring for Yourself at Home While Receiving Radiation Therapy

During your treatment planning session (also called simulation), we will draw purple-colored marks on your skin. They will outline the radiation treatment field (the area where the radiation will be). These purple marks are very important. Do not remove them before you are tattooed or before you have your last treatment.

Skin Care

The following instructions apply only to the skin in the treatment area.

- Wash the skin in the treatment area gently with lukewarm water. Blot your skin with a soft towel to dry. You may use a mild soap, if it does not contain perfumes or irritants. They can dry your skin.

- Do not apply any lotions, perfumes, or powders to the treatment area. These products can be irritating to the skin and cause a more severe reaction. Should you require a lotion to moisturize dry skin, see your doctor or nurse for a suggestion.

- If you normally use powder and would like to continue using it during treatment, use a light dusting of cornstarch in the treated area.

- Do not rub, scrub, or scratch the skin in the treatment area. Your skin will be dryer than usual and will peel and will be easily irritated. If your skin itches or becomes dry, tell your nurse.

- Check with your doctor or nurse first if you need to shave in the treatment area. If they allow you to shave, use an electric razor. Continue with the electric razor until any skin reaction has disappeared.

- Do not use hot water bottles, heating lights, electric heating pads, or hot packs on the treated areas.

- Keep the treated areas out of the sun. Make sure you do not sunburn throughout your treatment. Continue to avoid sunburns for at least one year after treatment has ended. Use a sun-blocking lotion that is at least a number 20 or greater, or cover the area with clothing.

- Skin reactions from radiation therapy are temporary and will begin to subside two to three weeks after therapy ends. Reactions generally begin two weeks after treatment and progress through to the end. Peak reactions may continue for two weeks after treatment ends and then begin to heal.

- If you develop a skin reaction, report it to your nurse or doctor. Keep your skin clean, dry, and open to air as much as possible. Wear only *loose-fitting* cotton clothing over the treatment area to prevent further irritation.

- Give special attention to areas where there are folds of skin. Skin in these areas is more likely to peel and become sore. Keep these areas clean and dry.

- If the skin in the treatment area becomes moist, sticky, or blistered, notify your doctor. You may be having a more severe skin reaction.

tissues, with subsequent formation of fibrotic tissue during the repair process.[62] In radioresistant cells as well as radiosensitive cells, additional tissue changes take place due to damage or destruction of the small blood vessels (arterioles, capillaries, venules). Subsequently, ischemia, cellular death, and tissue atrophy occur. The amount of tissue and organ damage is dependent on the richness of the blood supply and the amount of radiation effect on the vasculature.

It has been estimated that as many as 80% of women receiving pelvic radiation experience some *vaginal injury* as a result.[63] Patients with cancer of the cervix are at particular risk because of the high doses of radiation needed to adequately treat the tumor.[60] Exposure of the rapidly proliferating epithelial cells of the vaginal mucosa during high-dose external and internal radiation treatment, direct physical trauma to the vagina from applicator insertion, and cessation of estrogen production by the ovaries following surgery or exposure to radiation are the three identified causes of vaginal injury.[60,64,65] Of the three, the direct effect of radiation on the vaginal mucosa is the most significant. According to Brown, a series of radiation effects begins approximately one week after radiation therapy has been initiated.[65] At this time, a discharge develops containing transudates and sloughed substances including normal floral growth caused by radiation-induced changes within the vagina. Erythema and inflammation occur and may last from weeks to months. The vagina becomes pale, and a white radiation membrane and telangiectasia develop. Ulcerations and then adhesions form, particularly on the posterior and anterior surfaces of the upper third of the vagina and the external os of the cervix, where maximum amounts of radiation are delivered. The adhesions, if left unattended, lead to fibrosis and subsequent stenosis, shortening, constriction, or complete closure of the vagina.[60,65] When extreme vascular compromise is experienced, vascular necrosis may occur. Although the epithelium can take as long as two years following treatment to return to a more normal structure, it may never completely regain the normal status that existed prior to radiation.[66]

Clinical symptoms may be vaginal discharge, spontaneous or mechanically induced vaginal spotting or bleeding, pruritus, burning, pain, vaginal infections, and sexual dysfunction.[60,64] Medical management of the problem focuses on prevention. Early vaginal dilatation and the use of estrogen cream can significantly reduce the incidence of vaginal complications.[60,67] Conjugated estrogen creams, even though absorbed systemically, can be used safely unless contraindicated because the tumor is estrogen-dependent. Estrogen creams enhance regeneration of vaginal epithelial tissue and promote normal vaginal histology during the time they are used.[65,67] Once discontinued, the tissue reverts to the postirradiation status within several months. When infection is present, it is usually the result of alterations in vaginal environment caused by a decrease of vaginal glycogen, increased pH, and an imbalance of normal vaginal flora such as *Candida albicans*, *Gardnerella vaginitis*, and others. Systemic and topical antibiotics or antifungal medications are used to treat the infections, depending on the specific organisms and sensitivities involved.

Nursing as well as medical management of postradiation vaginitis and vaginal stenosis focuses on prevention through use of the vaginal dilator and lubricants. Vaginal dilatation using a plastic dilator, ranging from three times a week to daily depending on

TABLE 13.11

Patient Education: Vaginal Dilator

1. **What is a vaginal dilator?**
   A vaginal dilator is a plastic rod with a rounded end. The vaginal dilator comes in three sizes—small, medium, and large—because vaginas differ in size.

2. **Why must I use a dilator?**
   To prevent scarring of the vagina from treatment
   To keep the tissue soft and able to stretch
   To keep the vagina from closing up and preventing you from having sexual intercourse and exams by the doctor

3. **When do I start using a dilator?**
   Most doctors tell patients to begin 2–4 weeks after treatment.
   Your doctor wants you to start on _____.

4. **How often do I use the dilator?**
   Your doctor wants you to use the dilator at least 3 times each week. You can use it as often as every day if you wish.
   Do not stop using the dilator without your doctor's permission.

5. **Can I have intercourse instead of using a dilator?**
   Yes, you can have intercourse instead of using a dilator.
   OR
   You can use a dilator part of the time and have intercourse part of the time, as long as the two add up to the number of times that the doctor has told you to dilate each week.

6. **Will it hurt?**
   Both the vaginal dilator and intercourse may feel uncomfortable at first.
   Remember to:
   Use lots of lubricant.
   Go slowly at first. If it does not feel good, *stop* for a while and start again later.

7. **What kind of lubricant do I use?**
   Do not use anything with an oil base, such as Vaseline.
   Do use water-based lubricants or creams, such as K-Y Jelly, Replens, or Astro-Glide.

8. **How do I use a vaginal dilator?**
   Wash your hands and the dilator in warm, soapy water, then rinse and dry.
   Lubricate the dilator well.
   Lay on your back with the legs bent and apart.
   Slowly insert the *round* end upwards and toward the back, at an angle, as far as it will go without hurting.
   Close your knees together, straighten your legs, and relax.
   Keep the dilator in place for at least 10 minutes.
   Bend your knees and separate your legs.
   Slowly remove the dilator.
   Wash the dilator and your hands in warm, soapy water, then rinse, dry, and put away the dilator.

physician preference and hospital policy, is the generally accepted method of maintaining pliability of tissue and patency of the vaginal vault. Table 13.11 describes the rationale and procedure for use of the vaginal dilator.

Vaginal dryness is always present after pelvic radiation and requires use of a vaginal lubricator to enable more comfortable intercourse as well as to provide relief from the dryness, a frequent cause of burning, irritation, and pruritus. Table 13.12 provides a summary of common products available over the counter. Liberal lubrication must be used with dilator insertion and sexual intercourse to prevent trauma and pain. Some women use lubrication regularly, whether or not sexually active, to relieve symptoms of vaginal dryness. Unless contraindicated by the presence of an estrogen-dependent tumor, an estrogen cream, patch, or tablets may be prescribed to relieve vaginal dryness and associated symptoms. In any event, the nurse must stress the critical need to use lubrication and the vaginal dilator as prescribed to maintain vaginal health and patency for follow-up care. Involvement of a sex therapist or collaboration with another staff member or medical social worker to assist in a sexual evaluation is also helpful, particularly if the nurse is uncomfortable in addressing the issue. Sexual dysfunction is a common problem after radiation therapy and an important issue in patient care.

TABLE 13.12

Vaginal Lubricants

Type	Advantages	Disadvantages
Jelly	Inexpensive	Contains preservatives May cause "burning" "Messy" Applied with fingers
Vaginal Suppositories	Compact Easy to insert	Must allow time to melt if using before intercourse
Cream	Used 3 times per week Cartridge inserts like tampon Moisturizes tissue Long-lasting Does not require insertion before intercourse Company liberal with samples	Expensive Requires scheduled use, can be confusing Cream base
Viscous Liquid (Like Saliva)	Small, compact container Odorless, colorless, tasteless "Natural" feeling Company liberal with samples	Moderate cost Applied with fingers For best results, both partners use

When alterations, shortening, constriction, or stenosis of the vagina does occur, an attempt may be made to dilate the vagina. The process is often slow and painful. Smaller dilators, such as rectal dilators, may be used initially. Rectal dilators are shorter, come in a wide range of sizes, and are less threatening to many women. If dilatation is unsuccessful, vaginal reconstruction may be performed once the presence of persistent or recurrent disease has been eliminated. If surgery is undesirable, alternative methods of sexual practice are sometimes acceptable. Refer to Chapter 14 for a discussion of sexuality.

Chronic radiation enteritis appears from months to years following treatment and is a progressive disease. It is associated with inevitable ischemia of the bowel, deposition of collagen in the submucosa, atrophy of the mucosa, and fibrosis.[60,64] Ulceration, abscess, the formation of rectovaginal fistula, stenosis, and obstruction may occur as complications of the problem. The sigmoid colon and rectum are most frequently affected.

Initially, medical management is conservative. The patient is hospitalized, oral intake restricted, and the bowel is decompressed through insertion of a nasogastric tube to allow it to rest. Parenteral fluids and/or hyperalimentation is initiated to relieve dehydration and improve nutritional status. Medications are used, as in acute enteritis, to relieve diarrhea and cramping. Antibiotics and bile salt–sequestering (isolating) agents such as cholestyramine resin help relieve malabsorption. Should perforation or disease progression and obstruction, stenosis, or relentless nutritional depletion result, surgical intervention becomes the treatment of choice.

Nursing management deals with nutritional support, maintenance of skin integrity, symptom management, and emotional support. Generalized skin care is of extreme importance, as is local care of the perineal area, due to the poor nutritional status and likelihood of bed rest early in the treatment.

Fistula is a fairly common occurrence in gynecologic malignancies. Some common causes are cancer treatment (particularly surgery and radiation), preexisting bowel disease, and malignant tumors. Skin breakdown, offensive odors, and large amounts of drainage frequently present complicated problems requiring skillful nursing management. Fistula terminology and classification are often confusing but must be understood to provide effective management.

Fistulas can develop between two or more organs and present a problem, not only with drainage and odors, but with potential infection as well as protein depletion and electrolyte imbalance.

Colostomy and/or urinary diversions are often used to resolve fistulas requiring some type of containment system for drainage. Dressings and containment systems are also used when fistulas cannot be corrected. Careful evaluation of the defect and selection of an appropriate dressing or appliance are important. Because fistulas and colostomy or urinary diversions have significant psychological, psychosexual, and lifestyle implications, an effort to provide intense support is an essential part of patient care, whether the situation is temporary or permanent. Table 13.13 lists some community resources for support.

Vaginal vault necrosis is a severe complication of pelvic radiation. Although some response has been noted to estrogen cream (in tumors independent of estrogen), an-

TABLE 13.13	
Resources for the Patient Receiving Radiation Therapy	
Transportation	American Cancer Society
	American Red Cross
	Community agencies
	Community service groups
	Church groups/religious organizations
	Corporate angels
Lodging	Local hotels (special rates; occasionally free rooms)
	Family houses associated with hospital or clinics
	Private individuals
Literature	Cuker, D., & McCullough, V.E. (1993). *Coping with Radiation Therapy.* Chicago: Contemporary Books.
	McAllister, R., Horowitz, S., & Gilden, R. (1993). *Cancer.* New York: Harper-Collins.
	McGinn, K., & Haylock, P. (1993). *Women's Cancers.* Alameda, CA: Hunter House.
	Mullan, F., & Hoffman, J., eds. (1990). *An Almanac of Practical Resources for Cancer Survivors.* Mount Vernon, NY: Consumers Union, Inc.
	Radiation and You. NIH Publication No. 95-2227. Bethesda, MD: National Cancer Institute.
	Eating Hints. NIH Publication No. 94-2079. Bethesda, MD: National Cancer Institute.
Support	Medical social worker
	Pastoral care
	Hospital/clinic support groups
	Community support groups
	American Cancer Society
	I Can Cope
	I Can Surmount

tiseptic douches, and antibiotics, disease progression is common.[64] Exquisite pain unresponsive to narcotics, with resulting anorexia, malaise, weight loss, and depression are side effects that occur frequently. Later, hemorrhage, bowel and urinary tract fistulas, and severe depression may develop. Surgical debridement of necrotic tissue and skin grafting with nonradiated tissue are sometimes helpful. If fistula is also present, a diversional procedure (colostomy, urostomy, or exenteration) is necessary.

TABLE 13.14
Diagnostic Cluster

Diagnostic/Treatment Period

NURSING DIAGNOSIS

1. Decisional conflict related to insufficient knowledge of treatment options
2. Anxiety/fear related to insufficient knowledge of potential impact of condition and treatment on reproductive organs and sexuality
3. Grieving related to potential loss of fertility and perceived effects on lifestyle
4. Altered comfort related to effects of surgery, disease process, and immobility
5. Anxiety/fear related to insufficient knowledge of prescribed radiation therapy and necessary self-care measures
6. Anxiety/fear related to insufficient knowledge of prescribed gynecologic radiation implant: conventional afterloading procedure
7. Anxiety/fear related to insufficient knowledge of prescribed gynecologic radiation implant: remote afterloading procedure
8. Potential for infection related to immunosuppression neutropenia secondary to chemotherapy and/or radiation therapy
9. Potential for bleeding related to immunosuppression thrombocytopenia secondary to chemotherapy and/or radiation therapy
10. Potential alteration in skin integrity related to treatment modality and/or disease process
11. Potential for alteration in comfort related to side effects of therapy and/or disease process
12. Potential altered nutrition: less than body requirements related to nausea, vomiting, anorexia, and/or stomatitis
13. Potential for alteration in elimination: diarrhea related to radiation-induced enteritis
14. Potential for impaired elimination related to development of fistulae
15. Potential altered health maintenance due to insufficient knowledge of colostomy/ileostomy and/or ileal conduit
16a. Potential sexual dysfunction related to disease process, surgical intervention, fatigue, and/or pain
16b. Potential moderate or possible permanent alterations in sexual activity related to disease process, surgical intervention, fatigue, and/or pain
16c. Severe or permanent inability to engage in genital intercourse
17. Alteration in coping related to infertility
18. Potential altered health maintenance related to insufficient knowledge of dietary restrictions, medications, activity restrictions, self-care activities, symptoms of complications, follow-up visits, and community resources

✸ REFERENCES

1. Hoskins, W.J., Perez, C.A., & Young, R.C., eds. (1992). *Principles and Practice of Gynecologic Oncology* 2nd ed. Philadelphia: Lippincott.
2. Perez, C., & Brady, L., eds. (1992). *Principles and Practice of Radiation Oncology* 2nd ed. Philadelphia: Lippincott.
3. Perez, C., & Purdy, J. (1992). Biological and physical aspects of radiation oncology. In W.J. Hoskins, C.A. Perez, & R.C. Young, eds., *Principles and Practice of Gynecologic Oncology* 2nd ed. (pp. 217–288). Philadelphia: Lippincott.
4. Bucholtz, J. (1987). Radiation therapy. In C. Ziegfield, ed., *Core Curriculum for Oncology Nursing* (pp. 207–224). Philadelphia: Saunders.
5. Hilderley, L. (1992). Historical background and principles of teletherapy. In K. Hassey Dow and L. Hilderley, eds., *Nursing Care in Radiation Oncology* (pp. 3–15). Philadelphia: Saunders.
6. Glasgow, G., & Purdy, J. (1992). External beam dosimetry and treatment planning. In C. Perez & L. Brady, eds., *Principles and Practice of Radiation Oncology* 2nd ed. (pp. 208–267). Philadelphia: Lippincott.
7. Clarke, D., & Martinez, A. (1990). An overview of brachytherapy in cancer management. *Oncology, (4)*, 39–54.
8. Keegan, M., & Lanciano, R. (1992). Interstitial brachytherapy for gynecologic malignancies. *SGNO: Gynecol Oncol Nurs, 2*(3), 4–5.
9. Birk, C. (1992). Intraperitoneal chromic phosphate administration. *SGNO: Gynecol Oncol Nurs, 2*(3), 5–7.
10. Condra, K.S., Mendenhall, W.M., Morgan, L.S., Marcus, R.B. Jr. (1998). Consolidative ^{32}P after second-look laparatomy for ovarian carcinoma. *Radiat Oncol Invest, 6*(2),97–102.
11. Pattillo, R.A., Collier, B.D., Abdel-Dayem, H., et al. (1995). Phosphorus-32-chromic phosphate for ovarian cancer: I. Fractionated low-dose intraperitoneal treatments in conjunction with platinum analog chemotherapy. *J Nucl Med, 36*(1), 29–36.
12. Warren, S. (1935). Preliminary study of the effect of artificial fever upon hopeless cases. *Am J Roentgenol, 33*, 75.
13. Bicher, H., Wolfstein, R., Lewinsky, B., et al. (1986). Microwave hyperthermia as an adjunct to radiation therapy: Summary experience of 256 multifraction treatment cases. *Int J Radiat Oncol Biol Phys, 12*, 1667–1671.
14. Howard, G., Sathiaseelan, V., Freedman, L., et al. (1987). Hyperthermia and radiation in the treatment of superficial malignancy: An analysis of treatment parameters, response, and toxicity. *Int J Radiat Oncol Biol Phys, 3,* 1–8.
15. Hall, E., & Roizin-Towle, L. (1984). Biological effects of heat. *Cancer Res, 44*, 4708–4713.
16. Song, C. (1984). Effects of hyperthermia on blood flow and microenvironment: A review. *Cancer Res, 44,* 4721S.
17. Wotjas, F. (1992). Hyperthermia and radiation. In K. Hassey Dow & L. Hilderley, eds., *Nursing Care in Radiation Oncology* (pp. 307–319). Philadelphia: Saunders.
18. Tepper, J., & Calvo, F. (1992). Intraoperative radiation therapy. In C. Perez & L. Brady, eds., *Principles and Practice of Radiation Oncology* 2nd ed. (pp. 388–395). Philadelphia: Lippincott.
19. Smith, R. (1992). Intraoperative radiation therapy. In K. Hassey Dow & L. Hilderley, eds., *Nursing Care in Radiation Oncology* (pp. 295–319). Philadelphia: Saunders.
20. DiSaia, P,. & Creaseman, W., eds. (1993). *Clinical Gynecologic Oncology*. St. Louis, MO: Mosby.
21. DiSaia, P. (1992, February). Cancer in pregnancy. In L. Gossfeld, chair, *Ninth Annual Symposium of the Society of Gynecologic Nurse Oncologists*. Las Vegas, NV.
22. Grigsby, P.V., Kuske, R.R., Perez, C.A., et al. (1987). Medically inoperable stage I adenocarcinoma of the endometrium treated with radiotherapy alone. *Int J Radiat Oncol Biol Phy, 13*, 487.
23. Park, R., Grigsby, P., Muss, H., & Noris, H. (1992). Corpus epithelial tumors. In W.J. Hoskins, C.A. Perez, & R.C. Young, eds., *Principles and Practice of Gynecologic Oncology* 2nd ed. Philadelphia: Lippincott.
24. Morrow, C., & Townsend, D. (1987). *Synopsis of Gynecologic Oncology* 3rd ed. (pp. 483–491). New York: Wiley.
25. Randall, M., Evans, L., Greven, K., et al. (1993). Interstitial reirradiation for recurrent gynecologic malignancies: Results and analysis of prognostic factors. *Gynecol Oncol, 48*, 23–31.
26. Perez, C., & Grigsby, P. (1992). Vulva. In C. Perez & L. Brady, eds., *Principles and Practice of Radiation Oncology* 2nd ed. Philadelphia: Lipppincott.
27. Eisenkop, S., Lowitz, B., & Casiato, D. (1988). Gynecologic cancers. In D. Casciato & B. Lowitz, eds., *Manual of Clinical Oncology* 2nd ed. (pp. 166–188). Boston: Little, Brown.
28. Dembo, A. (1984). Radiotherapeutic management of ovarian cancer. *Semin Oncol, 11*, 238–250.
29. Dembo, A.J., Davy, M., & Stening, A. (1990). Prog-

nostic factors in patients with stage I epithelial ovarian cancer. *Obstet Gynecol, 75,* 263–273.

30. Potish, R. (1993). Radiotherapy for cancer of the ovary. In S. Rubin & G. Sutton, eds., *Ovarian Cancer* (pp. 375–389). New York: McGraw-Hill.

31. Mychalczak, B., & Fuks, Z. (1993). The role of radiotherapy in the management of epithelial ovarian cancer. In M. Markam & W.J. Hoskins, eds., *Cancer of the Ovary.* New York: Raven Press.

32. Dembo, A., Bach, R., Beal, F., et al. (1979). Ovarian carcinoma: Improved survival following abdominopelvic irradiation in patients with a complete pelvic operation. *Am J Obstet Gynecol, 134,* 793–800.

33. Horowitz, C., and Brady, L. (1992). Ovary. In C. Perez & L. Brady, eds., *Principles and Practice of Radiation Oncology* 2nd ed. (pp. 1221–1250). Philadelphia: Lippincott.

34. Landis, S.H., Murray, T., Bolden, S., Wingo, P.A. (1998). American Cancer Society: Cancer Statistics 1998. *CA Cancer J Clin, 48*(1), 6–30.

35. Fletcher, G. (1991). History of irradiation in the primary management of apparently regionally confined breast cancer. In K. Bland & E. Copeland, eds., *The Breast: Comprehensive Management of Benign and Malignant Disease* (p. 707). Philadelphia: Saunders.

36. Fletcher, G. (1988). Regaud lecture perspectives on the history of radiotherapy. *Radiother Oncol, 12,* 253–267.

37. Lichter, A. (1988). Technical aspects of the treatment of breast cancer with radiation therapy. In M. Lippman et al., *Diagnosis and Management of Breast Cancer* (p. 209). Philadelphia: Saunders.

38. Findly, P. (1988). Radiation therapy as a definitive treatment of breast cancer. In M. Lippman et al., *Diagnosis and Management of Breast Cancer.* Philadelphia: Saunders.

39. Mendenhall, N., Fletcher, G., & Million, R. (1991). Adjuvant radiation therapy following modified radical or radical mastectomy. In K. Bland & E. Copeland, eds., *The Breast: Comprehensive Management of Benign and Malignant Disease* (pp. 776–779). Philadelphia: Saunders.

40. Bonadona, G., Valsgusa, B., Rossi, A., et al. (1985). Ten year experience with CMF-based adjuvant chemotherapy in resectable breast cancer. *Breast Cancer Res Treat, 5,* 95–115.

41. Stefanich, D., Goldberg, R., Byrne, P., et al. (1985). Local regional failure in patients treated with adjuvant chemotherapy for breast cancer. *J Clin Oncol, 3,* 660–665.

42. Peters, W., Davis, R., & Shpall, E. (1990). Adjuvant chemotherapy involving high dose combination cyclophosphamide, cisplatin, and carmustine

(CPA/CDDP/BCNU) and autologous bone marrow support (ABMS) for stage II/III breast cancer involving 10 or more lymph nodes. *Proc ASCO, 9,* 22.

43. Lichter, A.S., Adler, D.D., August, D.A., et al. (1992). Breast cancer. In W.J. Hoskins, C.A. Perez, & R.C. Young, eds., *Principles and Practice of Gynecologic Oncology* 2nd ed. (pp. 827–890). Philadelphia: Lippincott.

44. McCall, A. (1992). Radiation therapy in the treatment of breast cancers. In J. Issacs, ed., *Textbook of Breast Disease* (pp. 265–276). St. Louis, MO: Mosby.

45. Fisher, B., Redmond, C., & Passion, R. (1989). Eight-year results of a randomized clinical trial comparing total mastectomy and lumpectomy with or without irradiation in the treatment of breast cancer. *N Engl J Med, 320,* 822–828.

46. Kuske, R.R., Bolton, J.S., Hanson, W. (1997). Radiation Therapy Oncology Group. RTOG 97–17. A Phase I/II Trial to Evaluate Brachytherapy as the Sole Method of Radiation Therapy for Stage I and II Breast Carcinoma.

47. Sorace, R., & Lippman, M. (1991). Locally advanced breast cancer. In M. Lippman et al., *Diagnosis and Management of Breast Cancer* (p. 272). Philadelphia: Saunders.

48. Goodman, M., & Hart, N. (1990). Breast cancer. In S. Groenwald, M. Frogge, M. Goodman, & C. Yarbro, eds., *Cancer Nursing: Principles and Practice* 2nd ed. (pp. 746–747). Boston: Jones and Bartlett.

49. McDonald, H. (1988). Reconstruction of the breast. In M. Lippman, A. Lichter, & D. Danforth, eds., *Diagnosis and Management of Breast Cancer* (pp. 480–481). Philadelphia: Saunders.

50. Scanlon, E. (1991). Breast cancer. In A. Hollieb, D. Fink, & G. Murphy, eds., *Clinical Oncology.* Atlanta: American Cancer Society.

51. Welch-McCaffrey, D. (1985). Evolving educational needs in cancer. *Oncol Nurs Forum, 12*(5), 62–65.

52. Derderian, A. (1987). Informational needs of recently diagnosed cancer patients, part II: Method and description. *Cancer Nurs, 10*(3), 156–163.

53. Derderian, A. (1987). Informational needs of recently diagnosed cancer patients, part I. *Cancer Nurs, 10*(2), 107–115.

54. Rotman, M., & Torpie, R. (1992). Supportive care in radiation oncology. In C. Perez & L. Brady, eds., *Principles and Practice in Radiation Oncology* 2nd ed. (pp. 1508–1516). Philadelphia: Lippincott.

55. Irvine, D., Vincent, L., Bubela, W., Thompson, L., & Graydon, J. (1991). A critical appraisal of the research literature investigating fatigue in the individual with cancer. *Cancer Nurs, 14*(4), 188–199.

56. Hilderley, L. (1992). Pain and fatigue. In K. Hassey Dow & L. Hilderley, eds., *Nursing Care in Radiation Oncology* (pp. 65–66). Philadelphia: Saunders.

57. Nail, L.M. (1990). Fatigue. In S. Groenwald, M. Frogge, M. Goodman, & C. Yarbro, eds., *Cancer Nursing: Principles and Practice* 2nd ed. (pp. 485–494). Boston: Jones and Bartlett.

58. Hilderley, L. (1990). Radiotherapy. In S. Groenwald, M. Frogge, M. Goodman, & C. Yarbro, eds., *Cancer Nursing: Principles and Practice* 2nd ed. (pp. 199–229). Boston: Jones and Bartlett.

59. McCarthy, C. (1992). Altered patterns of elimination. In K. Hassey Dow & L. Hilderley, eds., *Nursing Care in Radiation Oncology* (p. 126). Philadelphia: Saunders.

60. Lydon, J., Purr, S., & Goodman, M. (1990). Integumentary and mucus membrane alterations. In S. Groenwald, M. Frogge, M. Goodman, & C. Yarbro, eds., *Cancer Nursing: Principles and Practice* 2nd ed. (pp. 594–643). Boston: Jones and Bartlett.

61. Iwamoto, R. (1992). Altered nutrition. In K. Hassey Dow & L. Hilderley, eds., *Nursing Care in Radiation Oncology* (p. 99). Philadelphia: Saunders.

62. Rubin, P., Constine, L., & Nelson, D. (1992). Late effects of cancer treatment: Radiation and drug toxicity. In C. Perez & L. Brady, eds., *Principles and Practice of Radiation Oncology* 2nd ed. (pp. 124–128). Philadelphia: Lippincott.

63. Poma, P. (1980). Postirradiation vaginal occlusion: Nonoperative management. *Int J Obstet Gynecol, 18*, 90.

64. Byfield, J., & Lacey, C. (1987). Principles of radiation therapy. In C. Morow & D. Townsend, eds., *Synopsis of Gynecologic Oncology* 3rd ed. New York: Wiley.

65. Brown, D. (1991). Atrophic and postirradiation vaginitis. In B. Horowitz & P. Markham, eds., *Vaginitis and Vaginosis* (pp. 169–179). New York: Wiley.

66. Pithkin, R., & Vanboobis, L. (1971). Postirradiation vaginitis: An evaluation of prophylaxis and topical estrogen. *Radiology, 99*, 417–421.

67. McNally, J., Somerville, E., Miaskowski, C., & Rostad, M. (1991). *Guidelines for Oncology Nursing Practice* 2nd ed. Philadelphia: Saunders.

C H A P T E R   1 4

Sexuality and Fertility Issues

Lynn M. Gossfeld, RN, MSN
Mary Louise Cullen, RNP, MS

✻ INTRODUCTION

Sexuality is an integral part of our personalities, woven into the physical, psychological, cultural, and spiritual aspects of our lives. The experience of cancer poses many challenges and threats to all patients and their families. These threats may vary in intensity and duration and change over time for each individual. Women who have had a diagnosis of gynecologic or breast cancer experience a severe threat to their physical, psychological, and social well-being. Although the majority of patients are treated effectively, sexual functioning morbidity is the most probable area of life disruption for these women. Andersen has reported that upward of 90% of women with cancer may experience sexual dysfunction, with the highest rates among those with disease at a sexual body site.[1]

With aggressive, multimodal therapies and their resultant improved survival, there has been a shift in focus for the patient and clinician from the general effects of treatment to the long-term sequelae of cancer and its treatments. Over time, attention has turned to quality-of-life issues. However, until the past two decades, little attention was given to the sexual and fertility outcomes following the acute phase of diagnosis and treatment. Fortunately, researchers are now beginning to conduct prospective studies and develop comprehensive models and tools to assess sexual functioning in the cancer patient population.

✻ DEFINITION OF SEXUALITY

Human sexuality is a complex phenomenon that reflects an individual's personality and lifestyle. Sexuality, or sexual health, as defined by the World Health Organization (1975), is "the integration of the somatic, emotional, intellectual, and social aspects of sexual being in ways that are positively enriching and that enhance personality, communication, and love."[7] For many people, the ability to feel and act "sexy" verifies that they are living human beings. Sexuality is closely tied to the concepts of body image, self-esteem, and self-concept. It goes beyond the ability of the individual to engage in intercourse. Sexual functioning is affected by changes in appearance, mental states, and personal and social factors, and in the case of cancer, the effects of the disease process and treatments. Every woman is unique in the way she sees herself, how others relate to her, and how she communicates with others.

The nature of cancer and its treatment may temporarily or even permanently affect the sexual behavior of an individual. Foltz reported that the incidence, magnitude, and duration of sexual dysfunctions are dependent on the site of disease, treatment-associated injury determined by disease site, treatment modality, marital status, and age.[8] Sexual functioning and concerns vary throughout one's life span and cannot be assumed for any age group or extent of disease. Therefore, to prevent and treat sexual functioning morbidity, it is essential that the oncology nurse become familiar with sexual issues as they relate to cancer patients.

For some individuals, sexuality means feeling alive, and the cessation of sexual activity is the equivalent of letting go or dying. Sexuality is very personal and individualized. What is considered normal to one couple may be considered unacceptable behavior to another. A woman and her partner decide what is valuable in their love life, not what the media would have the public believe.

✱ NORMAL FEMALE SEXUAL RESPONSE CYCLE

The female sexual response cycle consists of four phases: desire, excitement, orgasm, and resolution. Desire begins when a person shows an interest in sex. Sexual desire is exhibited by sexual thoughts and fantasies or by finding a person attractive.[9]

The second phase, excitement, is the time when the woman feels sexually aroused. The sexual excitement phase may begin with physical or psychological stimulation. Excitement may be facilitated by focusing on erotic cues, such as books, films, and fantasies. Typically, touching and caressing feel much more intense and lead to increased excitement. Physiologically, widespread vasocongestion occurs, which leads to vaginal lubrication, enlargement of the clitoris, and engorgement of the uterus. The uterus rises out of its usual position in the pelvis. The vagina "balloons," becoming deeper and wider and creating an orgasmic platform in the lower one-third of the vagina. Blood pressure and heart rate increase and respirations become deeper. Some women describe feelings of "heaviness" and pelvic warmth when they are sexually aroused.[9]

Orgasm, or sexual climax, is the third phase of sexual response. Orgasm occurs when the maximum level of excitement has been achieved. During orgasm, rhythmic contractions of the uterus, orgasmic platform, and rectal sphincter occur, resulting in intense pleasure in the genital area. Women are unique in their ability to have multiple orgasms. Subjectively, orgasm crescendos into waves of pleasure and, ultimately, a feeling of release.[10]

The final phase of sexual response is resolution. During resolution, physiologic relaxation occurs and the body returns to its pre-excited state. Heart rate and blood pressure return to normal, the uterus returns to its position in the pelvis, the vagina shortens, and vasocongestion dissipates. A general feeling of contentment and relaxation occurs if orgasm was reached. Resolution occurs more slowly if orgasm was not achieved.

Human sexual response is a total body, vasocongestive, neuromuscular response mediated through the autonomic nervous system. Disruption of parasympathetic nerves and pelvic vasculature would delay physiologic response but would not destroy sexual function.[11]

❆ ALTERATIONS IN SEXUALITY FROM CANCER

Changes in sexuality caused by cancer are largely due to three main factors:

1. the disease process
2. the effects of treatment
3. the psychological sequelae

Sexual dysfunction may occur before cancer is diagnosed. Pain, vague discomfort, fatigue, and general malaise may contribute to a decrease in sexual desire and avoidance of love-making. Also, gynecologic cancers may manifest themselves through postcoital or abnormal bleeding, viral infections, vulvar pruritus, or malodorous vaginal discharge, which may be viewed as offensive and a sexual deterrent by a woman and her partner. With the progression of tumor growth, central and peripheral nerves may be affected, resulting in a loss of sensation and desire.[12] In addition, the impacts of a life-threatening illness can result in mood disturbances such as anger, fear, depression, and/or anxiety. Some women may view their disease as punishment for past sexual behaviors such as masturbation, abortions, or extramarital affairs.[13] Nurses can assist their patients in the psychosocial adjustment to their diagnosis by clarifying their understanding of the etiology of the disease and dispelling myths.

Effects of Treatment

The treatment modalities of surgery, chemotherapy, and radiation are given in an attempt to cure, arrest, or palliate cancer. Again, the side effects of these therapies depend on a number of factors: extent of disease, age, general health, dosage and mode of delivery, extent of surgery, and so forth. Table 14.1 is a synopsis of the potential effects on self-concept, anatomy and physiology, sexual functioning, and fertility by type of cancer and method of treatment.

Prevalence and Types of Sexual Dysfunction

Breast Cancer

Breast cancer patients have received extensive psychological study,[14] but the more specific effects of this cancer on sexuality are only now coming to light. Early research suggests that psychosocial sequelae of breast cancer and problems related to sexual function are primarily related to the devastating effect of radical amputation of the breast. Women have reported feeling lopsided, disfigured, disinterested in sex, and uncomfortable in situations of nudity. Maguire et al. found, in their prospective study of seventy-five breast cancer patients 65 years or younger and free of disease after treatment, that 40% indicated moderate to severe sexual problems four months after

TABLE 14.1

Possible Effects of Cancer Treatment on Female Sexuality and Fertility

Treatment	Self-Concept	Physiologic Changes	Sexual Functioning	Fertility
BREAST Mastectomy/Lumpectomy	Loss of self-esteem Loss of femininity Fear of rejection Disruption of body image	Removal of breast, axillary nodes, small amount of breast tissue Edema of upper extremities; pain Possible to reconstruct breast but decrease in sensation of breast, nipple	May see avoidance of sexual relationships Decrease in sexual desire Loss of possible erotic zone Breast reconstruction may restore feelings of wholeness	Not altered May be affected by adjuvant chemotherapy
GYNECOLOGIC SURGERY Radical Hysterectomy	Loss of self-esteem Loss of femininity and sense of wholeness as woman Disruption of body image Fear of rejection	Removal of uterus, cervix, supporting structures, upper one-third of vagina, pelvic lymph nodes Nerve, vascular disruption to pelvis May be possible to preserve ovarian function	May see decrease in sexual desire Possible painful intercourse with deep penetration Orgasm may have different quality	Sterility Consider IVF; gestational carrier if ovaries remain
Bilateral Oophorectomy	Loss of femininity and sense of wholeness as a woman Loss of self-esteem Disruption of body image Fear of rejection Reactions to early menopause	Removal of ovaries, fallopian tubes Menopausal symptoms in premenopausal patient: hot flashes, night sweats, decreased vaginal lubrication Symptoms may not occur if one ovary remains functioning or estrogen replacement therapy is given	Possible painful intercourse	Sterility via ovarian removal Candidate for IVF with donor oocyte

Procedure	Body Image / Psychosocial	Anatomical / Physical	Sexual Functioning	Fertility
Total Pelvic Exenteration	Profound disruption of body image Loss of self-esteem Loss of femininity Fear of rejection Social isolation	Removal of bladder, rectum, vagina, uterus, pelvic lymph nodes, fallopian tubes, ovaries Construction of urinary conduit and/or colostomy Possible vagina reconstruction	Inability to engage in sexual intercourse unless neovagina constructed; possible for neovagina to develop erotic sensitivity Possible decrease in sexual desire Decreased sexual activity Low arousability, sexual satisfaction	Sterility
Vaginectomy	Loss of self-esteem Disruption of body image Loss of femininity Fear of rejection	Removal of vagina Reconstruction of vagina possible but problems with size, malodorous discharge are common	Inability to engage in sexual intercourse unless neovagina constructed With neovagina, decreased vaginal lubrication resulting in painful intercourse Use of water-soluble lubricants, douches helps	Usually occurs when uterus removed during an exenteration If ovaries remain, candidate for IVF with gestational carrier
Radical Vulvectomy	Disruption of body image Loss of self-esteem Loss of femininity Fear of rejection, pain, punishment	Removal of all labial tissue, clitoris, groin lymph nodes, mons May cause introital stenosis Loss of fine sensory perception in vulva Possible lymphedema of lower extremities, restricted mobility in groin area	May lose arousal, orgasm capacity Erotic sensations may still occur in remaining genital area Decrease in sexual satisfaction May need to relearn how to reach orgasm	Unaffected
Wide Local Excision of the Vulva	Disruption of body image (but less than that seen in radical surgery) Loss of self-esteem Fear of rejection	Removal of minimal labial, subcutaneous tissue Retention of clitoris	Good function	Unaffected
Skinning Vulvectomy	Loss of self-esteem Fear of rejection	Usually good cosmetic results		
Conization of the cervix	Negative body image Fear of rejection	No loss Possibility of cervical stenosis or incompetent cervix	Rarely affected	Rarely affected May need intrauterine insemination if cervical mucus altered

(continued)

TABLE 14.1 *(continued)*

Possible Effects of Cancer Treatment on Female Sexuality and Fertility

Treatment	Self-Concept	Physiologic Changes	Sexual Functioning	Fertility
CHEMOTHERAPY	Loss of self-esteem Disruption of body image Loss of femininity Altered role function	Possible ovarian failure: irregular or no menstrual periods with decrease in estrogen levels Premature menopause: hot flashes, night sweats, decreased vaginal lubrication, vaginal atrophy Atrophy of endometrial lining of uterus Skin changes Alopecia Weight loss Nausea, vomiting Malaise, fatigue Diarrhea	Dependent on type of drug, dose, length of treatment, age Decreased sexual desire; usually returns when feeling well Painful intercourse	Related to type of drug, dose, length of treatment, age Often causes temporary or permanent sterility Teratogenic Potential for mutation of ova
RADIOTHERAPY Pelvic	Loss of self-esteem Disruption of body image	Thinning of vaginal lining Loss of vaginal elasticity (vaginal fibrosis, stenosis possible) Ovarian failure if ovaries not moved and shielded Diarrhea Skin changes Cystitis	Painful intercourse Decrease in sexual activity Decrease or loss of sexual desire, orgasm Fatigue, weakness contribute to sexual dysfunction	Possible ovarian failure Temporary or permanent sterility depending on total dose, volume of tissue irradiated, exposure time, age, prior fertility status Mutagenic Teratogenic
Breast	Loss of self-esteem Disruption of body image	Atrophy or swelling of breast; may change size or shape Skin changes Decrease in breast tissue sensitivity	Possible loss of an erotic zone	Unaffected

surgery, compared to 12% of the benign controls.[15] Retrospective studies estimate sexual disruption, reduced frequency of intercourse, or orgasmic dysfunction ranging from 21 to 39%.[16] However, other researchers have reported little change in sexual functioning[17] or improvement in sexual relationships after mastectomy.[18] More recent research indicates that only 10 to 20% percent of women with early stage breast cancer have major emotional problems.[19] In addition, two recent large studies of women who had mastectomy for early stage breast cancer showed that by one year postoperatively, they were as well adjusted emotionally and sexually as either healthy women or women who had surgery for benign problems.[20,21]

Because of the disfigurement from breast surgery, the impact of breast cancer on issues of body image, self-concept, and femininity have remained areas of great interest. More recent studies are focusing on the psychological impact of different treatment modalities, specifically breast-sparing and breast reconstruction procedures. Lumpectomy patients appear to have significantly less alteration in body image and sexual desire, more rapid resumption of sexual activity following therapy, and an overall lower incidence of sexual dysfunction compared to matched modified radical mastectomy patients.[22]

Empirically, breast cancer treatment impairs sexual response by:

- Threatening self-esteem and self-identity from loss of the breast and disfigurement
- Fear of rejection or loss of a partner
- Feeling less of a woman
- Threatening reproductive ability secondary to systemic therapy
- Threatening personal control
- Fear of becoming a burden to a loved one

The influence of these variables on sexual functioning has not yet been clarified.[23]

Cervical Cancer

Cervical cancer has received more attention with regard to sexual functioning than any other gynecological malignancy. Preinvasive disease of the cervix is common and highly curable, with minimal disruption of sexual function. Kilkku et al. reported on the sexual outcomes of sixty-four Finnish women who were treated by conization. There were no significant declines in frequency of sexual activity or sexual satisfaction.[24] In fact, some women reported an increase in activity as a result of decreased dyspareunia following treatment.

Most research has compared treatment with radical hysterectomy plus lymph node dissection to radiotherapy. There appears to be a higher incidence of sexual disruption after radiotherapy than after surgical treatment in retrospective studies.[25,26] Surgical treatment allows for the potential of ovarian preservation in premenopausal women. However, vaginal shortening occurs with the surgical removal of the upper one-third of the vagina. Although sexual feelings need not be altered following a radical hysterectomy, some women may measure their femininity by their ability to bear children. Either radiation or surgery may result in loss of childbearing capacities. However, ovaries may be retained after radical hysterectomy, offering a source for ova for in vitro fertilization and making surrogate parenting a possibility. Retained ovaries may continue hormonal function as well, but a high incidence of premature ovarian failure has been reported.[27] Loss of childbearing capacity could result in sexual dysfunction as exhibited by decreased sexual desire. For some women, their image as a woman is totally dependent on their ability to bear children. Infertility may therefore be taken as a severe assault to their femininity and influence their sense of wholeness. In addition, radiation causes physical changes, such as fibrosis of blood vessels, which causes decreased blood supply and increases the risk to tissue by trauma and infection. Pelvic irradiation can lead to a shortened and narrowed vagina, vaginal atrophy, and scarring. Vaginal shortening may contribute to feelings that the vagina is "too short" for intercourse. Reports of dyspareunia are common. Though it is generally believed that the sexual functioning outcome is better in the surgically treated group, data are conflicting. Most studies, which have been retrospective, have indicated the estimated loss or diminishment of sexual functioning to be from 6 to 19% for radical hysterectomy patients and from 44 to 79% for radiation therapy patients.[28,29]

Treatment with vaginal estrogen creams can improve vaginal epithelialization, and the use of oral estrogens can control symptoms of hot flushes. The use of water-soluble lubricants can lessen discomfort and provide encouragement to continue sexual intercourse, and this, in turn, has the added benefit of preventing vaginal adhesions.[30] Alternatively, regular use of a vaginal dilator with a water-soluble lubricant can prevent vaginal stenosis. Different positions may be helpful to enhance comfort. If the woman is in the superior position, she has greater control over the timing and degree of penetration. In cases where the ovaries could not be preserved, the woman experiences the effects of premature menopause, which include hot flushes, vaginal thinning, and a decrease in vaginal lubrication.

Total pelvic exenteration is considered at the time of diagnosis of a recurrence in a local area and for extensive disease that is resectable. It has the most profound, severe effects on body image and function because it involves removal of the uterus, tubes, ovaries, urinary bladder, rectum, and vagina. The creation of ostomies for urinary and fecal excretion further disrupt the woman's body image, self-esteem, and sexuality. Some women fear their partner's rejection, avoid resuming sexual activity because of the possibility of leakage, and may be uncomfortable with their appearance in the presence of their partners. Brown et al., in a study of fifteen women who had undergone pelvic exenteration, found that although 87% reported sexual activity to be pleasurable preoperatively, 73% indicated no interest in sexual activity postoperatively.[31] Andersen and Hacker reported a reduction in the frequency of sexual activity, low sexual arousal and satisfaction, and disruption of sexual confidence and body image in this population. However, these problems appear to be less distressing when a sexual partner is available and the patient has the desire to continue sexual activity.[32]

Exenteration also carries the implication of a final attempt at cure; therefore, the woman may be concentrating more on survival than on sexuality. The effects of vaginal reconstruction on sexuality and body image have recently been reported. Women who have not had reconstructive surgery cannot resume vaginal intercourse, yet women with neovaginas may not resume sexual activity because of persistent vaginal discharge, problems with the physical characteristics of the vagina (e.g., the cavity being either too large or too small), fears of pain or bleeding, or loss of sensation.[33] Forty women who had pelvic exenteration and reconstruction with muscle flaps reported only half had resumed intercourse usually within one year of surgery. These women most frequently reported concerns about feeling self-conscious about their ostomies, how they looked nude, and having difficulty with vaginal discharge and dryness. A number of women reported pain and lack of pleasure with intercourse.[34]

Endometrial and Ovarian Cancers

There have been few studies of the sexual functioning of patients following treatment of endometrial and ovarian cancers. Cochran et al. reported, in a retrospective study of twenty-two endometrial cancer patients and fourteen of their spouses, a significant decrease in the frequency of and satisfaction with sexual relations compared to their precancerous levels.[35]

The treatment of ovarian cancer involves the surgical debulking of tumor, hysterectomy, bilateral salpingo-oophorectomy, omentectomy, and lymph node dissection, followed by chemotherapy or possibly radiotherapy. The result of the combined therapy frequently influences sexual functioning. Fatigue, nausea, and malaise can diminish sexual desire as the woman focuses her energies on survival issues and the endurance of increasingly intense treatment regimens. Surgically induced menopause, loss of childbearing capacity, and the impact of a major life-threatening illness contribute significantly to the psychological recuperation of women with ovarian cancer.[23]

Vulvar Cancer

Vulvar cancer is rare and seen most frequently in older women. However, there has been an increased incidence of in situ vulvar carcinoma in a progressively younger population. Treatment for in situ disease of the vulva includes either wide local excision of the vulva, skinning vulvectomy, simple vulvectomy, laser vaporization, or chemotherapy (i.e., 5-FU cream). A retrospective study by Andersen et al. found significant disruption of sexual functioning, the magnitude of which is correlated to the extent of surgery.[36] Invasive disease of the vulva is typically treated with removal of all labial tissues, including the clitoris, and bilateral inguinal lymphadenectomy with or without removal of pelvic lymph nodes. Despite the mutilating effects of this therapy, there is a paucity of data on sexuality in these patients. Although the capacity for intercourse remains intact, substantial disfigurement of the genitals occurs, as well as decreased pelvic and genital sensitivity. Andersen and Hacker reported that in women treated with radical surgery, a limited capacity for sexual arousal was seen, although minimal diminution in sexual desire occurred.[37] But some women have reported orgasmic responsiveness despite removal of the clitoris at the time of vulvectomy. Negative feelings toward the physical changes in the woman's body may be attributed to severe dyspareunia as a result of a narrowed introitus. Andersen reported that as many as 50 to 90% of women may stop all sexual activity.[28] Andreasson et al. interviewed twenty-five women following vulvectomy and fifteen of their partners and found more than half the women had both sexual dysfunction and psychological problems. Although their partners reported no sexual dysfunction, half of them reported psychological problems.[38]

✳ NURSING ASSESSMENT OF SEXUAL DYSFUNCTION

Learning to Ask

Patients diagnosed with gynecologic cancer require an in-depth assessment of their sexual function and concerns. Lamb stated that assessment legitimizes the patient's sexual concerns, establishes an understanding of terminology, and determines the patient's understanding of her disease and treatment options, as well as the side effects of the proposed treatment and the effect it may have on body image, sexuality, and fertility.[13] Oncology nurses are in a position to evaluate and care for women with gynecologic cancers. Unfortunately, data indicate that the sexual knowledge and attitudes of professional nurses caring for oncology patients are deficient.[39]

Vincent et al. found that 80% of patients receiving cancer treatment desired more information regarding sex, although only 75% were willing to bring up the subject.[40] Nurses may be better able than any other health care professionals to establish the trusting relationship essential to providing sexual counseling. However, the nurse must recognize his or her own limitations, abilities, biases, and knowledge base and refer the patient to other personnel if uncomfortable in discussing the woman's sexual needs. Other nurses, clinical nurse specialists, social workers, or physicians are possible resources.

According to Schover and Fife, clinicians who undertake sexual counseling should meet the following three criteria:

1. Understand how each type of surgery affects the physiologic aspects of sexual function
2. Be able to respond to a patient's sexual questions and concerns without moralizing or judging
3. Know when a patient needs to be referred to a mental health professional for treatment of a serious psychiatric or sexual problem[41]

More detailed requisites essential for nurses to assess, plan, and counsel couples regarding sexuality are listed in Table 14.2. By critically evaluating his or her own feelings and attitudes toward sexuality in the oncology patient, the nurse will be better able to effectively incorporate the patient's sexual health in the care plan.

Nurses frequently feel inadequate and uncomfortable about providing advice and guidance regarding sexual issues. Certainly, the more knowledgeable a nurse becomes regarding sexual functioning, the more comfortable he or she will become in dis-

TABLE 14.2

Nurses' Requisites for Assessing, Planning, and Counseling Couples Regarding Sexuality

Acceptance of and comfort with one's own sexuality and that of others

Realization that sexuality and sexual expression are key elements of self-esteem

Knowledge of sexuality and sexual function and the effects of cancer and its therapy on this process

Awareness of one's attitudes, values, and beliefs regarding sexuality

Comfort with discussing sexual concerns with patients openly and honestly

Acceptance of couple's lifestyle, sexual activities, and preferences

Knowledge of sociocultural and religious tenets

Maintenance of confidentiality

Provision of adequate uninterrupted and unhurried time

Provision of opportunities for the couple to raise questions and resume discussion at a later date

Knowledge of personal limitations and resources for referral when needed

Source: Adapted with permission from Lamb, M. (1990). Psychosexual issues: The woman with gynecological cancer. *Seminars in Oncology Nursing, 6*(3), 237–243.

cussing it. Second, with each opportunity to intervene in sexual dysfunction issues, the nurse will continue to develop a style and repertoire with which he or she is comfortable. The suggestions in Table 14.3 may be helpful to nurses in obtaining sexual histories from patients.

What to Ask

Each woman has a unique set of sexual concerns. But young women may lack basic information about sexual function, have had less time to develop a stable sense of sexual identity, and may thus require additional time and information regarding sexual functioning. The older woman may be interested in sex but more reluctant to broach the subject with the physician. The single woman has special concerns regarding how she may be perceived by future partners, how to discuss her cancer treatment and its effects on sex with a new partner, dating issues, and whether she will be viewed as desirable.

Another area that warrants consideration is alternative lifestyles. Some lesbian women may be reluctant to discuss their sexual preference with their nurse or health care provider for fear that disclosure might adversely affect their care. By not being open, these women may unknowingly withhold information that is important to their medical problems and care. Again, the nurse must ensure that patient confidentiality is maintained.

TABLE 14.3
Nursing Guidelines in the Assessment of Sexual Functioning
1. Provide privacy, and create a nonthreatening atmosphere.
2. Ensure confidentiality.
3. Include the partner in the discussion whenever possible.
4. Begin with less sensitive issues once rapport is established.
5. Use dignified but simple language. Speak in clearly understood terms.
6. Ask open-ended questions to elicit information, and use active listening.
7. Use normalizing language to make the patient feel comfortable about revealing sexual material. Use a matter-of-fact approach.
8. Empower the patient to control how much she wishes to disclose about her sex life.

In any case, each woman should be assured that she will be able to find a comfortable and gratifying sex life after treatment.[19] The critical component of sexual counseling is to be consistently hopeful and positive.

When to Ask

Assessment of sexual function should be undertaken at the time of diagnosis. Although this is frequently the nurse's first encounter with the patient, it is the ideal time to obtain baseline information about sexual history and status. Questions regarding the patient's sexual well-being should be incorporated into the comprehensive nursing history. The briefest sexual history should include:

- Current sexual status
- Current relationship status
- Sexual history

When a more thorough evaluation is possible, inquiry into the patient's background, sexual attitudes, and cancer myths related to sexuality should be explored.[23] Kaplan's model for evaluating sexual problems may be helpful to nurses who are familiar with the medical model of history-taking.[42] It includes the following elements in the given sequence:

- Chief complaint—the patient's main sexual concern
- Sexual status—the current state of sexual functioning
- Medical status
    Current medical status
    Medical history
    Current medications (Tables 14.4 and 14.5)

TABLE 14.4
Medications That May Affect Sexual Response
Endocrine drugs, including hormones
Antihypertensive agents
Adrenergic receptor blockers (beta blockers)
Thiazide diuretics
Antipsychotic drugs
Tricyclic antidepressants (amitriptyline, imipramine) and serotonin reuptake inhibitors
Sedatives and hypnotics (lorazepam)
Antianxiety drugs
Narcotics (morphine, hydromorphone, codeine)
Alcohol
Amphetamines
Cocaine
Cannabis
Hallucinogens

- Family and psychosexual history
    - Previous sexual experience
    - Relationship history
    - Family attitudes
    - Cultural and religious beliefs
- Relationship assessment
    - Single / married / separated / divorced / widowed / remarried
    - Heterosexual / homosexual
    - Children
- Summary and recommendations
    - No treatment
    - Further discussion
    - Specific suggestions
    - Referral

When evaluating sexual function, it is also helpful to use the Triphasic Model.[23] This model categorizes sexual problems by the phase of the sexual response cycle (sexual desire, excitement, or orgasm) that is affected. Treatment can then be tailored to the phase-specific problem. For example, a decrease in sexual desire is commonly

TABLE 14.5	
Chemotherapy Agents That Affect Sexual or Reproductive Function	
Agent	*Complications*
Alkylating Busulfan Chlorambucil Cyclosphosphamide Melphalan Nitrogen mustard	Amenorrhea, oligospermia, azoospermia, decreased libido, ovarian dysfunction, erectile dysfunction
Antimetabolites Cytosine arabinoside 5-Fluorouracil Methotrexate	As for alkylating agents
Antitumor Antibodies Doxorubicin Plicamycin	As for alkylating agents
Plant Products Vincristine	Retrograde ejaculation, erectile dysfunction
Vinblastine	Decreased libido, ovarian dysfunction, erectile dysfunction
Miscellaneous Procarbazine Androgens Estrogens Progestins	As for alkylating agents Masculinization (women) Gynecomastia, acne Menstrual abnormalities, change in libido
Corticosteroids	Irregular menses, acne

Source: Krebs, L.U. (1990). Sexual and reproductive dysfunction. In S.L. Groenwald, M.H. Frogge, M. Goodman & C.H. Yarbro, eds., *Cancer Nursing: Principles and Practice* 2nd ed. (p. 570). Boston: Jones and Bartlett Publishers. Reprinted by permission.

seen during the active phase of cancer therapy, whereas lack of vaginal lubrication may occur after therapy. Therefore, for purposes of evaluation, Auchincloss proposed that the patient be asked about her experience with respect to each phase.[23] Table 14.6 offers a guide to the assessment and treatment of sexual dysfunction commonly seen in gynecologic cancers based on the Triphasic Model. Specific suggestions are included as nursing interventions for phase-specific problems. However, whenever an identified problem is beyond the realm of expertise for the nurse, a referral should be made to an appropriate therapist.

One other model that is frequently used for sexual counseling and intervention is the PLISSIT model.[43] The PLISSIT model consists of four stages of interventions:

1. *Permission.* First promoted when the nurse asks the patient about her sexual concern or suggests that it is an appropriate topic for discussion. Gives the patient permission to have (or not to have) sexual feelings.
2. *Limited information.* Continues to convey willingness to discuss sexuality and provides specific factual information to clarify concerns and misconceptions and eliminate myths.
3. *Specific suggestions.* Provided when support and limited information alone are inadequate. Follow-up is necessary to monitor effectiveness.
   - Suggestions include strategies for enhancing sexual expression.
   - Suggestions take into account the patient's and partner's values and attitudes toward sex.
   - Referral for intensive therapy is indicated if sexual concerns remain unresolved.
4. *Intensive therapy.* Requires referral when adequate progress is not being made at the other levels and more in-depth counseling is needed. Referral to a qualified sex therapist may be required to deal with:
   - Preexisting sexual problem
   - Reconstructive surgery

According to Dudas, the nurse may be able to assist patients with the majority of their concerns using the first three levels of intervention, whereas the more intensive therapy requires a qualified therapist.[44] The patient's sexual partner should be included in as many discussions as is feasible. It is important to establish the partner's acceptance of the situation, and it is important for the patient to feel she is not repulsive and that she will not be rejected.

Woods suggests three additional questions that may be helpful in assessing the woman's perception of how cancer has affected her:

1. Has this illness interfered with your role as a wife, mother, or worker?
2. Has this experience affected your feelings about yourself as a woman?
3. Has the cancer affected your ability to function sexually?[45]

Lamb and Woods propose an alternative technique called *unloading the question.* With this technique, the question is prefaced by a statement that encourages a range of possible responses.[46] For example, the nurse might state: "Some women have expressed concern that a radical hysterectomy will change their sex life. Do you have this concern?"

TABLE 14.6

Application of Triphasic Model to Assessment of Sexual Dysfunction in Gynecologic Cancer

Phase	Sexual Dysfunction	Relevance to Cancer Patients and Survivors	Interventions
DESIRE Sexual thoughts, fantasies, daydreaming, finding potential partner attractive	Inhibited sexual desire Loss of interest in sex Few or no thoughts about sex Negative (antisexual) attitudes about sex Anxious, panicky about sex Avoidance of sexual situations	Not unusual when patient is in active treatment After treatment, loss of desire may be related to the cancer itself, treatment side effects, psychological factors (depression, anxiety), partner issues Often requires longer treatment of couple by sex therapist because of prominent psychological component	Reassure sexual interest and drive are frequently decreased or absent during and possibly several weeks after therapy Encourage sexual activity during most desirable circumstances; goal is to rebuild sexual interest, confidence, response; establish what is comfortable, sexual via open communication Explore role of stress, fatigue. Encourage to set time aside
EXCITEMENT Vaginal lubrication, engorgement	Inhibited sexual excitement Impaired vaginal lubrication, engorgement	Requires thorough medical evaluation, including medication Common after surgery, irradiation to pelvis, or any treatment that causes ovarian loss or failure	Teach individual, couple exercises to gradually reintroduce relaxing, investigating new areas of stimulation

	Patient may complain of dry, sore vagina or painful intercourse	Touching, examination of affected areas introduced gradually; thorough gyn exam required to diagnose, treat dyspareunia
	May have psychological component even when physical cause is present	Prescribe possible medical treatment with estrogens (local or systemic) if not contraindicated
	Supportive partner is essential	Advise water-soluble lubricant for patient, partner
		Allow time for healing; vaginal fibrosis may require use of vaginal dilator
		Encourage more time for foreplay, creating relaxed atmosphere for intimacy
ORGASM Reflex muscle contractions associated with pleasure, pleasurable sensations	Inhibited female orgasm: anorgasmia	If clitoris removed, some women report orgasm with stimulation to remaining genitals, vagina; identify other areas of whole-body stimulation
	May be related to fatigue, depression, stress, medication, anxiety, surgery	Allow for longer, more direct stimulation of clitoris
		Address need for more time for arousal, relaxation, communication issues with partner

(continued)

TABLE 14.6 *(continued)*

Application of Triphasic Model to Assessment of Sexual Dysfunction in Gynecologic Cancer

Phase	Sexual Dysfunction	Relevance to Cancer Patients and Survivors	Interventions
OTHER	Dyspareunia: pain with intercourse	Leads to sexual avoidance unless treated promptly	Instruct in proper use of water-soluble lubricants, dilators (15–30 min. each day; should not hurt)
		Requires thorough gynecologic evaluation, treatment of cause (surgical change in vagina, irradiation changes, lack of estrogen)	Suggest use of vaginal estrogens, cream if permitted
		Practice "no painful sex" rule (i.e., no intercourse unless medical cause is adequately treated)	Suggest that change in position may help for shortened vagina after surgery (woman's thighs together, elevate woman's buttocks with a pillow to change angle, woman in superior position)
	Vaginismus: vaginal muscle spasm, making penetration painful or impossible	Response to pain or fear of pain with penetration	Teach progressive muscle relaxation
		Good prognosis with combined relaxation, sequenced penetration treatment, done by patient herself, then with partner	Teach Kegel interventions to increase awareness of vaginal muscles during penetration, intercourse

Source: Adapted with permission from Auchincloss, S. (1989). Sexual dysfunction in cancer patients: Issues in evaluation and treatment. In J. C. Holland & J. H. Rowland, eds., *Handbook of Psychooncology: The Psychological Care of the Patient with Cancer* (pp. 383–413). New York: Oxford University Press.

By initiating a conversation regarding sexual issues, the nurse conveys to the patient that this is an appropriate and important topic to be brought up during future visits. Certainly, the patient may be more concerned with her cancer diagnosis and fear of dying. However, if the woman perceives a warm, private, and sensitive atmosphere, she may be motivated to return with more definitive and intimate questions as she becomes more trusting and comfortable. Note that some patients do not wish or have no need to discuss sexual matters, though. The nurse should never force a discussion of sex on a patient. Let her know, however, that you are open to discussion if a problem arises. Finally, remember to bring up questions about sexual anxieties at all stages of disease and treatment. Sexual concerns frequently are vocalized at the three-, six-, and twelve-month follow-up evaluations.

Nursing Interventions

In summary, treatment for sexual dysfunction in gynecologic and breast cancer patients must be tailored to each individual and each diagnosis. Treatment may consist of only reassurance and education or may require intensive medical and psychological therapy.

Nurses should include the women's partner whenever possible in the plan of care from the beginning. Frequently, an active, caring partner is the key element in restoration of the patient's whole persona. In addition, psychosexual adjustment begins before surgery and requires a team approach involving the physician, nurse, social worker, dietician, and possibly enterostomal therapists and chaplain. The goal of rehabilitation is to return the woman to her home and occupation with the ability to deal with her altered body functions.

Resources

Gynecologic oncology nurses require a wide range of support systems to counsel women effectively in terms of sexuality. First, the woman must be knowledgeable about sexual response and sexual dysfunctions. Second, the nurse must have a referral network established in the hospital or community. When interventions must extend beyond simple strategies, nurses need to be able to refer to competent specialists trained in counseling couples with sexual dysfunctions. Health care personnel who may be properly trained in sexual counseling include social workers, psychiatric clinicians, and physicians. It is also important that the nurse formulate a referral base with a certified sex therapist in the community setting. National organizations, such as the American Association of Sex Educators, Counselors, and Therapists (AASECT), may be helpful in locating local sex therapists. Third, nurse training in sexuality is imperative. Nursing education can occur in a number of ways. Advanced-practice nurses in women's health can be good resources for staff by implementing programs to enhance the comfort with and increase the sexual knowledge of staff. Discussing sexual issues during nursing rounds, conducting other in-service programs devoted to the diagnosis and treatment of sexual dysfunction, and including the topic in care plans are additional possibilities.

❈ INFERTILITY

Gynecologic oncology nurses have a responsibility to provide holistic care to enhance the quality of life of their patient population. Frequently, because of high emotional stress and the rush to provide treatment, quality-of-life issues such as infertility are overlooked. Fertility problems can often be linked to substantial amounts of stress, a range of impairments to marital functioning, and reduced quality of life.[47] The impact of the loss of fertility on top of a diagnosis of cancer is monumental for most women. It is well documented that the woman who is given alternatives before a surgical procedure has a shorter hospital stay, better healing, and enhanced quality of life. Studies have shown that providing pretreatment psychological services increases reports of personal well-being and interpersonal functioning.[48]

The oncology nurse working with a woman who has fertility problems has the potential to make an impact on not only the quality of her life but also the evolution of her family. Inherent in this opportunity is the responsibility to ensure that such influence is, ideally, helpful, but at least not harmful.[49,50] Thus, the nurse must be realistic regarding the options available to the woman. Local and state regulations may have an impact on what options are available in the community or state. The nurse must also take into consideration the patient's and family's desires, opportunities, and expectations.

Overview of Assisted Reproductive Techniques

A number of assisted reproductive technologies (ART) are available. With basic knowledge and referral information about these, the oncology nurse is prepared to suggest realistic alternatives to the woman with fertility problems. Furthermore, referral to an infertility practice for further information and potential treatment can be more timely. See Table 14.7 for an outline of what fertility options may be available for women with different gynecologic cancers.

In Vitro Fertilization

The concept of in vitro fertilization (IVF) dates back to animal research in 1935, but it wasn't until 1978 that Edwards and Steptoe reported the first live birth of a human baby, Louise Brown, conceived by IVF, in England. The Jones Institute in Norfolk, Virginia, reported the first live birth in the United States in 1981. As of 1996, approximately 50,000 babies worldwide had been born as a result of IVF.[51]

Initially, IVF was designed to provide a reproductive mechanism for women who had no fallopian tube function.[52] Due to increased knowledge and success, however, other forms of infertility are now being treated by the process. Some examples include endometriosis, unexplained infertility, male infertility, immunological factors, and cervical factors. IVF and related technologies allow access to the microenvironment of the human oocyte, the subtleties of gamete interaction, and the intricacies of syngamy and early embryonic development.[53]

TABLE 14.7

Potential Fertility Options for Women with Gynecologic Cancers

Site	Stage/Histopathology	Fertility Options
Ovary	Stage Ia Favorable histologic type Borderline or well-differentiated epithelial ovarian cancer Young woman of low parity Cancer encapsulated and unruptured No surface excrescenses or adhesions No invasion of capsule or mesovarium Negative peritoneal washings Negative staging operation: omental biopsy, peritoneal biopsy, pelvic and periaortic node sampling, biopsy of opposite ovary Reliable follow-up Germ cell tumors (require chemotherapy)	Only one ovary removed, theoretically normal If one ovary is functioning but tube is not, IVF If both ovaries removed and uterus remains, IVF with donor oocytes
Cervix	Stage Ia1, Ia2, s/p cone biopsy (less than 3 mm invasion with no lymphovascular space involvement) Stage Ib, IIa, s/p radical hysterectomy with pelvic lymph node dissection (ovaries remain) versus radiation therapy	Desires children: cone biopsy with close follow-up versus simple hysterectomy IVF with gestational carrier Possible for ovary transposition (if radiation therapy indicated)
	Stage IIb, III, and IV Radiation and/or chemotherapy	Frozen embryo (IVF) (prior to treatment), implantation in gestational carrier Cryopreservation of ovarian tissue and oocytes
Gestational Trophoblastic Disease	Chemotherapy Hysterectomy	Normal IVF with gestational carrier

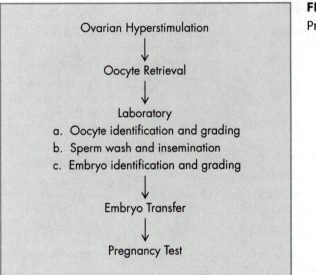

FIGURE 14.1.
Protocol for IVF.

The procedure of IVF is a relatively simple one, commonly done in an outpatient setting with mild sedation and minimal risk to the woman (Figure 14.1). After stimulation with ovulation-inducing medications, the woman's oocytes are collected from her ovaries through transvaginal, ultrasound-directed aspiration (Figure 14.2) and fertilized in the laboratory with her partner's or donor's sperm. Following early development, the embryo(s) are placed into her uterus via the cervix. This procedure, called *embryo transfer* (ET), is performed using a fine catheter attached to a sterile syringe containing the embryo(s) and culture media. If pregnancy ensues, the embryo(s) continues to develop naturally in the mother's uterus.

The 1995 clinical pregnancy statistics reported by the American Society for Reproductive Medicine (ASRM) for IVF are approximately 30% with a take-home baby rate of 22%.[51]

Gamete Intrafallopian Transfer

Gamete intrafallopian transfer (GIFT) is a technique developed in 1984 by Dr. Ricardo Asch. In this procedure, after ovarian stimulation, oocytes are removed from the woman's ovaries by aspiration via laparoscopy (Figure 14.3). The oocytes are loaded into a transfer catheter with sperm that have gone through a wash process and immediately transferred into the fimbriated end of the fallopian tubes (Figure 14.4). A woman must have at least one normal fallopian tube for this procedure. If fertilization occurs, the embryo(s) may travel through the fallopian tube to the uterus.

ASRM-reported GIFT statistics for 1995 were approximately a 34% clinical pregnancy rate and a 26% take-home baby rate.[51]

There are advantages and disadvantages to both procedures. The advantages of IVF include the following:

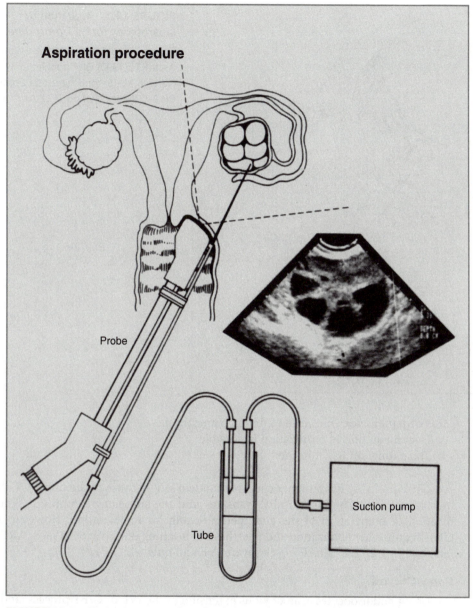

FIGURE 14.2. Aspiration procedure for IVF.

Source: Reproduced with permission from Sauer, M.V., & Paulson, R.J. (1989). Oocyte donation and ovarian failure. In *Contemporary Obstetrics & Gynecology, 34*(5), 128. Courtesy A. Michael Velthaus.

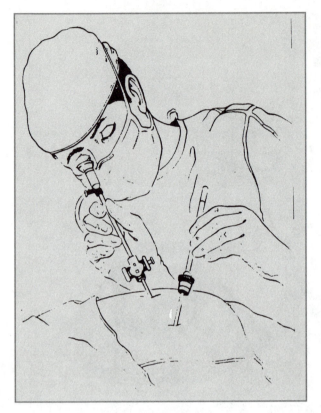

FIGURE 14.3. Aspiration by laparoscopy for GIFT procedure.

Source: Reproduced with permission from Asch, R.H. (1990). GIFT booklet (p. 5). Norwell, MA: Serono Symposia. Copyright © 1990, Serono Symposia, USA.

1. The patient does not need to undergo anesthesia.
2. Documentation of fertilization is possible.
3. Tubal function is not needed.

GIFT probably has a higher success rate than IVF because of the timing of blastocyst arrival in the uterus by tubal transport and the subsequent improved synchronization of preparation of the endometrial lining for implantation. However, since GIFT requires hospitalization and anesthesia it is falling out of favor in most ART centers. In 1995, 70% of all ART cycles were IVF and only 6% GIFT.[51]

Donor Oocytes

Using donor oocytes is an obvious extension of the IVF or GIFT process, and perhaps one of the most exciting. It means that women without functioning ovaries who have a normal uterus can now conceive. Following the common model for donor sperm, oocyte donation can be made anonymously, or known donors can be selected. While there are potential concerns with the use of known donors, no current data show that problems have occurred. Many programs in the United States require recip-

FIGURE 14.4. Catheter transfer of oocytes in the GIFT procedure.

Source: Reproduced with permission from Asch, R.H. (1990). GIFT booklet (p. 7). Norwell, MA: Serono Symposia. Copyright © 1990, Serono Symposia, USA.

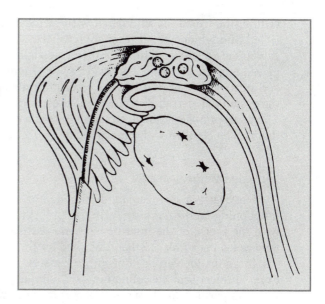

ients to identify their own donor; however, the use of anonymous donors is increasing. Many programs now have an extensive list of available anonymous donors.

Oocyte donation starts with the removal of eggs (through oocyte retrieval methods discussed above) from a donor after ovarian stimulation. Next, the donor oocytes are fertilized with the partner's sperm. Then either the gametes are transferred by the GIFT method to the fallopian tubes, or the resulting embryo(s) are transferred to the uterus of the recipient by the IVF procedure. The challenge of this procedure is the synchronization of the donor's and recipient's cycles. Hormone therapy is required for the recipient.

Screening of the donor varies from program to program. Current (1998) ASRM guidelines request that psychological, genetic, and serological testing (RH, syphilis, HIV, hepatitis B and C) be completed before initiation of oocyte donation. But as the technology evolves, these recommendations may change.[54]

To date, ART with oocyte donation is one of the most successful treatments performed in any infertility program. Pregnancy rates as high as 50% have been reported, though more commonly 33% of the procedures are successful.[49,50] Many young gynecologic oncology patients have lost one or both ovaries to borderline, early stage epithelial ovarian tumors, or germ cell tumors. Oocyte donation is a viable option for this patient population.

Surrogate Gestational Carrier

For a woman absent a uterus but with intact ovaries, a surrogate gestational carrier (host uterus) provides the only opportunity to have a biological child. In this procedure, the woman is stimulated with medication to produce oocytes. The eggs collected through oocyte retrieval are fertilized with her partner's sperm, then either the gametes are transferred into the surrogate's fallopian tubes (GIFT) or the embryo(s) is placed into the surrogate's uterus (ET). If synchronization of the cycles of the patient and surrogate is not possible, the resulting embryos may be frozen for later transfer to the gestational carrier. Currently, most couples are required to find their own carrier. The concept of gestational surrogacy introduces many social, ethical, and legal issues that will be clarified with time and experience.[55]

Surrogate Mother

Surrogacy, or surrogate motherhood, is an alternative when a woman has neither a functioning uterus nor ovaries. In this procedure, the surrogate mother is inseminated with the sperm of the infertile woman's partner. The male donor must complete extensive testing similar to that described for the oocyte donor.

Insemination can be done either intracervically or as an intrauterine (IUI) procedure. Intracervical insemination is a simple process. The sperm of the infertile woman's partner are drawn into a syringe and, with a speculum in place, deposited into the fertile mucus in the cervical os of the surrogate. With IUI, a speculum is placed in the vagina, the cervical os is identified, and using a very thin catheter, washed sperm are deposited directly into the uterine cavity of the surrogate. Both procedures need to be timed very carefully to coincide with ovulation.

The surrogate mother has a genetic link to the offspring, making the legal implications challenging and worrisome, as evidenced recently by the Baby M. case. There is, however, a biblical precedent for surrogate mothering. Jacob's wife, Rachel, was unable to bear a child, so she sent for her handmaiden and allowed her husband to sleep with her. The resulting offspring was considered Jacob and Rachel's child and was raised as such. Furthermore, according to the New York State Health Department's estimate of approximately 4,000 surrogate births since the late 1970s, only eleven documented cases involving custody of the child have gone to litigation, and in every case except one, custody has been awarded to the intended parents.[55]

Surrogate mother applicants, whether for gestational surrogacy or surrogate motherhood, undergo an extensive screening process. Most programs require that only women who have had successful, uncomplicated pregnancies with children of their own become candidates. Furthermore, it is desirable that candidates be motivated by factors other than money (e.g., the desire to help another or the view that surrogacy is a personally rewarding experience). After the initial interview, psychological testing is done on both potential candidates and their spouses. Intelligence, ability to understand treatment plans, reliability, self-esteem, coping mechanisms, support systems, and sensitivity are a few of the important screening criteria. Similar psychological screening is done on the infertile couple. Once psychological and medical screening is complete on all parties, they are matched and introduced, usually with the guidance of a psychologist. Ongoing psychological counseling is important to the outcome.

Cryopreservation and Embryo Donation

The human embryo has been successfully frozen at many stages of development. Stimulation of the ovary with medications during an IVF or GIFT cycle usually produces more oocytes than can be safely transferred at one time. For this reason, cryopreservation can offer a woman additional attempts at pregnancy without the necessity of repeating ovulation induction or egg retrieval. Another advantage of frozen embryo transfer (FET) is that transfer can occur at the time in a natural ovulatory cycle when endometrial receptivity may be improved. Cryopreserved embryo donation, where permitted by law, provides an opportunity for children in infertile couples who have no gametes of their own.

Approximately 14% of all ART cycles performed in 1994, or 7,103 cycles, used only frozen embryos. The success rate of frozen embryos is approximately 10% less than that for fresh embryos; this is in part because some embryos do not survive the thawing process. However, on average, fewer embryos are transferred in frozen cycles than in fresh cycles, and this may partly explain the lower success rate. In 1994 a total of 1,294 live-born infants resulted from 1,075 deliveries with known outcome. There were 1,259 normal infants, 34 with structural or functional defects, and with one unknown neonatal outcome.

Frozen embryos can be stored indefinitely, and approximately 75% of cryopreserved human embryos survive after thawing.[50] Like other aspects of ART, laws regarding human embryo freezing vary from state to state. Each program has well-defined legal contracts to protect both the patient and the medical community. Ownership and control of the embryos need to be decided before cryopreservation. Currently accepted practice in most states regarding legal ownership of embryos resulting from the fertilization of the wife's ova by the husband's sperm is that the embryos shall be considered the joint property of both partners.[56]

Autotransplantation of Cryopreserved Ovarian Tissue

A process currently undergoing clinical trials by a number of researchers, in both the United States and Great Britain, is the freezing of human ovarian tissue. Recent research by Gosden and colleagues, using animal tissue, offers the possibility for a more desirable approach to preserving reproductive potential in the female cancer patient. Gosden removed the ovaries from sheep, then froze thin slices of the cortical tissue. These slices of cortical tissue each contain thousands of oocytes. At a later date the tissue was thawed and replaced in the region of the residual ovarian site, near the fimbriated end of the fallopian tube. (See Figure 14.5). Since this is an autograft, there is no risk for immunological graft rejection. These sheep have since gone on to have normal ovulatory cycles and, more important, to bear and deliver normal offspring. Since eggs in slices of human ovarian tissue survive cryopreservation and thawing like animal ovaries, more research is imperative in this field. Female cancer patients have the potential to benefit greatly from this procedure since ovarian tissue could be frozen prior to any cancer treatment, much the same way as sperm are frozen and later thawed for use.

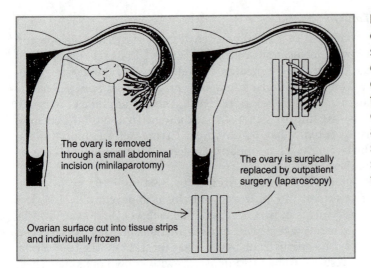

FIGURE 14.5. Ovarian cryopreservation involves surgical removal of the entire ovary. The ovarian cortex is processed into thin tissue strips for cryopreservation. When appropriate, the ovarian strips are thawed and surgically autografted next to the fallopian tube fimbria.

The ovary is removed through a small abdominal incision (minilaparotomy)

The ovary is surgically replaced by outpatient surgery (laparoscopy)

Ovarian surface cut into tissue strips and individually frozen

Current recommendations by the ASRM are that clinical trials be carried out according to the guidelines of each Institutional Review Board. Approved, written consent forms must be carefully presented and clearly understood, before signing, when a woman is offered this research protocol. Some female cancer patients have already had ovarian tissue frozen, but to date, none have had the tissue transferred back.[57,58]

Legal and Ethical Issues

The advent of ART has called into question some of our culture's most fundamental assumptions, beliefs, and practices with respect to how children are conceived. The ethical aspects of reproductive technology have raised debates since 1978, when IVF was first introduced. As recently as 1996, the Vatican formally denounced all ART as amoral. As techniques such as embryo-splitting to produce identical twins continue to grow more sophisticated, the debates will intensify.

According to Andrews and Jaeger, statutes, regulations, judicial decisions, and the constitutional protection of the right to privacy to make procreative decisions can profoundly influence which infertility services are offered and in what manner. The law shapes the standards by which health care professionals must practice and likewise influences the rights and responsibilities of both the infertile couple and society with respect to a resulting child.[59] To prevent misunderstandings, all parties must be fully informed about the legal situation in their jurisdiction. These disclosures should include legal uncertainties as well as what the law has already established.

It is impossible to discuss all the ethical and legal ramifications of ART here. In fact, laws are not well established and are changing rapidly. But ultimately, the decision regarding the use of ART lies with the individual or couple. Founded both in statutory and case law, the doctrine of informed consent protects the patient's decision making and right to control his or her own body. Informed consent requires education; the options that exist must be presented in a clear and concise manner, a challenge for the health care team.

Adoption or Child-Free Living

Two other options not often addressed by health providers are adoption and child-free living. These are frequently overlooked in the quest for family-building by ART.

In the United States, it is estimated that 2 to 4% of the population is adopted. Approximately 50,000 adoptions of nonrelated healthy children occur annually in the United States, with over 8,000 adoptions of foreign children taking place and 10,000 adoptions of children with special needs.[60] There are many different types of adoption—open and closed, private and agency, domestic and international, and special-needs adoptions. Advising a couple to contact an organization such as Resolve, Adoption Resources, or the National Committee on Adoption as soon as possible is extremely helpful. These organizations can inform couples of what is available, approximate costs, waiting times, risks and benefits, and what is legal in their state.

It is advisable to encourage couples to start pursuing adoption early in the infertility work-up, even if they are not yet committed to adoption. By doing so, the couple can learn what the racial, religious, and age restrictions are in various agencies, which should prevent confusion or disappointment concerning these issues.

The couple preparing for adoption due to gynecologic cancer has many feelings related to loss of genetic continuity and inability to experience pregnancy and birth. They need time to grieve these losses and encouragement to set realistic expectations for themselves. Advising them to spend time with people who respect them and to meet with both adoptive and nonadoptive families are also helpful interventions.

The possibility of child-free living should also be discussed early. Assurance by a health provider that this option is a viable one may remind the couple that they are valuable for more than just their reproductive potential. The nurse can suggest alternatives such as volunteering for children's activities, returning to school, starting a business, and traveling for the couple to consider. Open communication regarding what their life values are and prioritizing these values will enhance self-esteem. And, like the couple considering adoption, using resources such as Resolve and spending time with families committed to child-free living can help the couple to resolve their grief. Hopefully, once a couple comes to terms with the loss of childbearing capabilities and completes the grieving process, they will begin to develop realistic expectations for the future.

The Nurse's Role

The nurse's role in caring for the infertile oncology patient is multifaceted. Adviser, communicator, educator, counselor, and provider of support are the primary roles. The nurse must have the ability to listen and respond with empathy, recognizing and respecting the unique pain of the infertile woman and her partner. There may be no words to comfort someone whose life's dreams have recently been shattered by a diagnosis of malignancy and infertility. Nurses who have positive self-esteem and can acknowledge their own life sufferings and who possess an excellent knowledge base are best prepared to provide coping strategies in these cases.

According to Menning, such patients suffer intense emotional upheaval. They must learn to recognize, cope with, and resolve the feelings of denial, isolation, grief, anger, and depression.[61] The nurse must allow adequate time for verbalization of these feelings and for grieving. Reassurance that grief is normal and that it will take time for the process to be resolved must be repeated.

Widening the patient's support systems to include family, friends, social and religious services, and organizations such as Resolve are other important nursing strategies. Encouraging the couple to ask for support so that the systems may be beneficial in resolving grief and diffusing anger is an important nursing goal.

As for the patient considering ART, the following is a list of questions the nurse might answer:

1. What are the risks and benefits of the procedure?
2. What does our state allow; what is allowed in neighboring states?
3. How many IVF or GIFT cycles does the program complete per year?
4. What is the pregnancy rate; what is the take-home baby rate?

TABLE 14.8

References on Infertility

Becker, G. (1990). *Healing the Infertile Family: Strengthening Your Relationship in the Search for Parenthood.* New York: Bantam.

Corson, S.L. (1991). *Conquering Infertility: A Guide for Couples.* Englewood Cliffs, NJ: Prentice-Hall.

Greil, L.L. (1991). *Not Yet Pregnant: Infertile Couples in Contemporary America.* New Brunswick, NJ: Rutgers University Press.

Johnson, P.I. (1994) *Taking Charge of Infertility.* Indianapolis, IN: Prospective Press.

Karow, W.G. (1991). *A Baby of Your Own: New Ways to Overcome Infertility.* Dallas: Taylor.

Marrs, R., Block, L.F., & Silverman, K.K. (1997). *Dr. Richard Marr's Fertility Book.* New York: Dell Publishing.

Peoples, D., & Ferguson, H.R, (1998). *What to Expect When You're Experiencing Infertility.* New York: W.W. Norton.

Schover, L.R. (1997). *Sexuality and Fertility after Cancer.* New York: John Wiley and Sons.

Schwartz, L.L. (1991). *Alternatives to Infertility: Is Surrogacy an Answer?* New York: Brunner/Mazel.

Silber, S.J. (1998). *How to Get Pregnant with the New Technology.* New York: Warner Books.

5. What are the projected costs of the program?
6. How are the donors screened?
7. How long does it take to conceive; how many attempts must I consider?
8. What drugs will I receive, and what are potential side effects?
9. What is the time commitment for the various procedures?
10. How is the procedure done?
11. Will confidentiality be maintained?
12. What about medical insurance—who will be covered and who pays for it?
13. Should life insurance be purchased?
14. What is the incidence of miscarriage?
15. What is the risk of congenital anomalies?
16. What is the risk of HIV or other sexually transmitted diseases?
17. Should we tell the offspring, and if so, what?
18. What support systems are in place for us as a couple? as individuals?
19. After its birth, to whom does the child legally belong; must we adopt that child?
20. What is the chance a surrogate mother will refuse to relinquish a child?
21. What are the age limits of the program?
22. Are single women accepted into the program?

This list is not all-inclusive. Each couple will have their own set of questions and concerns. Referring a couple to a list of reading materials such as that in Table 14.8 adds to the nurse's armamentarium.

TABLE 14.9

Diagnostic Cluster

Diagnostic/Preoperative Period

NURSING DIAGNOSIS

1. Decisional conflict related to insufficient knowledge of treatment options
2. Anxiety/fear related to insufficient knowledge of potential impact of condition and treatment on reproductive organs and sexuality
3. Grieving related to potential loss of fertility and perceived effects on lifestyle

Postoperative/Treatment Period

NURSING DIAGNOSIS

1. Potential sexual dysfunction related to disease process, surgical intervention, fatigue, and/or pain
   a. Potential moderate or possible permanent alteration in sexual activity related to disease process, surgical intervention, fatigue, and/or pain
   b. Severe or permanent inability to engage in genital intercourse
2. Alteration in coping related to infertility

In addition, a directory recently compiled by Mary Partridge-Brown entitled *In Vitro Fertilization Clinics: A North American Directory of Programs and Services* lists 250 programs throughout the United States and Canada. This directory also provides the numbers of in vitro births over a three-year period, cost breakdown and insurance information, a description of each program's health professionals, and the restrictions involved. The book includes a description of each ART and is written for a layperson by a layperson. It can be located in local libraries or through the publisher, McFarland and Company, Inc.[62]

✺ SUMMARY

Nurses are in a unique position providing care for the woman undergoing evaluation and treatment for gynecologic and breast cancers. In the process of developing a therapeutic relationship, nurses can assess the woman's sexual and fertility needs, provide basic information regarding the effects of disease and possible effects of therapy, provide support, and promote hopefulness. As new treatment modalities evolve, it is essential that the nurse remain informed about how he or she can affect the patient's quality of life. It certainly seems appropriate to tackle infertility concerns and sexual dysfunctions just as aggressively as current treatment modalities aim for cure. The nurse can instill in the patient a sense of hope that sexual problems and fertility issues related to the disease and therapies are treatable and that it is indeed possible to feel feminine and sexually whole again.

✺ REFERENCES

1. Andersen, B.L. (1985). Sexual functioning morbidity among cancer survivors: Present status and future research directions. *Cancer, 55*(8), 1835–1842.
2. Andersen, B.L. (1993). Predicting sexual and psychologic morbidity and improving the quality of life for women with gynecologic cancer. *Cancer, 71*(4), 1678–1690.
3. Andersen, B.L., & Boffitt, B. (1988). Is there a reliable and valid self-report measure of sexual behavior? *Arch Sex Behav, 17*(6), 509–525.
4. Waterhouse, J., & Metcalfe, M.C. (1986). Development of the sexual adjustment questionnaire. *Oncol Nurs Forum, 13*(3), 53–59.
5. Bransfield, D.D., Horiot, J.C., & Nabid, A. (1984). Development of a scale for assessing sexual function after treatment for gynecologic cancer. *J Psychosoc Oncol, 2*(1), 3–19.
6. Anderson, B., & Lutgendorf, S. (1997). Quality of life in gynecologic cancer survivors. *CA Cancer J Clin, 47*(4), 218–225.
7. World Health Organization (1975). *Education and Treatment in Human Sexuality: The Training of Health Professionals* (Technical Report no. 572). Geneva: World Health Organization.
8. Foltz, A.T. (1987). The influences of cancer on self-concept and life quality. *Semin Oncol Nurs, 3*(4), 303–312.
9. Berek, J.S., & Andersen, B.L. (1992). Sexual rehabilitation: Surgical and psychological approaches. In W.J. Hoskins, C.A. Perez, & R.C. Young, eds., *Principles and Practice of Gynecologic Oncology* (pp. 401–416). Philadelphia: Lippincott.
10. Andersen, B.L., van der Does, J., & Anderson, B. (1992). Sexual morbidity following gynecologic

cancer. In M. Coppleson, ed., *Gynecologic Oncology: Fundamental Principles and Clinical Practice* (pp. 1481–1497). Edinburgh: Churchill Livingston.

11. Otte, D. (1990). Gynecologic cancers. In S.L. Groenwald, M.H. Frogge, M. Goodman, & C.H. Yarbro, eds., *Cancer Nursing: Principles and Practice* (pp. 845–888). Boston: Jones and Bartlett.

12. Chamorro, T. (1991). Cancer and sexuality. In S. Baird, ed., *A Cancer Source Book for Nurses* (pp. 141–149). Atlanta: American Cancer Society.

13. Lamb, M. (1990). Psychosexual issues: The woman with gynecologic cancer. *Semin Oncol Nurs, 6*(3), 237–243.

14. Bransfield, D.D. (1982). Breast cancer and sexual functioning: A review of the literature and implications for future research. *Int J Psych Med, 12*(3), 197–211.

15. Maguire, G.P., Lee, E.G., Bevington, D.J., et al. (1978). Psychiatric problems in the first year after mastectomy. *Br Med J, 1,* 963–965.

16. Andersen, B.L., & Jochimsen, P.R. (1985). Sexual functioning among breast cancer, gynecologic cancer, and healthy women. *J Consult Clin Psychol, 53*(1), 25–32.

17. Battersby, C., Armstrong, J., & Abrahams, M. (1978). Mastectomy in a large public hospital. *Aust NZ J Surg, 48*(4), 401–404.

18. Jamison, K.R., Wellisch, D.K., & Pasnau, R.O. (1978). Psychosocial aspects after mastectomy I: The woman's perspective. *Am J Psychol, 135*(4), 432–436.

19. Psychological Aspects of Breast Cancer Study Group (1987). Psychological Response to mastectomy: A prospective comparison study. *Cancer 59*(1), 189–196.

20. Vinokur, A.D., Threatt, B.A., Caplan, R.D. & Zimmerman, B.L. (1989). Physical and psychosocial functioning and adjustment to breast cancer: Long-term and follow-up of a screening population. *Cancer 63*(2), 394–405.

21. Shag, C.A., Ganz, P.A., Polinsky, M.L., et al. (1993). Characteristics of women at risk for psychosocial distress in the year after breast cancer. *J Clin Oncol 11*(4), 783–793.

22. Steinberg, M.D., Juliano, M.A., & Wise, L. (1985). Psychological outcome of lumpectomy versus mastectomy in the treatment of breast cancer. *Am J Psychol, 142*(1), 34–39.

23. Auchincloss, S. (1989). Sexual dysfunction in cancer patients: Issues in evaluation and treatment. In J.C. Holland & J.H. Rowland, eds., *Handbook of Psychooncology: The Psychological Care of the Patient with Cancer* (pp. 383–413). New York: Oxford University Press.

24. Kilkku, P., Grönroos, M., & Punnonen, R. (1982). Sexual function after conization of the uterine cervix. *Gynecol Oncol, 14*(2), 209–212.

25. Abitol, M., & Davenport, J. (1974). Sexual dysfunction after therapy for cervical carcinoma. *Am J Obstet Gynecol, 119*(2), 181–189.

26. Decker, W.H., & Schwartzman, E. (1962). Sexual function following treatment for carcinoma of the cervix. *Am J Obstet Gynecol, 83*(3), 401–405.

27. Andersen, B., LaPolla, J., Turner, D., et al. (1993). Ovarian transposition in cervical cancer. *Gynecol Oncol 49*(2), 206–214.

28. Andersen, B. (1986). Sexual difficulties for women following cancer treatment. In B. Andersen, ed., *Women with Cancer: Psychological Perspectives* (pp. 257–288). New York: Springer-Verlag.

29. Shover, L., Fife, M., & Gershenson, B. (1989). Sexual dysfunction and treatment for early stage cervical cancer. *Cancer, 63*(1), 204–212.

30. Jusenius, K. (1981). Sexuality and gynecologic cancer. *Cancer Nurs, 4*(6), 479–484.

31. Brown, R.S., Haddox, V., Posada, A., & Rubio, A. (1972). Social and psychological adjustment following pelvic exenteration. *Am J Obstet Gynecol, 114*(2), 162–171.

32. Andersen, B.L., & Hacker, N. (1983). Psychosexual adjustment following pelvic exenteration. *Obstet Gynecol, 61*(3), 331–338.

33. Andersen, B.L. (1987). Sexual functioning complications in women with gynecologic cancer: Outcomes and directions for prevention. *Cancer, 60*(8), 2123–2128.

34. Ratcliff, C.F., Gershenson, D.M., Morris, M., et al. (1996). Sexual adjustment in patients undergoing gracilis myocutaneous flap vaginal reconstruction in conjunction with pelvic exenteration. *Cancer 78*(10), 2229–2235.

35. Cochran, S., Hacker, N., Wellisch, D., & Berek, J. (1987). Sexual functioning after treatment for endometrial cancer. *J Psychosoc Oncol, 5*(2), 47–61.

36. Andersen, B., Turnquist, D., LaPolla, J., & Turner, D. (1988). Sexual functioning after treatment of in situ vulvar cancer: Preliminary report. *Obstet Gynecol, 71*(1), 15–19.

37. Andersen, B., & Hacker, N. (1983). Psychosexual adjustment after vulvar surgery. *Obstet Gynecol, 62*(4), 457–462.

38. Andreasson, B., Moth I., Jensen, S., & Bock, J. (1986). Sexual function and somatopsychic reactions in vulvectomy-operated women and their partners. *Acta Obstet Gynecol Scand, 65*(1), 7–10.

39. Fisher, S. (1985). Sexual knowledge and attitudes of oncology nurses: Implications for nursing education. *Semin Oncol Nurs, 1*(1), 63–68.

40. Vincent, C.E., Vincent, B., Greiss, F.C., & Linton E.G. (1975). Some marital-sexual concomitants of

carcinoma of the cervix. *South Med J, 68*(5), 552–558.

41. Shover, L., & Fife, M. (1986). Sexual counseling of patients undergoing radical surgery for pelvic or genital cancer. *J Psychosoc Oncol, 3*(3), 21–41.

42. Kaplan, H.S. (1983). *Evaluation of Sexual Disorders.* New York: Brunner/Mazel.

43. Annon , J.S. (1976). *Behavioral Treatment of Sexual Partners vol. 1: Brief Therapy.* Honolulu: Enabling Systems.

44. Dudas, S. (1990). Altered body image and sexuality. In S.L. Groenwald, M.H. Frogge, M. Goodman, & C.H. Yarbro, eds., *Cancer Nursing: Principles and Practice* 2nd ed. Boston: Jones and Bartlett.

45. Woods, N.F. (1979). *Human Sexuality in Health and Illness.* St. Louis, MO: Mosby.

46. Lamb, M., & Woods, N. (1981). Sexuality and the cancer patient. *Cancer Nurs, 4* (2), 137–144.

47. Andrews, F.M., Abbey, A., & Halman, L.J. (1992). Is fertility problem stress different? The dynamics of stress in fertile and infertile couples. *Fertil Steril, 57*(6), 1247.

48. Domar, A.D., Seibel, M.M., & Benson, H. (1990). The mind/body program for women with infertility. *Fertil Steril, 53*(2), 246.

49. Hahn, S. (1991). Caring for couples considering alternatives in family building. In C. Garner, ed., *Principles of Infertility Nursing* (p. 181). Boca Raton, FL: CRC Press.

50. Hahn, S. (1991). Caring for couples considering alternatives in family building. In C. Garner, ed., *Principles of Infertility Nursing* (p. 197). Boca Raton, FL: CRC Press.

51. American Society for Reproductive Medicine (1996). Assisted Reproductive technology in the U.S. and Canada: results from the American Society for Reproductive Medicine/Society for Assisted Reproductive Technology Registry. *Fertil Steril, 65*(5) 697.

52. Marrs, R.P., & Vargyas, J.M. (1986). Human in vitro fertilization: State of the art. In D.R. Mishell Jr. & V. Davajan, eds., *Infertility, Contraception &*

Reproductive Endocrinology (p. 565). Oradell, NJ: Medical Economics Company.

53. Navot, D., & Rosenwaks, Z. (1990). Ovum donation. In M.M. Seibel, ed., *Infertility: A Comprehensive Text* (p. 513). Norwalk, CT: Appleton & Lange.

54. American Society for Reproductive Medicine (1998). Guidelines for gamate and embryo donation. Fertility and Sterility. Supplement 3, Vol.70, No.4.

55. Handel, J.D., & Hanafin, H. (1989). Success rate of surrogate gestational pregnancies using in vitro fertilization donor oocytes (paper presented at VI World Congress on IVF, Jerusalem.)

56. Fugger, E.E. (1993). Clinical use of cryopreservation of the human embryo after in vitro fertilization (lecture presented at the Advanced Hands-On Workshop on Cryopreservation of Spermatozoa and Embryos—Postgraduate Course). Indianapolis: University of Indiana.

57. Gosden, R.G., Baird, D.T., Wade, J.C, et al. (1994) Restoration of fertility to oophorectomized sheep by ovarian autografts stored at -196 degrees C. *Hum Reprod 4* (9), 597-603.

58. Opsahl, M.S., Fugger, E.F., Sherins, R.J., Schulman, J.D. (1996) Preservation of reproductive function before therapy for cancer: New options involving sperm and ovary cryopreservation. *The Cancer Journal from Scientific American 3* (4), 189–191

59. Andrews, L.B., & Jaeger, A.S. (1990). Legal aspects of infertility. In M.M. Seibel, ed. *Infertility: A Comprehensive Textbook* (p. 539). Oradell, NJ: Medical Economics Company.

60. American Fertility Society (1991). *Adoption: A Guide for Patients.* Birmingham, AL: American Fertility Society.

61. Menning, B.E. (1980). The emotional needs of infertile couples. *Fertil Steril, 34*(4), 313–319.

62. Partridge-Brown, M. (1993). *In Vitro Fertilization Clinics: A North American Directory of Programs and Services.* Jefferson, NC: McFarland and Company.

Spirituality Issues

James C. Pace, RN, DSN, MDIV, ANP

✠ SPIRITUALITY, HEALTH, AND ILLNESS

Spirituality is as important a concept in nursing care as it is nebulous. According to Clark et al. (1991), "All disciplines have a problem defining spirituality and spiritual care, and applying these concepts in practice."[1] The ability to identify spiritual needs and provide appropriate interventions is of particular importance when dealing with people who have cancer because it has been suggested that this population is more focused on spirituality than is the general population.[2,3] Issues related to body image, mortality, quality of life, purpose in life, the meaning of life's experiences, the nature of hope, and a variety of coping strategies are all called into play when cancer becomes a part of one's existence and life course.

Nursing has long been an advocate of holistic care, incorporating the mind, body, and spirit into the object of care and attention. Davidson believes that a nursing model may be the best framework for studying spirituality.[1] Nursing has always been a forum for the comprehensive study of what it means to be involved in human relationships. In order to provide quality care, the nursing profession can add to the body of literature concerning spirituality by lending its views, research efforts, and findings to all that is needed and required for the provision of spiritual care.[1]

✠ SPIRITUALITY AND SPIRITUAL WELL-BEING

There are many definitions and terms used when discussing spirituality. As a part of the nursing diagnosis of "spiritual distress," the North American Nursing Diagnosis Association (NANDA) defines the human *spirit* as "the life principle which pervades a person's entire being and which integrates and transcends one's biological and psychosocial nature."[4] Millson and Dudley define spirituality as "pertaining to or consisting of spirit, soul, or incorporeal being, as distinguished from the physical being."[5] Spiritual well-being is comprised of several aspects: sense of purpose and meaning in life; sense of relationship with self, other(s), and a supreme being; and hope.[1,3,6] Burkhardt uses the term *spiriting* to encompass all the various terms relating to spirituality. She defines spirituality as "the unfolding of mystery through harmonious interconnectedness that springs from inner strength."[7]

Both Clinebell and Ellison have identified four categories of basic spiritual needs:

1. Meaning
2. Challenge in life
3. A reason for being
4. Continuing on in the face of adversity[8,9]

Clinebell; Ellison; Stuart et al.; and Clark et al. believe that increasing the sense of spiritual well-being assists in the integration of health and personality, and provides energy and direction to the whole person.[1,8,9,10] Ellison believes that spiritual well-being is present, in varying degrees, in everyone.[9]

People, by their very nature, need relationships: with self, others, friends, loved ones, and with a Supreme Other. "Harmonious interconnectedness," where the person feels in touch with a Supreme Being and others and feels positive links to the past, comfort with the present, and hope for the future, is suggested as another defining characteristic of spiritual well-being.[11]

Spirituality also involves our need for creativity with other people as well as with ourselves. People desire to be able to give something back to others and to be remembered as having done something worthwhile. Human beings desire freedom to choose which direction their lives take. To be creative means to be productive, to be capable, to be a living part of the world. To creatively exist is to be able to do, to think, to piece together, to build meaning. This meaning somehow affects the way the self views the world, as well as contributes to the lives of other people in some positive manner.

Another concept related in some manner to spiritual needs is the need for transcendence. Transcendence is the ability to move beyond the present moment, the here and now manifested in the physical expressions of life, to whatever and all that is beyond.[5,8,9,10,12,13] This movement toward "all that can be" gives new meaning and shape to one's life. The transcendent puts one in contact with the realization that there is indeed more. This "touching the veil," this experience of what can be, often leaves the person with a great sense of hope and meaning, not only to all that can be, but also to a more integrated sense of living in the present moment, in the here and now.

Hope is yet another facet of spirituality, and, as mentioned above, is often brought about by the transcendent. Hope is defined as "an inner power directed toward a new awareness and enrichment of 'being' rather than 'rational expectations.'"[14] A survey of terminally ill patients identified seven categories of hope-fostering strategies that parallel Clinebell's and Ellison's spiritual needs.[14] These included uplifting memories, an affirmation of worth, attainable aims, interpersonal connectedness and a spiritual base, lightheartedness, and "the personal attributes of determination, courage and serenity."[14] In a study by Herth, it was discovered that regardless of age, gender, ethnic origin, income, educational level, activity level, and fatigue level, all people experience hope. Hope exists in all people, at some level.[14]

Spiritual well-being is "a cornerstone of health" and believed to have impact on physical well-being.[10] A spiritually healthy person is known by many characteristics: He or she is hopeful, looks forward with expectancy to what is to come,[6] and most often has a positive attitude toward the self and others.[11]

Through the study of loneliness and its correlates, spiritual well-being has also been connected with overall quality of life. Loneliness has a negative relationship with quality of life, and spiritual well-being has a negative relationship with loneliness.[3,15,16,17]

✺ SPIRITUALITY AND RELIGIOSITY

Not until recent years has the construct of spirituality been considered in detail apart from the construct of religion/religiosity. For many years, it was assumed that religion and the spiritual realm were very similar, the same entity, or concepts that went hand-in-hand. However, research comparing the two constructs has found that although there indeed are many interconnecting themes, there are also some very important differences. Heriot conceptualizes spirituality as an "umbrella" under which can be found both religious and existential needs.[18] Religious needs are most often connected with a specific religion or a religious practice, while existential needs are those needs all people share regardless of the presence or absence of a religious background or belief.[15,18] Another way to conceptualize the difference between the two is to imagine a "map" (religion/religiosity) and "a journey" (spirituality) (Table 15.1).

Religion/Religiosity

Religion has often been viewed as an organized system of beliefs, rituals, and values—a patterned or structured set of beliefs that are expressed through behaviors, creeds, and/or catechisms. Fowler describes religion as the ideas that express the ultimate environment of one's faith.[19] Thus religion can be conceptualized as the "map" that allows followers to get from the "here" to the "there." Religion may be thought of as a set of lenses, a faith perspective, and a denominational approach to faith that gives the person an identity. It can also be thought of as a prescribed set of "rules," or operating procedures, that give one the means to come to an awareness of God/Other. For many people, religion provides the prime opportunity to go beyond the physical and come

---

TABLE 15.1

Comparison of Religiosity and Spirituality

Religiosity (The Map)	Spirituality (The Journey)

A "roadmap" that defines
    Beliefs
    Values
    Code(s) of conduct and ethics
	One's journey through life
	A personal quest to define
	    Meaning in life
	    Meaning of life

A tradition/system of worship that provides
    Rituals
    Answers
    Norms
	A dynamic relationship with that which transcends
	Always life-affirming and integrating

The roadmap and tradition Define
    What is to be believed
    How beliefs affect life
    Self-image and identity
	A capacity to know and be known
	A lifelong process of growth
	A constant process of taking in "truth" and then adding individual insight to arrive at a way of perceiving and acting in the world

to a greater awareness and knowledge of the transcendent. And it may be helpful for nurses to note that King and Speck found greater religiousness in women than in men.[20]

For many, religion is a source of happiness and contentment in life. Kushner asserts that religion gives people a way to find happiness, but that happiness is never the primary goal.[21] Happiness is a by-product of a life filled with a sense of purpose and meaning. Kushner also states that when a person has learned how to live (often one of the functions of religion), life itself is the reward.[21] He goes on to say that religion should not be expected to provide all the answers in life, but to give people the courage to find their own way.[21]

Spirituality

If religion can be thought of as the map, then spirituality may be best described as the journey. That is, a person's ever-evolving experience with life is that person's spiritual journey. It is very important to remember that agnostics and atheists have a spiritual perspective as well as religious people; belief in a Supreme Being is not a prerequisite for spirituality. Spirituality denotes a sense of direction (but can be the absence of one as well). In its most healthy sense, spirituality entails a connectedness to oneself, other people, and God. An individual's spirituality is never static. He or she continues to grow into and beyond what has been. Spirituality is always connecting with other people, getting to know oneself better, integrating the two, and reaching new conclusions about a Supreme Being or the transcendent and one's place in the world, in a perspective that somehow relates to the whole. Spirituality entails a person's worldview, or paradigm of how things "fit." As a result, spirituality provides a sense of meaning and purpose to the world and the person's place in it.

Joseph Campbell, the highly renowned scholar of the mythology of widely diverse cultures, describes the spiritual journey somewhat differently. In *The Power of Myth*, he states:

> People say that what we're all seeking is a meaning for life. I don't think that's what we're really seeking. I think that what we're seeking is an experience of being alive, so that our life experiences on the purely physical plane will have resonances within our own innermost being and reality, so we actually feel the rapture of being alive.[22]

In this sense, spirituality is a much more comprehensive construct than religion. It captures the "life journey" of every individual and may totally subsume religiosity, blend into and merge with religiosity, or be totally divorced from religiosity. There are indeed many people who want absolutely nothing to do with religion; yet, the same people may be very spiritual. Spirituality is ever-growing over time, shaped and molded by life experiences, decisions, joys, sorrows, victories, defeats, successes, and accomplishments. This integration of life experiences connects the individual with others and with the transcendent. Becoming, connecting, being, and creatively journeying seem to best capture the essence of the realm of spirituality. Spirituality can then be thought of as the *process* of getting from the "here" to the "there" and all that is learned in the meantime.

✳ NURSING AND SPIRITUALITY

Nursing care that integrates the spiritual dimension of care presents us with a nurse who is involved in a human relationship. This relationship is with another person who has come face to face with a significant life event that calls forth a new sense of meaning and purpose for her existence. Stiles describes this spiritual intervention as being "fully present to patients and families" and accompanied by excellent nursing care.[23] Qualities the nurse can demonstrate to provide better spiritual care include a supportive approach to the patient; what has been termed a sense of benevolence to the patient; awareness of the patient, self, and the impact of family and significant others; empathy; and nonjudgmental understanding.[24]

Granstrom studied the barriers to spiritual interventions by nurses.[10] Common barriers included different cultural and religious backgrounds of the nurse and patient; value differences regarding basic issues like illness, aging, and suffering; lack of personal spiritual awareness; fear of not being able to handle a discussion of spiritual ideas; and being unclear about the difference between religiosity and spirituality. In other words, the biggest barriers to providing spiritual care are the lack of awareness of one's own spirituality, the fear that this dimension calls forth a knowledge base in which the nurse is not competent, and perhaps a fear that encountering such discussions will be somehow misinterpreted.

Highfield believes there is a need for improved nurse–patient communication about spiritual needs and that nursing should become more aware of spirituality in general and patients' needs in particular.[2] Patients need clear, honest communication with their care providers.[6] Current nursing theories promoting "professional distance" and "objectivity" regarding patient care do not lend themselves to defining interventions for the patient in spiritual distress.[23]

Patients and nurses of course can be at different levels of self-discovery on their spiritual journeys at any given time. This difference can make planning appropriate interventions challenging.[10] Stepnick and Perry suggest that, for dying patients, whose spiritual focus is different from others', multiple types of nursing intervention are necessary to obtain positive outcomes.[25] Their combination of Kubler-Ross's stages of death and dying with Peck's process of spiritual development suggests ways to intervene with patients from all kinds of religious and nonreligious backgrounds and at all levels of faith.[25]

One study of oncology nurses found that over half incorrectly identified the patients' religion, and only 16% incorporated any kind of spiritual assessment into their care.[26] Highfield's study confirms the incidence of inaccurate spiritual assessment.[2] Whatever the reason, whether lack of time, lack of experience, or lack of confidence, the patient misses out on a potential source of support and the nurse misses an entire dimension of every person's being.[2,26]

It takes more than just education for a nurse to feel comfortable with spiritual issues. Introspection and an awareness of the nurse's own personal spiritual journey are required to integrate the spiritual domain into patient care. Lane identifies three steps in the spiritual growth of nurses:

1. Developing a "greater awareness of the spirit within self" in order to be a better listener for the patient
2. Opening the self by being totally present with the patient
3. Allowing the patient to share her feelings and emotions without reserve on the nurse's part

She also emphasizes the need for nurses to take care of their own spiritual needs; otherwise, providing this aspect of care can and will be emotionally draining.[27]

In several studies, however, nurses were found to be unsure of what constituted spiritual problems and spiritual interventions.[26,28,29] In some cases, a spiritual dimension of care was not identified, or religious aspects were taken into account but without reference to the existential domain.[26,29] Highfield and Cason found that oncology nurses placed greater emphasis on physical and psychosocial nursing care and that the patient's spiritual needs were identified infrequently.[28] It becomes obvious to the observer that nursing values give priority to those caring behaviors and greatly influence the care that is provided.[27,28]

✳ SPIRITUALITY AND LIFE-THREATENING ILLNESS

A person's spiritual outlook makes a tremendous difference to the process of both living and dying.[6] Spirituality functions as a resource during multiple losses and change.[12] The developmental tasks of those with a life-threatening illness include forgiveness of self and other(s), integrating past spiritual events, and planning and taking care of financial affairs.[6]

People with a life-threatening illness express spirituality differently from those who are not faced with such illness.[13] Spirituality appears to become a more personal and private experience after diagnosis of an illness that may progress over years, and finally be terminal. This more personal and private focus of living places less emphasis on the external expression of a belief system, for example, going to church, and gives more attention to the integration of beliefs and finding meaning and purpose in life's experiences. In Reed's study of their perceived needs, people with life-threatening illness identified arranging visits with clergy, having spiritual literature read to them, and providing time for involvement with family as the most important and helpful spiritual interventions provided by nurses.[13]

Ryan studied care-giver and nursing perceptions of the most and least helpful nursing behaviors in hospice care.[29] Interventions were classified as either physical or psychosocial; no spiritual dimension per se was identified. But three of the ten most helpful interventions by care givers could be considered "spiritual" in nature: listening to the patient, reducing fears, and answering questions honestly. Five of the ten most helpful interventions identified by hospice nurses could be considered "spiritual" in nature also: helping the patient to ventilate feelings, answering questions honestly, listening to the patient, allowing time for the primary care giver to ventilate feelings, and talking about such issues as death and dying. In a study by Zerwekh, the most common ways that hospice nurses met patients' spiritual needs were categorized as caring, guiding, and letting go.[30]

Where cancer is concerned, the illness trajectory is such that a patient is faced with a diagnosis, the impact of that diagnosis on life, the possibility of loss of control, and the beginning of realization of one's own mortality. These issues prompt many to look toward the spiritual for support and hope.[31] Spirituality often allows the patient to meet life in a way that is cushioned by previously built supports and the comfort of knowing the supports exist. Corless, however, suggests that much of current nursing care is based on a scientific paradigm.[32] She expresses concern as to whether spirituality can coexist with the scientific environment without being lost or relegated to second place. There needs to be room for hope, and for denial. A scientific approach often suggests that we must give patients "the facts" and help them to accept "the truth," but denial may be a functional and appropriate coping skill at that time.[32] As the old hospice adage goes, unless something is terribly wrong with where the patient is, that is perhaps where the patient needs to be.

IMPLICATIONS FOR NURSING

Nurses who are comfortable with spiritual interventions are definitely in the minority. Patients and their family members look to nurses for assistance with meeting some spiritual needs, needs many nurses may not recognize or feel prepared to deal with.[2,10,13,26,29] There are several options to help increase nurses' comfort with the provision of spiritual care in order to better meet the holistic needs of patients. Education that distinguishes between the traditional idea of "religion" and an ever-increasing knowledge base about all that comprises "spirituality" is an excellent place to begin. Other means to become more aware of the spiritual are arrived at by role-modeling, emotional and spiritual support for the evolving nurse, and giving nurses permission to express spiritual views.

Education about spiritual issues, both in nursing school and in practice, can increase the nurse's knowledge about the spiritual needs of her patients and the types of interventions that may be of help. Highfield and Cason suggested that nursing education needs to include content about spiritual intervention as a part of holistic care so that it becomes just another set of responses on the part of the nurse.[28] There are indeed times when the nurse is the only person available to provide spiritual support. If the teachable and reachable moment is lost, it may never surface to that same degree again. Adequate preparation to deal with such circumstances also enables the nurse to share a common language with other health care personnel who provide spiritual support: the social worker, chaplain, advanced practice nurse, physician, and ancillary staff members.

Nurses must give considerable thought to their own spiritual journeys before quality work can be hoped for with others. In order to do this, they must first be willing to compare and contrast the religious and the spiritual. Once the spiritual is recognized and nurtured within the self, it can be encountered in patients and a mutual journey can then begin. In a word, the recognition of the spiritual in the lives of patients allows nurses to learn the importance of "being with" patients rather than simply "doing for" them. There is much involved in spiritual care; it can be draining. But the rewards are many and there is much to gain.

✳ AREAS OF SPIRITUAL NEED AND RELATED INTERVENTIONS

How can the nurse identify the spiritual needs of any given patient in a way that can be helpful to the development of a plan of care? A sample spiritual assessment form such as that in Table 15.2, which can be filled out and added to anytime after a patient contact, may be a helpful starting point. And a method described by Speck may offer the best approach to understanding the patient's spiritual needs.[20] This approach is from the perspective of the patient's past, present, and future.

Encountering the Past

Every patient presents to the nurse with a past, a past that is a history, or a story to tell. It comprises the person's spiritual journey to date. The past frames who the person is today, how the person thinks, and how life's experiences have "packaged" the individual to this moment in time.

Thus the first spiritual intervention on the part of the nurse is simply a way of being, a way to "attend to" the person. It is the adoption of a philosophy of practice that insists on taking the time to be with and to journey with another for a reasonable amount of time. During this time, the nurse attempts to enter into the world of the patient to better understand the myriad circumstances that come together and contribute to the reason that the patient is now in the nurse's environment. Once the nurse puts this holistic orientation toward caring into practice, the second intervention is the ability to listen actively to the patient; and to listen in such a way that lends comfort to the person who is sharing what are, many times, intimate details about the past. Active listening is a difficult thing to do. The health care environment is not "consumer-friendly" when it comes to time. Increasingly, nurses are being called on to generate income based on the number of visits in any given day. Consequently, care must be a balance between the nurse's philosophy of care and the realities of today's job market.

A very important part of active listening is to acknowledge, commend, congratulate, and give positive feedback for all of those events in life that have contributed to

---

TABLE 15.2

A Sample of a Brief Spiritual Assessment Form

Person making assessment: _____ Patient: _____

Contact: _____ Date: _____

The patient/family/care giver is currently being visited by:

Minister: _____ Church/synagogue member: _____
Priest: _____ Other(s): _____
Rabbi: _____

Name and phone number of supporting/affiliated church/synagogue:

Patient/family/care giver perception of God/Divine Other:

Patient/family/care giver perception of life in relation to present illness:

Resources used by patient and/or family/care giver:

__Religious community __Scripture/writings   __Other
__Prayer   __Personal religious experience
__Hope   __Articles of faith: rosary, cross, other
__Prayer partner   __Friend(s)

Issues causing distress:
__Need for meaningful experience/philosophy of life
__Need for a sense of the transcendent/ultimate
__Need for trusting relationships: self__ other(s)__ health care team__ the world__ God__
__Need to vent anger
__Need for pain relief
__Need for hope
__Need to feel love/care
__Need for prayer__ sacraments:_____
__Other:

Plan, requests of patient/family/care giver:

Consults indicated:

well-being, that is, the memories that have built up and have contributed meaning and purpose. It is often such acknowledgments that are remembered far after the nurse–patient interaction. When memories are heard by the nurse, and heard in a way that the patient can identify with or relate to, they serve to call forth additional information. Conversations about the past might then elicit episodes that have been hurtful and have caused spiritual pain or distress.

Feelings of Guilt and/or Shame

Some events in a person's life may be associated with guilt or shame, the internalized sense that something wrong, bad, or evil is attributed *to the patient* by others. Such feelings may relate to past actions by the patient, the diagnosis or surgery, events caused by surgery, hospitalization, or interactions among people at various places over time. Shame may relate to such things as loss of hair as a result of chemotherapy or the presence of a newly created stoma. A person may feel guilty that she didn't want visitors while feeling bad. A person may feel shamed, unclean, or unattractive because of the loss of bowel and/or bladder control, disfiguring surgery, or any type of alteration in appearance.

In the midst of things done or left undone, when there is perceived, imagined, or actual harm associated with the past, it is important for the nurse to give considerable attention to the need for a realistic appraisal of the situation at hand, and then to lend some time to the need for forgiveness of the self, from others, and/or from God. Often there is some type of hurt associated with event(s) in the past. It is helpful to have that hurt identified and named, and the way the patient feels toward the event described as fully as possible. By recognizing the patient's feelings, seeing the incident through unbiased eyes, reflecting on the situation for a few needed moments, the nurse reaches out with love to the patient who has felt that hurt.

Often a patient feels let down by God, or that God has deserted her in time of real need. The person often feels that her faith has not been very strong, or not strong enough. Such feelings are associated with guilt over doubting God, or not being a strong enough person to bear up under "tests of one's faith." Those who experience doubt about their faith need encouragement that they are still acceptable to God in spite of doubts, uncertainties, and questions.

If a patient has lost her faith, she is likely to feel very isolated and alone. Often, it is the nurse who first models the behaviors that let the patient know she is still loved and accepted for who she has been and who she is now. Rituals, religious events and services, or referrals to others, particularly clergy, must not be imposed at this point. The patient should be allowed the time to work through all that has happened and to discover for herself what would help the most. Reassurance, support, gentle exploration, and being present with the person are the most important interventions at this point. Wanting to refer the patient to someone else may imply to the patient that the nurse wants to separate him- or herself from what has been shared. The patient may want you to say prayers she can no longer say, or read scripture that she can no longer look up; but maybe she simply wants to know that you will carry her needs in your heart and think about them during the course of the day. Perhaps a patient would like your suggestions as to whom she could talk the situation over with in more detail—a priest, rabbi, family member, social worker, or chaplain. Somehow an agreement should be reached as to how actively the patient wants the nurse to intervene at this time.

Issues of Trust

For many people, guilt and shame are nonspecific. Perhaps the patient let herself down. Perhaps family members let her down. Maybe God let her down. In any case, there is a strong possibility that health care, and caring professionals, also let the patient down in some way. Who can the patient trust?

It is helpful to remind the patient that we are all human, and as human beings, we never have been and never will be perfect. Humans are oftentimes very frail and vulnerable, and when our bodies let us down it reminds us that we are not perfect and are, finally, very mortal. But despite all the imperfections, there are indeed people who love us for who we are, not the person we wish we could be. We are still loved by other(s), by one's God, and, hopefully, by the self. The help of the ones who love the patient can provide her with the opportunities to reconcile the past with the present, come to grips with the real and the actual, and face the future with a renewed sense of hope and well-being.

For every person, religious or nonreligious, it is important for the nurse to seek to establish trust by giving clear and accurate information, following up on what is said or promised, providing reassurance that further treatment/help is available in some manner or form, and maintaining a consistency of care that eliminates conflicting signals and information.

Exploring the patient's past is the first key to spiritual health and well-being. Painful episodes in the past, guilt, feelings of loss, feelings of helplessness and powerlessness, feelings of shame, feelings of isolation, all need some form of reconciliation with the present. Old patterns, rituals, and faith practices from the past may be helpful to the patient and need reconnection. For other patients, the old may be abandoned for something new that seems more relevant and life-full. In any case, the past is slowly being reconnected with the present. Trust is the bridge that allows the person an opportunity to make this reconnection and allows past hurts and scars and breaks to begin to heal.

The Present

In the present, the patient may have a variety of spiritual needs, which can be broken down into several categories.

Anger

A person who has experienced cancer may be very angry with God, herself, the illness, family members, and the health care team. Often, the only one within reach or easily accessible is the nurse, who receives the bulk of the anger. The patient may lash out at the nurse with the specific purpose of causing hurt, thus unconsciously attempting to transfer her hurt to the health care provider. While it is never easy to endure this type of behavior, the nurse must realize that it is very helpful to the patient for the nurse to receive this anger and not reject her. It is only natural for the nurse to want to reject someone who is trying to inflict hurt and anger; but in so doing, the nurse may only serve to confirm that the person is bad and deserves to be ill. The nurse must continue to realize that, more often than not, the patient's anger is being thrown out at random rather than toward a specific individual. Behind the anger, there is a struggling person with desperate needs to understand why the illness has happened and what its nature, its cause, its predictability, its prognosis might be.

Suffering

In the early stage of illness, the patient may talk about pain. Pain, most often of a physiologic cause, is whatever the patient says it is. Pain has hope of relief, whether from aspirin, NSAIDs, opiates, TENS (transcutaneous electrical nerve stimulation) units, surgical procedures, stress therapy, chiropractic, massage, compresses, or something else. Suffering, on the other hand, has any number of meanings associated with it that seem to involve much more than just pain. Pain may be a part of suffering; but more to the point, suffering indicates some type of gradual loss and a growing sense of hopelessness. Suffering may be compounded by such things as fear, loneliness, hopelessness, isolation, lack of functional ability, and dread of what may yet be experienced.

Anger, Pain, Suffering, and Spiritual Health

In assessing the spiritual health of any given individual, it is not uncommon to find patients who have been able to discover ways of understanding their circumstances and living within the limits of what life provides. Perhaps it is a set of religious convictions that provides insight into the illness and allows for day-to-day coping to take place. Perhaps it is a philosophical belief system that provides answers. Experiencing serious illness allows some people to grow closer to God than ever before, and gives them new opportunities for appreciation of life's "simple" pleasures: the relief of pain for a few hours, the decrease of suffering, the relationship with a family member once estranged. Any of these processes of understanding may be backed up by a supportive network of family, friends, and other people who share the patient's belief system, including laity or local minsters who visit the sick in hospitals, hospices, and clinics.

In many circumstances, the belief pattern(s) of the patient may be very different from, and in some cases, clash very strongly with those of the nurse. Two or more different cultures with differing value systems may meet for the first time. In such situations, there is a great deal of doubt and anxiety on both sides of this health care relationship. The key to successful intervention lies in the ability of the nurse to enter into a holistic relationship in which he or she takes an active part in exploring the belief system of the patient while valuing her understanding and decision-making autonomy. The patient may find it reassuring to know that the nurse is also struggling to understand the issues related to health and illness. The willingness to explore the issues together may be very comforting and supportive. And it may be very affirming and meaningful for the two parties to pray together, if it feels right to do so. It should only take place *at the patient's invitation*. But if it happens, it can be a very meaningful moment that contributes to both nurse's and patient's well-being.

Additional Indicators of Spiritual Needs

In a study by Taylor et al., seventeen different spiritual need indicators, with accompanying examples, were identified for nurses.[33] These indicators are listed in Table 15.3. Spiritual care interventions implemented by nurses in these situations were also reviewed in the same study. They included verbal communication about spiritual or religious concerns; involving others in the patient's care (chaplains, clergy, other health care professionals, support people and groups); facilitating or initiating prayer; attending to the patient's family; providing or suggesting religious materials; serving as a therapeutic presence; touching the patient (holding a hand, touching an arm); and conveying a benevolent attitude (e.g., "being respectful, empathetic, supportive, and nonjudgmental").[33]

What Nurses Should Avoid

People who are in a difficult situation, such as the patient who is struggling with a faith issue, are a "captive audience" of sorts. There are health care providers who believe it their mission in life to bring people to a particular faith or understanding before a life-threatening event occurs. This is clearly an abuse of the spiritual care relationship. Another example of abuse is the nurse who believes that he or she can be all things to all people regardless of the patient's background or spiritual care need. Clearly, there are times to refer to another person, such as an ordained priest, deacon, healer, prayer partner, or someone else who is recognized by a particular organization as being a legitimate person of authority. Almost always this referral goes hand in hand with the permission of the patient. When a patient requests a healer, priest, rabbi, or prayer practitioner, the nurse should contact the chaplain of the hospital or hospice, or the local church or organization for further information and ways to intervene appropriately.

The Future

We are often told to live for today, to live as if there were no tomorrow. That may be good advice. Most people are also told that a chronic illness can give an appreciation of the "todays" of life that was not there previously. But there is always the possibility of a tomorrow and many more, and that is the patient's hope. Hope for the future can take many forms for the person with cancer: (1) hope that a new drug or treatment will be developed to prolong life, or add to quality of life, or lead to complete cure; (2) hope of being loved and sharing that love with other people; and (3) hope that a new sense of meaning in life will be discovered and that the mystery of death will lose its sting.

Some patients want their nurse's ideas about an afterlife, what research shows about near-death experiences and the "death surround." Is there a purgatory? Is there

TABLE 15.3

Patient Characteristics and Symptoms Indicating Spiritual Needs

Fear or Anxiety	Related to diagnosis, treatment, death, uncertainty, the future, night, prognosis, being alone, "letting go"; verbal or body language expresses fear, anxiety
Requests	For prayer or clergy; asking for guidance
Depression/Sadness/Grief	Grieving related to diagnosis or hospitalization
Discussion of Death Issues	Impending death; questioning if death will be painful; concerns about life after death
Hopelessness/Despair	Hopeless situation; having nowhere to turn; no hope of getting better; patients who appear in despair
Withdrawal/Aloneness	Withdrawal from family, friends, others
Recent Diagnosis or Treatment	A rough course of treatment ahead; new diagnosis, unable to receive effective treatment
Crying	Continuous tears; weeping
Anger	Frustrations; expressions of anger at self
Helplessness	Expressions of helplessness, not necessarily verbal; feelings of powerlessness over situation
Difficulty Coping	Denial; difficulty with acceptance; inappropriate coping; bargaining
Obvious Religious Clues	Reading Bible; watching religious programs; religious articles in plain view
Mention of God or Faith	Talking about religion or God; patient speaking about God's will; beseeching Allah, God, or Jesus for help
Family Issues	Overwhelmed with family conflict; lack of family support and understanding
Searching for Meaning	Asking Why? Why is this happening to me?; questioning faith
Guilt	Feeling guilty or at fault for their disease; guilt with how life has been lived
Restlessness/Difficulty Sleeping	If patient is restless and unable to say what she needs, sometimes prayer calms her; sleeplessness, fear of falling asleep

Source: Reproduced with permission from Taylor, E.J., Amenta, M., & Highfield, M. (1995). Spiritual care practices of oncology nurses. *Oncology Nursing Forum, 22*(1), 35.

a hell? Is there a continuation of life, as in reincarnation? Many patients are not as afraid of death as they are of the period that leads up to it: the possibility of pain, the potential for suffering, the loss of independence, the burden that may be placed on others. Patients may seek information about pain and symptom control, alternatives to hospital care, or information about the varieties of hospice care available. Making a will and discussing funeral arrangements may be issues that the patient wants to talk over with someone at 2 in the morning. Often, the patient who has been separated from the faith of her childhood suddenly requests to die with a priest (or a faith representative) present.

Thus the preparation for dying and death may entail more formal religious practices for some patients. This is often the time when the patient wishes to reconnect with the faith of her earlier life, or explore a new means of establishing a relationship between herself and whatever Higher Power she trusts. At this particular time, the nurse should recognize that each faith perspective has its own rituals and "helping acts," done by its own representatives, that are oriented toward the healing, sustaining, guiding, and reconciling of the person to the faith.[34] In most faiths, there are prayers and readings from sacred texts. Some faiths have sacramental acts that convey not only an inner meaning through an outer representational form (water, bread, wine, oil, the sign of a cross), but a source of strength that allows one to face the future with joy and hope. Some patients find it very helpful to make a "confession" before a potentially life-threatening event in order to seek forgiveness; some wish prayers to be said immediately before death. Such symbols and prayers are, in reality, "permissions granted" to the patient to let go; the future is bright and no longer holds fear. Religious and spiritual rites of passage also allow the patient the means to say goodbye to family members and to concentrate on the life that remains. Such situations also allow family members to take leave and say their goodbyes in a "safe" situation.

Hope, Healing, Cure, Miracle, and Spiritual Healing

Often, if asked, the patient, family, or care giver will put into words the hope for a cure. In the distant future, there is always the hope for a total and complete cure. This hope should never be taken away. The patient frequently asks the minister, priest, rabbi, friend, and/or nurse to pray for a cure. In some cases, the patient is asking for a miracle—the miracle of a cure, or the miracle of a total healing. These hopes and wishes are logical, rational, easily understood. In these events, it may be possible for nurses, as providers of care and fellows in the spiritual journey, to offer a way to reframe the picture. Perhaps healing does not necessarily have to imply the eradication of pain, suffering, or the existence of the diagnosis of the disease. Rather, it may mean a transformation in thinking in someone who has opened the way for the occurrence of the spiritual. In this sense, healing does indeed take place in the midst of miracles. A miracle is anything and everything that allows for the presence of the transcendent, whether God, Other, the experience of one's angel, or a brush with the divine.

In this perspective, a miracle does not necessarily contravene the law or order of the universe (though some miracles do). The traditional conception of a miracle as an event that breaks with the natural order of things is irreconcilable with our modern understanding of science and history. But miracles are, more often than not, events that proceed entirely lawfully but that upset a person's expectancies.[35] In this case, Macquarrie defines a miracle as an event "that excites wonder and in which God's presence and activity become known."[36] Miracles are spiritual phenomena, and as such they are mysterious; they are neither entirely definable nor comprehensible by our limited knowledge and understanding. The concept of a miracle could thus be characterized by ambiguity. In one sense, it can be viewed as a perfectly ordinary event; in another, it is an event that allows revelation of the transcendent.[36]

The goal of medicine is to heal the body, and the goal of psychosomatic medicine is to heal the emotions, which may in turn heal the body. But the goal of "spiritual medicine" is the health of the whole. Spiritual healing is ultimately directed toward wholeness. Spiritual healing is directed toward the spirit, yet also ultimately affects mind and body. However, wholeness does not necessarily entail absolute mental or physical wellness. "Becoming better is always more important than becoming well."[35] A "spiritual cure," in contradistinction to a cure by surgery or drugs, should always reflect an inward change, whether or not it is accompanied by an outer one also. A spiritual cure is characterized by an awakening of faith, a disclosure of the ultimate, the transcendent, or the Other. This is why miracles are often simple events that point beyond themselves to a new understanding of one's place in the world. And in the midst of spiritual cure, healing can and does take place. Perhaps the healing is an absence of pain, a decrease in fear, the desire to make things right with an estranged family member, or the realization that somehow things will be OK—not perfect, not the way the patient would like, certainly not the way things used to be, but somehow OK. When this occurs, the patient has arrived at a new place, armed with a new sense of hope and the knowledge that all kinds of miracles and cures take place all around us. At this place, a new sense of what it means to be "healthy" emerges. Health is always a state of becoming. Health implies much more than merely the presence or absence of disease. Health is a state of mind communicated by the spirit. Thus "healing" refers to all those acts and words that affirm life in a relationship to self, community, environment, and the Other. A healing environment offers the patient the chance of escaping all those ideas and images that serve to bind and limit. A spiritually healthy person is one who is finally able to affirm life and the relationships that create, reveal, and promote it.

✖ SUMMARY

The diagnosis of cancer changes the patient's life forever, causing her to confront her own mortality in some way. The nurse who cares for these patients confronts his or her own mortality an equal number of times. Times of crisis can usually be turned into opportunities for faith. Such opportunities can be a "best enemy" as well as a trusted friend. Maybe we have prayed with our patients, and they in turn have prayed for us. The intimacy of such moments can bring deep feelings, sometimes tears. Perhaps we have been asked about our own beliefs, or have only been wanted to simply listen to the patient's beliefs. At times we have sat in silence. And nurses often take a patient's needs and words and ways of life home in our hearts, never to discuss them with the patient. It never hurts to pray for a patient, even if she doesn't know it.

But the point of all this is that the core of every nursing care situation is that patients need someone who is genuine. They need the honest truth, not evasion, shallow platitudes, or empty reassurances. They feel most comfortable with other people who have faced the difficulties of life and have managed to find some meaning in their occurrence. If the nurse has not questioned and analyzed his or her own beliefs for the reassurances, doubts, and answers they provide, there is little of value to offer the patient who is forced to confront the ultimate truths and the uncertainties of all that comes thereafter. Because it is spirituality, in the end, that allows people the opportunities to live "in" their lives, find happiness and a sense of purpose and meaning, and to enjoy the "rapture" of life, whatever it might reveal and bring.

✳ REFERENCES

1. Clark, C., Cross, J., Deane, D., & Lowry, L. (1991). Spirituality: Integral to quality care. *Holistic Nurs Pract, 5*(3), 67–76.

2. Highfield, M. (1992). Spiritual healing of oncology patients: Nurse and patient perspectives. *Cancer Nurs, 15*(1), 1–8.

3. Miller, J. (1985). Assessment of loneliness and spiritual well-being in chronically ill and healthy adults. *J Prof Nurs, 1*(2) 79–85.

4. North American Nursing Diagnosis Association. (1986). *Classification of Nursing Diagnoses: Proceedings of the Sixth Congress* (p. 453). St. Louis, MO: Mosby.

5. Millison, M., & Dudley, J.R. (1992). Providing spiritual support: A job for all hospice professionals. *Hospice J, 8*(4), 53.

6. Moberg, D. (1982). Spiritual well-being of the dying. In G. Lesnoff-Caravaglia, ed., *Aging and the Human Condition*. Springfield, IL: Human Sciences Press.

7. Burkhardt, M. (1989). An analysis of spirituality. *Holistic Nurs Pract, 3*(3), 69–75.

8. Clinebell, H.J.J. (1966). *Basic Types of Pastoral Counseling*. Nashville, TN: Abingdon Press.

9. Ellison, C. (1983). Spiritual well-being: Conceptualization and measurement. *J Psychol Theol, 11*(4), 330–340.

10. Stuart, E., Deckro, J., & Mandle, C. (1989). Spirituality in health and healing: A clinical program. *Holistic Nurs Pract, 3*(3), 35–46.

11. Hunglemann, J., Kenkel-Rossi, E., Klassen, L., & Stollenwer, R. (1985). Spiritual well-being in older adults: Harmonious interconnectedness. *J Religion Health, 24*(2), 147–153.

12. Reed, P. (1987). Spirituality and well-being in terminally ill hospitalized adults. *Res Nurs Health, 10,* 335–344.

13. Reed, P. (1991). Preferences for spiritually related nursing interventions among terminally ill and not terminally ill hospitalized adults and well adults. *Appl Nurs Res, 4*(3), 122–128.

14. Herth, K. (1990). Fostering hope in terminally ill people. *J Adv Nurs, 15,* 1250–1259.

15. Paloutzian, R. (1983). *Invitation to the Psychology of Religion.* Glenview, IL: Scott, Foresman.

16. Paloutzian, R., & Ellison, C.W. (1982). Loneliness, spiritual well-being and the quality of life. In L. Peplau & D. Perlman, eds., *Loneliness: A Sourcebook of Current Theory, Research, and Therapy.* New York: Wiley.

17. Pace, J.C., & Stables, J.L. (1997). Correlates of spiritual well-being in terminally ill persons with AIDS and terminally ill persons with cancer. *J Assoc Nurses AIDS Care, 8*(6), 31–42.

18. Heriot, C. (1992). Spirituality and aging. *Holistic Nurs Pract, 7*(1), 22–31.

19. Fowler, J. (1981). *Stages of Faith: The Psychology of Human Development and the Quest for Meaning.* San Francisco: Harper & Row.

20. Speck, P.W. (1994). Spiritual issues in palliative

care. In D. Doyle, G.W.C. Hanks, & N. MacDonald, eds., *Oxford Textbook of Palliative Medicine* (p. 517–525). New York: Oxford University Press.

21. Kushner, H. (1986). *When All You've Ever Wanted Isn't Enough.* New York: Simon & Schuster.

22. Campbell, J., & Moyers, B. (1988). *The Power of Myth* (p. 4). New York: Doubleday.

23. Stiles, M. (1990). The shining stranger: Nurse–family spiritual relationship. *Cancer Nurs, 13*(4), 235–245.

24. Dickenson, C. (1975). The search for spiritual meaning. *Am J Nurs, 75*(10), 1789–1793.

25. Stepnick, A., & Perry, T. (1992). Preventing spiritual distress in the dying patient. *J Psychosoc Nurs, 30*(1), 17–24.

26. Sodestrom, K., & Martin, I.M. (1987). Patients' spiritual coping strategies: A study of nurse and patient perspectives. *Oncol Nurs Forum, 14*(2), 41–46.

27. Lane, J. (1987). The care of the human spirit. *J Prof Nurs, 3*(6), 332–337.

28. Highfield, M., & Cason, C. (1983). Spiritual needs of patients: Are they recognized? *Cancer Nurs, 6*(3), 187–192.

29. Ryan, P. (1992). Perception of the most helpful nursing behaviors in a home-care hospice setting: Care-givers and nurses. *Am J Hospice Palliative Care, 9*(5), 22–31.

30. Zerwekh, J. (1993). Transcending life: The practice wisdom of nursing hospice experts. *Am J Hospice Palliative Care, 10*(5), 26–31.

31. Belcher, A., & Dettmore, D. (1989). Spirituality and sense of well-being in persons with AIDS. *Holistic Nurs Pract, 3*(4), 16–25.

32. Corless, I. (1992). Hospice and hope: An incompatible duo. *Am J Hospice Palliative Care, 9*(3), 10–12.

33. Taylor, E.J., Amenta, M., & Highfield, M. (1995). Spiritual care practices of oncology nurses. *Oncol Nurs Forum, 22*(1), 31–39.

34. Clebsh, W.A., & Jaekle, C.R. (1967). *Pastoral Care in Historical Context.* New York: Harper.

35. Large, J.E. (1965). *The Church and Healing.* New York: Forward Movement Publications.

36. Macquarrie, J. (1977). *Principles of Christian Theology* 2nd ed. New York: Scribner.

Women and AIDS/HIV

Mitzie Fudge, RN, MSN

✳ INTRODUCTION

The first cases of autoimmune deficiency syndrome (AIDS) were reported in the United States in 1981 in a cohort of homosexual men whose presenting symptom was Kaposi's sarcoma. The cause of this debilitating and often fatal disease was discovered to be a retrovirus, human immunodeficiency virus (HIV). There are five known human retroviruses: HTLV-1, HTLV-2, HTLV-5, HIV-1, AND HIV-2. HTLV-1 and HTLV-5 are known to be associated with T-cell leukemia and lymphoma.[1] People at risk for HIV-2 are from a country where HIV-2 is endemic, such as West Africa, or are the sex partners of such people. HIV-2 is not prevalent in the United States.[2]

The HIV virus causes immunodeficiency through a cell-mediated immunity defect. The HIV virus changes its ribonucleic acid (RNA) to deoxyribonucleic acid (DNA) and invades a body cell, causing a number of cellular changes. The virus's ability to invade macrophages and monocytes allows it to be transported throughout the body.[3] The incubation period ranges from a few months to as long as seventeen years, with a median rate of ten years.[2] Viral replication increases substantially as the immune system deteriorates.[2]

✳ DIAGNOSIS

HIV is generally transmitted through contact with or exposure to body fluids of an infected person through intimate sexual contact, through parenteral exposure to blood or contaminated body fluids, and through perinatal transmission. Symptoms may be so mild that they may be missed; viral replication, however, remains active during all stages of infection. Patients' presenting symptom may be an acute retroviral syndrome characterized by fever, malaise, lymphadenopathy, and skin rash. These symptoms usually occur in the first few weeks after infection but before serum converts to a positive antibody test. It is possible that the initiation of antiretroviral therapy during this time can delay the onset of complications related to HIV infection and might improve prognosis.[2] See Figure 16.1

HIV infection is diagnosed by testing for the HIV-1 antibody. Testing is usually initiated by use of a screening test, such as the enzyme immunoassay (EIA) or enzyme-linked immunoabsorbent assay (ELISA). The ELISA has a sensitivity of 98.4 to 99.6%.[1] If this test returns reactive, the results are confirmed by a supplemental test such as the Western Blot (WB). If this test is confirmatory, the person is infected with HIV and is capable of transmitting the virus. One word of caution is that antibody tests cannot detect infection if exposure occurred within six months before the test.[2]

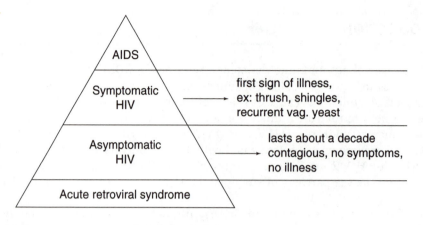

FIGURE 16.1. Course of HIV infection

Source: From Levine, A.M., Anastos, K., Bible, C., Cohen, M., Deely, M., Flexner, C., Greenblatt, R., Minkoff, H., and Young, M. (1998). Treatment strategies of HIV-infected women. *ARHP Clinical Proceedings.* October, 1998. Used with permission.

✖ PREVALENCE

Since the discovery of this virus, cases have increased at an alarming rate. With this increase has come an increase in the number of cases reported among women. Despite reports from the Centers for Disease Control and Prevention (CDC) in 1997 that the incidence of AIDS was on the decline in the United States, statistics indicate that women constitute the fastest-growing sector of the HIV population, with a rate of increase four times that found among men.[4] In 1985, women accounted for only 7% of the reported AIDS cases.[5] Since 1986, AIDS has been the leading cause of death in women aged 25–44 in New York City. In 1987, AIDS was identified as the eighth leading cause of death among women aged 15–44 in the United States. Between 1988 and 1989, newly reported cases increased by 29% in women as opposed to an 18% increase in cases reported in men. By 1990, women accounted for 11% of all cases reported in adults.[6] By 1994, women accounted for 18% of reported AIDS/HIV cases, and AIDS became the fourth leading cause of death in women aged 25–44.[5] By 1996, the estimated prevalence of AIDS among U.S. women was reported to have increased by 17% compared with only a 10% increase in men. Currently, women aged 15–44 comprise 84% of those infected with HIV, and AIDS is listed as the leading cause of death in women aged 25–44 in the United States.[7] See Figure 16.2.

Infection rates are reported to be higher among urban, African American, and Hispanic women.[8] These groups make up over 70% of all reported cases. African American women are reported to have an infection rate sixteen times higher than that of white women and a death rate nine times higher.[7]

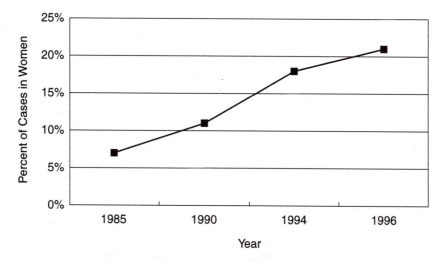

FIGURE 16.2. Prevalence of AIDS in the United States

Women from these three groups are those who many times have very little control over their own lives. They are not in a position to ask much of their male partners. They are more psychologically, economically, and socially dependent than men, and there is an imbalance of power between the women and their partners.[7]

The prevalence of HIV and the incidence of AIDS are higher in areas of lower socioeconomic status such as the urban inner city. Women in these areas are often single, have an annual income of less than $10,000, and have families to support. African American and Hispanic women make up a disproportionate percentage of lower socioeconomic groups in these areas in the United States. The lifestyle and culture of these women also subjects them to more of the risk factors that are associated with AIDS/HIV infection. These risk factors include injection drug use (IDU) and unprotected intercourse with multiple partners. These two risk factors have been identified as the primary modes of transmission of HIV in women.[7,9]

✳ TRANSMISSION

HIV is primarily transmitted by contact with infected body fluid. Body fluids that are most likely to be infected are blood and blood products, fluids contaminated with blood, and cerebrospinal fluid. HIV-1 has also been isolated from other body fluids such as breast milk, cervical secretions, semen, and vaginal fluid.

Women who are unaware of the risk of HIV infection to themselves may not see that they are participating in high-risk behaviors. These behaviors include sharing of needles through drug use, sexual activity that exposes open cuts or wounds to infected body fluids, prostitution, and anal, vaginal, or oral sex without the use of an appropriate barrier.[4]

In past reports, IDU was the most common mode of transmission of HIV, related to the sharing of contaminated needles. Also, women intravenous drug users are more likely to have infected sexual partners.

Non–intravenous drug use has also been identified with an increase in HIV infection, especially with the widespread use of "crack" cocaine, which is smoked. "Crack" users frequently exchange sexual favors for the drug. The encounters are frequently one-night stands and involve exposure to multiple sexual partners, increasing the women's risk of having contact with an infected partner. These women, therefore, may not see themselves as in a high-risk group or engaging in a high-risk activity.[10]

Heterosexual transmission of HIV is almost equal to that of transmission via IDU.[5] Women who live in an area of high injection drug use are at greater risk of contracting HIV, because they are more likely to encounter an infected male partner and more likely to trade sexual favors for drugs.

Seventy percent of wives of HIV-positive hemophiliacs are HIV-positive.[11] Women as a group may be less likely to practice "safe sex." Prostitutes have been known to forgo the use of a protective barrier to receive more money for their services. They may use protection with their clients and then not use protection with their regular partners to delineate between business and pleasure for themselves.[12]

Transfer of the virus seems to be more efficient from men to women than vice versa, putting women at greater risk for infection. It has been shown that a woman is ten times more susceptible to the virus during intercourse than a man. There is a higher concentration of HIV in semen because of the high number of lymphocytes, which leads to a higher concentration of the virus than is found in vaginal fluid or cervical secretions.[7] The anatomy and physiology of the female genital tract puts a woman at increased risk of infection. The vagina is a mucous membrane and is easily traumatized. Therefore, tiny cuts, tears, or sores that occur during intercourse give infected semen a route by which to enter the body.[4] The surface area of the vagina also leads to an increased risk of exposure. Because the vagina is a receptacle for semen, it can be exposed to HIV-infected semen for a longer period of time.[13]

Studies have shown that exposure to, and the presence of, sexually transmitted diseases (STDs) can facilitate the spread of HIV.[14] The virus has been detected in the exudate of genital ulcers in HIV-positive men and women. These ulcers are also known to bleed easily when irritated during sexual intercourse, exposing the partner to infected blood. The blood and exudate come into contact with the genital mucosa, which can be microscopically damaged from trauma, making an easy avenue for access of the virus to the body. Inflammatory STDs appear to cause increased shedding of the HIV virus. Therefore, people who do not have an open sore would not necessarily consider themselves to be contagious to their partner and therefore would not take the appropriate precautions. Ulcerative (i.e., genital herpes, syphilis) and nonulcerative STDs (i.e., chlamydia, candida) attract CD4+ lymphocytes to the ulcer surface or the surface of the endocervix. This attraction can disrupt the natural epitheleal and mucosal barrier, thus increasing a woman's susceptibility to infection.[10,14]

HIV can also be transmitted during the perinatal period. Mothers are often diagnosed only after a child is diagnosed with an AIDS-defining illness. Fifteen to 25% of infants born to untreated HIV-infected mothers are infected with HIV. The virus is transmitted through transplacental exposure and exposure to maternal blood and vaginal secretions at the time of delivery. The virus can also be transmitted after birth through the ingestion of breast milk from an infected mother.[2] Current studies have shown that treating the infected mother with Zidovudine (AZT) during late pregnancy and during labor and treating the infant for the first six weeks after birth reduces the risk of transmission to the infant to approximately 8%.[2,5]

Health care workers can be exposed to the virus in many settings. Anyone who has contact with blood or body fluids should always wear appropriate protective clothing, including gloves, gown, mask, and eye protection. Always wash your hands after exposure. If a needle stick should occur, the employee should be seen immediately in the employee health service or emergency department so that appropriate measures can be taken to prevent the spread of the virus.

✖ SYMPTOMS

Many clinical features should alert health care providers to the possibility that a patient may be HIV-positive. Some patients exhibit a type of viral syndrome that resembles mononucleosis or influenza as described earlier. They may complain of flulike symptoms—such as joint aches, fever, and sweats—that do not seem to go away with conventional treatment. Generalized lymphadenopathy may occur with or without the flulike symptoms. Patients may complain of dermatological manifestations, such as seborrhea or other similar skin conditions that arise without prior history. Unexplained weight loss, persistent fevers, anemia, or neutropenia should also make health care providers suspect a possible HIV infection.

Opportunistic infections are often a clinical feature of HIV infection. Because HIV infection is a chronic, systemic infection of lymphocytes, monocytes, and macrophages, it involves potentially every organ system in the body as the disease progresses. Opportunistic infections can quickly become life-threatening in the immunocompromised patient (Table 16.1).

Bacterial Infection

Mycobacterium avium is characterized by persistent fever, night sweats, fatigue, weight loss, abdominal pain, weakness, lymphadenopathy, and hepatosplenomegaly. Treatment consists of combination antibiotic therapy with a beta-lactam antibiotic and an aminoglycoside.

Fungal Infections

Candidiasis can affect the oral or vaginal tract. Symptoms include white patches on the tongue or buccal mucosa in oral infection. Vaginal symptoms include vulvar pru-

TABLE 16.1

Opportunistic Infections Related to HIV Infection

	Symptoms	Therapy	Other Info
Bacterial Infections			
Mycobacterium avium	Persistent fever, night sweats, fatigue, weight loss, abdominal pain, weakness, lymphadenopathy, hepatosplenomegaly	Combination antibiotic therapy with a beta-lactum antibiotic and an aminoglycoside	
Fungal Infections			
Candidiasis	Oral—white patches on the tongue or buccal mucosa Vaginal–vulvar pruritis, vaginal discharge	Appropriate antifungal therapy such as fluconazole, ketoconazole, or miconazole	May persist or be resistant to therapy
Cryptococcosis	Meningitis—headache, fever, progressive malaise, altered mental status, seizures pneumonia—fever, shortness of breath, cough	Amphotericin is the drug of choice	Causes side effects— fever, rigors, nausea, chills, vomiting, seizures, hypotension, bronchospasm
Histoplasmosis	Fever, weight loss, shortness of breath, lymphadenopathy	Appropriate antifungal therapy	
Protozoal Infections			
Pneumocystis	Fever, nonproductive cough, shortness of breath, weight loss, night sweats, fatigue	Trimethoprim-sulfamethoxazole, dapsone, or pentamidine	May be treated prophylactically
Cryptosporidiosis	Diarrhea, abdominal cramping, nausea, vomiting, fatigue, weight loss, dehydration	Symptom control	No known treatment

TABLE 16.1 *(continued)*			
	Symptoms	*Therapy*	*Other Info*
Protozoal Infections			
Toxoplasmosis	Altered mental status, seizures, fever, coma	Pyrimethamine plus sulfamethoxazole	
Viral Infections			
Cytomegalovirus	Retinitis—unilateral visual deficit or change Gastroenteritis—dysphagia, wasting, nausea, fever, diarrhea	Ganciclovir or foscarnet	
Herpes simplex (HSV)	Painful blisters or ulcers	Acyclovir	Recurrence is common

Adapted from Otto, S.E. *Oncology Nursing,* and Groenwald, S.L., Frogge, M. H., Goodman, M., & Yarbro, C.H. *Clinical Guide to Cancer Nursing.*

ritis and vaginal discharge. Treatment consists of an appropriate antifungal, such as fluconazole, ketoconazole, and miconazole; however, symptoms may persist and be resistant to therapy.

Cryptococcosis is characterized by either meningitis or pneumonia. Symptoms of meningitis include headache, fever, progressive malaise, altered mental status, and seizures. Symptoms of pneumonia include fever, shortness of breath, and cough. Treatment consists of appropriate antifungal therapy and antimicrobial therapy. Amphotericin B is the drug of choice. Side effects of this therapy include fever, chills, rigors, nausea, vomiting, hypotension, bronchospasm, and seizures, which may require intensive support. Nephrotoxicity is the major toxicity. Abelcet may be given if the patient does not respond to or cannot tolerate Amphotericin B.

Histoplasmosis is characterized by fever, weight loss, shortness of breath, and lymphadenopathy. Treatment consists of appropriate antifungal therapy as described above.

Protozoal Infections

Pneumocystis is probably the most familiar opportunistic infection associated with HIV. Pneumocystis is a pneumonia characterized by fever, nonproductive cough, shortness of breath, weight loss, night sweats, and fatigue. Treatment consists of trimethoprim-sulfamethoxazole, dapsone, or pentamidine. High-risk patients may be treated prophylactically.

Cryptosporidiosis symptoms include diarrhea, abdominal cramping, nausea, vomiting, fatigue, weight loss, and dehydration. Treatment consists of symptom control; there is no known treatment for this species at present.

Toxoplasmosis is encephalitis characterized by altered mental status, seizures, fever, and coma. Treatment consists of pyrimethamine plus sulfamethoxazole.

Viral Infections

Cytomegalovirus is characterized by retinitis or gastroenteritis. Symptoms of retinitis include a unilateral visual deficit or change. Gastrointestinal symptoms include dysphagia, wasting, nausea, fever, and diarrhea. Treatment consists of ganciclovir or foscarnet.

Herpes simplex (HSV) symptoms include painful blisters or ulcers. Acyclovir is the drug of choice to treat HSV. Recurrence is common.[1,16]

Gynecologic symptoms are often the first sign of HIV infection in women because other signs and symptoms may be attributed to other problems as described above. Candidal vaginitis of new onset or increasing frequency may be the earliest sign of HIV infection in a woman. Symptoms such as oral thrush, oral hairy leukoplakia, or herpes zoster (shingles) should trigger further investigation into a woman's risk for HIV. Women who do not respond to usual and customary treatment or who have a particularly severe infection such as candidiasis, genital herpes, genital warts, or recurrent pelvic inflammatory disease should be suspect for HIV infection.[5]

Human papillomavirus (HPV) is considered to be an opportunistic infection in HIV-positive women, with the clinical course more accelerated and the therapeutic response to treatment decreased. HPV is found 35–50% more often in HIV-positive women than in HIV-negative women. Symptomatic women are more likely to have multifocal and genital involvement than are asymptomatic HIV-infected women. After treatment, HIV-positive women are more likely to have persistent or recurrent disease. The goal of treatment is to remove existing warts, prevent recurrence, maintain normal anatomy, and preserve optimal genital functioning.[17]

✖ AIDS-RELATED MALIGNANCIES

Patients who are immunocompromised because of infection with HIV-1 are at an increased risk for developing a malignancy. Thirty to 70% of people with AIDS develop a malignancy. The most common ones include Kaposi's sarcoma (KS), non-Hodgkin's lymphoma, primary CNS lymphoma, and invasive squamous cell carcinoma of the cervix.[16]

Kaposi's Sarcoma

Kaposi's sarcoma (KS) is the most common neoplasm in the HIV-infected patient. Kaposi's sarcoma is more predominant in homosexual and bisexual men, but it has been seen (rarely) in women. Etiologic factors may include a sexually transmitted agent or an infection with a virus such as cytomegalovirus (CMV). CMV has been found in KS lesions.

KS is characterized by multicentric skin lesions that may be found on any area of the body. The pigmentation of these lesions ranges from brown to violet. The lesions may be raised nodules, or they may be flat. They are usually painless. Suspicious lesions should be biopsied.

Visceral and lymphatic involvement may be seen late in the disease process. Progressive disease results in enlarging lesions, severe edema, protein-losing enteropathy, and respiratory distress. The edema results from the lymphatic involvement with compromised lymphatic drainage and blood circulation. Gastrointestinal involvement leads to protein-losing enteropathy and the accumulation of ascites. Ascites can further impair lymphatic drainage and blood circulation, especially from the lower extremities, leading to further edema. Respiratory distress is related to lung involvement of the lesions, but can also be related to accumulation of ascites leading to reduced diaphragmatic expansion and generalized edema.[1,16]

Treatment of KS is aimed at controlling the tumor without further compromising the patient's immune system. Radiation therapy is often used for the local control of lesions. Chemotherapeutic agents, either alone or in combination, may be beneficial; however, they can lead to further compromise of the immune system. Some patients have responded to Interferon therapy. Those who have responded to this therapy have CD4 counts higher than $200/mm^3$, no symptoms of fever, night sweats, or weight loss; and no prior AIDS diagnosis.[16] Curative therapy for KS does not yet exist, but the disease itself is rarely life-threatening. Most patients succumb to opportunistic infection related to the profound immunodeficiency of HIV infection.

Although KS is seen less frequently in women, the negative impact on body image can further isolate the female patient. The visible skin lesions announce to the world that she has AIDS.

Non-Hodgkin's Lymphoma

Non-Hodgkin's lymphoma (NHL) has been reported to be present in at least 33% of AIDS patients.[16] The most common symptom of NHL is painless lymphadenopathy involving the abdominal nodes. Presenting symptoms may include fever, chills, and weight loss. Patients usually have advanced disease, which involves extranodal sites. These sites include the central nervous system, bone marrow, bowel, and anorectum. Peripheral lymphadenopathy may be absent. Symptoms may include vague abdominal discomfort, back pain, gastrointestinal symptoms, or ascites.[1] The majority of patients have high-grade lymphoma.

Patients are diagnosed by a positive biopsy of a suspicious mass and are staged by the use of several diagnostic tests (blood counts, chest X-ray, CT scan, lumbar puncture, etc.) that evaluate all areas of the body. Bone-marrow involvement is common in HIV-infected patients, resulting in the need for bone-marrow biopsy early in the diagnostic work-up. Treatment is determined by the grade of the tumor. Chemotherapy or radiation may be used to treat intermediate-grade tumors. High-grade tumors are generally treated with combination chemotherapy and CNS prophylaxis. Prognosis is poor. Median survival ranges from four to seven months.

Central Nervous System Lymphoma

Central nervous system (CNS) lymphoma occurs most often in immunocompromised patients. It is a rare malignancy accounting for only 0.3–2% of newly diagnosed lymphomas. The cell of origin is the same as the one that causes NHL.

Patients who have primary CNS lymphoma may have presenting symptoms of confusion, lethargy, memory loss, alteration in personality or behavior, hemiparesis, aphasia, or seizures and focal neurologic symptoms. CT scans and magnetic resonance imaging (MRI) are used to identify single or multiple discrete lesions. Because these symptoms can be found in other CNS disorders, laboratory tests and titers should be done to rule out other diseases such as toxoplasmosis and syphilis. Neither radiation nor chemotherapy treatment seems to have any effect on survival rates. Prognosis is poor, with survival of approximately 2.5 months.[1,16]

Cervical Cancer

Cervical cancer resulting from HPV infection in HIV-infected women is potentially fatal and is the most serious gynecologic disease these women experience. HIV-infected women often present with advanced disease and do not respond to conventional treatment. Their response and prognosis are directly related to the severity of their immunosuppression and their CD4 count. The female patient infected with HIV-1 who is diagnosed with cervical cancer should be treated according to the stage of her disease. However, it should be noted that her response to treatment does not equal that of the HIV-negative patient. Radical hysterectomy and pelvic lymphadenectomy may be performed safely in the patient with early disease. Women with profound immunodeficiency are more likely to have lymph node involvement and have a higher recurrence rate and death rate with shorter intervals between recurrence.[1] Patients with advanced disease should be treated with chemotherapy or radiation therapy; however, careful monitoring is needed to observe for hematologic toxicities. Drugs of choice include cisplatin, bleomycin, and vincristine.[1] (see Chapter 3.)

Cervical Intraepithelial Neoplasia

Women who are immunosuppressed appear to be at greater risk of developing neoplastic changes of the lower genital tract than are those in the general population.

Women with HIV have a higher prevalence of cervical intraepithelial neoplasia (CIN) and human papillomavirus (HPV) related to their immunocompromised state, up to ten times that of women attending family planning clinics in the United States.[18] CIN has been shown to occur in HIV-infected women at five to ten times the expected rate. These women also have a higher incidence of cervical cancer; however, the usual risk factors do not correlate with the HIV-infected population. Asymptomatic HIV-positive women with a CD4 count greater than 400 are less likely to have high-grade lesions than are women with profound immunodeficiency.

CIN needs to be identified and followed more aggressively in the HIV-positive patient. The CDC recommends that HIV-infected women have an initial exam and Pap smear. If this exam and Pap test are negative, then the Pap test should be repeated in six months. If these are within normal limits, the patient may go to annual follow-up. If the Pap test returns with severe inflammation or reactive cellular changes, it should be repeated in three months. If a squamous intraepithelial lesion or the presence of atypical squamous cells of undetermined significance is identified, the patient should undergo colposcopy and biopsy if indicated by exam.[19] Appropriate therapy should be instituted when the results are obtained (see Chapter 2).

✖ TREATMENT

In 1993, the CDC revised the classification system for HIV infection and case definition for AIDS (Table 16.2). This revised system has allowed the CD4+ lymphocyte count to be used with certain disease states to identify when and what type of treatment is to be rendered. This was done because therapy had been shown to be most effective within certain levels of immune dysfunction. Included in the clinical categories of this definition were vulvovaginal candidiasis, cervical intraepithelial neoplasia, and pelvic inflammatory disease. Included in the AIDS case definition was invasive cervical carcinoma.[18]

There has been much controversy over the antiretroviral treatment of asymptomatic patients. The CDC has identified certain risks and benefits for early treatment of asymptomatic patients. Benefits include control of viral replication and mutation, which helps to reduce the viral burden. Progressive immunodeficiency is prevented, leading to potential maintenance or reconstitution of a normal immune system. Early treatment delays the progression to AIDS, therefore allowing for prolongation of life. Early initiation of treatment decreases the risk of drug toxicity.

As with all benefits to treatment, there are potential risks to early initiation of therapy. Quality of life may be reduced because of adverse drug events. Drug resistance may develop early in the disease, thus limiting the future choice of therapy. Because of limited experience, the long-term effects of toxicity on the body are not known. The duration of effectiveness of current therapies is also unknown.[20]

Treatment should be offered to the asymptomatic patient with a CD4+ count <500/mm^3. If such a patient has a CD4+ count >500/mm^3, many experts would delay

TABLE 16.2		
AIDS-Defining Illnesses		
The definition of AIDS includes that an individual be infected with HIV and have one or more of the following disorders:		
Opportunistic Infections	*Cancers*	*Other Symptoms*
Pneumocystis carinii pneumonia (PCP) Mycobacterium avium complex (MAC) Cryptosporidiosis	Kaposi's sarcoma High-grade B-cell lymphoma Cervical cancer	AIDS dementia syndrome AIDS wasting syndrome Recurrent bacterial pneumonia CD4 cells less than $200/mm^3$ or less than 14%

Source: Adapted from Treatment Strategies for HIV-infected Women, AHRP Clinical Proceedings, October, 1998, p. 5.

treatment and observe. Symptomatic patients (those with fever, thrush, etc.) should be treated no matter what their CD4+ count is.

AZT was the first, and is still the most widely used, antiretroviral medication. New drugs have been developed that appear to prolong life, slow progression of the disease, and increase quality of life.

The primary goal of antiretroviral therapy is to reduce viral replication to undetectable levels. The preferred regimen is a combination of two nucleoside reverse transcripterase inhibitors (NRTIs) and one potent protease inhibitor (PI). Drugs in the NRTI category include Zidovudine (AZT), Didanosine (ddl), Zalcitabine (ddC), Stavudine (d4T), and Lamivudine (3TC). Drugs in the PI category include Indinavir, Ritonavir, Saquinavir, and Nelfinavir. These drugs are known for drug interactions and patients need to be monitored closely.[20]

Barriers to Prevention and Treatment

Prevention is best brought about through education of health care providers and the public. One of the biggest barriers to prevention and treatment is the attitudes and beliefs patients hold about those in the health care profession.

Studies have identified barriers to seeking treatment and therapy. These barriers include the overall poor treatment of women by the health care system, women's inability to obtain health care insurance, inaccessibility of transportation to receive care, inability to find care for dependent children while seeking care, and inability to access health care providers and facilities because of lack of resources.[21,22]

Efforts must focus on preventing the spread of the disease. This is a two-part process. The first part entails identifying those at risk—IV drug users, prostitutes, those participating in unprotected sexual activities, and women in low-income and minority groups. Identification can be made by taking adequate medical and social histories. This history should include the following:

1. Menstrual history—should include age at menarche; interval, flow, duration of menses; date of last menstrual period; any recent changes, amenorrhea, dysmenorrhea, PMS, any history of toxic shock
2. Sexual history—history of abuse, incest, rape, or trauma; age at first sexual activity; any current abusive situation; male or female sexual partners (or both); sex for drugs or money; knowledge and practice of safe sex; partner's HIV status
3. Obstetrical history—number of pregnancies and outcomes of each pregnancy, history of breastfeeding, complications during pregnancy and delivery, HIV status of children, desire for future pregnancy
4. Gynecologic history—STDs, PID, UTI, vaginitis, any gynecologic surgeries or conditions
5. Family medical history—any history of cancer, heart disease, CVA, renal disease
6. Personal medical history—review of systems; previous history of cancer, heart disease; thyroid, liver, or renal disease; also any prior surgery
7. Health maintenance and habits—frequency of exams including Pap smears, mammograms, and follow-up of abnormal results; breast self-exam; female hygiene and use of feminine products; nutrition; exercise; and tobacco, alcohol, and substance abuse
8. Social history—marital status, employment, living conditions, transportation

After identifying women at risk, barriers need to be overcome, including attitudinal and organizational barriers. Attitudinal barriers prevent women from seeking care. They include lack of motivation, cultural isolation, fatalism, mores, superstitions, and fears. Organizational barriers include inability to seek care, lack of health insurance, lack of transportation, lack of health care providers, and lack of health care facilities.[22]

To break these barriers, nurses need to be aware of these issues and be able to counsel the patient appropriately. A nurse can gain a patient's trust by listening nonjudgmentally and showing caring and compassion. Simple behaviors, such as using language the patient understands and relates to or using a gentle touch, send a message of openness and caring.

Once you have established trust you can help these women to gain access to health care for screening and treatment. Referrals need to be made to the appropriate neighborhood clinics, family planning clinics, public health facilities, drug treatment programs, and medical specialists. Working with case managers to find funds for care and medications and to gain access to clinical trials, transportation, and child care can increase access to care. Peers may serve as positive role models and as a credible source of information because they communicate in a language the patient is more likely to understand.[7]

SUMMARY

Nurses need to be leaders and advocates for women with HIV. Nurses need the knowledge and tools to empower these women to take control of their lives. Women with HIV need to be educated in the importance of safer sexual practices and the need to be able to say no to drug and alcohol use. They need help to overcome the fear of abandonment, withdrawal of economic support, and threat of physical violence if they suggest that their partners practice safe sex with them.

When society first learned about HIV, it was known as a "man's" disease. As time has progressed, it has shown to have a much greater impact on women than anyone thought possible. It is important for nurses to keep abreast of information about this disease as it relates to women; its impact on women's health is changing every day. New treatments are being developed and research in the area of women with this disease is increasing. Being knowledgeable about how HIV impacts women is one of the best ways that nurses can begin to help them.

REFERENCES

1. Otto, S.E. (1997). HIV and related cancers. *Pocket Guide to Oncology Nursing* (pp. 241–252). St. Louis: Mosby. 241–252.
2. Centers for Disease Control and Prevention. (1998a). Guidelines for treatment of sexually transmitted diseases. *MMWR, 47*(RR–1), 11–16.
3. Edge, V., & Miller, M. (1994). Acquired immune deficiency syndrome (pp. 135–136). *Women's Health Care.* St. Louis: Mosby, 135–136.
4. Katz, D.A. (1997). The profile of HIV women: A challenge to the profession. *Soc Work Health Care, 24*(3–4), 127–134.
5. Klaus, B.D. (1995). Recognizing and managing HIV infection in women. *Nurse Pract, 20*(12), 52–53.
6. Smeltzer, S.C., & Whipple, B. (1991). Women with HIV infection: The unrecognized population. *Health Values, 15,* 41–48.
7. Gaskins, S.W. (1997). Heterosexual transmission of HIV in women. *J Assoc Nurses AIDS Care, 8*(6), 84–87.
8. van Servellen, G., Sarna, L., & Jablonski, K.J. (1998). Women with HIV: Living with symptoms. *West J Nurs Res, 20*(4): 448–464.
9. Cohen, M. (1997). Natural history of HIV infection in women. *Obstet Gynecol Clin North Am, 24*(4), 743–758.
10. Jones, L. and Catalan, J. (1989). Women and HIV disease. *Br J Hosp Med, 41,* 526–538.
11. Provencher, D., Valme, B., Averette, H. E. Ganjel, P., Donato, D., Penalver, M., & Sevin, B.U. (1988). HIV status and positive Papanicolau screening: Identification of a high-risk population. *Gynecol Oncol, 32,* 184–188.
12. Wenstrom, K.D., & Gall, S.A. (1989). HIV infection in women. *Obstet Gynecol Clin North Am, 16,* 627–643.
13. Campbell, C.A. (1995). Male gender roles and sexuality: Implications for women's AIDS risk and prevention. *Soc Sci Med, 41*(2), 197–210.
14. Centers for Disease Control and Prevention. (1998) HIV prevention through early detection and treatment of sexually transmitted diseases—United States. *MMWR 14* (RR-12), 2–3.
15. Zidovudine for the prevention of HIV transmission from mother to infant. (1994, April 29). *MMWR, 43*(16), 285–287.
16. Groenwald, S.L., Frogge, M.H., Goodman, M., & Yarbro, C.H. (1998). Aids-related malignancies. *Clinical Guide to Cancer Nursing* (pp. 315–322) 4th ed. Boston: Jones and Bartlett.
17. Colletta, L. (1997). Human papillomavirus in the woman with HIV. *Women's Health,* (October), 16–21.
18. Centers for Disease Control and Prevention. (1993). Revised classification system for HIV infection and expanded surveillance case definition for AIDS

among adolescents and adults. *MMWR, 41* (RR–17), 1–19.

19. Saglio, S.D., Kurtzman, J.T., & Radner, A. B. (1996). HIV infection in women: An escalating health concern. *Am Fam Physician 54*(5), 1541–1556.

20. Centers for Disease Control and Prevention. (1998). Report of the NIH panel to define principles of therapy of HIV infection and guidelines for the use of antiretroviral agents in HIV-related adults and adolescents. *MMWR, 47*(RR–5), 50, 68, 70, 71–78.

21. Misener, T.R., & Sowell R.L. (1998). HIV-infected women's decisions to take antiretrovirals. *West J Nurs Res, 20*(4), 431–437.

22. Foster, H. W. Jr. (1997). Women's health care for the coming millennium. *J Fla Med Assoc, 84*(6): 358–363.

Controversies in Breast Cancer

Randolph E. Gross, MS, RN, CS, AOCN

✖ INTRODUCTION

Despite, or perhaps because of, tremendous technological advances in the prevention, screening, diagnosis, and treatment of breast cancer, many controversies exist that affect the care of women. At the core of these controversies is a lack of complete understanding of the origin of breast cancer and its unpredictability as a disease entity. The current recommendations for screening, prevention, and treatment are founded on the relatively extensive information on the role that age, diet, genetics, environment, and hormones play in the development of human breast cancer. However, the plethora of research has yielded various and conflicting data and results. Women rely on health care practitioners to interpret the current literature and provide them with information and recommendations based on their individual medical and family histories. This chapter addresses several of the controversies in which nursing can have an impact in patient care.

✖ INTERPRETATION OF RISK FACTORS FOR BREAST CANCER

Much attention has been focused on the risk for breast cancer and how to prevent the development of the disease. Myriad studies have been conducted worldwide in an attempt to identify a single common risk factor or a combination of risk factors, but a clear and definitive answer remains elusive. Many individual, social, and environmental variables affect the risk for breast cancer. Because of our highly mobile and technical society, comparison and interpretation of data can be difficult and fraught with further questions.

Risk Factors

Table 17.1 summarizes the known risk factors for breast cancer. Two established risk factors are being female and getting older, with the majority of risk beginning after age 50.[1] Other major factors such as a benign breast biopsy with a diagnosis of atypical hyperplasia or lobular carcinoma in situ (LCIS) also increase risk, but to varying degrees, and treatment of these conditions lacks definitive standards.[2] Another risk factor is the identification of a family history of breast or ovarian cancer, which increases risk; the extent of that risk, however, is also an issue of discussion, debate, and ongoing research. The most confusing and controversial of all these factors is the identification of the BRCA1 and BRCA2 gene mutations and how genetic testing and subsequent possible treatments can be incorporated into women's health care.

Minor risk factors such as reproductive history, the influence of endogenous and exogenous hormones, and lifestyle issues (tobacco usage, alcohol consumption, dietary fat and soy intake, and the effect of exercise) have some impact on risk, but to various and lesser degrees. Many of these minor factors are consistent with our

TABLE 17.1

<table>
<tr><td colspan="3" align="center">Factors Associated with Breast Cancer</td></tr>
<tr><td>*Major Risk*</td><td>*Minor Risk*</td><td>*Protective*</td></tr>
<tr><td>Being female</td><td>Nulliparity</td><td>Breastfeeding</td></tr>
<tr><td>Being over 50 years old</td><td>First childbirth after age 30</td><td>Regular exercise</td></tr>
<tr><td>Atypical hyperplasia</td><td>Alcohol consumption
(>2 drinks a day)</td><td>First childbirth before
age 30</td></tr>
<tr><td>LCIS</td><td></td><td></td></tr>
<tr><td>BRCA1 or BRCA2</td><td>ERT?</td><td></td></tr>
<tr><td></td><td>Excessive intake of dietary fat?</td><td></td></tr>
<tr><td></td><td>Use of birth control pills</td><td></td></tr>
</table>

lifestyles and environment in North America, and women, the media, clinicians, and researchers focus much attention on these issues and their relation to breast cancer risk.

For example, although dietary influences are a major concern and focus for women, researchers have been unable to prove a strong correlation between dietary intake and breast cancer development. The use of hormone products and the influence of exercise are other minor risk factors that receive much attention. To further complicate the picture, only 30 to 40% of diagnosed breast cancer patients have attributable and identifiable risk factors.

Determining Individual Risk

Identifying the women who are at higher risk than others for the development of breast cancer is more clear-cut because of current research efforts and an overall increase in public awareness. Individual variables affect the picture for each woman, however. Less clear is the degree of risk involved in treatment recommendations once determined to be high risk. When a women is identified as having one of the major risk factors (atypia, LCIS, family history, or BRCA1/BRCA2 gene mutation), she can be presented with various treatment options that range from long-term surveillance to possible risk-reducing surgery to chemoprevention through the use of drugs.

The diagnosis of atypical hyperplasia or LCIS commonly occurs after a breast biopsy for a change in breast tissue (typically seen on screening mammogram). Atypical hyperplasia is an abnormal increase in the ductal or lobular cells within the breast and increases a woman's risk of developing an invasive breast cancer approximately 10 to 20% over a period of ten years. The risk is greater for premenopausal women and tends to decrease after menopause. A diagnosis of LCIS increases a woman's risk of developing an invasive breast cancer 25 to 40% over a period of twenty-five years, and this risk does not diminish over time.[3]

For women with a family history of breast or ovarian cancer, the risk is less clear. The amount of risk depends on the number of first- and second-degree relatives affected by the disease and the age of the family member at diagnosis. Also relevant are how closely related these relatives are to the patient and, to some degree, their prognosis with the disease itself. The risk increases greatly when there is a strong and significant breast cancer history: multiple first-degree relatives (parent, sibling, or child of either sex), an early-age diagnosis, and bilaterality.[4]

At present, researchers think that approximately 5 to 10% of breast cancer today is linked to either the BRCA1 or BRCA2 gene mutation.[5] Furthermore, these two gene mutations have possible links to the development of ovarian cancer, cancer of the colon and prostate, and even pancreatic cancer. However, breast cancer in general is most likely a genetic disease, and hypotheses exist that possibly 80% of breast cancer diagnosed before the age of 50 has some genetic link.[6] These cancers are believed to be linked to other gene mutations that have not yet been identified through genetic research.

Abnormalities in the BRCA1 and BRCA2 genes lead to a different degree of risk. A woman who carries the BRCA1 gene mutation has a risk of developing breast cancer ranging from 50 to 90% and a risk for developing ovarian cancer that ranges from 20 to 60%. A woman who carries the BRCA2 gene mutation has a 20 to 60% risk of developing breast cancer, but a lesser risk of ovarian cancer, approximately 15 to 30%. Also, it is thought that the BRCA2 gene may play a role in the development of cancer of the male breast.[7]

This broad statistical range demonstrates the lack of clarity in predicting risk, which makes treatment issues and decisions so difficult. The process of identifying women who carry these genetic alterations also is very controversial. These two gene mutations can be identified through a blood test, which was made available in 1995. Selecting appropriate women for such genetic testing is crucial, as it is not a test to take lightly.

A number of emotional, social, and physical consequences exist for any woman who undergoes genetic testing. Counseling should be mandatory before any testing for either of these gene mutations, because women should be aware of the risks and benefits of testing, as well as the risks and benefits of both a positive and negative result. A positive result can cause tremendous anxiety and fear, unleash the possibility of discrimination in employment and insurability, and cause a woman to search for answers that may not be available. A negative result can produce survivor guilt in an individual with a strong family history and indicates only that a woman should follow established screening guidelines. The possibility does exist that a negative result, in the context of a significant family history, means that another gene mutation not yet discovered may be the cause. The results of genetic testing can also affect family members, since they may or may not want to know such risk-related information. The decision to pursue genetic testing has to be made carefully, and women should be asked what changes they would make once they knew the results, whether positive or negative.

Treatment Options for High-Risk Women

Once a woman has been determined to be at high risk for the development of breast cancer, she must sort through her options, which consist of long-term surveillance, risk-reducing surgery, or chemoprevention. Each option is complex and has its own associated issues.

Long-term surveillance, the most conservative and least controversial option, is a model of intervention consisting of a multidisciplinary team to meet the woman's needs.[8] A breast specialist who provides the woman with frequent clinical exams (usually every three, four, or six months depending on her risk factors) usually heads this type of program. Mammography services are usually a component of such programs, with radiologists who specialize in reading mammograms of both high-risk women and those with breast cancer.

Nursing services usually focus on educating patients regarding breast self-exam along with answering questions related to being at high risk. Nutritional education is integral to any program for high-risk women. Controversies abound about many dietary issues, and the literature provides no clear answers on issues such as dietary fat, herbal products, vitamin supplements, soy, and alcohol consumption. Access to services such as smoking cessation programs, genetic counselors, and psychosocial resources is also part of a long-term surveillance program.

Risk-reducing surgery is another option for women who are at high risk. Some women mull over the option of a bilateral total mastectomy (removal of 98% of breast tissue from each side) to decrease their risk and possibly a bilateral oophorectomy to decrease their risk for ovarian cancer. Each option has its own controversies. The bilateral mastectomy can be performed for a woman at any age, but a woman must consider the risks and benefits of such a procedure along with the resultant effects on her relationships and lifestyle.

Breast reconstruction is an option for a woman who considers this procedure, but the reconstructed breast will never be the same as what she had; her scars are visible when she is undressed and sensations are changed. Furthermore, the literature is scant on the actual benefit of such a procedure; few longitudinal data have been kept on women who have had such a procedure. A recent study suggests, however, that women can reduce their risk of developing breast cancer by 90% and their risk of dying from breast cancer by 80% through prophylactic mastectomy.[9] Moreover, there is some thought in the research community that if an at-risk woman were to actually get breast cancer, with the current survival rates for early-stage localized disease at 97%, her life span would not be greatly altered.[10]

Another issue to consider is that being at high risk is not a guarantee that a woman will get breast cancer in her lifetime, indicating the prophylactic surgery may be unnecessary, and many women actually overestimate their true risk for breast cancer.[11] However, despite education and extensive psychosocial support from the multidisciplinary team, some women continue with persistent, unrealistic fear and anxiety. The surgery can be a therapeutic option to alleviate the anxiety that accompanies being at high risk. This point underscores how important it is for women considering this surgery to have a psychological assessment before the procedure.[12]

A prophylactic oophorectomy to decrease the possibility of developing ovarian cancer is an option for women who have the BRCA1 or BRCA2 gene mutation. Because an increased risk for ovarian cancer is associated with these two gene mutations, ovarian cancer has no proven method for screening, it is difficult to diagnose until its later stage, and survival rates are low, this procedure may also be a viable option. Premenopausal women who elect to have a prophylactic oophorectomy, however, face immediate symptoms from surgical menopause (hot flashes and vaginal dryness) and sequelae (increased risk for heart disease and osteoporosis). Estrogen replacement therapy (ERT) is an option, but with it comes the increased risk of breast cancer (unless the patient has had a prophylactic mastectomy). There is also conflicting evidence on ERT and its associated risks (discussed later in this chapter).

Another caveat to prophylactic oophorectomy is that it provides no guarantee against ovarian cancer. The actual risk after such surgery, however, is believed to be minimal.[13]

Any woman who considers prophylactic surgery also needs to consider the pyschosocial pieces of the puzzle. Important issues relate to the woman's perception of her breasts or ovaries to her esteem and body image. Whether the surgery will affect personal relationships and sexual functioning is an important issue for the woman to examine with her partner. If she is single, issues of future dating are paramount.

Chemoprevention is the third option that women at high risk can consider. Currently, the only FDA-approved drug for chemoprevention is tamoxifen (Nolvadex). The results of the Breast Cancer Prevention Trial released in April 1998 indicate that tamoxifen reduces the incidence of breast cancer by 45% when compared with placebo.[14] In November 1998, the FDA approved tamoxifen as a chemopreventive drug for high-risk women.

Chemoprevention with tamoxifen, however, has risks and side effects. The main risks include an increase in the possibility of the development of endometrial cancer, blood clots, and subsequent pulmonary embolus and the possibility of cataract formation and macular degeneration. The main side effects from the drug mimic those of menopause; approximately 45 to 60% of women actually experience bothersome hot flashes and, to a lesser extent, another potential side effect—vaginal dryness or discharge.[15] Weight gain, nausea, and depression are less common, but possible, side effects. The benefits with the drug include prevention of bone resorption, thereby protecting a woman from osteoporosis, and a reduction in cholesterol levels, possibly decreasing her risk of atherosclerosis and subsequent coronary artery disease.

Another drug that shows promise for chemoprevention is raloxifene (Evista), but it is not FDA approved for prevention of breast cancer. Raloxifene, a drug structurally similar to tamoxifen, is indicated for the prevention of osteoporosis. A clinical trial that examined the drug's effects showed an incidental decrease in breast cancer cases in women who took the drug.[16] This incidental finding has received much attention, but until further studies clarify these data, raloxifene is indicated only for osteoporosis prevention. A large study is planned for the coming decade; the STAR trial (the study of tamoxifen and raloxifene) will enroll 23,000 women and compare which drug is a more efficacious preventive.

A nurse's key intervention for women at increased risk is to provide information about their options and discuss their concerns about the risks and benefits of each choice. Providing concrete ways to explore their options, such as talking with other women who have undergone similar decision making and providing written educational materials, can help with this process. Also, reinforcing appropriate screening behaviors, lifestyle and behavior modifications, and risk reduction is another nursing intervention for women at risk. Anxiety management is an important consideration; unlike a cancer diagnosis, which peaks in crisis and resolution, the label "high risk" is one a woman carries throughout her lifetime. Reinforcing positive coping strategies is essential. No easy answer exists for at-risk women, and education and psychosocial support remain the focus for helping them.

✳ CONTROVERSIES IN BREAST CANCER SCREENING

Breast cancer screening provides for early detection, better treatment options, and subsequently increased survival rates when diagnosis occurs. How to best screen the women in the general public has some clear guidelines along with some controversial issues.

Table 17.2 identifies the reasons women avoid screening. Nurses can be influential in increasing adherence to screening by informing the public through education and outreach. Target audiences, such as minority groups and women in rural areas, need information and access to screening. Furthermore, research has shown that social support can have a positive impact on obtaining screening.[17]

Mammography

In conjunction with an annual clinical examination by a health care provider and a woman's own monthly self-exam, mammography has become standard for women in the screening of breast cancer. Its sensitivity approaches 90%.

Recently, many have focused attention on the appropriate age to begin screening. Much of the focus examined the usefulness of mammography for women between the ages of 40 and 50; previous recommendations had been confusing and vague for providers and women themselves. After much debate, discussion, and review of the literature, the National Cancer Institute (NCI) and the American Cancer Society (ACS) have come to the conclusion that mammography for women should begin by age 40 and continue yearly thereafter.[18] The reason for the controversy lies in the fact that breast cancer risk increases significantly after the age of 50. Women between 40 and 50 years of age have a 25% chance of a false-negative or incomplete evaluation because the breast tissue of younger women is so dense.

TABLE 17.2
Reasons Women Avoid Breast Cancer Screening
Lack of physician or health care provider recommendation
Misconception that, without symptoms, there is no need for screening
Lack of awareness about mammography, BSE, and yearly clinical exams
Cost or lack of health insurance
Fear of cancer detection
Fear of radiation exposure
Fear of pain associated with the procedure
Inability to speak English or lack of fluency in English
Cultural beliefs and values not consistent with preventive medical care
Lack of social support for screening
Inconvenience associated with life responsibilities (work, child care, etc.)

In women over the age of 50, the false-negative rate is only 10%.[20] This finding serves mainly to emphasize the importance of combining self-exam and clinical exam for breast cancer screening. On the question of the age at which a woman should have a baseline mammogram, in 1997, the NCI and ACS conceded that it should be done between the ages of 35 and 40 and then yearly after that.

Ultrasonography

The use of ultrasonography as a screening tool for breast cancer has sparked an ongoing debate among health care professionals. Ultrasound is useful in the diagnosis of breast problems identified through either mammographic findings or clinical exam. This procedure can identify whether a mass is fluid filled (if so, it is most likely a cyst, which is a benign process) or a solid lesion (which would require some form of diagnostic procedure, usually a biopsy). The controversy rises, however, when ultrasonography is used for routine screening.

For women with dense breasts (typically younger women or women on hormone replacement), mammography can be of limited use in detecting a mass, lesion, or microcalcifications; the chance of a missed finding is approximately 25%.[21] Figure 17.1 shows the difference between a dense and a fatty breast.

For women with dense breasts, a screening ultrasound can aid in the possible early diagnosis of a cancer; it is a painless procedure that poses no risk of radiation exposure.[22] It can significantly increase the accuracy of screening for breast cancer in this subset of women. A drawback, however, is that ultrasonography is more likely to detect areas that may need further investigation, usually a biopsy to prove they are benign. If implemented on a more routine and widescale basis as an adjunct to mam-

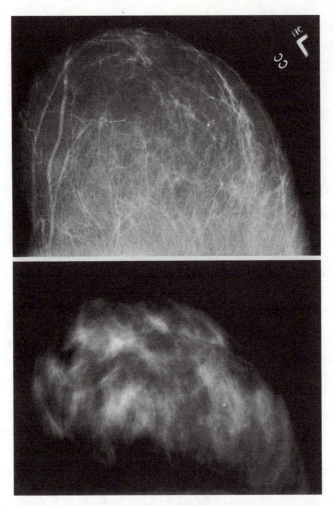

FIGURE 17.1. Comparison of (*top*) dense breast tissue and (*bottom*) fatty breast tissue.

mography, this procedure and subsequent biopsies could significantly increase the costs of screening.[23] Further research will help to define the role of sonography in screening for breast cancer.

Nurses' Role in Breast Cancer Screening

For screening to be effective in the early detection of breast cancer, women in our society need to follow the suggested guidelines. Nurses can be influential in guiding women to have mammography, do breast self-exam (BSE), and have a yearly clinical exam. Providing education and enabling women to have access to resources are two interventions in which nursing has been very successful already. Nursing research into the areas of compliance, BSE performance, and motivations and barriers to screening will provide important further insight into these issues.

✳ SENTINEL LYMPH NODE BIOPSY AND AXILLARY LYMPH NODE DISSECTION

Axillary lymph node dissection has been the standard for staging, prognosis indication, and determination of adjuvant treatments in women with breast cancer.[24] This procedure is usually done in conjunction with the surgical treatment of the breast (either complete removal or a limited resection) as the definitive surgery. The procedure, however, usually requires general anesthesia and has been associated with various chronic morbidities (lymphedema, pain, neuropathies, and impaired mobility). Because of early detection of breast cancer through enhanced usage of screening over the last two decades, approximately 60–70% of women with Stage I breast cancer have negative axillary lymph nodes at the time of surgery.[25] This statistic led to the idea that dissection was perhaps unnecessary for a select subset of surgical patients, and other ways of identifying the nodal status could be developed.

The introduction of the sentinel lymph node biopsy in breast cancer treatment began in the mid-1990s after the procedure was shown to reduce the number of lymph node dissections in patients with malignant melanoma.[26] The procedure identifies the presence of the sentinel node with a scan called a *lymphoscintigram*. A radioactive blue dye that turns the sentinel node blue is injected immediately before the surgery. If biopsy of the sentinal node is negative, the patient requires no further axillary surgery and the surgeon proceeds with the breast surgery. If the node is positive for cancer, then the patient undergoes the standard axillary dissection. Patients are prepared prior to the surgery for this either/or scenario.

Breast surgeons explored the use of this procedure and found that the sentinel lymph node (the primary node that drains the breast) is an accurate predictor of the rest of the lymph nodes in the axillary region. Early studies indicate that the accuracy rate for women with Stage I tumors (2 cm or less) approached 98%, but for women with Stage II tumors (2 cm or greater) the rate dropped to 82%.[27] Currently a number of studies continue to further define the population of women who will benefit from the procedure, the best technique, and the pathologic accuracy of this approach. However, because of significant early research results, the sentinel lymph node biopsy is now being offered to women with tumors 2 cm or less as an alternative to standard lymph node dissections.

The benefits of this procedure to the patient are several: it involves a less extensive surgery than standard dissection, with less time in the hospital, fewer complications, no need for a surgical drain, and a decrease in the associated morbidities. Table 17.3 compares patient expectations for the two procedures.

Controversies do exist over this procedure, however, the most prominent one being the issue of lymphedema. Women who have had standard axillary dissections face a 15% risk for lymphedema. They are taught special hand and arm care to decrease the possibility of its development.[28]

No data exist on the risk of lymphedema for women with sentinel lymph node biopsy. Since lymphedema can occur months or even years after surgery, the question arises of what we should teach our patients who have undergone this procedure. The-

<table>
<tr><td colspan="3" align="center">**TABLE 17.3**</td></tr>
<tr><td colspan="3" align="center">Sentinel Node Biopsy Compared with Axillary Lymph Node Dissection</td></tr>
</table>

Patient Expectations	*Sentinel Node Biopsy without Axillary Dissection*	*Sentinel Node Biopsy with Axillary Dissection*
Length of hospital stay	Discharge same day	Discharge after 24–48 hours
Pain/discomfort	Minimal	Varies, but some to be expected
Drain management	No—but there is a possibility of seroma formation several days after procedure	Yes—instruction to be provided before discharge home
Range of Motion and Exercises	Usually no impact on range of motion, but exercises may be needed if discomfort is present	Limited range of motion, but with exercise regimen, full range of motion returns in 4–6 weeks
Sensations in affected extremity	No—some initial numbness possible, but it resolves within short period	Yes—to be expected after procedure; they usually increase and persist for several months afterward
Hand and arm care instruction	No—risk for lymphedema is minimal to nonexistent	Yes—prevention of injury or infection to the affected extremity is necessary to decrease the possibility of developing lymphedema
Incision care	May shower second day after procedure and wash incisions with soap and water	Showering, incision and dressing care dependent on surgeon preference

Source: Adapted with permission from CJON

oretically, the risk for lymphedema is believed to be minimal; however, there has nonetheless been a disruption within the axillary tissues, which potentially could cause altered collateral circulation, thus increasing the risk.

Nursing research in this area of patient care is needed to answer several questions related to sentinel node biopsy: (1) Is there an increased risk in patients for the development of lymphedema, (2) can certain factors be identified within this population that increase risk, and (3) is there a subset of patients that requires special hand and arm care similar to that taught to women with the standard axillary dissections?

Nursing standards of care need to be developed for this new technology and, at present, no consensus exists. Nurses can have an impact on this care issue through investigation.

✖ SHORT-TERM HOSPITAL STAY FOR BREAST CANCER SURGERY

The trend in the past decade has been to shorten the length of hospital stay for women who undergo breast cancer surgery (mastectomy procedures and axillary lymph node dissections). Most institutions have limited stays to 24–48 hours for these procedures, and the care that was traditionally provided during longer stays in the hospital now takes place in the ambulatory setting.[29] Benefits of short-term hospital stays include a decrease in costs, which has been the driving force behind this change in health care delivery, and an increase in patient independence, which enhances self-esteem and recovery.

For patients to receive appropriate care, however, the health care system requires a structure that provides for adequate preoperative and postoperative education and access to health care professionals for questions and concerns and the reporting of possible complications, usually through telephone contact. Most patients find satisfaction with a short-term stay, as long as they are prepared to manage the sequelae of surgery (management of the drainage device, pain, and recovery needs).

Meeting these patients' psychosocial needs becomes the challenge. In the past, the hospital stay provided a buffer for patients to adjust to the diagnosis and surgical treatment before returning to their life activities.[30] Also, in the hospital setting, patients usually found support from other women who had undergone the same or similar surgeries. With shortened stays, the buffer is eliminated along with proximity to other breast cancer patients, unless the patient seeks it through outpatient support groups.

Another drawback of short-term stay is that patients must rely on care providers outside the health care system, usually family or friends, to assist in care needs and recovery. Referrals to home care nursing agencies have filled this postsurgical care gap. Home care nurses, however, though quite knowledgeable about many illnesses, may not have the same specialized skills and knowledge as the hospital-based nurses who have cared for these patients. Additionally, insurance may not cover an adequate number of home care visits—a problem for patients who require additional care after their short-term stay. At present, ambulatory care nurses are required to fill this gap.

Nurses need to address these various issues to ensure that breast cancer surgical patients' care needs are met after discharge. They must provide adequate instruction prior to surgery through individual teaching sessions or group classes and reinforce content with written materials. Assessing the patient's resources for assistance at home needs to occur before admission for the surgery and referrals to home care agencies made at the appropriate time to ensure a visit within twenty-four hours of discharge. Telephone follow-up by either the ambulatory nurse or the discharge nurse is necessary to make sure the patient has adjusted to the transition from hospital to home and also to identify any care issues that may have arisen since the discharge.[31]

Ongoing contact by telephone may be necessary before and even after the postoperative visit with the surgeon. The psychosocial adjustment after surgery requires assessment also. The patient's adjustment to the surgical site, body image changes, overall cancer prognosis and further treatment issues, and awareness of postoperative sensations and other expectations all require follow-up from the ambulatory setting; many of these issues used to be addressed in the inpatient setting. Providing the patient with access to support groups also becomes necessary, since the benefits of psychosocial support of other breast cancer survivors cannot be overlooked.

As short-term stays for breast cancer surgery become standard in our health care system, the shift in care requires organization and resources. Nurses play a key role in helping patients recover outside the hospital setting.

HORMONE REPLACEMENT IN BREAST CANCER SURVIVORS

Estrogen replacement therapy (ERT), a controversial issue for women in the general population, has received a great deal of attention from the media, health care providers, researchers, and the women affected by it. The risks and benefits of using estrogen products after menopause have been debated and health care providers cannot come to consensus on these issues. The beneficial effects of ERT are now being explored in women who have survived breast cancer.[32]

Beneficial Effects of ERT

The hot flashes, night sweats, and insomnia that 75% of women experience as a result of estrogen deficiency can greatly interfere with the quality and function of life. Many women seek relief through estrogen replacement.[33] ERT has been demonstrated to quickly alleviate these symptoms of menopause. Furthermore, urogenital atrophy along with lack of vaginal lubrication, urinary frequency, urgency, and urge incontinence can also be problematic and distressing for women. These symptoms lead women to seek relief, and ERT is the most common form of prescribed treatment for women in the general population.

In addition to these immediate effects, ERT has been proved to decrease a woman's risk for cardiovascular disease by 20 to 50%.[34] By lowering levels of low-density lipoproteins (LDL) and raising those of high-density lipoproteins (HDL), ERT improves cardiovascular status, thus providing protection against heart disease, the leading cause of death for women in our society. This beneficial effect has been another primary reason for using ERT. It also has a beneficial effect in osteoporosis prevention, another health problem for women in our society. ERT can prevent the bone loss that occurs due to age and decreased estrogen levels, resulting in a 50% reduction in osteoporotic-associated fractures.[35]

Possible Risks of ERT

A risk of developing endometrial cancer exists for the woman with an intact uterus who takes ERT unopposed by progesterone. The addition of progesterone either as a supplement or in combination form with the estrogen has mostly resolved this issue. The risk for breast cancer, however, remains controversial. Some studies have shown an increase in risk for the development of breast cancer, as much as 30–80% greater than in nonusers of ERT,[36] while other studies contradict this finding,[37] suggesting that there is no increase in risk. Moreover, some researchers suggest that it is not ERT itself that increases risk, but rather the overall exposure to both endogenous hormones and exogenous hormone products. This thought only complicates matters for patients in their understanding and decision making.

Decision Making for Women in the General Population

Because of the associated risk for the development of breast cancer, many women are concerned about taking ERT. Since approximately 46% of women in the general population are at greater risk for heart disease, and osteoporosis affects 50% of women by the age of 75, there are definite benefits to taking ERT. The lifetime risk for a hip fracture equals that of the combined risks for breast and gynecologic cancers.[38] The lifetime risk for breast cancer is 10% for women without risk factors.[39] The decision to take ERT is not an easy one. All the factors need to be explored; family history of both heart disease and osteoporosis along with the family history for cancer should be considered. Also, the individual risk factors for each disease need to be considered (see Table 17.4).

The nurse's role within this process focuses on allowing a woman to verbalize her concerns about the risks and benefits and on clarifying misconceptions. Also, educating her on reducing risk for these diseases through diet, exercise, smoking cessation, and decreased alcohol consumption allows a woman to see that alternative choices are available. Furthermore, by providing referral to a nutritional specialist, the issues of diet can be further illuminated, specifically dietary fat reduction, calcium supplementation, and the use of other vitamins and herbal products. Providing the woman with written information and education materials or access to the numerous sites on the Internet about what is known can also be helpful. Informing a symptomatic woman that nonhormonal methods are available to manage the symptoms of menopause helps her to understand she has a choice (see Table 17.5).

Given all this information, a woman can make her decision about whether or not to use ERT. One of the most important considerations in this issue is the family history; a history of heart disease or osteoporosis would lead many women toward ERT, but a family history of breast cancer may cause some women to avoid this option. The nurse can be an influential component in this important process in helping the woman to make a decision by clarifying misconceptions, illuminating alternatives, and allowing her to identify and address her concerns.

TABLE 17.4
Risk Factors for Cardiovascular Disease and Osteoporosis

Risk Factors for Cardiovascular Disease	Risk Factors for Osteoporosis
Obesity	Caucasian and Asian racial heritage
Smoking	Estrogen deficiency
Family history of cardiovascular disease or hypertension	Early menopause, usually iatrogenic
	Thin body frame
Hypercholesterolemia	Prolonged immobilization
Diabetes mellitus	Sedentary lifestyle
Sedentary lifestyle	Alcoholism
High-fat diet	Family history of osteoporosis
	Smoking
	Deficiency in dietary calcium
	Chronic renal disease
	Medications (steroids, heparin)

ERT and Breast Cancer Survivors

Because of the beneficial effects of ERT and the resultant effects of menopause from either aging or cancer treatments, health care professionals and women have been considering ERT in cancer survivors. Heart disease remains the leading cause of death in long-term cancer survivors,[40] and ERT can decrease this possible occurrence. Also, premature menopause due to chemotherapy is associated with more intense symptoms. However, many data support a strong association between estrogen exposure (both endogenous and exogenous) and breast cancer development.[38] Also, blocking estrogen exposure, either through oophorectomy or use of tamoxifen, is a proven method to increase survival outcomes for women with breast cancer.[41]

Some studies have been done on breast cancer survivors who have received ERT with a suggestion that its usage has not affected disease recurrence,[42] and other studies suggest that no good data exist for this issue, as many of the studies have confounding variables.[40] Long-term prospective randomized studies are needed to provide more definitive information on this subject.

Until more information becomes available through research, most oncologists and gynecologists still view ERT in breast cancer survivors with extreme caution, but it is an option in certain individual cases.[43] Clearly outlining the risks and benefits to a woman is necessary, if ERT is a consideration.

The nurse's role within this dilemma is similar to that for women within the gen-

TABLE 17.5

Nonhormonal Management of Menopause

Menopausal Problems	Alternative Considerations

Vasomotor
  Hot flashes
  Sweats
  Flushing
  Palpitations
	Clonidine, megestrol acetate, belladonna alkaloids, fluoxetine hydrochloride, phytoestrogen, soy, vitamins E and B_6, biofeedback/relaxation techniques

Urogenital
  Vaginal dryness
  Painful intercourse
  Frequent urinary tract infections
	Vaginal lubricants/moisturizers, vaginal estrogen creams, vaginal estrogen ring device, vitamin E suppository

Osteoporosis
  Increasing bone fractures
  (especially hip and vertebrae)
	Biphosphonates, calcium supplements, calcitonin, diet, weight-bearing exercise

Heart Disease
  Hyperlipidemia
  Cardiovascular vessel disease
	Cholesterol-reducing drugs, low-fat diet, exercise program

Somatic
  Generalized, diminished well-being
  Depression
  Sleep disturbances
  Memory problems
	Medications, herbal preparations, short-term use of antidepressants

Source: Reprinted with permission from ONF

eral population, but the issues may be different. Fear of recurrence may cause a woman to avoid ERT, while bothersome and problematic symptoms that may affect the quality of life may facilitate a decision to take ERT. Assisting in symptom management and identifying alternatives to the use of ERT are important interventions for the nurse to provide. Patient education and supportive counseling throughout this process are necessary.

❀ BREAST CANCER AND PREGNANCY

Another controversial issue is pregnancy after breast cancer. Since 10 to 20% of women diagnosed with breast cancer are of childbearing age, pregnancy has become an issue for certain women who have survived the disease. The decision to have children is often delayed in our society for personal, professional, and educational reasons. This becomes a quality-of-life issue, because many women want to resume their life roles after completing breast cancer treatment. For young women, especially those whose menstrual cycles return after they have completed adjuvant treatment, childbearing and becoming a mother are of paramount importance.

A woman's hormonal milieu is a well-documented potential risk factor for the development of breast cancer.[1] Prolonged exposure to uninterrupted menstruation due to early menarche, late menopause, nulliparity, and pregnancy after age 30 all have a possible effect on the development of breast cancer. Therefore, estrogen exposure from pregnancy, with hormone levels 1,000 times greater than a menstrual cycle, has been presented with a theoretic significantly increased risk of recurrence. The limited number of studies and small numbers of patients included in the analyses leave this issue unresolved.[44]

The studies that have explored the issue of pregnancy safety after breast cancer show no increase of risk of recurrence.[45] This finding could be due to collection bias, meaning women who did become pregnant and subsequently did or did not survive because of recurrent cancer were not identified for data analysis. Also, to date, no prospective studies explore this issue. Based on theoretic principles and laboratory and research data, the intense gestational hormones could stimulate micrometastases, an issue of great concern. Ethical issues that present themselves within this discussion are the possibility that the disease could recur at some time after the birth of the child, and its potential effects on the child's development—such as the mother's ongoing treatment which would distract her from childrearing or even the possibility that the child may grow up without a mother because of her death from breast cancer.

Without good long-term data, physicians are left in a quandary as what to recommend for women. Many oncologists recommend waiting two to three years after completing treatment before becoming pregnant. The majority of recurrences occur within this time frame, so by waiting women theoretically have a lesser chance of recurrence. However, some data suggest that no increased risk occurred for women who had a child less than two years after diagnosis.[46] Such a discussion should also include other alternatives to pregnancy for women to consider, such as adoption or engaging the service of a surrogate mother.

The role of the nurse for women who are considering pregnancy after completion of treatment focuses on acting as a sounding board for all these issues. Once the woman and her partner have been presented with the information on the risks and benefits, helping the woman and her partner explore their personal values, beliefs, and concerns is key. Clarifying misconceptions and answering questions as women struggle with this issue is an important aspect of nursing care. For some women, the inability to have a child because of iatrogenic infertility or the choice due to concern about recurrence stimulates grief, loss, and a period of adjustment. The nurse's supportive approach and identification of positive coping strategies can facilitate the patient's movement through this period. Possible referrals to psychosocial resources and counseling, such as psychiatry, support groups, or community resources, may be necessary.

✳ SUMMARY

As women deal with these controversies related to breast cancer, nurses need to keep updated on current information so they can provide accurate information and education. Also, listening to the concerns that surround these issues is necessary, as this intervention helps to guide women in some resolution with one choice or another. Furthermore, only further scientific and medical research can help to provide additional information that may elucidate these issues for these women. Nursing research that explores how women deal with these issues, patterns of coping and decision making, and symptom management is warranted.

✳ REFERENCES

1. Vogel, V.G. (1996). Assessing women's potential risk of developing breast cancer. *Oncology, 10*(10), 1451–1461.
2. Osbourne, M., & Borgen, P. (1993). Atypical ductal and lobular hyperplasia and breast cancer risk. *Surg Oncol Clin North Am, 2*(1), 1–11.
3. Kinne, D. (1993). Lobular carcinoma in situ. *Surg Oncol Clin North Am, 2*(1), 65–73.
4. Bilimoria, M., & Morrow, M. (1995). The woman at increased risk for breast cancer: Evaluation and management strategies. *CA Cancer J Clin, 45*(5), 263–278.
5. Tranin, A.S. (1996). Genetics and breast cancer risk. In K.H. Dow, ed., *Contemporary Issues in Breast Cancer* (pp. 3–18). Boston: Jones and Bartlett.
6. Hughes, K.S., & Roche, C.A. (1996). How do we apply genetic testing for breast cancer susceptibility to clinical practice? *Surg Oncol, 62,* 155–157.
7. Lessick, M., Wickham, R., & Rehwalt, M. (1997). Breast and ovarian cancer: genetic update and implications for nursing. *Medsurg Nursing, 6*(6), 341–352.
8. Gross, R.E., Van Zee, K.J., & Heerdt, A.S. (1997). The special surveillance breast program: A model of intervention for women at high risk for breast cancer. *J NY State Nurses Assoc, 28*(4), 9–12.
9. Hartmann, L.C., Schaid, D.J., Woods, J.E., et. al. (1999). Efficacy of a bilateral mastectomy in women with a family history of breast cancer. *N Engl J Med, 340*(2), 77–84.
10. Schrag, D., Kuntz, K.M., Garber, J.E., et. al. (1997). Decision analysis: Effects of prophylactic mastectomy and oophorectomy on life expectancy among women with BRCA1 and BRCA2 mutations. *N Engl J Med, 336*(20), 1465–1471.
11. Gagnon, P., Massie, M.J., Kash, K.M., et. al. (1996). Perception of breast cancer risk and psychological distress in women attending a surveillance program. *Psycho-Oncology, 5,* 259–269.
12. Baron, R.H., & Borgen, P.I. (1997). Genetic susceptibility testing for breast cancer: Testing and primary prevention options. *Oncol Nurs Forum, 23*(4), 461–468.
13. Weitzel, J.N., & MacDonald, D.J. (1998). Genetic testing for ovarian cancer risk. *Quality of Life—A Nursing Challenge, 6*(4),101–108.
14. Fisher, B., Costantino, J.P., Wickerham, D.L., et. al. (1998). Tamoxifen for prevention of breast cancer: Report of the national surgical adjuvant breast and bowel project p-1 study. *J Natl Cancer Inst, 90*(18), 1371–1388.
15. Pasacreta, J.V., & McCorkle, R. (1998). Providing accurate information to women about

tamoxifen therapy for breast cancer: Current indications, effects, and controversies. *Oncol Nurs Forum, 25*(9).

16. Cummings, S.R., Norton, L., Eckert, S., et al. (1998). Raloxifene reduces the risk of breast cancer and may decrease the risk of endometrial cancer in postmenopausal women. Two-year findings from the Multiple Outcomes of Raloxifene Evaluation (MORE) trial (abstract). *Proc Am Soc Clin Oncol, 17:* 2a.

17. McCance, K.L., Mooney, K.H., Field, R., & Smith, K.R. (1996). Influence of others in motivating women to obtain cancer screening. *Cancer Pract, 4*(3), 141–155.

18. National Institutes of Health. (1997). Consensus statement: Breast cancer screening for women ages 40–49. 15(1).

19. Gail, M.H., & Rimer, B.K. (1998). Risk-based recommendations for mammographic screening for women in their forties. *J Clin Oncol, 16*, 3105–3114.

20. Kolb, T.M., Lichy, J., & Newhouse, J.H. (1998). Occult cancer in women with dense breasts: Detection with screening US: Diagnostic yield and tumor characteristics. *Radiology, 207*, 191–199.

21. Harris, R., & Leininger, L. (1995). Clinical strategies for breast cancer screening: Weighing and using the evidence. *Ann Intern Med, 122*(7), 539–547.

22. Farria, D.M., Mund, D.F., & Bassett, L.W. (1995). Evaluation of missed cancers using screening mammography. *Am J Radiol, 126*, 1645.

23. Brown, D.W., French, M.T., Schweitzer, M.E., et.al. (1999). Economic evaluation of breast cancer screening. *Cancer Pract, 7*(1), 28–33.

24. Tyler, T. (1998). The medical management of breast cancer. *Prim Care Practitioner, 2*(2), 176–183.

25. Guiliano, A.E., Barth, A.M., Spivack, B., et. al. (1996). Incidence and predictors of axillary metastasis in T1 carcinoma of the breast. *J Am Coll Surg, 183*, 185–189.

26. Morton, D.L., Wen, D.R., Wong, J.H., et. al. (1992). Technical detail of intraoperative lymphatic mapping for early stage melanoma. *Arch Surg, 127*, 392–399.

27. O'Hea, B.J., Hill, A., El-Shirbiny, A.M., et. al. (1998). Sentinel lymph node biopsy in breast cancer: Initial experience at Memorial Sloan-Kettering Cancer Center. *J Am Coll Surg, 186*, 423–427.

28. Marcks, P. (1997). Lymphedema: Pathogenesis, prevention, and treatment. *Cancer Pract, 5*, 32–38.

29. Burke, C.C., Zabka, C.L., McCarver, K.J., et al. (1997). Patient satisfaction with 23-hour "short stay" observation following breast cancer surgery. *Oncol Nurs Forum, 24*(4).

30. Gross, R.E. (1998). Current issues in the surgical treatment of early stage breast cancer. *Clin J Oncol Nurs, 2*(2), 55–63.

31. Young Summers, B.L., & Chisholm, L.M. (1997). Opportunities and challenges for oncology nursing in ambulatory cancer care. *Oncology Nursing Updates: Patient Treatment and Support, 4*(1).

32. DiSaia, P.J. (1996). Hormone replacement in the gynecologic and breast cancer patient. *Cancer Control, 3*(2), 101–106.

33. Appling, S.E. (1996). Hormone replacement therapy: Helping your patient decide. *Med-Surg Nurs, 5*(5), 370–373.

34. Smith, H.O., Kammerer-Doak, D.N., Barbo, D.M., et. al. (1996). Hormone replacement therapy in menopause: A pro opinion. *CA Cancer J Clin, 46*(6), 343–363.

35. Smith, A., & Hughes, P.L. (1998). The estrogen dilemma. *Am J Nurs, 98*(4), 17–20.

36. Colditz, G.A., Hankinson, S.E., Hunter, D.J., et. al. (1995). The use of estrogens and progestins and the risk of breast cancer in postmenopausal women. *N Engl J Med, 332*(24), 1589–1593.

37. Stanford, J.L., Weiss, N.S., Voight, L.F., et. al. (1995). Combined estrogen and progestin hormone replacement therapy in relation to risk of breast cancer in middle-aged women. *JAMA, 274*(2), 137–142.

38. Woods, N.F. (1996). Cancer risk controversies: Women' exposure to exogenous ovarian hormones. *Oncology Nursing Updates: Patient Treatment and Support, 2*(1), 1–16.

39. Appling, S. (1996). One in nine: Risks and prevention strategies for breast cancer. *Med-Surg Nurs, 5*(1), 62–64.

40. Snyder, G.M., Sielsch, E.C., & Reville, B. (1998). The controversy of hormone-replacement therapy in breast cancer survivors. *Oncol Nurs Forum, 25*(4).

41. Jaiyesimi, I.A., et.al. (1995). The use of tamoxifen for breast cancer: Twenty-eight years later. *J Clin Oncol, 13*(2), 513–529.

42. Cobleigh, M.A. (1997). Hormone replacement therapy in breast cancer survivors. *Diseases of the Breast Updates, 1*(2), 1–10.

43. American College of Gynecologists Committee on Gynecological Practice. (1994). Estrogen replacement therapy in women with pre-viously treated breast cancer. *Int J Gynaecol Obstet, 45,* 184–188.

44. Canty, L. (1997). Breast cancer risk: Protective effect of an early first full-term pregnancy versus increased risk of induced abortion. *Oncol Nurs Forum, 24*(6).

45. Surbone, A., & Petrek, J.A. (1997). Childbearing issues in breast carcinoma survivors. *Cancer, 79*(7), 1271–1277.

46. Baron, R.H. (1994). Dispelling the myths of pregnancy-associated breast cancer. *Oncol Nurs Forum, 21*(3), 507–512.

CHAPTER 18

Complementary and Alternative Medicine

Giselle J. Moore-Higgs, ARNP

✖ INTRODUCTION

One of the most impressive qualities of the human psyche is its ability to withstand severe personal tragedy successfully. Despite serious setbacks, such as personal illness or the death of a family member, most people facing such tragedy achieve a quality of life or level of happiness equivalent to or even exceeding their prior level of satisfaction.[1] Not everyone readjusts, of course,[2] but most do, and furthermore they do so substantially on their own. The theory of cognitive adaptation suggests that when an individual has experienced a personally threatening event such as an illness, the readjustment process focuses around three themes: a search for meaning in the experience, an attempt to regain mastery over the event in particular and one's life more generally, and an effort to enhance one's self-esteem—to feel good about oneself again despite the setback.[3]

Cancer, as a collective of over 100 diseases, is a chronic illness. It is expected to become the major cause of death in the United States by the year 2000. Traditionally, a cancer diagnosis has been regarded as a death sentence marked by pain and the loss of functional independence. With the advent of new diagnostic and therapeutic technology, cancer has been reconceptualized as a chronic disease characterized by episodic acute morbidities.[4] Working from the theory of cognitive adaptation, logic would indicate that cancer survivors may also enter a period of readjustment, attempt to gain mastery over the diagnosis and the outcome of treatment, to regain control over their lives including quality of life, and to enhance their self-esteem. Strategic decisions of cancer survivors may include the use of complementary and alternative medicine (CAM) practices, either as "alternatives" to traditional cancer treatment (chemotherapy, surgery, and radiation therapy) or as a complementary or adjuvant therapy.

With the amount of information available to the public and a recent drive to integrate CAM therapies into orthodox Western medicine clinical paths, health care providers must be aware of the potential benefits and risks associated with these therapies. This chapter provides an overview of the current understanding of CAM practices and provide nurses with a method for evaluating research and guiding patients to the appropriate resources.

✖ OVERVIEW OF CAM PRACTICES

The popularity and availability of CAM has increased significantly in the United States during the past fifteen years. Eisenberg et al. conducted a national survey to determine the prevalence, costs, and patterns of use of unconventional therapies, such as acupuncture and chiropractic.[5] They found the frequency of use of these therapies was far higher than previously reported: 33.8% of respondents reported use of at least one unconventional therapy in the past year, and one-third of these respondents reported visits to a "provider" for the therapy. The latter group had made an average of nineteen visits to such providers during the preceding year, at an average charge of $27.60 per visit. In a follow-up study by Eisenberg et al., 42.1% of adult American respondents reported use of at least one of sixteen alternative therapies during the previous year, an increase of 8.3% (P ≤.001) from the 1993 report.[6] The probability of users visiting an alternative medicine practitioner increased from 36.3% to 46.3% (P = .002). Modalities such as relaxation techniques, herbal medicine, massage, homeopathy, and energy healing all gained in popularity during the past decade. Visits to alternative therapy practitioners continued to outpace visits to primary care providers, and adult Americans spent more than $27 billion for treatment.[6]

These data are similar to those analyzed from a general probability sample (N = 3450) of the 1994 Robert Wood Johnson Foundation National Access to Care Survey. The survey indicated that nearly 10% of the population of the United States saw a professional in 1994 for at least one of the following four therapies: chiropractic, relaxation techniques, therapeutic massage, or acupuncture.[7] Among individuals with cancer, research indicates that anywhere from 9% to 94% of patients choose CAM practices along with orthodox Western medicine.[8] The extensive range of percentages is the result of widely varied definitions of terms and methods of data collection.

It has been speculated that a multiplicity of reasons lies behind the increased popularity of alternative therapies. They include a rise in chronic disease, greater access to health information, reduced tolerance for paternalism, and increasing demands for quality of life.[9] Eisenberg et al. found that 42% of all alternative therapies used were exclusively attributed to treatment of existing illness, whereas 58% were used, at least in part, to "prevent future illness from occurring or to maintain health and vitality."[6]

CAM practices stress the importance of the holistic approach: seeing the mind and body as inseparable and capable of self-repair if the individual is ready to take an active part in his or her own healing and general welfare.[10] Recently, acceptance of the concept of CAM has taken hold within orthodox Western health care. Originally initiated by congressional mandate in 1992 as the Office of Alternative Medicine, the National Center for Complementary and Alternative Medicine (NCCAM) was established in 1998 under provisions of the Omnibus Appropriations Bill.[11]

The mandate stated that the center's purpose was to "facilitate the evaluation of alternative medical treatment modalities" to determine their effectiveness. The mandate also provided for a public information clearinghouse and a research training program. The stated mission of the NCCAM is to conduct and support basic and applied research and training and disseminate information on complementary and alternative medicine to practitioners and the public. The fiscal year budget in 1993 was $2 million and has dramatically increased to an estimated $50 million in 1999.[11] The NCCAM has six functional areas: extramural affairs, research database and evaluation, clearinghouse and media relations, international and professional liaison, research development and investigation, and intramural research training.[11]

In recent years, the rising costs of health care and the concern that some testing and treatment practices are unnecessary or inappropriate have stimulated a critical appraisal of health care practices and the development of clinical guidelines. The development of practice guidelines in CAM has been limited because of lack of relevant outcomes data from well-designed clinical trials. Now, with more CAM practices being evaluated by accepted research methods, measurable and objective end points, and meaningful patient outcomes, more insurers, hospitals, medical schools, and nursing schools are incorporating CAM into their networks.

A reflection of this move into the mainstream is the expert panel recommendations for the integration of CAM into medical and nursing education. Held in 1996, the panel was cosponsored by the USUHS and NCCAM. The recommendations of the blue-ribbon panel entail the following:[12]

1. Medical and nursing education should include information about complementary practices.
2. Medical and nursing education about each complementary practice should include information about the discipline's philosophical/spiritual paradigm, scientific foundation, educational preparation, practice, and evidence of efficacy and safety.
3. National centers of excellence should continue to be developed to foster collaboration among complementary practitioners, nurses, and physicians and to promote synergy among education, research, and clinical practice.

Another example of the move into the mainstream was the November 11, 1998, issue of the *Journal of the American Medical Association (JAMA)*, as well as all of the AMA Archives journals, which featured alternative medicine as the theme of their annual coordinated issues. The editors received more than 200 manuscript submissions for *JAMA* alone, with many more received by the Archives journals' editors. As a result, they published eighty articles and editorials across the ten journals, covering thirty topics from sixteen countries.[9] An example of the type and quality of the research was the inclusion of the results of six randomized trials of alternative therapies evaluating procedures such as chiropractic manipulation and moxibustion published in *JAMA*.

Definition and Classification System

The definition of CAM is open to some interpretation and discussion even though many of the therapies have millions of followers and many CAM practices have existed longer than current conventional nursing and medical practices.[13] During a conference held by the OAM in April 1995, the Panel on Definition and Description defined CAM as follows:

> Complementary and alternative medicine (CAM) is a broad domain of healing resources that encompasses all health systems, modalities, and practices and their accompanying theories and beliefs, other than those intrinsic to the politically dominant health system of a particular society or culture in a given historical period. CAM includes all such practices and ideas self-defined by their users as preventing or treating illness or promoting health and well-being. Boundaries within CAM and between the CAM domain and the domain of the dominant system are not always sharp or fixed.[14]

Aakster proposed a conceptual framework for defining what is considered CAM and defined CAM therapies as those that seek to internally and externally balance opposing forces while focusing on body language that indicates disruptive forces or restorative processes.[15] Within this framework, CAM diagnoses are considered functional, and treatment focuses on strengthening constructive forces, with the individual as an active participant in regaining health (see Table 18.1).

Terms used to refer to "unconventional" health care include *natural* and *alternative health care. Unorthodox, nonstandard, complementary,* and *adjunctive therapy* are other terms. Whatever they are called, when viewed from a Western nursing and/or medicine perspective, practitioners and recipients of CAM usually agree that these therapies are outside what is practiced in orthodox Western health care systems.

A classification system was developed by the NCCAM to assist in prioritizing applications for research grants in CAM. The system was adapted from *Alternative Medicine: Expanding Medical Horizons,* a report prepared under the auspices of the Workshop on Alternative Medicine held in September 1992.[16] It is divided into seven major categories and includes examples of practices or preparations in each category. Within each category, medical practices that are not commonly used, accepted, or available in conventional medicine are designated as CAM. Those practices that fall mainly within the domains of conventional medicine are designated as behavioral medicine. Practices that can be either CAM or behavioral, depending on their application, are designated as "overlapping." Descriptions of the seven major categories follow.

Mind–Body Medicine

Mind–body medicine involves behavioral, psychological, social, and spiritual approaches to health. It is divided into four subcategories: mind–body systems; mind–body methods; religion and spirituality; and social and contextual areas. Table 18.2 provides a list of the various systems and methods within each subcategory. *Mind–body systems* involve whole systems of mind–body practice that are used largely as primary interventions for disease. They are rarely delivered alone; instead, they are used in combination with lifestyle interventions or are part of a traditional medical system. *Mind–body methods* include individual modalities used in mind–body approaches to health. These approaches are often considered conventional practice and overlap with CAM only when applied to medical conditions for which they are not usually used. The *religion and spirituality* subcategory includes those nonbehavioral aspects of spirituality and religion that examine their relationship to biological function of clinical conditions. *Social and contextual areas* refers to social, cultural, symbolic, and contextual interventions that are not covered in any other areas.[16]

Alternative Medical Systems

Alternative medical systems involve complete systems of theory and practice that have been developed outside the Western biomedical approach. This category is divided into four subcategories: acupuncture and Oriental medicine; traditional indigenous systems; unconventional Western systems; and naturopathy. Table 18.3 provides a list of the various disciplines within each subcategory. *Oriental medicine* encom-

TABLE 18.1

Therapeutic Approaches of Alternative Medical Traditions

Tradition	Somatic Approaches	Herbal and Nutritional Approaches	Energetic Approaches
Oriental medicine	Acupressure Oriental massage Chi kung Tai chi	Chinese herbs Dietary guidance	Acupuncture Moxibustion Acupressure Tai chi Chi kung
Ayurveda	Massage Pranayama Yoga	Ayurvedic herbs Dietary guidance	Pranayama Massage Meditation
Homeopathy	None	None	Homeopathic remedies
Naturopathic medicine	Variety of manipulative therapies, massage and body work Hydrotherapy	Both Eastern and Western herbal medicine Dietary guidance	May use methods from all traditions
Mind–body medicine	Exercise, yoga, chi kung, tai chi, and other self-directed practices	Compliance with dietary guidelines provided by other traditions	Imagery Biofeedback Relaxation Meditation Breath therapy Chi kung, tai chi Autogenic training Hypnosis Psychotherapy Group support
Osteopathic medicine	Osteopathic manipulation of all the bones, tissues, and organs of the body	Depends on the individual practitioner's training and interests	Depends on the individual practitioner's training and interests
Chiropractic	Chiropractic manipulation of skeletal system and soft tissue	Depends on the individual practitioner's training and interests	Depends on the individual practitioner's training and interests
Massage therapy and bodywork	Traditional European Contemporary Western Structural Functional Movement integration Oriental Energetic (non-Oriental) Other approaches	None	Energetic methods of bodywork (Oriental and non-Oriental)

Reproduced with permission: Collinge, W. (1996). *The American Holistic Health Association Complete Guide to Alternative Medicine* (p. 310). New York: Warner Books.

TABLE 18.2			
Mind–Body Medicine			
Subcategory	CAM	Behavioral Medicine	Overlapping
Mind–body methods	Yoga Internal qi gong Tai chi	Psychotherapy Meditation Imagery Hypnosis Biofeedback Support groups	Art therapy Music therapy Dance therapy Journaling Humor Body psychotherapy
Religion and spirituality	Confession Nonlocality Nontemporality Soul retrieval Spiritual healing "Special" healers		
Social and contextual areas	Caring-based approaches 　　Holistic nursing 　　Pastoral care		Placebo Explanatory models Community-based 　　Alcoholics Anonymous 　　Native American "sweat" 　　rituals

Data taken from: National Center for Complementary & Alternative Medicine, NIH. Classification of Alternative Medicine Practices. Available at http://nccam.nih.gov/nccam/what-is-cam/classify.shtml. Accessed 5/14/99.

passes a wide range of treatment modalities referred to in classical texts as "the five branches." These include acupuncture and moxibustion, herbal medicine, tui na (Oriental body work), nutritional therapy, and internal exercise (meditation, qi gong). *Traditional indigenous systems* include major indigenous systems of medicine other than acupuncture and traditional Oriental medicine. Many of these systems have been developed within a specific culture, such as Native American medicine. *Naturopathy* is an eclectic collection of natural systems and therapies.[16]

Lifestyle and Disease Prevention

The *lifestyle and disease prevention* category is concerned with integrated approaches for the prevention and management of chronic disease in general or the common determinants of chronic disease. This category involves theories and practices designed to prevent the development of illness, identify and treat risk factors, or sup-

TABLE 18.3

Alternative Medical Systems

Acupuncture and Oriental Medicine	Traditional Indigenous Systems	Unconventional Western Systems
Acupuncture	Native American	Homeopathy
Herbal formulas	Ayurvedic	Functional medicine
Diet	Unani-tibbi, SIDDHI	Environmental medicine
External and internal qi gong	Kampo	Radiesthesia
Tai chi	Traditional African	Psionic medicine
Massage and manipulation (tui na)	Traditional Aboriginal	Cayce-based systems
Acupotomy	Curanderismo	Kneipp "classical" homeopathy
	Central and South American practices	Orthomolecular medicine
	Psychic surgery	Radionics
		Anthroposophically extended medicine

Data taken from: National Center for Complementary & Alternative Medicine, NIH. Classification of Alternative Medicine Practices. Available at http://nccam.nih.gov/nccam/what-is-cam/classify.shtml. Accessed 5/14/99.

port the healing and recovery process. It is divided into three subcategories: clinical preventative practices, lifestyle therapies, and health promotion. *Clinical preventative practices* are unconventional approaches used to screen for and prevent health-related imbalances, dysfunction, and disease. These practices include electrodermal diagnostics, medical intuition, chirography, functional cellular therapy, enzyme measures, and panchakarma. *Lifestyle therapies* consist of complete systems of lifestyle management that include behavioral changes, dietary changes, exercise, stress management, and addiction control. To be classified as CAM, the changes in lifestyle must be based on a nonorthodox system of medicine, be applied in unconventional ways, or be applied across non-Western diagnostic approaches. *Health promotion* involves laboratory and epidemiological research on healing, the healing process, health promotion factors, and autoregulatory systems.[16]

Biologically Based Therapies

Biologically based therapies comprise natural and biologically based practices, interventions, and products. Many overlap with conventional medicine's use of dietary supplements. This category is divided into four subcategories: phytotherapy or herbalism; special diet therapies; orthomolecular medicine; and pharmacological, biological, and instrumental interventions. Table 18.4 provides a list of the various products and methods within each subcategory. *Phytotherapy* or *herbalism* addresses plant-

TABLE 18.4

Biologically Based Therapies

Phytotherapy	Special Diet Therapies	Orthomolecular Medicine	Pharmacological, Biological, and Instrumental
Individual Herbs	Pritikin	Ascorbic acid	Coley's toxins
Ginkgo biloba	Ornish	Carotenes	Antineoplastons
Hypericum	McDougall	Tocopherols	Cartilage
Garlic	Gerson	Folic acid	EDTA
Ginseng	Kelly-Gonzales	Niacin	Ozone
Echinacea	Wigmore	Niacinamide	H_2O_2
Saw palmetto	Livingston-Wheeler	Panothenic acid	Hyperbaric oxygen
Utica diocia (nettle)	Atkins	Pyridoxine	IAT
Kava-kava	Diamond	Riboflavin	714X
Hawthorn	Vegetarian	Thiamine	MHT-68
Witch hazel	Fasting	Vitamins A, D, and K	Gallo immunotherapy
Bilberry	High fiber	Biotin	Cone therapy
Ginger	Macrobiotic	Choline	Revici system
Aloe vera	Mediterranean	Sadenosylmethionine	Enzyme therapies
Capsicum	Paleolithic	Calcium	Cell therapy
Feverfew	Asian	Magnesium	Enderlin products
Green tea	Natural hygiene	Selenium	T/Tn vaccine
Tea tree oil		Potassium	Bee pollen
Licorice root		Taurine	Induced-remission
Yohimbe		Lysine	therapy
Valerian		Tyrosine	Apitherapy
Bee pollen		Gamma-oryzanol	Neural therapy
Cat's claw		Iodine	Electrodiagnostics
Evening primrose		Iron	Iridology
Dong quai		Manganese	Chirography
Fenugreek		Molybdenum	Special funtional tests
Marsh mallow		Boron	Bioresonance
Psyllium		Silicon	MORA device
Tumeric		Vandium	
Mistletoe		Co-enzyme Q10	
Mohania aquifolium		Carnitine	
Oleum		Glutamine	
Menthae piperitea		Phenylalanine	
(peppermint oil)		Glucosamine sulfate	
		Chondroitin sulfate	
Combinations		Lipoic acid	
Padma 28		Amino acids	
Essiac		Phosphatidylserine	
JCL 2306		Melatonin	
Hoxey		DHEA	
Saw palmetto and		Glandular Product	
pygeum africanium		Fatty Acids	
		Medium-chain	
		triglycerides	

Data taken from: National Center for Complementary & Alternative Medicine, NIH. Classification of Alternative Medicine Practices. Available at http://nccam.nih.gov/nccam/what-is-cam/classify.shtml. Accessed 5/14/99.

derived preparations that are used for therapeutic and preventive purposes. These may be individual herbs or combinations of herbs. *Special diet therapies* includes dietary approaches and special diets that are applied as alternative therapies for risk factors or chronic disease in general. *Orthomolecular medicine* refers to products used as nutritional and food supplements (and not covered in other categories). These products are used for preventive or therapeutic purposes and are usually used in combinations and at higher doses. *Pharmacological, biological,* and *instrumental interventions* include products and procedures applied in an unconventional manner that are not covered in other categories.[16]

Manipulative and Body-Based Systems

Manipulative and body-based systems involve manipulation and/or movement of the body and have three subcategories: chiropractic medicine, massage and body work, and unconventional physical therapies.[16] Specific therapies are listed within each subcategory in Table 18.5.

Biofield Medicine

Biofield medicine involves systems that use subtle energy fields in and around the body for medical purposes. Examples of these therapies include therapeutic touch,

---

TABLE 18.5

Manipulative and Body-Based Systems

Massage and Body Work	Unconventional Physical Therapies
Osteopathic manipulative therapy (OMT)	Hydrotherapy
Cranial-sacral OMT	Diathermy
Swedish massage	Light and color therapies
Applied kinesiology	Heat and electrotherapies
Reflexology	Colonics
Pilates method	Alternate-nostril breathing techniques
Polarity	
Body psychotherapy	
Trager body work	
Alexander technique	
Feldenkreis technique	
Chinese tui na massage and acupressure	
Rolfing	

Data taken from: National Center for Complementary & Alternative Medicine, NIH. Classification of Alternative Medicine Practices. Available at http://nccam.nih.gov/nccam/what-is-cam/classify.shtml. Accessed 5/14/99.

mariue, healing science, reiki, healing touch, huna, natural healing, external qi gong, SHEN, and biorelax.[16]

Bioelectromagnetics

Bioelectromagnetics refers to the unconventional use of electromagnetic fields for medical purposes.[16]

Why People Choose CAM Therapies

Only a few studies have investigated in depth people's motives for choosing unorthodox or complementary medicine. Although some studies document failures or general mistrust of orthodox medicine as the main reasons for turning to complementary medicine, others conclude that the decision to try alternative medicine is not necessarily true disappointment with conventional medicine but rather an endeavor to do everything possible for one's own health.

Vincent and Furnham asked 250 patients to complete a questionnaire rating twenty potential reasons for seeking complementary treatment.[17] The most strongly endorsed reasons were "because I value the emphasis on treating the whole person"; "because I believe complementary therapy will be more effective for my problem than orthodox medicine"; "because I believe that complementary medicine will enable me to take a more active part in maintaining my health"; and "because orthodox treatment was not effective for my particular problem." Five factors were identified, in order of importance: a positive valuation of complementary treatment, the ineffectiveness of orthodox treatment for the complaint, concern about the adverse effects of orthodox medicine, concerns about communication with doctors and, of least importance, the availability of complementary medicine. Schar and colleagues found that patients indeed regard complementary medicine as a complement.[18] Longer-lasting consultation and a better doctor–patient relationship were also favorable aspects of CAM. Other identified motives were a critical attitude on the patient's part to modern civilization and the growing symbolic value of health. The choice may also be related to the nature of the disease, and as a general rule it is chronic problems that are dealt with by complementary medicine.

Although all CAM practitioners do not share a common epistemology, they do tend to share a common set of principles in regard to the role of the patient in treatment and the patient/provider relationship. These common principles probably account to a large degree for the popularity of complementary practices. They include:

1. Focus on patients' "felt needs" rather than diagnosed needs
2. Attention to patients' emotional states, tastes, and behavioral patterns
3. Expectation that patients are not passive recipients but active participants in treatment
4. View of the body as an integrated organism (physical, mental, and emotional) prone to self-regulation and self-healing
5. Viewing treatment as a process

6. Promotion of the use of a variety of therapeutic options for the purposes of prevention and treatment.[19]

Lerner suggests that people with cancer who are seeking CAM are "more deeply engaged than the average patient in their fight for recovery" and are most likely to remain under the care of their allopathic physicians while using CAM.[20] Others have found that individuals with recurrent disease may make greater attempts to remain in control than when they faced their initial diagnosis, may be frustrated with the apparent lack of effectiveness of conventional therapies, or may identify conventional therapies as mutilating or poisonous and therefore see CAM therapies as an option.[21]

Several studies have also identified possible predictors of alternative health care use. Astin surveyed 1,035 individuals throughout the United States.[22] The response rate was 69%. The following variables emerged as predictors of alternative health care use: more education; poorer health status; a holistic orientation to health; any of the following health problems: anxiety, back problems, chronic pain, urinary tract problems; classification in a cultural group identifiable by its commitment to environmentalism; commitment to feminism; and interest in spirituality and personal growth psychology medicine.

✖ THE USE OF CAM PRACTICES IN WOMEN'S HEALTH

As mentioned earlier, numerous studies have found that users of complementary medicine tend to be female, with higher education, from the upper middle class, and aged between 30 and 50. These users tend to have postmaterialistic value priorities, holistic interpretive models of health and disease, and want to share in decision making on treatment questions. The women's health movement of the 1970s (in concert with the community health movement) was influential in the development of the modern alternative health movement.[19] Female health workers turned to many forms of self-care and alternative treatments and practiced an integrative concept of care, often referred to as "whole mind and body health." It is probably accurate to suggest that a significant proportion of women with gynecologic and breast malignancies will have experienced CAM practices in their adult life, either before, during, or after their cancer diagnosis.

Women's experiences may determine their choice of CAM health providers. Women who are victims of sexual and or physical assault and women who have perceived that they have been mistreated in health care encounters are likely to seek out nontraditional providers who are prone to be more interested in and responsive to the woman's personal history, emotions, and felt needs.[19] Lesbians often feel that their concerns go unaddressed in medical settings that assume heterosexuality, and therefore they tend to prefer a holistic approach to women's health.[23] Lesbians tend to use alternative types of health care including self-care, acupuncture, naturopathic medicine, and homeopathy.

Although no known data look specifically at women's use of CAM in the United States, it is possible to speculate on what groups of women might be frequent utilizers, based on gender-specific illness patterns and what is generally known about the utilization of CAM.[19] Women have long used alternative therapies for certain gynecological problems. One example is the use of natural substances such as lactate gel and commercial yogurt to relieve symptoms from recurrent bacterial vaginosis. Dysmenorrhea, mood swings, bloating, and other symptoms associated with premenstrual syndrome have been reported to respond to a variety of herbal substances and blends. Nonhormonal alternatives, including soy and flaxseed dietary supplements, are used by women for many menopausal symptoms including hot flashes, decreased libido, malaise, and vaginal dryness as well as osteoporosis. Depression, anxiety, headaches, insomnia, and substance abuse are also major health care problems for which treatments such as acupuncture and herbal therapies are commonly used.

Few studies have been conducted about the use of CAM practices among women with gynecologic malignancies. Munstedt et al. conducted a survey of the various unconventional methods used by women with gynecologic malignancies.[24] Of 206 respondents, 80 (38.8%) used unconventional therapies. The researchers found mistletoe extracts (50%), trace minerals (46%), megavitamins (39%), and enzymes (22%) were the most common. The perceived etiology of the cancer appeared to determine the choice of treatment. Users of CAM suffered significantly more from conventional therapy, had less faith in their doctors, and felt more nervous and emotionally unstable after the diagnosis of cancer.

A CAM approach may be appropriate for a number of symptoms related to breast and gynecologic malignancies and their treatment. Symptoms associated with menopause, depression, insomnia, anxiety, pain, and postoperative discomfort due to scarring and fibrosis may be reduced through dietary, herbal, relaxation, biofeedback, and body-work therapies. Unfortunately, very little research confirms the efficacy of many of these therapies, and much of the knowledge is anecdotal. Three specific examples of CAM therapies that are currently receiving a significant amount of research attention in clinical trials are phytoestrogens, relaxation techniques, and herbal therapy.

Phytoestrogens

Phytoestrogens represent a family of plant compounds that have been shown to have both estrogenic and antiestrogenic properties. A variety of these plant compounds and their mammalian metabolic products have been identified in various human body fluids and fall under two main categories: isoflavones and ligans. A wide range of commonly consumed foods, including soy and flax products, contain appreciable amounts of these different phytoestrogens. Accumulating evidence from molecular and cellular biology experiments, animal studies, and, to a limited extent, human clinical trials suggests that phytoestrogens may potentially offer health benefits related to cardiovascular diseases, cancer (including endometrial cancers), osteoporosis, and menopausal symptoms.

These potential health benefits are consistent with the epidemiological evidence that rates of heart disease, various cancers, osteoporotic fractures, and menopausal symptoms are more favorable among populations that consume plant-based diets, particularly among cultures with diets that are traditionally high in soy products.[25] In addition to current clinical trials evaluating efficacy, information is needed to standardize dosage as well as provide accurate safety and efficacy labeling.

Relaxation Techniques

A number of techniques are available to elicit a relaxation response, including yoga, guided imagery, meditation, and hypnosis. Researchers have attempted to evaluate the role of these techniques for a variety of symptoms with mixed results. In a recent study, Irvin et al. investigated the efficacy of elicitation of the relaxation response for the treatment of menopausal hot flashes and concurrent psychological symptoms.[26] The results demonstrated a significant reduction in hot-flash intensity ($p < 0.05$), tension–anxiety ($p < 0.05$), and depression ($p < 0.05$) in the relaxation response group.

Although this research is promising, several questions still need to be answered. Additional research should focus on the best relaxation methods to use, how to teach these methods to different groups of women, how frequently these relaxation skills should be used and for how long, and how long the effect lasts.

Herbal Therapy

Herbs are used by women around the world for a variety of reproductive health problems. All indigenous cultures have developed knowledge of local plants and foods that can be used to promote health and cure illness.[27] Beal speculates that perhaps one reason women tend to try using herbal treatments for reproductive problems is that many of the clinical issues that arise are functional problems, such as failure of cyclic events or adjustments of physiologic events, rather than infection or surgical emergencies. A number of herbs have been described in the literature as having some benefit in reducing premenstrual syndrome and menopausal symptoms, as well as depression and insomnia. They include black cohosh, ginseng, dong quai, chaste tree berry, licorice root, fennel seed, and red clover.

Most of the current research on herbal therapies is focused on efficacy. Information regarding dose, frequency, long-term effects, and potential drug and food interactions will also be necessary. Herbal products can have serious toxic effects also. There are several issues related to this topic.[28]

- Some products have ingredients that can produce serious harmful consequences, including direct effect on body organs, incompatibility with other medications or foods, and electrolyte imbalance.
- Some products are promoted as cures for illnesses they do not cure.
- Certain herbs are sold to achieve "legal highs" that can cause cardiac and neural toxicity with subsequent death.

- Some herbal products are fake or highly contaminated.
- Some products contain something other than what is indicated on the label.
- Some products are sold by promoters who make claims based only on unverified, scantly anecdotal evidence.

With the extraordinary number of herbals and blends as well as the number of "new companies" developing products, it is crucial that individuals who are planning to use herbal therapies visit a trained herbalist or physician who practices Oriental medicine. In addition, they should carefully evaluate the ingredients of all products and stay with reputable herbal manufacturers.

✳ CLINICAL PRACTICE GUIDELINES

Because the safety and efficacy of most CAM practices remain largely unknown, advising patients who use or seek CAM treatments presents a professional challenge. Eisenberg proposed a step-by-step strategy whereby conventionally trained medical providers and their patients can proactively discuss the use or avoidance of CAM therapies.[29] This strategy involves a formal discussion of patient preferences and expectations, the maintenance of a symptom diary, and follow-up visits to monitor for potentially harmful situations. In the absence of professional medical and legal guidelines, the proposed management plan emphasizes patient safety, the need for documentation in the patient record, and the importance of sharp decision making.

For a health care provider and consumer, three principal issues arise when considering the use of a CAM therapy. First is the development of a departmental or office policy regarding the sanctioning of CAM therapies. The second principle is the selection of a therapy, and the third is the selection of an appropriate provider.

Policy Development for CAM Referrals

The development of an office or departmental policy regarding the integration of CAM therapies in clinical practice provides a written code of conduct that each member can follow in the recommendation and referral of patients to CAM providers. The policy, based on careful review of the research, provides a resource to members, reflects the perspective of the department, and provides a safeguard for patients and practitioners. The policy should include the following:

- Identification of the overall goal of the policy
- Identification of CAM practices that have been carefully selected after review of the available research
- Identification of specific symptoms or diseases that may benefit from CAM
- Procedure for referral and documentation of referral
- Procedure for evaluation and documentation of outcome of CAM therapy

- List of established CAM practitioners whose credentials and practice have been carefully evaluated
- Process for annual review of policy and updating list of practitioners
- Procedure for filing professional complaint in case of malpractice or injury

Choosing a CAM Therapy

Choosing a CAM therapy, whether for personal use or to enhance the therapeutic role, entails thorough investigation of potential risks and benefits. It is important to critically evaluate the research data available. Collinge recommends that the following questions be addressed when considering CAM:

- What underlying theories, principles, or beliefs guide this tradition's understanding of health and illness?
- Variations within the tradition: Are there different forms of practice of specialties within this tradition? How are they identified?
- Procedures and techniques: What kinds of procedures and techniques is the patient most likely to encounter?
- Scientific support: What scientific support is there for this tradition's methods, principles, and effectiveness?
- Strengths and limitations: With what kinds of illnesses is this tradition most and least effective?
- The practitioner–patient relationship: What kind of personal attention and support can the patient expect from a practitioner?
- Evaluating personal results: How will the patient's progress and the effectiveness of treatment be evaluated? Are there any objective measures or tests?
- Relationship to other forms of medicine: Does this tradition exclude other forms of medicine? Will it interfere or can the patient combine it with another tradition?
- Costs: How expensive are consultations, procedures, and medicines? What about insurance coverage?
- Choosing a practitioner: What credentials should the patient look for in choosing a practitioner of this tradition?[30]

Choosing a CAM Practitioner

Considerable changes have occurred in the delivery of health care in the United States over the past fifteen years. During this time, statutory activity related to alternative medicine has been growing. Because of state regulations allowing physicians to go beyond conventional forms of treatment and explore the healing potential of CAM, a form of "turf" protection has resulted. Some states have regulated educational requirements and licensure for some practices such as acupuncture and massage, but not for others such as reflexology. The result is a significant opportunity for overlap of practices with little uniformity among state laws. For example, the language of the current nurse practice acts neither prohibits nor actively promotes alternative medicine practices.

TABLE 18.6

Sources of CAM Information

Alexander Technique International
1692 Massachusetts Ave., 3rd Floor,
Cambridge, MA 02138
888-321-0856
617-497-2242, 617-497-2615 Fax
www.ati.net.com

American Association of
Naturopathic Physicians
601 Valley Street, Ste. 105
Seattle, WA 98109
206-298-0126
206-298-0129 Fax
www.naturopathic.org

American Botanical Council
P.O. Box 144345, Austin, Texas 78714-4345
512-926-4900, 512-926-2345 Fax
www.herbalgram.org

American Chiropractic Association
1701 Clarendon Blvd., Arlington, VA 22209
800-986-4636, 703-243-2593 Fax
www.amerchiro.org

American Herbalist Guild
P.O. Box 70, Roosevelt, UT 84066
435-722-8434, 435-722-8452 Fax
www.health.net/herbalists

American Herbal Pharmoacopia
(Monographs)
Box 5159
Santa Cruz, CA 95063
831-461-6317, 831-438-7410 Fax
www.herbal-ahp.org

American Holistic Medical Association
4101 Lake Boone Trail, Ste. 201.
Raleigh, NC 27607
703-556-9245
www.holisticmedicine.org

American Holistic Nurses' Association
P.O. Box 2130, Flagstaff, AZ 86003-2130
1-800-278-AHNA
www.ahna.org

American Massage Therapy Association
820 Davis Street, Ste. 100,
Evanston, IL 60201-4444
847-864-0123, 847-864-1178 Fax
www.amtamassage.org

Feldenkrais Guild of North America
524 Ellsworth St. S.W., P.O. Box 489
Albany, OR 97321-0143
800-775-2118
541-926-0981, 541-926-0572 Fax
www.feldenkrais.com

Food and Drug Administration
FDA (HFE-88)
5600 Fishers Lane, Rockville, MD 20857
888-INFO-FDA
www.fda.gov

International Council of Reflexologists
P.O. Box 17356, San Diego, CA 92177-7356
619-275-1011 Tel/Fax
www.reflexology.org

National Center for Complementary &
Alternative Health (NIH) Clearinghouse
P.O. Box 8218
Silver Spring, MD 20907-8218
888-644-6226, 301-495-4957 Fax
www.nccam.nih.gov

National Certification Board for
Therapeutic Massage and Bodywork
8201 Greensboro Drive, Ste 300
McLean, VA 22102
800-296-0664
703-610-9015, 703-610-9005 Fax
www.ncbtmb.com

National Certification Commission for
Acupuncture and Oriental Medicine
11 Canal Center Plaza, Ste. 300
Alexandria, VA 22314
703-548-9004, 703-548-9079 Fax
www.nccaom.org

TABLE 18.6 *(continued)*

Sources of CAM Information

National Center for Homeopathy 801 North Fairfax Street, Ste. 306, Alexandria, VA 22314 703-548-7790, 703-548-7792 Fax nchinfo@igc.org	Quackwatch P.O. Box 1747, Allentown, PA 18105 610-437-1795 www.quackwatch.com
National Council Against Health Care Fraud P.O. Box 1276, Loma Linda, CA 92354-9983 www.ncahf.org	The Center for Mind–Body Studies 5225 Connecticut Avenue, NW, Ste. 414 Washington, DC 20015 202-966-7338, 202-966-2589 Fax
Planetree Health Resource Center 98 N. 17th Street, San Jose, CA 95112 408-977-4549 www.planetreesanjose.org	The Council on Naturopathic Medical Education P.O. Box 11426, Eugene, OR 97440-3626 541-484-6028 www.cnme.org
Reflexology Association of America 4012 Rainbow Blvd., Box K585 Las Vegas, NV 89103-2059 www.reflexusa	The Rolf Institute of Structural Integration 205 Canyon Blvd., Boulder, CO 80302 303-449-5903, 303-449-5978 Fax www.rolf.org

Primary care clinicians may provide some integrative therapies directly (massage therapy, guided imagery, therapeutic touch, acupressure) after additional training and practice. However, many integrative therapies require years of intensive education and training (Oriental medicine, chiropractic). Most primary care providers will need to refer to competent providers for these services. In these instances, the health care provider should know the educational, practice, and credentialing requirements for each of the professions in order to identify competent providers. Most states have licensing requirements for chiropractors, homeopathists, naturopathic healers, and acupuncturists. Table 18.6 provides a list of sources for CAM information including major credentialing groups for practitioners in integrative therapies.

In 1993, the Royal College of Nursing issued a consumer checklist to help patients feel more confident about choosing a CAM practitioner. Some of the points they identified are:

- What are the therapist's qualifications and how long was the training?
- Is the therapist a member of a recognized, registered body with a code of practice?
- Can the therapist provide the address and telephone number of this organization to check?
- Is the therapy covered by the patient's insurer or HMO?
- Can a physician delegate care to the therapist?
- Is this the most appropriate CAM therapy for the particular problem?

TABLE 18.7

Recommended CAM Reading Materials

Complementary & Alternative Medicine: Legal Boundaries and Regulatory Perspectives. (1998). Written by Michael H. Cohen. Baltimore: Johns Hopkins University Press.

Dr. Susan Love's Hormone Book. (1997). Written by Susan M. Love, MD. New York: Random House.

PDR for Herbal Medicines. (1998). Montvale, NJ: Medical Economics Company.

Professional's Handbook of Complementary and Alternative Medicines. (1999). Written by Charles W. Fetrow and Juan R. Avila. Springhouse Publishing Company.

The Alternative Medicine Handbook: The Complete Reference Guide to Alternative and Complementary Therapies. (1999). Written by Barrie R. Cassileth. New York: W.W. Norton & Company.

The American Holistic Health Association Complete Guide to Alternative Medicine. (1996). Written by William Collinge. New York: Warner Books

The Breast Cancer Prevention Diet. (1998). Written by Robert B. Arnot. Boston: Little, Brown and Company.

Women's Bodies, Women's Wisdom: Creating Physical and Emotional Health and Healing. (1998). Written by Christiane Northrup. Bantam Doubleday Dell Publishers.

Women's Encyclopedia of Natural Medicine: Alternative Therapies and Integrative Medicine (2nd ed.). (1999). Written by Tori Hudson. Keats Publishers.

- Does the therapist send a letter to the physician advising of any treatment the patient received?
- Are the patient records confidential?
- What is the cost of the treatment?
- How many treatments will be needed?
- What insurance coverage does the therapist have?[31]

Nursing Role in CAM

Nurses and other health care providers, especially those who work in women's health, need to know much more about CAM for a number of reasons:

- Most women will use complementary therapies at some time in their lives.
- Women use CAM most often as an adjunct to, rather than in place of, orthodox Western medicine and therefore the potential exists for interactive effects.
- The practice of CAM is growing very quickly, especially in health promotion, mind–body connection, and attention to the effects of patient/provider communication.[19]

To provide safe care that nurtures healing on all levels (physical, emotional, and spiritual) as well as to encourage patients to be active participants in decisions related to their care, nurses should be able to alert patients to side effects associated with some CAM therapies and encourage the use of beneficial complementary therapies. Swanson and Facione recommend the following clinical practice tips developed while working with women with breast cancer:

- Establish a trusting rapport with the patient during your first contact.
- Ask what CAM practices the patient is currently using or has used in the past. Avoid a judgmental attitude.
- Openly and frequently endorse the patient's right to freedom of informed choice.
- Do a thorough and comprehensive ongoing assessment of side effects during treatment, focusing on the patient's ability to function in various roles and settings. Encourage the patient to keep a journal or diary and review it often with her.
- Collaboratively develop an assessment tool that you can both use to evaluate risks and benefits of CAM practices she may choose to use.
- Carefully evaluate all of the products for safety.
- Learn more about CAM practices and artfully integrate this knowledge into your practice.[32]

✖ SUMMARY

CAM use among adults and children is outpacing current research evaluation of many of these methods. In addition, there are no FDA regulations for vitamin, herbal, and nutritional supplements; many "new and improved" substances are introduced to the public every year that have not been investigated and are primarily for the financial gain of the promoter. It is the responsibility of all health care providers to familiarize themselves with the most common CAM practices and read the efficacy research as it is published. In addition, health care providers should assist patients to become informed consumers by providing resources about a particular CAM practice or practitioner. Until there is a sufficient research foundation to support CAM practices, the health care provider and consumer must rely on anecdotal information and personal experience. It is important that they work together to reduce the risk of individual morbidity and mortality.

✖ REFERENCES

1. Turk, D.C. (1979). Factors influencing the adaptive process with chronic illness: Implications for intervention. In E.G. Sarason & C.D. Speilberger (eds.), *Stress and Anxiety* (vol. 6), Washington, D.C.: Hemisphere.
2. Silverman, R.L., & Wartman, C.B. (1980). Coping with undesirable life events. In J. Garber & M.E.P. Seligman, eds., *Human Helplessness:*

Theory and Applications. New York: Academic Press.
3. Taylor, S.E. (1983). Adjustment to threatening events: A theory of cognitive adaptation. *Am Psychol, 38*(11), 1161–1173.
4. Dorsett, D.S. (1991). The trajectory of cancer recovery. *Scholarly Inquiry for Nursing Practice, 5*(3), 175–184.

5. Eisenberg, D.M., Kessler, R.C, Foster, C., et al. (1993). Unconventional medicine in the United States: Prevalence, costs, and patterns of use. *N Engl J Med, 328*(4), 246–252.

6. Eisenberg, D.M., Davis, R.B., Ettner, S.L., et al. (1998). Trends in alternative medicine use in the United States, 1990–1997: Results of a follow-up national survey. *JAMA, 290*(18), 1569–1575.

7. Paramore, L.C. (1997). Use of alternative therapies: Estimates from the 1994 Robert Wood Johnson Foundation National Access to Care Survey. *J Pain Symptom Manage, 13*(2), 83–89.

8. Montbriand, M.J. (1994). An overview of alternate therapies chosen by patients with cancer. *Oncol Nurs Forum 21*(9), 1547– 1554.

9. Marcus. C.L. (1999). Alternative medicine: The AMA reviews scientific evidence. *Clin Rev 9*(2), 87–90.

10. Shealy, C.N., & Thomas, R. (eds.) (1996). *The Complete Family Guide to Alternative Medicine.* New York: Barnes & Noble Books.

11. National Center for Complementary & Alternative Medicine, NIH. General Information. Available at http://nccam.nih.gov/nccam/about/general.shtml. Accessed 5/14/99.

12. *Complementary Alternative Medicine,* July 1996, Volume III, Number 2. Silver Spring, MD: Office of Alternative Medicine Clearinghouse.

13. Huebscher, R.R. (1994). What is natural/alternative health care? *Nurse Pract Forum, 5*(2), 66–71.

14. Panel on Definition and Description, CAM Research Methodology Conference, April 1995. (1997). Defining and describing complementary and alternative medicine. *Alternative Therapies in Health and Medicine, 3*(2), 49–57.

15. Aakster, C.W. (1986). Concepts in alternative medicine. *Soc Sci Med, 22*(2), 265–273.

16. National Center for Complimentary & Alternative Medicine, NIH. Classification of Alternative Medicine Practices. Available at http://nccam.nih.gov/nccam/what-is-cam/classify.shtml. Accessed 5/14/99.

17. Vincent, C., & Furnham, A. (1996). Why do patients turn to complementary medicine? An empirical study. *Br J Clin Psychol, 35*(Pt. 1), 37–48.

18. Schar, A., Messerli-Rohrbach, V., & Schubarth, P. (1994). Conventional or complementary medicine: What criteria for choosing do patients use? [Article in German] *Schweiz Med Wochenschr Suppl, 62*, 18–27.

19. Burg, M.A. (1996). Women's use of complementary medicine. Combining mainstream medicine with alternative practices. *J Fla Med Assoc, 83*(7), 482–488.

20. Lerner, M. (1994). *Choices in Healing: Integrating the Best of Conventional and Complementary Approaches to Cancer.* Cambridge: MIT Press.

21. Zaloznik, A.J. (1994). Unproven (unorthodox) cancer treatments: A guide for health care professionals. *Cancer Pract, 2*(1), 19–24.

22. Astin, J.A. (1998). Why patients use alternative medicine: Results of a national study. *JAMA, 279*(19), 1548–1553.

23. Trippet, S.E., & Bain, J. (1992). Reasons American lesbians fail to seek traditional health care. *Health Care for Women International, 13*(2), 145–153.

24. Munstedt, K., Kirsch, K., Milch, W., et al. (1996). Unconventional cancer therapy—Survey of patients with gynecological malignancy. *Arch Gynecol Obstet, 258*(2), 81–88.

25. Tham, D.M., Gardner, C.D., & Haskell, W.L. (1998). Clinical review 97: Potential health benefits of dietary phytoestrogens: A review of the clinical, epidemiological and mechanistic evidence. *J Clin Endocrinol Metab, 83*(7), 2223– 2235.

26 Irvin, J.H., Domar, A.D. , Clark, C., et al. (1996). The effects of relaxation response training on menopausal symptoms. *J Psychosom Obstet Gynaecol, 17*(4), 202–207.

27. Beal, M.W. (1998). Women's use of complementary and alternative therapies in reproductive health care. *J Nurse Midwifery, 43*(3), 224–234.

28. Cassileth, B.R. (1998). Complementary and alternative therapies. *Oncology Nursing Updates, 5*(4), 1–11.

29. Eisenberg, D. M. (1997). Advising patients who seek alternative medical therapies. *Ann Intern Med, 127*(1), 61–69.

30. Collinge, W. (1996). *The American Holistic Health Association Complete Guide to Alternative Medicine* (p. 310). New York: Warner Books.

31. Complementary Therapies in Nursing Special Interest Group. (1993). *Consumer checklist for complementary therapies.* London: Royal College of Nursing.

32. Swanson, S.A., & Facione, N. (1998). Complementary alternative medicine practices in women with breast cancer. *Am J Nurs,* (suppl), 34–39.

INDEX